Review of Surgery for

ABSITE AND BOARDS

Review of Surgery for
ABSITE AND BOARDS

THIRD EDITION

EDITORS

Christian de Virgilio, MD, FACS
Chair
Department of Surgery
Harbor-UCLA Medical Center
Torrance, California;
Co-Chair
College of Applied Anatomy;
Professor of Surgery
UCLA School of Medicine
Los Angeles, California

Areg Grigorian, MD
Assistant Clinical Professor of Surgery
Department of Surgery
Division of Trauma, Burns and Critical Care
University of California, Irvine
Orange, California

ASSOCIATE EDITORS

Amanda C. Purdy, MD
Surgical Resident Physician
Department of Surgery
Harbor-UCLA Medical Center
Torrance, California

Eric O. Yeates, MD
Resident Physician
Department of Surgery
University of California, Irvine
Orange, California

Naveen Balan, MD
Surgical Resident
Department of Surgery
Harbor-UCLA Medical Center
Torrance, California

ILLUSTRATOR

Stephanie Cohen, MD
Surgical Resident
Beth Israel Deaconess Medical Center
Boston, Massachusetts

ELSEVIER

ELSEVIER

1600 John F. Kennedy Blvd.
Ste 1800
Philadelphia, PA 19103-2899

REVIEW OF SURGERY FOR ABSITE AND BOARDS, THIRD EDITION ISBN: 978-0-323-87054-2

Notice

Practitioners and researchers must always rely on their own experience and knowledge in evaluating and using any information, methods, compounds, or experiments described herein. Because of rapid advances in the medical sciences, in particular, independent verification of diagnoses and drug dosages should be made. To the fullest extent of the law, no responsibility is assumed by Elsevier, authors, editors, or contributors for any injury and/or damage to persons or property as a matter of products liability, negligence or otherwise, or from any use or operation of any methods, products, instructions, or ideas contained in the material herein.

Previous editions copyrighted 2018 and 2010.

Content Strategist: Jessica McCool
Content Development Specialist: Shweta Pant
Publishing Services Manager: Shereen Jameel
Project Manager: Beula Christopher
Design Direction: Ryan Cook

Printed in India.
Last digit is the print number: 9 8 7 6 5 4 3 2

Working together
to grow libraries in
developing countries

www.elsevier.com • www.bookaid.org

To my family, who always support me, and to all students of surgery, who motivate and inspire me to always keep learning the art and science of medicine.

—Christian de Virgilio

I would not be where I am today if it wasn't for my mentors. Dr. de Virgilio—you are the reason I love surgical education. Dr. Demetriades, you taught me trauma surgery but more importantly, you taught me how to be an effective and inspiring teacher. Dr. Inaba, you have taught me how to be an effective leader both inside and outside the operating room. Dr. Nahmias, you have taught me how to be an academician and researcher. And to my loving wife, Rebecca Grigorian—a superhero mom and physician! Thank you all!

—Areg Grigorian

Contributors

Mark Archie, MD
Assistant Clinical Professor of Surgery
Department of Surgery
Harbor-UCLA Medical Center
David Geffen School of Medicine at UCLA
Los Angeles, California

Naveen Balan, MD
Surgical Resident
Department of Surgery
Harbor-UCLA Medical Center
Torrance, California

Jeremy M. Blumberg, MD
Chief of Urology
Harbor-UCLA Medical Center;
Associate Professor of Urology
David Geffen School of Medicine at UCLA
Los Angeles, California

Nina M. Bowens, MD
Assistant Professor
Department of Surgery
David Geffen School of Medicine at UCLA;
Associate Program Director, Vascular Surgery Program
Division of Vascular and Endovascular Surgery
Harbor-UCLA Medical Center
Torrance, California

Caitlyn Braschi, MD
Resident Physician
Department of Surgery
Harbor-UCLA Medical Center
Torrance, California

Formosa Chen, MD, MPH
Health Sciences Assistant Clinical Professor
Department of Surgery
David Geffen School of Medicine at UCLA
Los Angeles, California

Kathryn T. Chen, MD
Assistant Professor
Department of Surgery
Harbor-UCLA Medical Center
Torrance, California

Christine Dauphine, MD, FACS
Vice Chair, Education
Department of Surgery
Harbor-UCLA Medical Center
Torrance, California;
Professor of Surgery
David Geffen School of Medicine at UCLA
Los Angeles, California

Christian de Virgilio, MD, FACS
Chair
Department of Surgery
Harbor-UCLA Medical Center
Torrance, California;
Co-Chair
College of Applied Anatomy;
Professor of Surgery
UCLA School of Medicine
Los Angeles, California

Benjamin DiPardo, MD
Resident
Department of Surgery
UCLA
Los Angeles, California

Richard Everson, MD
Assistant Clinical Professor of Surgery
Department of Surgery
Harbor-UCLA Medical Center
David Geffen School of Medicine at UCLA
Los Angeles, California

Mytien Goldberg, MD
Assistant Clinical Professor of Surgery
Department of Surgery
Harbor-UCLA Medical Center
David Geffen School of Medicine at UCLA
Los Angeles, California

Areg Grigorian, MD
Assistant Clinical Professor of Surgery
Department of Surgery
Division of Trauma, Burns and Critical Care
University of California, Irvine
Orange, California

Joseph Hadaya, MD, PhD
Resident Physician
Department of Surgery
David Geffen School of Medicine at UCLA
Los Angeles, California

Danielle M. Hari, MD, FACS
Division Chief, Surgical Oncology
Department of Surgery
Harbor-UCLA Medical Center;
Associate Professor
Department of Surgery
David Geffen School of Medicine at UCLA
Los Angeles, California

Dennis Kim, MD
Trauma Medical Director
Island Health Trauma Services
Victoria, British Columbia, Canada

Catherine M. Kuza, MD, FASA
Assistant Professor
Department of Anesthesiology, Division of Critical Care
Keck School of Medicine of the University of Southern
 California
Los Angeles, California

Steven L. Lee, MD, MBA
Professor and Chief
Pediatric Surgery
UCLA Mattel Children's Hospital
Los Angeles, California

John McCallum, MD, MPH
Assistant Professor
Department of Surgery
Harbor-UCLA Medical Center
Torrance, California

Michael A. Mederos, MD
Resident Physician
Department of Surgery
UCLA
Los Angeles, California

Alexandra Moore, MD
Surgery Resident
Department of Surgery
UCLA
Los Angeles, California

Jeffry Nahmias, MD, MHPE
Associate Professor
Department of Surgery
University of California, Irvine
Orange, California

Kristofer E. Nava, MD
Department of General Surgery
Western Michigan University Homer D. Stryker School
 of Medicine
Kalamazoo, Michigan

Junko Ozao-Choy, MD, FACS
Vice Chair, Research
Department of Surgery
Harbor-UCLA Medical Center
Torrance, California;
Associate Professor of Surgery
David Geffen School of Medicine at UCLA
Los Angeles, California

Joon Y. Park, MD
Surgery Resident
Department of Surgery
David Geffen School of Medicine at UCLA
Los Angeles, California

Beverley A. Petrie, MD, FACS, FASCRS
Professor of Surgery
Department of Surgery
David Geffen School of Medicine at UCLA
Los Angeles, California;
Assistant Chief
Division of Colon and Rectal Surgery, Department of Surgery
Harbor-UCLA Medical Center
Torrance, California

Amanda C. Purdy, MD
Surgical Resident Physician
Department of Surgery
Harbor-UCLA Medical Center
Torrance, California

Shonda L. Revels, MD, MS
Assistant Professor
Department of Surgery
UCLA
Los Angeles, California

Jordan M. Rook, MD
Resident Physician
Department of Surgery
David Geffen School of Medicine at UCLA
Los Angeles, California

Saad Shebrain, MBBCh, MMM, FACS
Program Director, Associate Professor of Surgery
Department of Surgery
Western Michigan University Homer Stryker M.D. School
 of Medicine
Kalamazoo, Michigan

Eric R. Simms, MD
Chief
Division of General, Bariatric and Minimally Invasive Surgery,
Assistant Program Director of Surgery Residency
Department of Surgery
Harbor-UCLA Medical Center
Torrance, California

Veronica Sullins, MD
Assistant Clinical Professor of Surgery
Department of Pediatric Surgery
David Geffen School of Medicine at UCLA
Los Angeles, California

Maria G. Valadez, MD
General Surgery Resident
Department of Surgery
Harbor-UCLA Medical Center
Torrance, California

**Luis Felipe Cabrera Vargas, MD, MACC, FACS,
 MACCVA, MFELAC**
President of the Future Surgeons Chapter of the Colombian
 Surgery Association,
Professor of the Universidad Javeriana and Universidad El Bosque,
Fellow of Vascular Surgery of the Universidad Militar Nueva
 Granada
Bogotá, Colombia

Zachary N. Weitzner, MD
Resident Physician
Department of Surgery
UCLA
Los Angeles, California

James Wu, MD
Assistant Clinical Professor of Surgery
Department of Surgery
UCLA Medical Center
David Geffen School of Medicine at UCLA
Los Angeles, California

Tajnoos Yazdany, MD
Vice Chair of Education
Program Director, Obstetrics and Gynecology Residency,
Chief and Program Director, Female Pelvic Medicine and
    Reconstructive Surgery,
Associate Professor
David Geffen School of Medicine at UCLA
Harbor-UCLA Medical Center
Torrance, California

Eric O. Yeates, MD
Resident Physician
Department of Surgery
University of California, Irvine
Orange, California

Amy Kim Yetasook, MD
MIS and Bariatric Surgeon
Department of Surgery
Harbor-UCLA Medical Center
Torrance, California;
Assistant Professor
Department of Surgery
David Geffen School of Medicine at UCLA
Los Angeles, California

Foreword

It is an honor to write the foreword to the third edition of *Review of Surgery for ABSITE and Boards* by one of the foremost surgical educators of our time, Dr. Christian de Virgilio. This book grew out of his initial informal attempts to improve ABSITE scores among his own residents at Harbor-UCLA. Over the years, this effort has grown and expanded, including collaborators from multiple institutions, to produce a book that has become an essential tool in the surgical resident's armamentarium.

The most valuable aspect of this book, in my humble opinion, is that in addition to questions testing pure "didactic" knowledge—factoids the resident is expected to learn by rote and memorize—there are many clinical questions that require an advanced level of cognitive effort. Here, the learner is expected to synthesize anatomic and physiologic knowledge within a clinical context and exercise surgical judgment based on probabilities of different outcomes. Too often, books specifically targeted at passing multiple-choice examinations tend to skip the latter, in favor of questions that have easy answers—hence the common surgical aphorism that there are more exam questions on the clinical presentation of MEN-2 syndrome than patients with this disease! Writing questions that test esoteric minutiae is easy; writing questions that promote further reading and study of complex surgical scenarios is much harder. I applaud Dr. de Virgilio and his colleagues for reaching this higher goal, while still including the "knowledge-regurgitation" questions that are an inevitable part of the standardized exam process.

Each question is followed by a thoughtful explanation of the right answer, with accompanying references, to provide a brief summary of essential relevant knowledge. The newest edition also includes a summary of "high-yield" principles at the beginning of each chapter, which will further enhance the goal of rapid dissemination of essential information on a given topic.

In addition to serving as a valuable training tool for the in-service examination, it is our hope that this book will also inspire the resident to augment their learning by delving into relevant sections of textbooks and online resources, including videos and podcasts—all part and parcel of the total educational package freely available to modern surgical trainees. The breadth and depth of multimedia education available today is enormous, compared to what I had as a resident; conversely, the volume of knowledge and technical skills new surgeons are expected to learn and master has also increased significantly.

The doubling of scientific knowledge, in medicine and surgery, is now occurring at an exponential pace, and we need all the help we can get to keep up! I am grateful to Dr. de Virgilio and his colleagues for continuing to invest the effort necessary to update this wonderful book, so it can continue to serve as a vital resource for present and future surgeons.

Sharmila Dissanaike, MD, FACS, FCCM
Peter C. Canizaro Chair,
University Distinguished Professor of Surgery,
Texas Tech University Health Sciences Center
Lubbock, Texas

Preface

We are thrilled about this third edition of *Review of Surgery for ABSITE and Boards,* created to help students of surgery prepare for the American Board of Surgery In-Training (ABSITE) and the American Board of Surgery (ABS) Qualifying (written) Examination. The original inspiration for the book stemmed from a surgery review program we developed at Harbor-UCLA Medical Center, designed to stimulate the residents to read, improve performance on the ABSITE, and enhance their likelihood of passing the ABS examinations on the first try. We were inspired to hear that the first two editions proved to be a valuable resource.

With that in mind, we have strived to make the 3rd edition even better with some exciting updates and changes. Areg Grigorian and I have added three new Assistant Editors to our team, Drs. Amanda Purdy, Eric Yeates, and Naveen Balan. All are surgical residents; Drs. Purdy and Balan at Harbor-UCLA and Dr. Yeates at UC Irvine. We handpicked them because of their outstanding record of accomplishment in test taking and question writing and their demonstrated strong interest in surgical education. We have also added numerous residents and surgical educators from around the country (and even one from Colombia) as contributing authors. Another important new feature is that we added a summary of high-yield information at the beginning of each chapter. We feel this will serve as a rapid-fire way to brush up on key points. We have also added new, high-yield questions to remain up-to-date with the ever-changing and dynamic field of surgery.

Finally, we have added illustrations from an incredibly talented surgical illustrator, Dr. Stephanie Cohen, who is a surgical resident at Beth Israel Deaconess. We loved her work so much that we asked her to make a drawing for the cover!

The cover illustration, which combines elements of art, music, and anatomy, reminds us that Surgery is both an art and a science. To master the arts requires tremendous dedication. Excellent surgical knowledge is one characteristic that is paramount to becoming an outstanding surgeon. This requires a lifelong commitment to reading and then testing your knowledge. We believe that the ideal way to acquire knowledge is to create a year-round reading program. Strive to read daily, even if just for 15 minutes.

As with the original version, we believe that the greatest value of our book lies in the design of the questions and the robust responses. The questions are intended to make you think (try not to get frustrated if you miss many of them!). We provide in-depth explanations for why we feel the correct answer is right and why the incorrect answers are wrong. Please be aware that no textbook or review book has all the answers. Some questions and answers may be controversial. If you disagree with a question or think you found an error, we would love to hear back from you (our emails are cdevirgilio@lundquist.org and agrigori@uci.edu). We sincerely hope you find our review book useful.

Christian de Virgilio and Areg Grigorian

Acknowledgments

We would like to acknowledge the efforts of Elsevier for the timely preparation and publication of this review book, in particular Jessica McCool, Content Strategist, who helped with the development of this book and supported it throughout production, and the contributions made by Shweta Pant, Senior Content Development Specialist, Beula Christopher, Senior Project Manager, and Ryan Cook, Book Designer. In addition, we would like to thank the surgery faculty and residents at Harbor-UCLA and UC Irvine Medical Centers who assisted in the production and inspiration of this project.

Contents

PART II: MEDICAL KNOWLEDGE

Abdomen—General

NAVEEN BALAN, AREG GRIGORIAN, AND CHRISTIAN DE VIRGILIO

1

ABSITE 99th Percentile High-Yields

I. Enhanced recovery after surgery (ERAS) – associated with a lower overall complication rate, although there is no difference in surgical complications or mortality

A. Preoperative optimization
1. Includes preadmission patient education on analgesia management after OR, control of medical comorbidities, smoking cessation, prehabilitation, nutritional care, and correction of anemia
2. Ideal patient is ASA 1 or 2, ambulatory, good nutritional status; absolute contraindication is urgent surgery, ASA 4–6, severely malnourished, or immobile

B. Intraoperative management
1. Standard anesthesia protocol, minimizing intraoperative fluids, preventing intraoperative hypothermia, maintain normal serum glucose, minimally invasive approach (when feasible), avoid routine use of drains

C. Postoperative care
1. Avoid routine use of nasogastric (NG) tubes, multimodal analgesia to minimize opioid use, use of epidurals in laparotomy cases, use of TAP (transversus abdominis plane) blocks, early urinary catheter discontinuation, and early mobilization

QUESTIONS

1. A 56-year-old male undergoes laparoscopic peritoneal dialysis (PD) catheter placement. Several months later the patient comes to the emergency department reporting problems with his PD catheter. He reports that he can instill dialysate without difficulty but is unable to withdraw fluid through the catheter. His abdomen is distended and he has mild abdominal pain. He is afebrile and not tachycardic. What is the next best step?

    A. Prompt removal of PD catheter
    B. Abdominal x-ray
    C. Instill tPA through the catheter
    D. Intraperitoneal antibiotics
    E. Intravenous antibiotics

2. A 24-year-old male undergoes laparotomy for an anterior abdominal stab wound with peritoneal violation. A small perforation of the transverse colon is repaired primarily. While examining the small bowel, an antimesenteric diverticulum is found 10 cm proximal from the ileocecal junction. It is 3 cm in diameter, 3 cm in height, and there is a fibrous band extending from the diverticulum to the abdominal wall. There is no palpable abnormality adjacent to the diverticulum and no evidence or history of GI bleeding. What is the appropriate management of the diverticulum?

    A. Obtain additional imaging postoperatively
    B. Diverticulectomy
    C. Biopsy
    D. Observation
    E. Segmental resection

3. Which of the following is true about intraabdominal hypertension (IAH) and abdominal compartment syndrome (ACS)?
   A. Diagnosis of ACS is established when intraabdominal pressure is greater than 20 mmHg
   B. Intraabdominal hypertension is defined as intraabdominal pressure >12 mmHg
   C. Neuromuscular blockade reduces mortality in patients with ACS
   D. Paracentesis is contraindicated in patients with IAH
   E. Cerebral perfusion is increased in ACS

4. Which of the following is true regarding omental torsion?
   A. Secondary torsion is more common than primary
   B. If surgery is necessary, management consists of detorsion and omentopexy
   C. Treatment is usually observation with pain control
   D. The pain is usually in the left lower quadrant of the abdomen
   E. It typically produces purulent-appearing peritoneal fluid

5. The most common organism isolated from the infected peritoneal fluid of a patient with a PD catheter is:
   A. Beta-hemolytic streptococcus
   B. Enterococcus
   C. Escherichia coli
   D. Coagulase-negative staphylococcus
   E. Coagulase-positive staphylococcus

6. A 70-year-old woman presents with progressive abdominal pain and abdominal distention with nonshifting dullness. A CT scan demonstrates loculated collections of fluid and scalloping of the intraabdominal organs. At surgery, several liters of yellowish-gray mucoid material are present on the omentum and peritoneal surfaces. Which of the following is true about this condition?
   A. There is no role for surgical resection
   B. It is most commonly of ovarian origin
   C. There is a strong genetic influence
   D. It is more common in males
   E. Cytoreductive surgery may be of benefit

7. The most common cause of a retroperitoneal abscess is:
   A. Diverticulitis
   B. Appendicitis
   C. Renal infection
   D. Tuberculosis of the spine
   E. Hematogenous spread from a remote location

8. A 50-year-old male with cirrhotic ascites secondary to hepatitis C presents with fever, elevated white blood cell count, and abdominal pain. He has a history of esophageal varices. He has been on the liver transplant list for 6 months. Paracentesis was performed and cultures were sent. A single organism grows from the culture. Which of the following is true regarding this condition?
   A. It is most likely due to appendicitis
   B. Prophylactic use of fluoroquinolone can be used to prevent this condition
   C. In adults, nephrotic syndrome is the most common risk factor
   D. In children, *E. coli* is the most common isolate
   E. He will likely need an exploratory laparotomy

9. A 74-year-old male presents to clinic hoping to have his reducible umbilical hernia repaired secondary to increasing but intermittent pain and discomfort. Two days before his clinic visit, he had been discharged from the hospital for unstable angina, for which he underwent balloon angioplasty with placement of a bare metal coronary artery stent (BMS). When should his surgery be scheduled?
   A. 2 weeks
   B. 1 month
   C. 2 months
   D. 6 months
   E. 1 year

10. Which of the following is true regarding abdominal incisions and the prevention of incisional hernias?
    A. A 4:1 suture:wound length is the current recommended closure length
    B. There is no difference in hernia occurrence between a running closure and an interrupted closure
    C. A permanent monofilament suture is preferred in the closure of the fascia in a running fashion
    D. Prophylactic use of mesh after open aortic aneurysm surgery is not efficacious
    E. A 1-cm bite between each stitch is the recommended distance during abdominal closure

11. A 55-year-old obese male presents to the hospital for his bariatric sleeve gastrectomy procedure. His comorbidities include diabetes and hypertension, and he states he was diagnosed with "walking pneumonia" 2 weeks ago and placed on antibiotics, which he has finished. Which of the following would not be beneficial if the SCIP measures for preoperative and postoperative care are followed?
    A. Placing the patient on an insulin sliding scale to keep glucose levels between 80 and 120 mg/dL
    B. Clipping the patient's abdominal hair with an electric shaver before operating
    C. Administering anticoagulation on postoperative day 1
    D. Administering antibiotics within 1 hour of surgery
    E. Discontinuing antibiotics by postoperative day 1

12. A 32-year-old female who is 24 weeks pregnant presents to the emergency department with acute onset of abdominal pain, fever, and vomiting. She states that the pain woke her up in the middle of the night with sudden onset of epigastric pain that is now diffuse. She has no vaginal bleeding and fetal monitoring demonstrates normal vitals for the fetus. Upon physical exam, the patient has diffuse tenderness with guarding throughout the abdomen, worse in the epigastric region. Pelvic examination is normal. She has a leukocytosis of 15,000 cells/L. Abdominal x-ray series shows some dilated bowel loops but no other findings. What is your next step in management of this patient?
    A. Abdominal ultrasound
    B. CT scan of the abdomen/pelvis with contrast
    C. Admit and observe with serial abdominal exams
    D. Exploratory laparotomy
    E. Diagnostic laparoscopy

13. Which of the following is true regarding a rectus sheath hematoma?
    A. If located above the umbilicus, it is more likely to resemble an acute intraabdominal process
    B. If located below the umbilicus, it is more likely to cause severe bleeding
    C. The majority are associated with a history of trauma
    D. Operative drainage is the treatment of choice in most cases
    E. Angiographic embolization is not useful

14. A woman presents with a firm, enlarging mass on her abdominal wall. After appropriate workup, she is diagnosed with a desmoid tumor. Which of the following is true about this condition?
    A. There is a high rate of metastasis without proper treatment
    B. The chance of local recurrence is low after appropriate intervention
    C. These tumors tend to enlarge during menopause
    D. They occur most commonly in women after childbirth
    E. These tumors arise from proliferative chondroblastic cells

15. Which of the following is true regarding retroperitoneal sarcomas?
    A. They are best managed by enucleation
    B. Prognosis is best determined by histologic grade
    C. Fibrosarcomas are the most common type
    D. Lymph node metastasis is common
    E. Radiation therapy is often curative for small sarcomas

16. A 75-year-old female with recently diagnosed atrial fibrillation, for which she was given an anticoagulant, presents with sudden onset abdominal pain unrelated to oral intake. Surgical history is remarkable for a total hip arthroplasty 3 years ago. Her physical exam is significant for a tender, palpable abdominal wall mass above the umbilicus that persists during flexion of abdominal wall muscles. The mass is most likely related to which of the following?
    A. A malignancy
    B. Bleeding from the superior epigastric artery
    C. Occult trauma
    D. An intraabdominal infection
    E. Bleeding from the inferior epigastric artery

ANSWERS

1. B. PD catheters can become malpositioned postoperatively despite intraoperative confirmation of proper placement. Instilling dialysate in the peritoneal cavity without the ability to remove it may lead to abdominal distention and mild pain. The first step for a suspected malpositioned PD catheter that may have been flipped or kinked is to obtain a KUB. If the catheter appears malpositioned, then a reasonable next step would be to return to the OR for diagnostic laparoscopy to reposition the catheter. For catheters that are clogged (resistance to instilling dialysate through the catheter or inability to instill fluid), tPA can be used (C). Omentopexy or omentectomy can also be helpful in cases of a malfunctioning catheter due to obstruction. Peritonitis is a common complication of PD and accounts for 50% of technical failures. This complication presents with abdominal pain, fever, and cloudy dialysate. The initial management involves intraperitoneal antibiotics, most commonly vancomycin, which cures 75% of cases without discontinuation of PD (D). Patients who continue to become increasingly septic may require intravenous (IV) antibiotics as well (E). Any fungal infection of PD requires prompt removal of the catheter (A).

Reference: Miller M, McCormick B, Lavoie S, Biyani M, Zimmerman D. Fluoroscopic manipulation of peritoneal dialysis catheters: outcomes and factors associated with successful manipulation. *Clin J Am Soc Nephrol*. 2012;7(5):795–800.

2. B. This patient has a Meckel diverticulum. This is a true intestinal diverticulum that results from the failure of the vitelline duct to obliterate during the fifth week of fetal development. It is the most common congenital anomaly of the GI tract. Pancreatic heterotopia is found in a minority of cases. The most common heterotopic tissue found in resected specimens is gastric mucosa, which can lead to ulcer formation and GI bleeding. Meckel with gastric mucosa is located at the antimesenteric border; however, ulceration occurs in the opposite mesenteric border of the ileum. Symptomatic cases require surgical intervention. The management of an incidentally discovered asymptomatic Meckel diverticulum during abdominal exploration is a controversial topic. Recently, it has been suggested to selectively intervene on patients with risk factors, namely age <50, male sex, large diverticulum >2 cm in diameter, presence of heterotopic tissue, palpation of abnormal nodules, or presence of fibrous bands. This patient has three indications for removal including age <50, male sex, and fibrous band (D). The ectopic tissue in a Meckel diverticulum secretes acid leading to ulcer formation in the adjacent ileum. Thus a segmental bowel resection should be performed in cases of GI bleeding to include the diverticulum (E). Otherwise, a simple diverticulectomy is appropriate. Routine use of 99mTc-pertechnetate scans in asymptomatic patients is not indicated (A). Biopsy of a Meckel diverticulum is not typically required; however, the most common cancer in Meckel is carcinoid (C, D).

Reference: Blouhos K, Boulas KA, Tsalis K, et al. Meckel's diverticulum in adults: surgical concerns. *Front Surg*. 2018;5:55.

3. B. IAH is defined as an intraabdominal pressure >12 mmHg. This is assessed by measuring the bladder pressure while the patient is paralyzed. ACS is defined by IAH >20 mmHg AND evidence of end-organ malperfusion (i.e., oliguria) (A). Patients who are mechanically ventilated often have high peak pressures. Primary ACS occurs most commonly after surgical procedures associated with massive resuscitation and tense fascial closure. Secondary ACS is due to medical conditions such as ascites or conditions requiring resuscitation without an abdominal procedure (i.e., significant burn injury). Nasogastric decompression and neuromuscular blockade are conservative measures to treat IAH but neither has been proven to significantly reduce mortality (C). Reducing IAH with paracentesis should be performed first in secondary ACS due to ascites (D). In refractory cases and all other cases of ACS, decompressive laparotomy should be performed expeditiously to lower mortality. The pathophysiology of ACS involves compression of the IVC, which can lead to elevated SVC pressures, and in turn increased intracranial pressures resulting in decreased cerebral perfusion pressures (E).

Reference: Muresan M, Muresan S, Brinzaniuc K, et al. How much does decompressive laparotomy reduce the mortality rate in primary abdominal compartment syndrome?: a single-center prospective study on 66 patients. *Medicine (Baltimore)*. 2017;96(5):e6006.

4. A. It is important to be aware of omental torsion because it readily mimics an intraabdominal perforation. Because it is typically very difficult to diagnose preoperatively, the diagnosis is most often made at surgery. Torsion of the omentum describes a twisting of the omentum around its vascular pedicle along the long axis. Primary torsion, in which case there is no underlying pathology, is extremely rare. Secondary torsion is much more common, and the torsion is usually precipitated by a fixed point such as a tumor, an adhesion, a hernia sac, or an area of intraabdominal inflammation. Omental torsion is much more common in adults in their fourth or fifth decade of life. Children with torsion are typically obese, likely contributing to a fatty omentum that predisposes to twisting. Other factors that predispose a patient to torsion include a bifid omentum and a narrowed omental pedicle. In primary omental torsion, the twisted omentum tends to be localized to the right side; thus, it is most commonly confused with acute appendicitis, acute cholecystitis, and pelvic inflammatory disease (D). Complicating the diagnosis is the fact that the omentum itself tends to migrate and envelop areas of inflammation. Laparoscopy is ideal for establishing the diagnosis and excluding other etiologies. Treatment is to resect the twisted omentum, which can often be infarcted at the time of surgery, and to correct any other related condition that may be identified (B, C). The finding of purulent fluid would suggest another diagnosis because it is not consistent with omental torsion. The fluid usually seen is serosanguinous (E).

References: Chew DK, Holgersen LO, Friedman D. Primary omental torsion in children. *J Pediatr Surg*. 1995;30(6):816–817.

Sánchez J, Rosado R, Ramírez D, Medina P, Mezquita S, Gallardo S. Torsion of the greater omentum: treatment by laparoscopy. *Surg Laparosc Endosc Percutan Tech.* 2002;12(6):443–445.

Young TH, Lee HS, Tang HS. Primary torsion of the greater omentum. *Int Surg.* 2004;89(2):72–75.

5. D. Coagulase-negative staphylococci (*Staphylococcus epidermidis*) is by far the most common cause of peritoneal catheter–related infections (A–C). *Staphylococcus aureus* is coagulase positive (E). Another defining feature of *S. aureus* is that it is catalase positive. The diagnosis is made by a combination of abdominal pain, development of cloudy peritoneal fluid, and an elevated peritoneal fluid white blood cell count greater than 100/mm³. Initial treatment consists of intraperitoneal antibiotics, which seem to be more effective than IV antibiotics for a total of 2 weeks. If the infection fails to clear based on abdominal examination, clinical picture, or persistent peritoneal fluid leukocytosis, then the catheter needs to be removed and a temporary hemodialysis catheter will need to be inserted. *S. aureus* and gram-negative organism infections are less likely to respond to antibiotic management alone.

6. E. Pseudomyxoma peritonei is a rare process in which the peritoneum becomes covered with semisolid mucus and large loculated cystic masses. There is no familial predisposition (C). A useful classification derived from a large series uses two categories: disseminated peritoneal adenomucinosis (DPAM) and peritoneal mucinous carcinomatosis (PMCA). DPAM is histologically a benign process and is most often due to a ruptured appendix. In one large series, appendiceal mucinous adenoma was associated with approximately 60% of patients with DPAM. In patients classified as PMCA, the origin was either a well-differentiated appendiceal or intestinal mucinous adenocarcinoma (B). Pseudomyxoma peritonei is most common in women aged 50 to 70 years (D). It is often asymptomatic until late in its course. Symptoms are often nonspecific, but the most common symptom is increased abdominal girth. Physical examination may demonstrate a distended abdomen with nonshifting dullness. Management is surgical, with cytoreduction of the primary and secondary implants, including peritonectomy and omentectomy (A). If there is a clear origin at the appendix, a right colectomy should also be performed. If the origin appears to be the ovary, total abdominal hysterectomy with bilateral salpingo-oophorectomy is recommended. The recurrence rate is very high (76% in one series).

References: Gough D, Donohue J, Schutt AJ, et al. Pseudomyxoma peritonei: long-term patient survival with an aggressive regional approach. *Ann Surg.* 1994;219(2):112–119.

Hinson FL, Ambrose NS. Pseudomyxoma peritonei. *Br J Surg.* 1998;85(10):1332–1339.

Ronnett BM, Zahn CM, Kurman RJ, Kass ME, Sugarbaker PH, Schmookler BM. Disseminated peritoneal adenomucinosis and peritoneal mucinous carcinomatosis: a clinicopathologic analysis of 109 cases with emphasis on distinguishing pathologic features, site of origin, prognosis, and relationship to "pseudomyxoma peritonei." *Am J Surg Pathol.* 1995;19(12):1390–1408.

7. C. Primary retroperitoneal abscesses are secondary to hematogenous spread while secondary retroperitoneal abscesses are related to an infection in an adjacent organ. The most common source of retroperitoneal abscesses is secondary, with renal infections accounting for nearly 50% of all

cases. Hematogenous spread is not a significant contributing factor for secondary retroperitoneal abscesses (E). Other common causes include retrocecal appendicitis (B), perforated duodenal ulcers, pancreatitis, and diverticulitis (A). In rare cases, patients may have Pott disease, which is a disseminated form related to tuberculosis (D). Patients typically present with back, pelvic, flank, or thigh pain with associated fever and leukocytosis. Flank erythema may be present. Kidney infections often have gram-negative rods such as *Proteus* and *E. coli.* Treatment consists of broad-spectrum antibiotics and drainage, and identification of the source. If the abscess is simple and unilocular, then CT-guided drainage is the treatment of choice. Operative drainage may be required for complex abscesses.

8. B. Spontaneous (primary) bacterial peritonitis (SBP) is defined as bacterial infection of ascitic fluid in the absence of any surgically treatable intraabdominal infection. Patients usually present with fever, diarrhea, and abdominal pain, but if severe enough, they will also have altered mental status, hypotension, hypothermia, and a paralytic ileus. However, 13% of patients will be completely asymptomatic. Treatment is with antibiotics alone. Prophylactic antibiotics (with fluoroquinolones) to prevent SBP should be considered in high-risk patients with cirrhosis, ascites, and history of gastrointestinal bleeding (as in the present case). Patients with cirrhosis who have low ascitic fluid protein (<1.0 g/dL) and those with a serum bilirubin greater than 2.5 mg/dL should also be started on prophylactic antibiotics. Opsonic or bactericidal activity of ascitic fluid is related to protein concentration. One of the key features of primary peritonitis is that the isolate is usually a single organism and that organism usually is not an anaerobe. Secondary peritonitis refers to peritonitis in the setting of a bowel perforation. Thus, polymicrobial or anaerobic cultures should raise suspicion for bowel perforation (A) and secondary peritonitis (E). In adults, the most common pathogens in SBP are the aerobic enteric flora *E. coli* and *Klebsiella* (C). In children with nephrogenic or hepatogenic ascites, group A *Streptococcus*, *S. aureus*, and *Streptococcus pneumoniae* are common isolates (D). The diagnosis is made by paracentesis demonstrating more than 250 neutrophils/mm³ of ascitic fluid in the presence of a correlating clinical presentation. This should be evaluated before initiating antibiotics because cultures will return falsely negative. An active infection is considered a contraindication for liver transplantation.

References: Bell RB, Seymour NE. Abdominal wall, omentum, mesentery, and retroperitoneum. In: Brunicardi FC, Andersen DK, Billiar T, et al., eds. *Schwartz's principles of surgery.* 8th ed. New York: McGraw-Hill; 1990:1317–1328.

Runyon BA. Monomicrobial nonneutrocytic bacterascites: a variant of spontaneous bacterial peritonitis. *Hepatology.* 1990;12(4 Pt 1):710–715.

Turnage RH, Li B, McDonald, JC. Abdominal wall, umbilicus, peritoneum, mesenteries, omentum and retroperitoneum. In: Townsend CM Jr, Beauchamp RD, Evers BM, Mattox KL, eds. *Sabiston textbook of surgery: The biological basis of modern surgical practice.* 17th ed. Philadelphia: W.B. Saunders; 2004:1171–1198.

9. B. Good communication between the cardiologist and surgeon is essential before performing coronary interventions in a patient who requires surgery. Coronary revascularization before elective surgery is not recommended if the patient has asymptomatic coronary artery disease (CAD). However, in the setting of an acute coronary syndrome (acute myocardial infarction [MI], unstable angina), a percutaneous coronary intervention (PCI) is recommended before surgery. The options are to perform balloon angioplasty alone or add a bare metal stent (BMS) or a drug-eluting stent (DES). The DES is the best long-term option, but it requires a longer delay of surgery. Thus, the decision of which to use depends on the urgency of the subsequent operation (urgent, time sensitive, or elective) and the feasibility of operating with antiplatelet agents on board. If the operation is urgent (within 2 weeks), a PCI with balloon angioplasty may be best because the waiting period for surgery is 2 weeks (A). If the operation is time sensitive (2–6 weeks), a BMS is a better option because it is less likely to suddenly occlude as compared with angioplasty alone. However, one should wait 1 month before performing surgery (C). Because this patient has a relatively symptomatic hernia, the operation is time sensitive. Finally, if a DES is placed, the recommendation is to wait 6 months before performing surgery (D, E).

References: Fleisher LA, Fleischmann KE, Auerbach AD, et al. 2014 ACC/AHA guideline on perioperative cardiovascular evaluation and management of patients undergoing noncardiac surgery: a report of the American College of Cardiology/American Heart Association Task Force on Practice Guidelines. *J Am Coll Cardiol.* 2014;64(22):e77–e137.

Guyatt GH, Akl EA, Crowther M, Gutterman DD, Schünemann HJ, American College of Chest Physicians Antithrombotic Therapy and Prevention of Thrombosis Panel. Executive summary: antithrombotic therapy and prevention of thrombosis, 9th ed: American College of Chest Physicians Evidence-Based Clinical Practice Guidelines [published corrections appear in *Chest.* 141(4):1129].

Dosage error in article text. *Chest.* 2012;142(6):1698.

Dosage error in article text]. *Chest.* 2012;141(2 suppl):7S–47S.

Livhits M, Ko CY, Leonardi MJ, Zingmond DS, Gibbons MM, de Virgilio C. Risk of surgery following recent myocardial infarction. *Ann Surg.* 2011;253(5):857–864.

10. A. The material and the surgical technique used to close an open abdomen are important determinants of the risk of developing an incisional hernia. The European Hernia Society has recently come out with guidelines recommending that a small bite closure be performed using at least a 4:1 suture:wound length during closure. It has also been shown that running closure is superior to an interrupted closure (B). Prophylactic use of mesh during closure has been shown to be efficacious after open aortic aneurysm surgery because of the high rate of incisional hernia (D). A randomized control trial looking at small bites compared to large bites has recently been performed, looking at 560 patients who received either small, 5-mm bites 5 mm apart or large, 1-cm bites 1 cm apart. They found a statistically significant reduced rate of hernia occurrence in the small bite group, which is now the recommended bite size and length (E). A slowly absorbable monofilament suture (polydioxanone suture [PDS]) has been shown to also be the recommended suture in abdominal closure (C).

References: Deerenberg EB, Harlaar JJ, Steyerberg EW, et al. Small bites versus large bites for closure of abdominal midline incisions (STITCH): a double-blind, multicentre, randomised controlled trial. *Lancet.* 2015;386(10000):1254–1260.

Muysoms FE, Antoniou SA, Bury K, et al. European Hernia Society guidelines on the closure of abdominal wall incisions. *Hernia.* 2015;19(1):1–24.

11. A. The Surgical Care Improvement Project (SCIP) is a national quality partnership of organizations interested in improving surgical outcomes that began in 2006. Care is taken by all institutions to follow the recommendations by the Joint Commission because all these outcomes are documented and measured quarterly. The core measures include giving antibiotics within 1 hour of surgery (D) and discontinuing within 24 hours (E), Foley catheter removal by postoperative day 2, and hair removal by clipping on the day of surgery. Shaving the hair off has been shown to increase the risk of infection (B). Other beneficial measures include being on appropriate venous thromboembolism (VTE) prophylaxis within 24 hours of surgery and glucose control. The importance of glucose control and surgical outcomes has been well established; however, in 2009, the NICE-SUGAR trial demonstrated that strict glucose control was actually associated with worse outcomes. It is now widely accepted that the goal should be to keep glucose levels below 180 mg/dL (C).

Reference: NICE-SUGAR Study Investigators, Finfer S, Chittock DR, et al. Intensive versus conventional glucose control in critically ill patients. *N Engl J Med.* 2009;360(13):1283–1297.

12. B. Fear of radiation exposure during pregnancy should not take precedence over quickly establishing the correct diagnosis and initiating treatment. Based on the patient's acute onset of symptoms and location, the presentation is concerning for peritonitis, potentially due to a perforated viscus, such as a peptic ulcer, or a closed-loop bowel obstruction. In this situation, the best next step would be to perform a computed tomography (CT) scan of the abdomen (A, C–E). As a general rule, the care of the patient, not the fetus, should take first priority. Based on the National Guideline Clearinghouse, expeditious and accurate diagnosing should take precedence over risk of ionizing radiation. The effects of radiation exposure on the fetus depend on the gestational age and the amount of radiation. In general, the earlier the gestational age, the greater the risk. High dose (>10 rads) exposure early in pregnancy (within the first 4 weeks) can lead to fetal demise. However, such a high exposure exceeds the dose of typical imaging (abdominal x-ray is 200 mrad while abdominal and pelvic CT is about 3–4 rads). Between 8 and 15 weeks' gestation, high-dose (>10 rads) radiation can lead to intrauterine growth retardation and central nervous defects. Beyond 15 weeks (as in the present case), there do not appear to be any deterministic effects (dose-dependent events such as fetal loss, congenital defects) on the fetus. Stochastic effects (those that are not dose dependent), such as the subsequent risk of cancer or leukemia, are increased with exposure of 1 rad or more. The risk is about 1 cancer for every 500 exposures. Conversely, if the pregnant patient with an acute abdomen progresses to peritonitis and bowel perforation, the risk of fetal demise is very high. Thus, the risk of fetal miscarriage is higher with visceral perforation than with radiation exposure, and therefore all measures should be taken for an accurate diagnosis. Magnetic resonance imaging (MRI) is considered a good imaging option in pregnancy; however, its use in the emergent setting may be limited by its availability. Ultrasound is also useful but would be more useful if the patient presented with right upper quadrant pain (suspected biliary disease) or right lower quadrant pain (suspected appendicitis).

Reference: Khandelwal A, Fasih N, Kielar A. Imaging of acute abdomen in pregnancy. *Radiol Clin North Am.* 2013;51(6):1005–1022.

13. B. Rectus sheath hematomas are clinically significant because of the fact that they can easily be mistaken for an intraabdominal inflammatory process. The etiology is an injury to an epigastric artery within the rectus sheath. In most cases, there is no clear history of trauma (C). Particularly in the elderly who are taking oral anticoagulants, these typically occur spontaneously. Patients frequently describe a sudden onset of unilateral abdominal pain, sometimes preceded by a coughing fit. In one series, 11 of 12 patients were women, and in another series, all 8 were women, with an average age in the sixth decade. Below the arcuate line, there is no aponeurotic posterior covering to the rectus muscle. Therefore, hematomas below this line can cross the midline, causing a larger hematoma to form, and then cause bilateral lower quadrant pain resembling a perforated viscus. On physical examination, a mass is often palpable. The Fothergill sign is the finding of a palpable abdominal mass that remains unchanged with contraction of the rectus muscles. This helps distinguish it from an intraabdominal abscess, which would not be palpable with rectus contraction. The diagnosis is best established with a CT scan, which will demonstrate a fluid collection in the rectus muscle. The hematocrit should be closely monitored. Once the diagnosis is established, management is primarily nonoperative and consists of resuscitation, monitoring of serial hemoglobin/hematocrit levels, and reversal of anticoagulation (D). However, one should be cautious with reversal of anticoagulation, as stable patients may benefit from continued anticoagulation (e.g., recent mechanical valve). On rare occasions, angiographic embolization may be necessary (E). Surgical management, while rarely necessary, would involve ligation of the bleeding vessel and evacuation of the hematoma.

References: Berná JD, Zuazu I, Madrigal M, García-Medina V, Fernández C, Guirado F. Conservative treatment of large rectus sheath hematoma in patients undergoing anticoagulant therapy. *Abdom Imaging.* 2000;25(3):230–234.

Zainea GG, Jordan F. Rectus sheath hematomas: their pathogenesis, diagnosis, and management. *Am Surg.* 1988;54(10):630–633.

14. D. Desmoid tumors are unusual soft-tissue neoplasms that arise from fascial or fibro-aponeurotic tissue. They are proliferations of benign-appearing fibroblastic cells with abundant collagen and few mitoses (E). Desmoid tumors do not metastasize (A); however, they are locally aggressive and have a very high local recurrence rate reaching almost 50% (B). They have been associated with Gardner syndrome (intestinal polyposis, osteomas, fibromas, and epidermal or sebaceous cysts) and familial adenomatous polyposis (FAP), which is why patients should be scheduled for a colonoscopy soon after diagnosis. In sporadic cases, surgical trauma appears to be an important cause. Desmoid tumors may develop within or adjacent to surgical scars. Patients with FAP have a 1000-fold increased risk of the development of desmoid tumors. Desmoids are more common in women of childbearing age, tend to occur after childbirth, and may be linked to estrogen. Oral contraceptive pills (OCP) have also been found to be associated with the occurrence of these tumors, whereas antiestrogen medications may lead to shrinkage. They've been reported to shrink after menopause (C).

Patients are typically in their third or fourth decade of life and present with pain, a mass, or both. They are classified as either extra abdominal (extremities, shoulder), abdominal wall, or intraabdominal (mesenteric and pelvic). There are no typical radiographic findings, but MRI may delineate muscle or soft-tissue infiltration and is required in larger tumors to delineate anatomic relations before surgical intervention. Core needle biopsy often reveals collagen with diffuse spindle cells and abundant fibrous stroma, which may suggest a low-grade fibrosarcoma; however, the cells lack mitotic activity. An open incisional biopsy of lesions larger than 3 to 4 cm is often necessary. Wide local excision with negative margins is indicated for symptomatic desmoid tumors. Nonresectable or incidentally found, asymptomatic, intraabdominal desmoid tumors (even if resectable) should be treated with nonsteroidal antiinflammatory agents (e.g., sulindac) and antiestrogens, which have met with objective response rates of 50%. In regard to adjuvant therapy, recent retrospective reviews have seen significant reductions in recurrence with radiation combined with surgery and even with radiation alone. More research is necessary for the use of chemotherapy agents, but it has been seen that when cytotoxic chemotherapy agents are used in inoperable desmoid tumors, there is a 20% to 40% positive response. The aggressive nature of these tumors and high rate of occurrence make desmoid tumors the second most common cause of death in patients with FAP, after colorectal carcinoma.

References: Ballo MT, Zagars GK, Pollack A, Pisters PW, Pollack RA. Desmoid tumor: prognostic factors and outcome after surgery, radiation therapy, or combined surgery and radiation therapy. *J Clin Oncol.* 1999;17(1):158–167.

Hansmann A, Adolph C, Vogel T. High dose tamoxifen and sulindac as first-line treatment for desmoid tumors. *Cancer.* 2004;100(3):612–620.

Janinis J, Patriki M, Vini L, Aravantinos G, Whelan JS. The pharmacological treatment of aggressive fibromatosis: a systematic review. *Ann Oncol.* 2003;14(2):181–190.

Nuyttens JJ, Rust PF, Thomas CR Jr, Turrisi AT 3rd. Surgery versus radiation therapy for patients with aggressive fibromatosis or desmoid tumors: a comparative review of 22 articles. *Cancer.* 2000;88(7):1517–1523.

15. B. Most retroperitoneal tumors are malignant and comprise approximately half of all soft-tissue sarcomas. The most common sarcomas occurring in the retroperitoneum are liposarcomas, malignant fibrous histiocytomas, and leiomyosarcomas (C). Approximately 50% of patients will have a local recurrence and 20% to 30% will end up having distant metastases. Lymph node metastases are rare (D). Retroperitoneal sarcomas present as large masses because they do not typically produce symptoms until their mass effect creates compression or invasion of adjacent structures. Symptoms may include gastrointestinal hemorrhage, early satiety, nausea, vomiting, and lower extremity swelling. Retroperitoneal sarcomas have a worse prognosis than nonretroperitoneal sarcomas. The best chance for long-term survival is achieved with an en bloc, margin-negative resection. Tumor stage at presentation, high histologic grade, unresectability, and grossly positive resection margins are strongly associated with increased mortality rates. Tumor grade is the most significant predictor of outcome. Complete surgical resection is the most effective treatment for primary or recurrent retroperitoneal sarcomas (A, E). Surgical cure can be limited because the margins are often compromised by anatomic constraints. There is no difference in survival between those who had a resection with a grossly positive margin and those with inoperable tumors. Unlike extremity sarcomas, external beam radiation therapy is limited for retroperitoneal malignancies because there is a low tolerance for radiation to surrounding structures. Postoperative and intraoperative radiation therapy have been shown to reduce local recurrence, but further studies are needed to determine if this leads to improved survival.

Reference: Lewis JJ, Leung D, Woodruff JM, Brennan MF. Retroperitoneal soft-tissue sarcoma: analysis of 500 patients treated and followed at a single institution. *Ann Surg.* 1998;228(3):355–365.

16. B. This patient was recently diagnosed with atrial fibrillation and started on oral anticoagulants. One should suspect a rectus sheath hematoma in older patients taking anticoagulants who present with the clinical triad of acute abdominal pain, an abdominal wall mass, and anemia. The mass is palpable even during flexion of abdominal wall muscles, helping to differentiate this from an intraperitoneal process (Fothergill sign) (D). In a review of 126 patients by Mayo Clinic, anticoagulation was associated with 70%. Above the arcuate line, the etiology is often related to a lesion to the superior epigastric artery within the rectus sheath (E). In most cases, there is no clear history of trauma (C). In particular, in the elderly who are taking oral anticoagulants, they typically occur spontaneously. The most common treatment for patients with rectus sheath hematomas is rest, analgesics, and blood transfusions as necessary. In general, coagulopathies are corrected; however, continuing anticoagulation may be prudent in select patients (e.g., biomechanical valve, recent saddle embolus). In extreme cases, angioembolization may be required.

References: Alla VM, Karnam SM, Kaushik M, Porter J. Spontaneous rectus sheath hematoma. *West J Emerg Med.* 2010;11(1):76–79.

Cherry WB, Mueller PS. Rectus sheath hematoma: review of 126 cases at a single institution. *Medicine (Baltimore).* 2006;85(2):105–110.

Abdomen—Hernia

AMANDA C. PURDY AND AMY KIM YETASOOK

2

ABSITE 99th Percentile High-Yields

I. Abdominal Wall Hernia
   a. From skin to peritoneum: skin → fascia of Camper → fascia of Scarpa → external oblique → internal oblique → transversus abdominis → transversalis fascia → preperitoneal fat → peritoneum
   b. Superior to arcuate line:
      1. Anterior sheath comprised of aponeurosis of external oblique and the anterior half of the aponeurosis of internal oblique
      2. Posterior sheath comprised of aponeurosis of transversus abdominis and aponeurosis of the posterior half of internal oblique; posterior sheath not present inferior to arcuate line
   c. Ten to 15% of all incisions will develop into ventral (incisional) hernia; wound infection after surgery doubles risk of a hernia development
   d. Midline epigastrium is a physiologic area of weakness in the abdomen where patients can develop diastasis recti and/or epigastric hernia; risk factors include pregnancy and weight gain
   e. Diastasis recti: attenuation of linea alba causing rectus muscle separation; when the rectus contract, a bulge appears in the upper midline abdomen; no fascial defect, not a hernia

II. Umbilical Hernias
   a. Pediatric umbilical hernias
      1. Congenital defect, repair by age 5 or sooner if symptomatic
   b. Umbilical hernias in adults
      1. Acquired defect, increased intraabdominal pressure causes weakening of transversalis fascia and of the umbilical ring
      2. Women are 3 times more likely to develop umbilical hernias than men (due to pregnancy), and up to 90% of women develop an umbilical hernia during pregnancy; incarceration occurs more in men
      3. Cirrhotic patients with uncomplicated umbilical hernias should be medically optimized before undergoing elective surgical repair; this includes free water restriction, diuretics, and large volume paracentesis (with infusion of albumin); mesh can be used

III. Inguinal Hernias
   a. Cremaster muscle fibers arise from internal oblique muscle, inguinal ligament from external oblique muscle; the internal oblique and transversalis fascia form the internal ring of the inguinal canal; the conjoint tendon is the lower common aponeurosis of the internal oblique and the transversus abdominis
   b. Though widely believed as true, there is little evidence to support physical activity with inguinal hernia development; inguinal hernias have increased type 3 collagen and decreased type 1 collagen
   c. During dissection, an indirect hernia sac is found on the anteromedial aspect of spermatic cord
   d. The genital branch of the genitofemoral nerve supplies sensation to the mons and labia majora in women, and in men it supplies motor to the cremaster and sensation to the scrotum; it runs within the spermatic cord and exits via the deep inguinal ring

e. The iliohypogastric nerve arises from the first lumbar branch and travels between the transversus abdominis and the internal oblique muscles

f. The ilioinguinal nerve runs anterior to the spermatic cord in men or round ligament in women and passes through the superficial inguinal ring; supplies sensation to the upper medial thigh

g. Pediatric inguinal hernias (due to a congenital failure of the processus vaginalis to close):
   1. Repair only requires high ligation of the hernia sac (ligation at the internal ring)

IV. Hernia Repair
   a. Open repair
      i. Open repair with mesh (<10% recurrence rate)
         1. Lichtenstein repair (tension free): mesh is sutured medially to the transversus abdominis arch, and the lateral edge of mesh is sutured to the inguinal ligament; mesh should overlap 2 cm over pubic tubercle and 2 to 4 cm lateral to the internal ring
      ii. Open repair without mesh (30%–50% recurrence rate)
         1. Bassini repair: the conjoint tendon is sutured to the inguinal ligament with interrupted, nonabsorbable sutures
         2. McVay repair: the conjoint tendon is sutured to Cooper ligament (also called the pectineal ligament); need to expose Cooper ligament by incising transversalis fascia and entering preperitoneal space; relaxing incision has to be made in the anterior rectus sheath; repairs both inguinal and femoral hernias
         3. Shouldice repair: the transversalis fascia is incised and reapproximated, 4-layer closure with running suture
   b. Laparoscopic repair
      i. Best option for recurrent hernias (previously treated with an open approach), bilateral hernias, and obese patients; contraindicated in patients with large scrotal hernias or who have undergone prior extensive lower abdominal or pelvic surgery
      ii. Mesh fixation inferior to the iliopubic tract and lateral to the epigastric vessels (triangle of pain) is avoided because of the risk of injury to the lateral femoral cutaneous nerve; similarly, avoid fixation below the internal ring, which is bordered laterally by spermatic vessels and medially by vas deferens (triangle of doom), as this risks injury to the external iliac artery and vein
      iii. The two laparoscopic procedures: transabdominal preperitoneal (TAPP) and totally extraperitoneal (TEP) repair
         1. TAPP: the peritoneal space is entered at umbilicus, peritoneum overlying inguinal floor is dissected away as a flap, hernia is reduced, mesh is fixed over internal ring opening in the preperitoneal space, and peritoneum is reapproximated; can also examine contralateral side
         2. TEP: the preperitoneal space is developed w dissecting balloon inserted between posterior rectus sheath and rectus abdominis and directed toward pelvis inferior to arcuate ligaments; other ports inserted into preperitoneal space without ever entering peritoneal cavity; advantage here is that you never open peritoneum so no mesh exposure to abdominal organs, so less adhesions
   c. If chronic groin pain after hernia surgery, perform a pelvic MRI; risk of chronic groin pain after hernia repair is 15% to 20%
   d. Most common location for breakdown of laparoscopic hernia repair is the medial portion of the mesh; often because the mesh is too small or that it was not appropriately attached medially

V. Femoral Hernia
   a. Femoral triangle: femoral vein laterally, adductor longus medially and inguinal ligament superiorly
   b. Boundaries of femoral canal: superior (inguinal), medial (lacunar ligament), lateral (femoral vein), and posterior or floor (iliacus and psoas tendon; fascia of pectineus)
   c. All femoral hernias should be repaired as they have a 15% to 20% risk of strangulation

VI. Miscellaneous Hernias

a. Obturator hernia: Howship-Romberg sign is internal thigh pain with external rotation; repair for obturator hernia should be an abdominal approach as this allows access to the defect and reduction of contents, may require incision of the obturator membrane

b. Petit hernia is bound by latissimus dorsi, iliac crest, and external oblique muscle; Grynfeltt hernia is bound by sacrospinous muscle, internal oblique, and the 12th rib

c. Spigelian hernia is defect through Spigelian fascia, which is area between semilunar line and lateral border of rectus abdominis; majority occur just below arcuate line where no posterior rectus sheath exists

d. A sports hernia is not a true hernia; it is a weakness of the inguinal floor developing in those with significant physical activity (athletes); pressure is placed on the genital branch of the genital femoral nerve and can lead to chronic groin pain; on exam, there may be tenderness with palpation of the inguinal floor through the external ring, but no hernia is identified with Valsalva

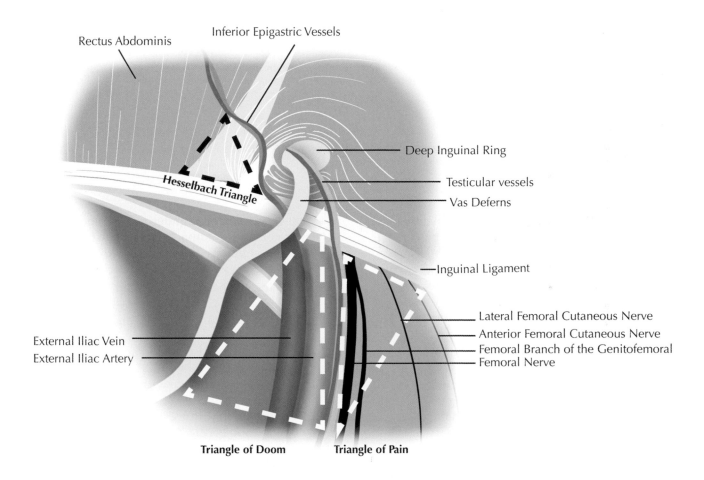

The "triangle of doom" contains the external iliac vessels, and is bounded by the vas deferens medially, spermatic vessels laterally and the peritoneal fold inferiorly. The "triangle of pain" is an "V"-shaped area with its apex pointing toward the deep inguinal ring bound anteriorly by the inguinal ligament and the spermatic vessels posteromedially. Hesselbach triangle is the space where a direct hernia could occur. It is an area of weakness bordered by the rectus abdominis medially, the inferior epigastric vessels laterally, and the inguinal ligament inferiorly. An indirect hernia occurs laterally to the inferior epigastric vessels through the deep inguinal ring. A femoral hernia occurs inferior to the inguinal ligament, lateral to the lacunar ligament and medial to the femoral vein.

Fig. 2.1

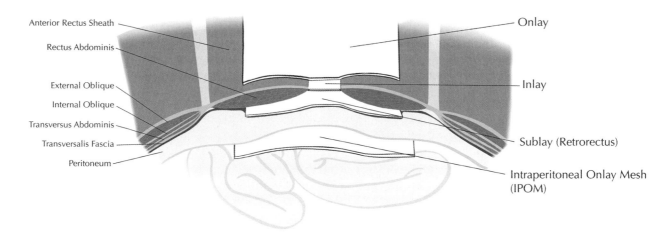

Onlay Hernia repairs secure hernia mesh to the fascia anteriorly. They have the highest recurrence rate and rate of seroma formation of all ventral hernia repairs.
Inlay Hernia repairs position the mesh between the edges of the fascia.
Sublay Hernia repairs (retrorectus repairs) have the lowest incidence of recurrence and the mesh is placed over the transversalis fascia but under the rectus abdominus muscle.
Intraperitoneal onlay mesh repairs are placed in the abdominal cavity beneath the peritoneum.

Fig. 2.2

QUESTIONS

1. A 45-year-old woman with diabetes mellitus and a BMI of 35 kg/m^2 presents to clinic for an intermittent, painful bulge in her mid-abdomen over an old midline laparotomy scar. On exam, there is a reducible midline bulge with a 7 by 3 cm fascial defect. She would like to proceed with surgery. What is the most appropriate management?
   A. Physical therapy referral for abdominal wall strengthening
   B. Open hernia repair with onlay mesh
   C. Open hernia repair with sublay mesh
   D. Laparoscopic hernia repair with mesh
   E. Component separation and primary repair

2. A 55-year-old man with a history of abdominoperineal resection for rectal cancer two years ago has intermittent pain and fullness next to his colostomy that is sometimes associated with nausea and vomiting. On exam, his colostomy appears healthy, and no bulge is palpated. CT demonstrates a loop of bowel superficial to the fascia that is adjacent to the stoma. What is the best management?
   A. Primary repair of parastomal hernia
   B. Relocate the colostomy
   C. Repair with prosthetic mesh
   D. Repair with biologic mesh
   E. Reassurance and return precautions

3. A 30-year-old patient underwent exploratory laparotomy for trauma. Which of the following closure techniques is associated with the lowest risk of developing an incisional hernia?
   A. Placing stitches 1 cm apart and 1 cm from the fascial edge
   B. Placing sutures 5 mm apart and 5 mm from the fascial edge
   C. Placing stitches 1 cm apart and 5 mm from the fascial edge
   D. Using running suture with a suture to wound length ratio of 2:1
   E. Using running suture with a suture to wound length ratio of 3:1

4. A 60-year-old woman with chronic kidney disease is undergoing elective peritoneal dialysis catheter placement. At her preoperative appointment, she is noted to have a small, nontender, reducible inguinal hernia. She says it has been there for years and that it does not bother her. What is the most appropriate management?
   A. Peritoneal dialysis catheter placement alone
   B. Inguinal hernia repair with mesh with peritoneal dialysis catheter placement 6 weeks later
   C. Inguinal hernia repair without mesh with peritoneal dialysis catheter placement 6 weeks later

D. Concurrent inguinal hernia repair with mesh and peritoneal dialysis catheter placement

E. Concurrent inguinal hernia repair without mesh and peritoneal dialysis catheter placement

5. The genital branch of the genitofemoral nerve:
   A. is typically found anteriorly on top of the spermatic cord
   B. provides sensation to the base of the penis and inner thigh
   C. typically lies on the anterior surface of the internal oblique muscle
   D. if cut will result in ipsilateral loss of cremasteric reflex
   E. often intermingles with the iliohypogastric nerve

6. Which of the following is true regarding hernia anatomy?
   A. Poupart ligament is formed from the anteroinferior portion of the external oblique aponeurosis
   B. The cremaster muscle arises from the transversus abdominis muscle
   C. The genital branch of the genitofemoral nerve passes through the superficial ring
   D. The femoral branch of the genitofemoral nerve innervates the cremasteric muscle
   E. Indirect hernias most often arise within the borders of the rectus muscle, inferior inguinal ligament, and inferior epigastric artery

7. Which of the following is true regarding the arcuate line?
   A. It is usually located a few centimeters above the umbilicus
   B. Below this line, the internal oblique aponeurosis splits
   C. Below this line, the rectus muscle lies on the transversalis fascia
   D. Below this line, the posterior rectus sheath is thinner
   E. Below this line, the external oblique muscle does not contribute to the anterior rectus sheath

8. A 55-year-old male presents with a painful bulge in the left groin that first appeared several months ago. His surgical history includes a right-sided open inguinal hernia repair. Upon examination you also note a bulge in the right groin over his previous incision. Both masses are reducible. Which of the following is true regarding this patient's condition?
   A. Open repair is preferred
   B. In laparoscopic repair, failure to tack the mesh lateral to the inferior epigastric vessels can lead to recurrence through the internal ring

C. Violation of the peritoneum during a totally extraperitoneal (TEP) repair requires conversion to an open or transabdominal preperitoneal (TAPP) approach

D. Persistent numbness or pain of the lateral thigh is more common with open versus laparoscopic repair

E. Laparoscopic repair will prevent him from developing a femoral hernia in the future

9. A 28-year-old male patient is asking for advice on whether to pursue open mesh repair or TEP repair of a newly diagnosed, reducible right-sided inguinal hernia. What can you tell the patient about these two methods of repair?
   A. Chronic pain is reduced with an open mesh repair
   B. Operative time is not significantly different between the two
   C. TEP repair is associated with a quicker return to work and normal activities
   D. Open mesh repair is associated with a higher rate of intraoperative complications
   E. Recurrence is relatively common (>25%) no matter which method is chosen

10. One hour after laparoscopic repair of a left inguinal hernia, the patient complains of severe burning groin pain. Which of the following is the most appropriate recommendation?
    A. Immediate return to the OR for laparoscopy
    B. Nonsteroidal antiinflammatory drugs
    C. Neurontin
    D. Opioid analgesia
    E. Inject groin region with local anesthetic

11. Ischemic orchitis after inguinal hernia repair is most often due to:
    A. Too tight a reconstruction of the inguinal ring
    B. Preexisting testicular pathology
    C. Inadvertent ligation of the testicular artery
    D. Completely excising a large scrotal hernia sac
    E. Anomalous blood supply to the testicle

12. A 45-year-old man presents with an asymptomatic right inguinal hernia. It is easily reduced with gentle pressure. Which of the following is true about this condition?
    A. The likelihood of strangulation developing is high without surgery
    B. Without surgery, intractable pain will most likely develop
    C. Waiting until symptoms develop is a reasonable alternative to surgery
    D. Laparoscopic repair is the best option
    E. If the hernia is small, there is a lower chance of incarceration

13. A 5-month-old previously full-term male infant presents with a tender left groin mass that has been present for the past several hours. There is slight erythema over the skin. He is afebrile and his labs are normal. Which of the following is the best next step?
    A. Attempt manual reduction, and if successful, schedule surgical repair when infant reaches 1 year of age
    B. Attempt manual reduction, and if successful, immediately take to the operating room for surgical repair
    C. Attempt manual reduction, and if successful, schedule repair in 2 days
    D. Attempt manual reduction, and if successful, schedule left-sided surgical repair with contralateral groin exploration in 2 days
    E. Take immediately to the operating room for operative repair

14. Which of the following best describes umbilical hernias in children?
    A. They have a significant risk of incarceration.
    B. Repair is indicated once an umbilical hernia is diagnosed
    C. Repair should be performed if the hernia persists beyond 6 months of age
    D. Most close spontaneously
    E. Repair should be performed only if the child is symptomatic

15. Which of the following is true regarding umbilical hernias in adults?
    A. Most are congenital
    B. Repair is contraindicated in patients with cirrhosis
    C. Strangulation is less common than in children

D. Small, asymptomatic hernias can be clinically observed
E. Primary closure has recurrence rates similar to those of mesh repair

16. Which of the following is true regarding femoral hernias?
    A. They are the most common hernia in females
    B. The Cooper ligament is considered the anterior border of the femoral canal
    C. They are lateral to the femoral vein
    D. Repair involves approximating the iliopubic tract to the Cooper ligament
    E. A Bassini operation is considered an appropriate surgical option

17. A 55-year-old woman presents with a painless abdominal wall bulge. She reports a successful diet and exercise program and has lost almost 40 kg over the past 2 years. However, she is worried because yesterday when she was sitting up in bed, she noticed an upper midline abdominal bulge that looks like a large ridge between her rib cage and belly button. On physical exam the bulge becomes visible when she lifts her head off the bed. Which of the following is true regarding her condition?
    A. Surgical repair should be done immediately before signs of incarceration develop
    B. There are both congenital and acquired etiologies
    C. A strict regimen of abdominal wall exercises usually results in complete resolution
    D. The defect is limited to the transversalis fascia
    E. Typically these defects contain only preperitoneal fat

ANSWERS

1. D. This patient has a symptomatic ventral incisional hernia. The best option for repair in this patient with multiple risk factors for perioperative infection (diabetes and obesity) is laparoscopic hernia repair with mesh. Compared to open incisional hernia repair, laparoscopic repair has a lower incidence of surgical site infection and is the best option for patients at risk for postoperative infection (C–D). Open and laparoscopic ventral hernia repairs with mesh have similar recurrence rate. Component separation is a technique where the anterior rectus sheath is incised 2 cm lateral to the semilunar line in order to primarily close large defects while minimizing tension. This is unnecessary in this case, as the defect is only 3 cm wide, and a minimally invasive technique is more appropriate (E). Abdominal wall strengthening exercises are the primary repair for rectus diastasis, which is an attenuation of the linea alba in the superior abdominal wall without a true hernia. This patient has a hernia, as evidenced by fascial defect on physical exam (A).

Reference: Guidelines for laparoscopic ventral hernia repair. SAGES. Published June 7, 2016. https://www.sages.org/publications/guidelines/guidelines-for-laparoscopic-ventral-hernia-repair

2. C. This patient has a parastomal hernia. Although the incidence of parastomal hernias is higher with end ostomies than with loop ostomies, this may simply be due to loop ostomies getting reversed more often, and sooner than end ostomies that are more often permanent. The majority of parastomal hernias are asymptomatic and do not require intervention. However, this patient is experiencing symptoms with intermittent bowel obstruction and should undergo repair (E). The best option for management of a symptomatic parastomal hernia is to take the ostomy down if appropriate. Unfortunately, this is not an option for this patient with a prior abdominoperineal resection (APR). The next best option is repair of the hernia with synthetic mesh using the Sugarbaker technique, where intraperitoneal mesh covers the entire defect, and the bowel leading to the ostomy enters laterally between the mesh and abdominal wall. Biologic mesh is associated with higher recurrence rates compared to prosthetic mesh (D). It may be considered for patients with significant contamination. Primary repair of parastomal hernias has been largely abandoned due to unacceptable recurrence rates of up to 70% (A). Ostomy relocation solves the problem at hand (the current symptomatic parastomal hernia); however, it is inferior to repair with mesh as there is a high risk of developing another parastomal hernia at the new ostomy site (B).

Reference: Hansson BM, Slater NJ, van der Velden AS, et al. Surgical techniques for parastomal hernia repair: a systematic review of the literature. *Ann Surg.* 2012;255(4):685–695.

3. B. After vertical midline abdominal incision, approximately 10% to 20% of patients develop incisional hernias. Randomized controlled trials have shown that small (5 mm) fascial bites 5 mm apart have a significantly lower rate of developing incisional hernia than large (1 cm) bites 1 cm apart (A, C). Also, a suture to wound length ratio of at least 4:1 is associated with less tension and a decreased incidence of incisional hernia development (D, E).

References: Deerenberg EB, Harlaar JJ, Steyerberg EW, et al. Small bites versus large bites for closure of abdominal midline incisions (STITCH): a double-blind, multicentre, randomised controlled trial. *Lancet (London, England).* 2015;386(10000):1254–1260.

Millbourn D, Cengiz Y, Israelsson LA. Effect of stitch length on wound complications after closure of midline incisions: a randomized controlled trial. *Arch Surg.* 2009;144(11):1056–1059.

4. D. Conditions that increase intraabdominal pressure (cystic fibrosis, chronic lung disease, ventriculoperitoneal shunts, constipation, and peritoneal dialysis) are associated with higher risk for developing an inguinal hernia. Patients with small asymptomatic hernias are at risk for developing symptoms as their hernias enlarge during peritoneal dialysis. Therefore, everyone undergoing peritoneal dialysis should be examined for presence of abdominal hernias preoperatively. If a hernia is found, the patient should undergo concurrent herniorrhaphy at the time of peritoneal dialysis catheter placement (A–C). Hernia repair should be done with mesh, as mesh is associated with decreased recurrence rates and are safe in patients undergoing peritoneal dialysis (E).

Reference: Chi Q, Shi Z, Zhang Z, Lin C, Liu G, Weng S. Inguinal hernias in patients on continuous ambulatory peritoneal dialysis: is tension-free mesh repair feasible? *BMC Surg.* 2020;20(1):310.

5. D. The genitofemoral nerve arises from the L1-L2 level. The genital branch innervates the cremaster muscle and sensation to the side of the scrotum and the labia. It is responsible for the cremasteric reflex. In women, it accompanies the round ligament of the uterus. The genital branch of the genitofemoral nerve is part of the cord structures. It lies on the iliopubic tract and accompanies the cremaster vessels (B). The ilioinguinal nerve lies on top of the spermatic cord (A). It innervates the internal oblique muscle and is sensory to the upper medial thigh adjacent to the genitalia. The nerve can sometimes splay out over the cord, making dissection difficult. The iliohypogastric and ilioinguinal nerves arise from the T12-L1 level and intermingle. They provide sensation to the skin of the groin, the base of the penis, and the upper medial thigh. The iliohypogastric nerve lies on the internal oblique muscle (C), provides sensory innervation from the skin overlying the pubis, and does not intermingle with the genitofemoral nerve because they cross different paths (E).

Reference: Wantz GE. Testicular atrophy and chronic residual neuralgia as risks of inguinal hernioplasty. *Surg Clin North Am.* 1993;73(3):571–581.

6. A. Poupart ligament is another name for the inguinal ligament. The inguinal ligament is formed from the anteroinferior portion of the external oblique aponeurosis folding back on itself. It extends from the anterosuperior iliac spine to the pubic tubercle, turning posteriorly to form a shelving edge. The cremaster muscle fibers arise from the internal oblique muscle and surround the spermatic cord (B). The genital branch of the genitofemoral nerve passes through the deep ring (C), whereas the ilioinguinal nerve passes through the superficial ring. The genital branch innervates the cremaster muscle, whereas the femoral branch controls sensation to the upper lateral thigh (D). Indirect hernias arise lateral to the inferior epigastric vessels, whereas direct hernias arise medial to the inferior epigastric vessels. The lateral border of the rectus muscle, inferior inguinal ligament, and inferior epigastric artery define the borders of Hesselbach triangle and define the location of a direct hernia (E).

7. C. The arcuate line is located below the umbilicus, typically one-third the distance to the pubic crest (A). Between the costal margin and the arcuate line, the anterior rectus sheath is made up of a combination of the aponeurosis of the external and internal oblique muscles. The posterior sheath is made up of a combination of the aponeuroses of the internal oblique and transverse abdominal muscles. Below the arcuate line, the anterior sheath is made up of the aponeuroses of all three abdominal muscles (E). The internal oblique aponeurosis splits above the arcuate line to envelop the rectus abdominis muscle (B). There is no posterior sheath below the arcuate line (D), and the transversalis fascia therefore makes up the posterior aspect of the rectus abdominis muscle.

8. E. This patient has bilateral inguinal hernias, one of which is recurrent and should be offered a laparoscopic repair. The advantages of this include the ability to visualize both sides through a single incision and a potentially easier surgery in the setting of recurrence. It also protects the patient from developing a femoral hernia since the femoral canal is covered by the mesh. Of note, femoral hernias are known to develop after open inguinal hernia repair. They develop on average sooner than a typical recurrence, suggesting that the original hernia was in fact a femoral one and was missed at the original surgery. The two laparoscopic approaches include TEP and TAPP. TEP involves dissecting a plane in the preperitoneal space, which may actually be advantageous when compared to TAPP because intraabdominal adhesions are avoided (A). This does not hold true for prior pelvic surgery as the preperitoneal space may be obliterated in these patients, necessitating a TAPP. If the peritoneum is violated during TEP, it is important to repair the defect to prevent adhesion formation postoperatively, but it is not mandatory to convert to a different technique (C). Though there are few absolute contraindications to laparoscopic hernia surgery, bowel ischemia with perforation or sepsis precludes the use of mesh, which is required in both TEP and TAPP. Tacking of the mesh in either laparoscopic approach can reduce mesh migration but should be avoided lateral to the epigastric vessels and inferior to the iliopubic tract to avoid placement in the "triangle of doom" or the "triangle of pain," which contains the external iliac vessels and several nerves (lateral femoral cutaneous and femoral branch of genitofemoral, respectively) (B). Injury to these nerves is relatively specific to laparoscopic repairs (D).

Reference: Fischer JE. *Fischer's mastery of surgery.* Wolters Kluwer Health/Lippincott Williams & Wilkins; Chicago, IL, 2012.

9. C. The preferred initial approach for an uncomplicated inguinal hernia is still actively debated within the surgical community. The LEVEL-trial specifically compared TEP repair versus open mesh repair and demonstrated reduced pain in the immediate postoperative period and earlier return to work. However, this came at the expense of longer operating room times and higher intraoperative complication rates (B, D). This seems to be consistent with the results of a *New England Journal of Medicine (NEJM)* study from 2004 comparing open mesh repair to all methods of laparoscopic mesh repair. However, they diverge on reported recurrence rates, with the *NEJM* study favoring open repair (recurrence of 4% versus 10.1%) while the LEVEL-Trial showed equivalent recurrence rates (3.0% for open and 3.8% for TEP) (E). The LEVEL-Trial also indicated an equivalent prevalence of chronic pain, which was not one of the outcomes in the *NEJM* article (A).

References: Langeveld HR, van't Riet M, Weidema WF, et al. Total extraperitoneal inguinal hernia repair compared with Lichtenstein (the LEVEL-Trial): a randomized controlled trial. *Ann Surg.* 2010;251(5):819–824.

Neumayer L, Giobbie-Hurder A, Jonasson O, et al. Open mesh versus laparoscopic mesh repair of inguinal hernia. *N Engl J Med.* 2004;350(18):1819–1827.

10. A. Severe groin pain developing in the recovery room following laparoscopic hernia repair is most likely due to a stapling/tacking injury to a nerve. If this complication is suspected, the patient should return to the operating room to remove the offending tack. Acute groin pain is most likely from injury to the ilioinguinal nerve. However, the most commonly injured nerve during laparoscopic hernia repair is the lateral femoral cutaneous nerve (provides sensation to the lateral thigh). Injecting the groin with local anesthetic may not relieve the pain and if it works, it will only be a temporary measure (E). Medical therapy is not appropriate if the suspected etiology is irritation of the nerve secondary to stapling/tacking (B–D). Chronic groin pain may occur in 10% to 25% of patients 1 year after surgery. The etiology is

thought to be entrapment of the nerve during surgery or postoperative scarring. Chronic groin pain is best worked up with MRI. If conservative management does not resolve the pain, operative exploration and division of the nerve(s) have met with success. The ideal approach in the setting of hernia reoperation after open repair is to enter a space in which the tissue planes have not been violated. The preferred management is a laparoscopic retroperitoneal triple neurectomy, which allows a single staged approach to access the ilioinguinal, iliohypogastric, and genitofemoral nerves.

11. D. Ischemic orchitis is thought to develop as a result of thrombosis of veins of the pampiniform plexus, leading to testicular venous congestion. It has thus been termed congestive orchitis. The precise etiology of ischemic orchitis is unclear. The most commonly identified risk factor is extensive dissection of the spermatic cord. This occurs particularly when a patient has a large hernia sac, and the entire distal sac is dissected and excised. As such, it is recommended that the sac instead is divided and the distal sac left in situ. In addition, the cord should never be dissected past the pubic tubercle. The presentation is that of a swollen, tender testicle, usually 2 to 5 days after surgery. The testicle is often high riding. This may eventually progress to testicular atrophy. Scrotal duplex ultrasonography has been shown to be useful in evaluating the perfusion of the testicle after hernia repair. However, it does not change the management of ischemic orchitis. Management is expectant. In the past, attempts to reexplore the groin were undertaken to try to loosen the inguinal ring, but this was not successful (A). The blood supply to the testicle is via the testicular artery, but there are rich collaterals including the external spermatic artery and the artery to the vas. Thus, inadvertent ligation of the testicular artery does not typically lead to this complication (C). Preexisting testicular pathology (B) or anomalous blood supply (E) to the testicle is not thought to contribute to ischemic orchitis following inguinal hernia repair. However, ischemic orchitis can occur more frequently in recurrent inguinal hernia surgery using the anterior approach; thus, the laparoscopic approach should be considered for recurrent hernias.

References: Holloway B, Belcher HE, Letourneau JG, Kunberger LE. Scrotal sonography: a valuable tool in the evaluation of complications following inguinal hernia repair. *J Clin Ultrasound.* 1998;26(7):341–344.

Wantz GE. Testicular atrophy and chronic residual neuralgia as risks of inguinal hernioplasty. *Surg Clin North Am.* 1993;73(3):571–581.

12. C. A large prospective randomized study in men demonstrated that watchful waiting for patients with asymptomatic or minimally symptomatic inguinal hernias is an acceptable option for surgery (D). The patients were followed for as long as 9 years. Acute hernia incarceration without strangulation developed in only one (0.3%) patient, and acute incarceration with bowel obstruction developed in only one (A). Approximately one-fourth of the watchful waiting group eventually crossed over to receive surgical repair due to increased hernia-related pain (B). Smaller hernias tend to have a smaller neck, placing them at higher risk for developing incarceration (E).

Reference: Fitzgibbons RJ Jr, Giobbie-Hurder A, Gibbs JO, et al. Watchful waiting vs repair of inguinal hernia in minimally symptomatic men: a randomized clinical trial. *JAMA.* 2006;295(3):285–292.

13. C. The vast majority of inguinal hernias in children are the indirect type due to a persistent patent processus vaginalis. Approximately 1% to 5% of children can develop an inguinal hernia. However, the incidence increases in preterm infants and those with a low birth weight. Right-sided hernias are more common, and 10% of hernias diagnosed at birth are bilateral. Incarceration is a more serious problem in pediatric patients than in adults. Emergent operation on an infant with an incarcerated hernia can be very challenging. Thus, it is preferable to try to reduce the hernia, which is successful in 75% to 80% of cases, allow the inflammation to subside over several days, and then perform the repair semielectively. The routine use of contralateral groin exploration is not widely supported (D). For elective cases, one option is to perform laparoscopy via the hernia sac to look for a contralateral hernia and, if found, proceed to repair. If there are any signs of strangulation (e.g., leukocytosis, fever, elevated lactate), then manual reduction should be avoided, and the patient should be taken immediately to the operating room for surgical intervention (E). In the patient described, though the skin is erythematous, there are no signs of systemic toxicity. Methods to achieve reduction include the use of intravenous (IV) sedation, Trendelenburg positioning, ice packs, and gentle direct pressure. Reduction without subsequent surgery is not appropriate. That being said, infants with anemia and history of prematurity are at significantly increased risk of postoperative apnea and would require overnight monitoring.

Reference: Özdemir T, Arıkan, A. Postoperative apnea after inguinal hernia repair in formerly premature infants: impacts of gestational age, postconceptional age and comorbidities. *Pediatr Surg Int.* 2013;29(8):801–804.

14. D. In children, umbilical hernias are congenital. They are formed by a failure of the umbilical ring to close, causing a central defect in the linea alba. Most umbilical hernias in children are small and will close by 2 years of age, particularly if the defect is less than 1 cm in size. As such, repair is not always indicated at the time of diagnosis (B). Additionally, the decision to perform an elective repair is not solely determined by the presence of symptoms (E). If closure does not occur by age 4 or 5 years, elective repair is then considered a reasonable option (C), even if the patient is asymptomatic. If the hernia defect is large (>2 cm) or the family is bothered by the cosmetic appearance, repair should be considered. Although umbilical hernias in children can incarcerate, this is very rare (A). If the child presents with abdominal pain, bilious emesis, and a tender, hard mass protruding from the umbilicus, immediate exploration and hernia repair are indicated.

15. D. Unlike in children, umbilical hernias in adults are usually acquired (A). Risk factors are any conditions that increase intraabdominal pressure, such as pregnancy, obesity, and ascites. Overall strangulation of umbilical hernias in adults is uncommon, but it occurs more often than in children (C). Small, barely palpable and asymptomatic hernias can be followed clinically. Larger or symptomatic hernias should be repaired. In patients with cirrhosis and ascites, the markedly increased pressure causes the skin overlying the hernia to become thin and eventually ischemic. One of the most catastrophic complications in this setting is rupture of the hernia through the ischemic skin, leading to peritonitis and death. Thus, patients with cirrhosis and ascites should undergo repair if there is evidence that the skin overlying the hernia is thinning or becoming ischemic (B). However, repair should be delayed until after medical management of the ascites. If medical management fails and the skin over the hernia is thinned and tense, then a transjugular portosystemic shunt should be considered before repair. Alternatively, if the patient is a candidate for liver transplant, the hernia can be repaired during the transplantation. Umbilical hernias have historically all been repaired by primary closure. Borrowing from the low recurrence rates using mesh for inguinal hernias, umbilical hernias are now more frequently being repaired using mesh, particularly those with large defects. A recent prospective, randomized study compared primary closure with mesh repair. The early complication rates such as seroma, hematoma, and wound infection were similar in the two groups. However, the hernia recurrence rate was significantly higher after primary suture repair (11%) than after mesh repair (1%) (E). Some authors are now advocating for the routine use of mesh for all adult umbilical hernias in the absence of bowel strangulation.

References: Arroyo A, García P, Pérez F, Andreu J, Candela F, Calpena R. Randomized clinical trial comparing suture and mesh repair of umbilical hernia in adults. *Br J Surg.* 2001;88(10):1321–1323.

Belghiti J, Durand F. Abdominal wall hernias in the setting of cirrhosis. *Semin Liver Dis.* 1997;17(3):219–226.

16. D. Femoral hernias occur more commonly in females and have a high risk of incarceration. However, the most common overall hernia in females is an indirect inguinal hernia (A). Bowel entering a femoral hernia passes down a narrow femoral canal. This is because the femoral ring, which serves as the entrance for the femoral canal, is very rigid and unyielding. Thus, the fixed neck of a femoral hernia is prone to pinching off the bowel, putting the patient at risk for incarceration. The borders of the femoral canal are as follows: inguinal ligament (anterior) (B), Cooper ligament (posterior), femoral vein (lateral), and Poupart ligament (medial). Femoral hernias occur most commonly lateral to the lymphatics and medial to the femoral vein, within the empty space (C). It is important to recognize that femoral hernias pass deep (posterior) to the inguinal ligament. As such, repairs to the inguinal ligament (such as a Bassini operation and standard mesh repair) will not obliterate the defect (E). The femoral hernia can be fixed either through a standard inguinal approach or directly over the bulge using an infrainguinal incision. The essential elements of femoral hernia repair include dissection and removal of the hernia sac and obliteration of the defect in the femoral canal. This can be accomplished by either approximation of the iliopubic tract to the Cooper ligament or by placement of prosthetic mesh.

Reference: de Virgilio C, Frank PN, Grigorian A, eds. *Surgery: a case based clinical review.* Springer; 2015.

17. B. It is important to understand the difference between epigastric hernias and diastasis recti because the former is a true hernia, which should be repaired, and the latter is a benign condition. Diastasis recti is caused by increased separation of the rectus abdominis muscles and a relative thinning of the linea alba, which can mimic a hernia. The condition can be acquired, such as in multiparous women where the repeated stretching of the abdominal wall causes the rectus muscles to separate, or congenital, secondary to more lateral attachment of the rectus muscles at birth. Classically, patients present after recent weight loss because this allows for the lesion to be visible. There is no risk for strangulation in diastasis recti because all of the facial layers are intact (A, D). Though several methods of surgical repair have been described, these are mainly cosmetic. In general, all that is required is reassurance and abdominal wall exercises to help strengthen the musculature—though complete resolution in adults is unlikely (C). In contrast, epigastric hernias are true hernias and represent a true defect in the linea alba. They are generally small and contain either preperitoneal fat or part of the falciform ligament (E). They arise from defects in the fascia in locations where neurovascular bundles perforate through. Though small, they can cause significant pain because of compression of the nerves traveling through the defect. There is some evidence to suggest that diastasis rectus may increase the risk for development of an epigastric hernia and will make primary repair of epigastric hernias more challenging. Of note, patients with diastasis recti are at increased risk of abdominal aortic aneurysms.

References: Brunicardi FC, Andersen DK, Schwartz SI. *Schwartz's principles of surgery.* 10th ed. McGraw-Hill Education.

Köhler G, Luketina RR, Emmanuel K. Sutured repair of primary small umbilical and epigastric hernias: concomitant rectus diastasis is a significant risk factor for recurrence. *World J Surg.* 2015;39(1):121–126.

Townsend CM, Jr, Beauchamp RD, Evers BM, Mattox KL, eds. *Sabiston textbook of surgery: the biological basis of modern surgical practice.* 17th ed. Philadelphia, PA: W.B. Saunders; 2004.

Abdomen—Biliary

AMANDA C. PURDY AND DANIELLE M. HARI

3

ABSITE 99th Percentile High-Yields

I. Physiology
   A. Bile consists of water, bile salts, phospholipids, and cholesterol
   B. Primary bile acids (cholic & chenodeoxycholic acids) become secondary bile acids when dehydroxylated by gut bacteria (lithocholate and deoxycholate acids)
   C. Mechanism of bile concentration in the gallbladder: active transport of NaCl into gallbladder mucosal cells, passive absorption of water

II. Cholecystitis, Choledocholithiasis, and Cholangitis
   A. Acute calculous cholecystitis: gallbladder inflammation due to gallstone impacted in the neck; management is NPO, IV antibiotics, resuscitation, laparoscopic cholecystectomy
   B. Acute acalculous cholecystitis: usually seen in critically ill patients in the ICU; US demonstrates gallbladder wall thickening, pericholecystic fluid, with no stones; HIDA if US is equivocal, tx is IV antibiotics, resuscitation, and percutaneous cholecystostomy tube if critically ill versus laparoscopic cholecystectomy if stable for surgery
   C. Choledocholithiasis: may have obstructive jaundice; elevated direct bilirubin, may have transaminitis; US demonstrates gallstones, dilated CBD, +/− stone in the CBD (sensitivity only 50%); tx is ERCP followed up by laparoscopic cholecystectomy
      1. If intraoperative cholangiogram is positive for choledocholithiasis: first attempt to flush the stone with saline; if it doesn't work try flushing after giving 1 mg IV glucagon (relaxes sphincter of Oddi); if stones don't clear, options include:
         a) Postoperative ERCP
         b) Transcystic CBD exploration—best for small stones, large cystic duct, or small CBD; generally preferred over transductal CBD exploration because it avoids a CBD incision
         c) Transductal CBD exploration—best for large stones (>8–10 mm), large CBD, proximal stones (above cystic duct), choledochotomy made anterior to avoid vasculature laterally
   D. Acute ascending cholangitis: Charcot triad (RUQ pain, fever, jaundice) presents in about 20%; Reynolds pentad adds hypotension and confusion; RUQ US: +/− gallstones, dilated CBD, elevated direct BR; tx is IV antibiotics, fluid resuscitation, pressors if in septic shock, followed by ERCP or percutaneous transhepatic cholangiography (PTC) tube placement after resuscitation; laparoscopic cholecystectomy during same admission if due to gallstones
   E. Mirizzi syndrome: large stone in the gallbladder neck compresses the common hepatic duct (CHD), can cause CHD stricture or fistula between the gallbladder and CHD; usually presents similar to cholecystitis and diagnosed during cholecystectomy; manage with cholecystectomy

III. Choledochal cysts
   A. Due to an anomalous pancreaticobiliary junction, with a fused, long common pancreaticobiliary channel allowing pancreatic enzymes to reflux into the biliary tree leading to inflammation and cystic degeneration

B. More common in females and those of Asian descent, 60% diagnosed before age 10
C. First step in workup is US but MRCP is best for diagnosis and preop planning
D. Associated with cholangiocarcinoma and gallbladder cancer; type III has very low risk of malignancy; management for all types besides type III is surgical to decrease subsequent malignancy risk
   1. Management is based on location (described by Todani Classification):
   2. Type I (fusiform dilation, most common): cyst excision, Roux-en-Y hepaticojejunostomy, cholecystectomy
   3. Type II: cyst excision, primary closure, cholecystectomy
   4. Type III: endoscopic sphincterotomy and cyst unroofing
   5. Type IVa: cyst excision, partial hepatectomy, Roux-en-Y hepaticojejunostomy, cholecystectomy
   6. Type IVb: cyst excision, Roux-en-Y hepaticojejunostomy, cholecystectomy
   7. Type V (Caroli disease): if only in one lobe of the liver—hepatic resection and cholecystectomy; if bilobar or unresectable—liver transplant

IV. Gallbladder Polyps
   A. Polypoid lesions of the gallbladder: cholesterolosis (most common, cholesterol-laden macrophages in the lamina propria), adenomatous polyp (risk for gallbladder cancer)
   B. Indications for cholecystectomy for gallbladder polyps: symptomatic, polyp >10 mm, primary sclerosing cholangitis, and polyp of any size
   C. If cholecystectomy is not indicated, should follow patient with serial US in 6 to 12 months

V. Gallbladder Adenocarcinoma (most common biliary malignancy)
   A. Risk factors: gallstones, gallbladder polyp >10 mm, porcelain gallbladder with selective mucosal calcification (as opposed to transmural calcification)
   B. May present similarly to cholecystitis, often diagnosed on pathology after cholecystectomy
   C. Management:
   1. T1a (into lamina propria) → cholecystectomy
   2. >T1b (into muscularis) OR >N1 → cholecystectomy, segment IVb & V hepatectomy, portal lymphadenectomy (port site resection not indicated); followed by adjuvant chemotherapy (gemcitabine and cisplatin)
   3. If positive cystic duct margin, need extrahepatic bile duct resection and hepaticojejunostomy

VI. Cholangiocarcinoma
   A. Risk factors: primary sclerosing cholangitis, ulcerative colitis, choledochal cyst, liver fluke infection
   B. Can present with painless jaundice; suspect in patient with focal bile duct stenosis without history of biliary surgery or pancreatitis; best imaging is MRCP
   C. Unresectable if distant metastasis, which includes multifocal hepatic disease and lymph node mets beyond the porta hepatis
   D. For potentially resectable cholangiocarcinoma, start with diagnostic laparoscopy; goal of surgery is negative margins; all surgery includes portal lymphadenectomy; management depends on location:

Location/Classification			Management
Lower 1/3 of extrahepatic bile duct			Whipple
Middle 1/3 of extrahepatic bile duct			Resection, hepaticojejunostomy
Upper 1/3 of bile duct *AKA Klatskin tumor Further classified with the Bismuth classification:*	Type I	CHD (not to the confluence)	If localized to one side—hemi-hepatectomy, extrahepatic bile duct excision, Roux-en-Y hepaticojejunostomy
	Type II	CHD to the confluence	
	Type IIIa	CHD + RHD	
	Type IIIb	CHD + LHD	If unresectable hilar tumor ≤3cm without nodal disease or distant mets—evaluate for transplant
	Type IV	CHD + RHD + LHD	

VII. Bile duct injuries (incidence 0.3%–0.8%, most commonly due to cystic duct stump leak)
   A. Risk of bile duct injury higher with laparoscopic cases and elective (not emergent/urgent cases)
   B. Principles of management: control sepsis, drain bile collections, and establish secure biliary drainage
   C. Marked laboratory abnormalities are not typical; bilirubin may be elevated due to systemic resorption; US is initial imaging study, +/− HIDA
   D. In immediate postop period, treat with IV antibiotics, fluid resuscitation, percutaneous drainage and ERCP with stent placement and/or sphincterotomy as this is sufficient for majority of cases; if not, percutaneous transhepatic catheter required; if leak has not healed in 6 to 8 weeks, biliary reconstruction is considered with Roux-en-Y hepaticojejunostomy
   E. If discovered intraoperatively, repair only indicated if adequate hepatobiliary surgical experience is available; otherwise, wide drainage and referral to higher level of care

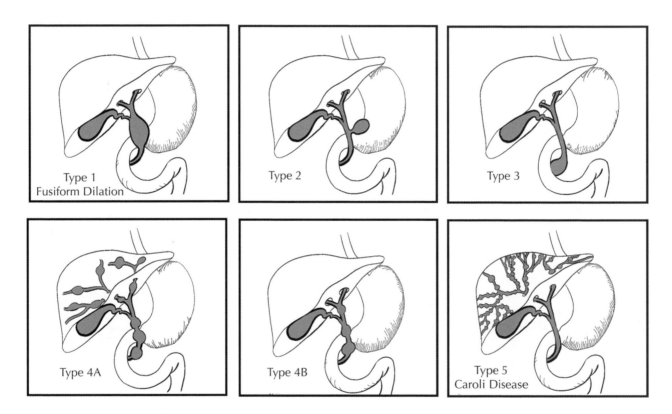

Type 1 biliary cysts are classically managed with resection of the extrahepatic cyst and Roux-en-Y hepaticojejunostomy. Type 2 cysts are managed with simple excision. Type 3 cysts may be observed or treated with endoscopic sphincterotomy if symptomatic. Type 4A are treated with resection of the extrahepatic cyst, partial hepatectomy, and Roux-en-Y hepaticojejunostomy. Type 4B cysts are treated with resection of the extrahepatic cysts and Roux-en-Y hepaticojejunostomy. The ultimate management for Type 5 cysts is liver transplantation.

Fig. 3.1 Biliary Cysts.

Questions

1. A 10-year-old boy with sickle cell disease presents with right upper quadrant pain, nausea, vomiting, fever, and yellowing of the eyes for the past day. He denies dark urine or light stool. On exam, he is febrile, hemodynamically stable, and has a positive Murphy sign. He has leukocytosis, elevated alkaline phosphatase, and elevated unconjugated bilirubin. On ultrasound, there are gallstones, pericholecystic fluid, and gallbladder wall thickening, and CBD diameter is 4 mm. After starting IV fluid resuscitation and IV antibiotics, what is the next step?
   A. MRCP
   B. ERCP
   C. Percutaneous transhepatic cholangiography
   D. Laparoscopic cholecystectomy
   E. Cholecystostomy tube

2. A 25-year-old woman is undergoing elective laparoscopic cholecystectomy for symptomatic cholelithiasis. When removing the gallbladder from the fossa, a 2-mm tubular structure is completely transected and is leaking bile. The structure appears to come from the liver fossa and enter directly into the gallbladder. What is the most appropriate management?
   A. Laparoscopic clip placement
   B. Repair over a T-tube
   C. Roux-en-Y hepaticojejunostomy
   D. Immediate transfer to a hospital with a hepatobiliary surgeon
   E. Complete cholecystectomy and plan for postoperative ERCP

3. A 45-year-old male presents with hematemesis two weeks after a motor vehicle accident in which he suffered a liver injury that was managed nonoperatively. Laboratory values are significant for an elevated total bilirubin and alkaline phosphatase, as well as significant anemia. This patient is most likely to have which of the following?
   A. Arterioportal vein fistula
   B. Arteriohepatic vein fistula
   C. Arterial pseudoaneurysm
   D. Portal venous pseudoaneurysm
   E. Cavernous hemangioma

4. Which of the following patients should be offered a cholecystectomy?
   A. A 40-year-old woman with an incidentally discovered 6-mm gallbladder polyp
   B. A 30-year-old man with asymptomatic gallstones undergoing gastric bypass
   C. A 65-year-old woman with asymptomatic gallstones and an incidentally discovered porcelain gallbladder with selective mucosal calcification
   D. A 50-year-old man with a history of diabetes and asymptomatic gallstones
   E. A 12-year-old boy with sickle cell disease and asymptomatic gallstones

5. Which of the following is true regarding bile and gallstones?
   A. The primary bile acids are deoxycholic and lithocholic acid
   B. The primary phospholipid in bile is lecithin
   C. Cholecystectomy decreases bile salt secretion
   D. Brown pigmented gallstones are more likely to be found in the gallbladder versus the CBD
   E. Bile consists of an equal part of bile salts, phospholipids, and cholesterol

6. Which of the following is true regarding the gallbladder?
   A. It passively absorbs sodium and chloride
   B. In the setting of cholelithiasis, cholecystokinin (CCK) can cause gallbladder pain that waxes and wanes
   C. It harbors an alkaline environment
   D. Glucagon can help empty the gallbladder
   E. Its contraction is inhibited by vagal stimulation

7. A 75-year-old woman presents to the emergency department with a 2-day history of nausea, feculent vomiting, and obstipation. Her blood pressure on admission is 80/60 mm-Hg, and her heart rate is 120 beats per minute, both of which normalize after fluids. Plain films reveal distended loops of small bowel with air–fluid levels and air in the biliary tree. Which of the following is the best management option?
   A. Small bowel enterotomy with removal of the gallstone plus
   B. Small bowel enterotomy with removal of the gallstone
   C. Small bowel enterotomy with removal of the gallstone followed 8 weeks later by cholecystectomy and takedown of fistula
   D. Small bowel resection to include area of impacted gallstone
   E. Small bowel resection to include area of impacted gallstone plus cholecystectomy and takedown of the fistula

8. Jaundice with absent urine urobilinogen is most consistent with:
   A. Hepatitis
   B. Cirrhosis
   C. Hemolysis
   D. Biliary obstruction
   E. Sepsis

9. Which of the following is true regarding bile and gallbladder disease?
   A. Primary bile acids are formed by deconjugation
   B. Bile acids are passively absorbed in the terminal ileum
   C. Bile acids are responsible for the yellow color of bile
   D. Bile duct stones occurring 1 year after cholecystectomy are considered primary common duct stones
   E. In between meals, gallbladder emptying is stimulated by motilin

10. Which of the following is true regarding biliary anatomy?
   A. The right hepatic duct tends to be longer than the left and more prone to dilation
   B. Venous return from the gallbladder is most often via a cystic vein to the portal vein
   C. Heister valves have an important role in the gallbladder's function as a bile reservoir
   D. The CBD and pancreatic duct typically unite outside the duodenal wall
   E. The arterial supply to the CBD derives primarily from the left hepatic and right gastric arteries

11. Ultrasonography of the gallbladder reveals a polypoid lesion. This most likely represents:
   A. a cholesterol polyp
   B. adenomyomatosis
   C. a benign adenoma
   D. adenocarcinoma
   E. an inflammatory polyp

12. Which of the following is the correct pairing of anatomic structure and direction for retraction during a laparoscopic cholecystectomy?
   A. Gallbladder fundus laterally
   B. Gallbladder infundibulum laterally
   C. Gallbladder body laterally
   D. Gallbladder infundibulum cephalad
   E. Gallbladder fundus medially

13. Hydrops of the gallbladder:
   A. Poses a significantly increased risk of malignancy
   B. Is due to a stone impacted in the cystic duct
   C. Typically starts with an enteric bacterial infection
   D. Is associated with marked right upper quadrant tenderness
   E. Results in the gallbladder getting filled with bile-stained fluid

14. During a laparoscopic cholecystectomy for symptomatic cholelithiasis, the surgeon inadvertently transects the CBD. An experienced hepatobiliary surgeon is available. The best choice for operative repair is:
   A. End-to-end CBD anastomosis
   B. Choledochoduodenostomy
   C. Choledochojejunostomy
   D. Hepaticoduodenostomy
   E. Hepaticojejunostomy

15. The most common cause of benign bile duct stricture is:
   A. Ischemia from operative injury
   B. Chronic pancreatitis
   C. Common duct stones
   D. Acute cholangitis
   E. Sclerosing cholangitis

16. A 45-year-old man has a 50% total body surface area third-degree burn. Fever, marked leukocytosis, and right upper quadrant pain develop on hospital day 7. His blood pressure is 130/80 mm-Hg, and his heart rate is 110 beats per minute. Ultrasonography shows a distended gallbladder with gallbladder wall thickening and sludge. However, it is negative for gallstones. Antibiotics are initiated. The next step in management would consist of:
    A. Laparoscopic cholecystectomy
    B. Computed tomography
    C. Hepatobiliary iminodiacetic acid (HIDA) scan
    D. Percutaneous cholecystostomy
    E. Upper endoscopy

17. During laparoscopic cholecystectomy, bile appears to be emanating near the junction of the CBD and cystic duct. Upon conversion to open cholecystectomy, the injury is noted to be a 3-mm longitudinal tear in the anterolateral distal common hepatic duct. The duct itself measures 7 mm in diameter. Management consists of:
    A. Primary repair of the injury without a T tube
    B. Primary repair of the injury over a T tube
    C. Primary repair of the injury with a T tube placed through a separate choledochotomy
    D. Hepaticojejunostomy
    E. Choledochoduodenostomy

18. Which of the following statements is true regarding the use of intraoperative cholangiography (IOC) during laparoscopic cholecystectomy?
    A. It helps prevent inadvertent incision of the common bile duct (CBD)
    B. It is the best way to identify clinically significant common duct stones
    C. Routine use is justified because of its ability to identify anatomic anomalies of the hepatic ducts
    D. Routine use is helpful to ensure complete removal of the gallbladder and cystic duct
    E. Routine use is unnecessary

19. An 80-year-old patient presents with nausea, fever, and right upper quadrant pain and tenderness. Ultrasonography reveals gallstones as well as air in the wall of the gallbladder. His temperature is 103.5°F and blood pressure is 70/40 mm-Hg. Medical therapy is initiated, and pressors are needed to maintain blood pressure. Which of the following is true regarding this condition?
    A. Metronidazole is an important antibiotic choice
    B. Emergent cholecystectomy is indicated
    C. Urgent percutaneous drainage is preferred over cholecystectomy
    D. The most common organism is an anaerobic gram-negative rod
    E. Perforation of the gallbladder is rare

20. Which of the following best describes the role of preoperative biliary drainage before a Whipple procedure in a patient with obstructive jaundice?
    A. It has been shown to decrease the rate of cholangitis
    B. It has been shown to increase the rate of wound infections
    C. It should be performed routinely if the bilirubin level is greater than 8 mg/dL
    D. It has been shown to shorten the hospital stay
    E. It has been shown to decrease the mortality rate

21. A 35-year-old Chinese man presents with a fever of 103.5°F, right upper quadrant pain, and jaundice. Laboratory values are significant for a white blood cell count of 15,000 cells/L, an alkaline phosphatase level of 400 U/L, and a serum bilirubin level of 3.8 mg/dL. Magnetic resonance cholangiopancreatography (MRCP) demonstrates a markedly dilated CBD, markedly dilated intrahepatic ducts with several intrahepatic ductal strictures, and multiple stones throughout the ductal system. Which of the following is true regarding this condition?
    A. It is associated with close contact with dogs and sheep
    B. It is more commonly associated with black pigment stones versus brown pigment stones
    C. It more commonly affects males
    D. Metronidazole is able to resolve the majority of cases
    E. Initial treatment is with endoscopic retrograde cholangiopancreatography and transhepatic cholangiography

22. A 65-year-old woman presents with symptoms and signs of acute cholecystitis and undergoes an uneventful laparoscopic cholecystectomy. On postoperative day 7, the pathology report indicates a superficial gallbladder carcinoma that invades the perimuscular connective tissue. There is no evidence of distant metastasis on subsequent imaging. Which of the following would be the best management?
    A. Radiation and chemotherapy
    B. Observation
    C. Reoperation with resection of liver segments IVB and V
    D. Reoperation with resection of liver segments IVB and V and regional lymph node dissection
    E. Reoperation with resection of liver segments IVB and V, regional lymph node dissection, and resection of all port sites

23. A 24-year-old male presents with acholic stools and cola-colored urine. Alkaline phosphatase is 2000 IU/L, AST is 78 IU/L, ALT is 88 IU/L, and total bilirubin is 2.1 mg/dL. Liver biopsy demonstrates periductal concentric fibrosis around macroscopic bile ducts. He is positive for perinuclear antineutrophil cytoplasmic antibody (p-ANCA). Which of the following is true about this condition?
    A. It is more commonly associated with Crohn disease than it is with ulcerative colitis
    B. Cancer antigen (CA) 19-9 levels should be determined
    C. Endoscopic retrograde cholangiopancreatography (ERCP) will predominantly demonstrate irregular narrowing of the intrahepatic biliary tree
    D. Symptoms are often well controlled with medical management
    E. It is more common in females

24. Which of the following is a feature of gallbladder cancer?
    A. Speckled cholesterol deposits are found on the gallbladder wall
    B. There are thickened nodules of mucosa and muscle
    C. Gallbladder cancer is more common in males
    D. It is more likely to be accompanied by large gallstones compared with smaller ones
    E. Cancer invading muscularis layer is managed with cholecystectomy alone

25. Choledochal cyst disease is thought to be caused by an abnormality of the:
    A. Bile duct smooth muscle
    B. Bile composition
    C. Bile duct adventitia
    D. Pancreaticobiliary duct junction
    E. Bile duct mucosa

26. On CT scan, a type I choledochal cyst appears to be adherent to the posterior wall of the portal vein. Management consists of:
    A. Partial excision of the cyst, leaving posterior wall behind, and cholecystectomy with Roux-en-Y hepaticojejunostomy
    B. Complete excision of the cyst, cholecystectomy, and hepaticojejunostomy
    C. Partial excision of the cyst, fulguration of posterior cyst mucosa, and cholecystectomy with Roux-en-Y hepaticojejunostomy
    D. Observation
    E. Roux-en-Y cyst jejunostomy

27. Which of the following is the best management of a localized Klatskin tumor?
    A. Pancreaticoduodenectomy (Whipple procedure)
    B. Resection of the entire extrahepatic biliary tree with hepatic resection if necessary
    C. Resection of the middle third of the biliary tree with hepaticojejunostomy
    D. Chemotherapy
    E. Radiation followed by chemotherapy

28. Which of the following is true regarding cholangiocarcinoma?
    A. The majority are intrahepatic
    B. Bismuth-Corlette type I cholangiocarcinoma occurs above the confluence of the right and left hepatic ducts
    C. Most patients benefit from adjuvant chemoradiation after surgical intervention
    D. It arises from malignant transformation in hepatocytes
    E. Resection with biliary-enteric bypass is considered appropriate management in patients with early disease

Answers

1. D. This patient with sickle cell disease has acute calculous cholecystitis and should undergo laparoscopic cholecystectomy after fluid resuscitation and initiation of antibiotics. Signs that point to acute cholecystitis in this case include: fever, positive Murphy sign, leukocytosis, and ultrasound findings of gallstones, gallbladder wall thickening, and pericholecystic fluid. MRCP is reasonable if there is concern for possible choledocholithiasis. However, it is important to distinguish obstructive jaundice from jaundice from hemolytic anemia (as seen in this patient) (A). Although this patient has jaundice, his labs show an increased *unconjugated* bilirubin. He also does not have dark urine or acholic stools, and CBD diameter is normal. This is more consistent with hemolytic anemia than with obstructive jaundice (in which you would expect conjugated bilirubinemia, dark urine, acholic stools, and CBD dilation). This young patient with sickle cell disease has chronic hemolysis, which likely led to development of pigmented gallstones, and now cholecystitis. Sepsis can trigger increased hemolysis in patients with sickle cell disease and is responsible for his perceived increased jaundice since symptom onset. ERCP would be an appropriate choice if there is a very high suspicion for choledocholithiasis or ascending cholangitis; however, there is no evidence of biliary obstruction in this case (B). Percutaneous transhepatic cholangiography can also be used to decompress the biliary tree, which is not indicated in this case (C). Cholecystostomy tube can be considered in patients with cholecystitis that are too unstable to undergo cholecystectomy, which is not true in this case (E).

2. A. Ducts of Luschka are small ducts that originate in the gallbladder fossa and drain directly into the gallbladder, as described in this question. When transected, they can cause bile leaks. When discovered intraoperatively, the duct should be clipped or oversewn. More commonly these are diagnosed postoperatively as a fluid collection at the gallbladder fossa (biloma) and should be drained percutaneously and an ERCP with sphincterotomy and stent placement should be performed to encourage bile flow into the duodenum (E). Primary repair over a T-tube and Roux-en-Y hepaticojejunostomy are the appropriate treatment for common bile duct injuries (with <50% luminal injury and >50% luminal injury, respectively), which is not what is described in this case (B, C). If a common duct injury occurs at a hospital without a surgeon who is experienced in biliary reconstruction, the surgeon should place wide drains and then arrange transfer to a referral center. However, that is not necessary in this case (D).

References: Mercado MA, Domínguez I. Classification and management of bile duct injuries. *World J Gastrointest Surg.* 2011;3(4):43–48.

Spanos CP, Syrakos T. Bile leaks from the duct of Luschka (subvesical duct): a review. *Langenbecks Arch Surg.* 2006;391(5):441–447.

3. C. Hemobilia is a rare condition and presents with a classic (Quinke) triad of upper gastrointestinal bleeding (hematemesis), combined with jaundice and right-sided upper abdominal pain. It is most often a result of iatrogenic injury of the right hepatic artery (more common if there is an aberrant right hepatic artery off the superior mesenteric

artery) during laparoscopic cholecystectomy but may also occur following blunt and penetrating traumatic injuries. The underlying lesion is typically an arterial pseudoaneurysm that has a connection with the biliary tree (hence the jaundice). It can also occur in association with gallstones, tumors, inflammatory disorders, and vascular disorders. Treatment in most instances involves angiographic embolization of the artery (thus angiography is most likely to be the therapeutic study of choice). Endoscopy may show blood coming from the ampulla of Vater but will not typically be therapeutic (because the bleeding is coming from a hepatic artery pseudoaneurysm). The remaining answer choices are not thought to play a role in hemobilia (A, B, D, E).

References: Ahrendt SA, Pitt HA. Biliary tract. In: Townsend CM, Jr, Beauchamp RD, Evers BM, Mattox KL, eds. *Sabiston textbook of surgery: the biological basis of modern surgical practice.* 17th ed. Philadelphia: W.B. Saunders; 2004:1597–1642.

Bloechle C, Izbicki JR, Rashed MY, et al. (1994). Hemobilia: presentation, diagnosis, and management. *Am J Gastroenterol.* 1994;89(9):1537–1540.

Croce MA, Fabian TC, Spiers JP, Kudsk KA. Traumatic hepatic artery pseudoaneurysm with hemobilia. *Am J Surg.* 1994;168(3):235–238.

Nicholson T, Travis S, Ettles D, et al. Hepatic artery angiography and embolization for hemobilia following laparoscopic cholecystectomy. *Cardiovasc Radiol.* 1999;22(1):20–24.

4. C. Asymptomatic patients who are incidentally discovered to have gallstones usually do not require surgery because the lifetime risk of developing symptoms is <5%. There are, however, certain indications for cholecystectomy in asymptomatic patients. These include gallbladder polyps ≥10 mm and a porcelain gallbladder with selective mucosal calcification of the gallbladder because both have and associated malignancy risk (A). Historically, all patients with porcelain gallbladder underwent cholecystectomy because of the malignancy risk. It is now understood that the risk is not as high as originally thought, and only selective mucosal calcification is associated with malignancy risk, while transmural calcification is not. More extensive intramural deposits cause mucosal sloughing, which reduces the rate of adenocarcinoma, while the selective calcification yields to a continued inflammatory stimulus. Thus, a stronger recommendation for prophylactic cholecystectomy is made for the selective mucosal calcification pattern in an asymptomatic patient. Patients with cholelithiasis undergoing gastric bypass are at increased risk for developing gallstones because of rapid weight loss. However, most do not develop symptoms requiring cholecystectomy, and prophylactic cholecystectomy in these patients is not indicated (B). Diabetes is also not an indication for cholecystectomy in the absence of symptoms (D). Patients with conditions that cause hemolytic anemia, such as sickle cell disease and hereditary spherocytosis, are at increased risk of developing pigmented gallstones. However, surgery for asymptomatic cholelithiasis in these patients is only recommended if they are undergoing another abdominal operation (such as splenectomy for children with hereditary spherocytosis [E]).

References: Warschkow R, Tarantino I, Ukegjini K, et al. Concomitant cholecystectomy during laparoscopic Roux-en-Y gastric bypass in obese patients is not justified: a meta-analysis. *Obes Surg.* 2013;23(3):397–407.

Overby DW, Apelgren KN, Richardson W, Fanelli R, Society of American Gastrointestinal and Endoscopic Surgeons. SAGES guidelines for the clinical application of laparoscopic biliary tract surgery. *Surg Endosc.* 2010;24(10):2368–2386.

5. B. Bile consists of bile salts, phospholipids, and cholesterol in the following concentrations: 80%, 15%, and 5%, respectively (E). Normally, more than 95% of bile salts are reabsorbed by the enterohepatic circulation and negative feedback accounts for replacement of the 0.5 g loss of bile salts in the stool. The primary bile acids are cholic acid and chenodeoxycholic acid. The secondary bile acids are lithocholate and deoxycholate acids (A). Cholecystectomy has minimal effect on bile acid secretion but does increase enterohepatic circulation of bile salts (C). Pigment stones get their characteristic color from calcium bilirubinate. Brown pigment gallstones occur more commonly in the setting of biliary stasis such as cholangitis and tend to form in the CBD. Black pigment stones are associated with hemolytic disorders and are more likely to be found within the gallbladder (D).

Reference: Oddsdottir M, Hunter JG. Gallbladder. In: Brunicardi FC, Andersen DK, Billiar TR, et al., eds. *Schwartz's principles of surgery.* 8th ed. New York: McGraw-Hill; 2005:1187–1200.

6. D. The gallbladder concentrates and stores bile. It does so by rapidly absorbing sodium and chloride against a concentration gradient by active transport and passive water absorption (A). The epithelial cells of the gallbladder secrete mucous glycoproteins and hydrogen ions into the gallbladder lumen. The secretion of hydrogen ions acidifies the bile, increasing calcium solubility, and thus preventing its precipitation as calcium salts (C). Inflammation of the gallbladder mucosa seems to affect the ability to secrete hydrogen ions, making the bile more lithogenic. Vagal innervation stimulates contraction of the gallbladder (E). CCK causes steady and tonic contraction. The term *biliary colic* is a misnomer because postprandial gallbladder pain secondary to cholelithiasis does not wax and wane but rather stays constant for up to several hours (B). The more appropriate term is *symptomatic cholelithiasis.* The gallbladder normally fills by contraction at the sphincter of Oddi at the ampulla of Vater. In contrast, glucagon relaxes the sphincter of Oddi and creates the path of least resistance allowing the gallbladder to empty into the duodenum.

References: Ahrendt SA, Pitt HA. Biliary tract. In: Townsend CM, Jr, Beauchamp RD, Evers BM, Mattox KL, eds. *Sabiston textbook of surgery: the biological basis of modern surgical practice.* 17th ed. Philadelphia, PA: W.B. Saunders; 2004:1597–1642.

Oddsdottir, M, Hunter, JG. Gallbladder. In: Brunicardi FC, Andersen DK, Billiar TR, et al., eds. *Schwartz's principles of surgery.* 8th ed. New York: McGraw-Hill; 2005:1187–1200.

7. B. The presentation is consistent with gallstone ileus. *Gallstone ileus* is a misnomer because it is actually a type of mechanical small bowel obstruction. It occurs more commonly in elderly females (>70 years). The most specific study to help confirm diagnosis is a CT scan showing air in the biliary tree. It usually results from a large gallstone (>2.5 cm) that has eroded through the gallbladder into the adjacent duodenum and causing air in the biliary tree, creating a cholecystoduodenal fistula (the most common type of biliary fistula). Less commonly, the fistula can be between the gallbladder and the colon (hepatic flexure) or the stomach. The stone typically lodges in the narrowest portion of the gastrointestinal tract—the distal ileum, near the ileocecal valve. The diagnosis of gallstone ileus is made preoperatively in only approximately half of cases because a history of biliary disease may be absent, pneumobilia may not be seen, the gallstone may not be visualized, or the abdominal radiographic findings may be nonspecific. Because many of these patients are elderly, have other major comorbidities, and are often markedly dehydrated, initial surgical management should focus on relieving the obstruction. This is best accomplished by a transverse enterotomy proximal to the palpable stone and stone removal (C–E). It is also important to run the small bowel because a significant portion of patients will have more than one gallstone. Leaving the fistula does not seem to lead to significant morbidity on long-term follow-up. Most surgeons would not recommend taking the patient back at a later time for fistula takedown. A resection of the small bowel is usually not necessary.

References: Ahrendt SA, Pitt HA. Biliary tract. In: Townsend CM, Jr, Beauchamp RD, Evers BM, Mattox KL, eds. *Sabiston textbook of surgery: the biological basis of modern surgical practice.* 17th ed. Philadelphia: W.B. Saunders; 2004:1597–1642.

Rodríguez-Sanjuán JC, Casado F, Fernández MJ, Morales DJ, Naranjo A. Cholecystectomy and fistula closure versus enterolithotomy alone in gallstone ileus. *Br J Surg.* 1997;84(5):634-637.

Tan YM, Wong WK, Ooi LLPJ. A comparison of two surgical strategies for the emergency treatment of gallstone ileus. *Singapore Med J.* 2004;45(2):69–72.

Halabi WJ, Kang CY, Ketana N, Lafaro KJ, Nguyen VQ, Stamos MJ, Imagawa DK, Demirjian AN. Surgery for gallstone ileus: a nationwide comparison of trends and outcomes. *Ann Surg.* 2014;259(2):329–35.

8. D. Bilirubin is the result of the breakdown of old red blood cells into heme. Heme is broken down into biliverdin and then bilirubin. Bilirubin is bound to albumin in the circulation, but as it reaches the liver, it is conjugated and eventually enters the gastrointestinal tract. In the gastrointestinal tract, it is deconjugated into urobilinogen by bacteria. Some urobilinogen gets reabsorbed in the gut, returns to the liver, and is excreted in the urine, where it is eventually converted to urobilin, giving urine its yellow appearance. The remaining urobilin is oxidized to stercobilin in the intestines, giving stool its brown appearance. In the presence of biliary obstruction, less bilirubin enters the gut, less urobilinogen is made, and therefore less appears in the urine. Less stercobilin is made and therefore the stools turn pale. Hemolysis would generate an increase in bilirubin and a corresponding increase in urobilinogen in the gut and in the urine (C). The remaining answer choices do not play a significant role in bilirubin metabolism (A, B, E).

Reference: Ahrendt SA, Pitt HA. Biliary tract. In: Townsend CM, Jr, Beauchamp RD, Evers BM, Mattox KL, eds. *Sabiston textbook of surgery: the biological basis of modern surgical practice.* 17th ed. Philadelphia: W.B. Saunders; 2004:1597–1642.

9. E. Cholesterol that has been conjugated with taurine or glycine is considered a primary bile (cholic and chenodeoxycholic acid). Secondary bile acids are a result of bacterial deconjugation in the gastrointestinal tract (A). Although bile acids are passively absorbed along the entirety of the small intestine, they are actively absorbed only in the terminal ileum (B). Bile acids are colorless, and the yellow hue of bile is a result of the pigmented biliverdin (breakdown product of bilirubin) that is also found in bile (C). Bile duct stones occurring after 2 years are considered primary common duct stones and are often pigmented (D). During the fasting state, gallbladder emptying is stimulated by motilin.

Reference: Luiking YC, Peeters TL, Stolk MF, et al. Motilin induces gall bladder emptying and antral contractions in the fasted state in humans. *Gut*. 1998;42(6):830–835.

10. D. The left hepatic duct is longer than the right and is more likely to be dilated in the presence of distal obstruction (A). The spiral Heister valves within the cystic duct do not have any true valvular function (C). In approximately three-fourths of individuals, the CBD and the main pancreatic duct unite outside the duodenal wall and traverse the duodenal wall as a single duct. The blood supply to the CBD runs along the lateral and medial walls at the 3 and 9 o'clock positions and comes from the right hepatic artery and retroduodenal artery (off gastroduodenal artery) (E). Thus, a transverse hemitransection of the duct will likely interrupt the blood supply and render a repair prone to ischemia and stricture. Venous return of the gallbladder is typically drained directly to the parenchyma of the liver (B).

Reference: Oddsdottir, M, Hunter, JG. Gallbladder. In: Brunicardi FC, Andersen DK, Billiar TR, et al., eds. *Schwartz's principles of surgery*. 8th ed. New York: McGraw-Hill; 2005:1187–1200.

11. A. Most polypoid lesions of the gallbladder are benign, and of these, cholesterol polyps are the most common. They are usually small (<10 mm), pedunculated, and multiple. They are usually seen in association with cholesterolosis. Ultrasound imaging often demonstrates hyperechoic foci with a comet tail artifact; unlike gallstones, these foci don't produce shadowing. Adenomyomatosis polyps are the second most common (B). They appear as sessile polyps that cause focal thickening of the wall. Inflammatory polyps are the third most common (E). All three are benign and are pseudopolyps. Adenomas and adenocarcinomas of the gallbladder are generally larger than 10 mm. However, distinguishing between a benign and a malignant polyp on ultrasonography is generally not reliable (C, D). Thus, when a polyp is found on ultrasound, the general indications for cholecystectomy are (1) a symptomatic polyp, (2) a polyp in association with gallstones, (3) a polyp larger than 6 mm, and (4) patient age over 50. For asymptomatic gallstone polyps that do not meet the above criteria, the recommended management is follow-up ultrasound in 6 months.

References: Ahrendt SA, Pitt HA. Biliary tract. In: Townsend CM, Jr, Beauchamp RD, Evers BM, Mattox KL, eds. *Sabiston textbook of surgery: the biological basis of modern surgical practice*. 17th ed. Philadelphia: W.B. Saunders; 2004:1597–1642.

Myers R, Shaffer E, Beck P. Gallbladder polyps: epidemiology, natural history and management. *Can J Gastroenterol*. 2002;16(3):187-194.

Shinkai H, Kimura W, Muto T. Surgical indications for small polypoid lesions of the gallbladder. *Am J Surg*. 1998;175(2):114–117.

12. B. A total of four trocar sites is typically placed during laparoscopic cholecystectomy: (1) a 5-mm umbilical port for the laparoscope, (2) a 12-mm epigastric port for dissection and retrieval of the specimen, (3) a 5-mm right-sided subcostal port, and (4) an additional 5-mm port inferior and lateral to the subcostal port. The 5-mm ports allow graspers to retract the gallbladder fundus superiorly (A, E) and infundibulum, or the neck, laterally. This is the ideal positioning to achieve the "critical view" and prevent CBD injury because it allows the cystic duct to remain perpendicular to the CBD. Excess cephalad retraction of the gallbladder infundibulum shifts the cystic duct in line with the CBD and is considered the most common cause of CBD injury (D). The gallbladder body should not be used as a retraction site (C).

13. B. When a gallstone becomes impacted in the cystic duct, the typical course is that acute cholecystitis will develop in the patient. Less frequently, an acute infection does not develop in the patient even though the cystic duct remains obstructed. In this situation, bile within the gallbladder becomes absorbed, but the gallbladder epithelium continues to secrete glycoprotein (mucus). The gallbladder becomes distended with mucinous material (E). This is known as hydrops. The gallbladder may be palpable but does not create the Murphy sign (D). Hydrops of the gallbladder may result in edema of the gallbladder wall and perforation. Although hydrops may persist with few consequences, cholecystectomy is generally indicated to avoid complications. Hydrops of the gallbladder does not significantly increase the risk for malignancy (A). Although this can subsequently become infected, enteric bacterial infection is not typically responsible for the development of hydrops (C).

Reference: Oddsdottir, M, Hunter, JG. Gallbladder. In: Brunicardi FC, Andersen DK, Billiar TR, et al., eds. *Schwartz's principles of surgery*. 8th ed. New York: McGraw-Hill; 2005:1187–1200.

14. E. The majority of common bile duct injuries occur iatrogenically during laparoscopic cholecystectomy in patients with relatively benign gallbladder disease (e.g., symptomatic cholelithiasis, acute cholecystitis). The management of an intraoperative bile duct injury depends on the type of injury and the clinical setting. If a small lateral injury (<50%) is created in the CBD, this can be repaired by closing the ductotomy over a T tube and leaving a drain. Conversely, if the common bile duct is transected, this results in an interruption in the blood supply to the duct and attempts at primary repair will inevitably lead to stricture formation and recurrent episodes of cholangitis (A). Thus, if a transection is recognized intraoperatively, and an experienced hepatobiliary surgeon is available, it is best to repair it immediately and to do so with a biliary enteric bypass. Because most of these injuries will be in the common bile duct, the best option is to perform a hepaticoenterostomy (B, C). A critical element of the repair is to perform a tension-free, mucosa-to-mucosa duct enteric anastomosis. Hepaticoduodenostomy has largely been abandoned for benign liver disease due to ongoing enteric reflux (D). It is also more technically challenging to perform because it is difficult to reach the duodenum to the hepatic duct; thus most surgeons prefer a Roux-en-Y hepaticojejunostomy. If an experienced hepatobiliary surgeon is not available, the best option is to drain the area, place transhepatic catheters, and refer the patient to higher level of care. If the injury is discovered postoperatively and there has been a long delay, the best option is to perform transhepatic drainage and delay primary repair for 6 to 8 weeks to allow the inflammation to subside.

References: Ahrendt SA, Pitt HA. Biliary tract. In: Townsend CM, Jr, Beauchamp RD, Evers BM, Mattox KL, eds. *Sabiston textbook of surgery: The biological basis of modern surgical practice.* 17th ed. Philadelphia: W.B. Saunders; 2004:1597–1642.

MacFadyen BV Jr, Vecchio R, Ricardo AE, Mathis CR. Bile duct injury after laparoscopic cholecystectomy: the United States experience. *Surg Endosc.* 1998;12(4):315–321.

Narayanan SK, Chen Y, Narasimhan KL, Cohen RC. Hepaticoduodenostomy versus hepaticojejunostomy after resection of choledochal cyst: a systemic review and meta-analysis. *J Pediatr Surg.* 2013;48(11):2336–2342.

15. A. Most benign bile duct strictures are iatrogenic and are due to a technical error during cholecystectomy, such as excessive use of cautery, incorrect placement of a surgical clip, and overly aggressive dissection near the CBD, all of which may be the result of unclear anatomy (B–E). Regardless of the cause, the eventual response is fibrosis and stricture formation. As many as three-fourths of injuries that lead to strictures are not recognized at surgery, and as many as one-third occur 5 years or more after the operation. The majority of iatrogenic strictures are short and occur in the common bile duct and can present with an episode of cholangitis. The workup consists of ultrasonography, which will detect dilated ducts proximal to the stricture, a computed tomography scan to look for masses, and endoscopic retrograde cholangiography (ERCP) with endoscopic ultrasound (EUS), which can be both diagnostic and therapeutic. EUS can be helpful in detecting a tumor within the bile duct. During ERCP, a brushing of the bile duct should be taken for cytology to rule out a malignancy. Management of focal benign strictures by a biliary enteric bypass or stenting remains debatable because of the lack of randomized trials and the lack of good long-term follow-up with stenting. The primary concern with stenting is that the strictures may become obstructed and lead to recurrent cholangitis. Given the much less invasive nature of stenting, strong consideration should be given to this approach. If recurrent obstructive symptoms subsequently develop, a biliary enteric bypass should be performed.

References: Ahrendt SA, Pitt HA. Biliary tract. In: Townsend CM, Jr, Beauchamp RD, Evers BM, Mattox KL, eds. *Sabiston textbook of surgery: the biological basis of modern surgical practice.* 17th ed. Philadelphia: W.B. Saunders; 2004:1597–1642.

Chun K. Recent classifications of the common bile duct injury. *Korean J Hepatobiliary Pancreat Surg.* 2014;18(3):69–72.

Costamagna G, Shah SK, Tringali A. Current management of postoperative complications and benign biliary strictures. *Gastrointest Endosc Clin N Am.* 2003;13(4):635–648.

Lopez RR, Jr, Cosenza CA, Lois J, et al. Long-term results of metallic stents for benign biliary strictures. *Arch Surg.* 2001;136(6):664–669.

Oddsdottir M, Hunter, J. G. Gallbladder. In: Brunicardi FC, Andersen DK, Billiar TR, et al., eds. *Schwartz's principles of surgery.* 8th ed. New York: McGraw-Hill; 2005:1187–1200.

Siriwardana HPP, Siriwardena AK. Systematic appraisal of the role of metallic endobiliary stents in the treatment of benign bile duct stricture. *Ann Surg.* 2005;242(1):10–19.

16. A. The presentation is consistent with acalculous cholecystitis. The initial study of choice is ultrasonography, which can be performed at the bedside. Findings to confirm the diagnosis would include thickening of the gallbladder wall, sludge (as in this patient), and pericholecystic fluid. If the ultrasound findings are negative and the patient is not critically ill, the next study would be a HIDA scan with sincalide or morphine. A positive study finding would demonstrate nonfilling of the gallbladder with visualization of the tracer in the liver and small bowel. Morphine decreases the rate of false-positive HIDA scan results because it leads to sphincter of Oddi contraction and thus increases the likelihood of filling of the gallbladder in the absence of cholecystitis. A HIDA scan is not recommended in critically ill patients in whom a delay in therapy can be potentially fatal (C). Acalculous cholecystitis requires urgent intervention, preferably cholecystectomy. The procedure can be attempted laparoscopically; however, there is a higher chance of finding gangrenous cholecystitis and needing to convert to open. If the patient is too ill for surgery, percutaneous ultrasonography or CT-guided cholecystostomy is the treatment option of choice (B, D). Upper endoscopy is not indicated (E).

Reference: Ahrendt SA, Pitt HA. Biliary tract. In: Townsend CM, Jr, Beauchamp RD, Evers BM, Mattox KL, eds. *Sabiston textbook of surgery: the biological basis of modern surgical practice.* 17th ed. Philadelphia: W.B. Saunders; 2004:1597–1642.

17. B. All of the provided options are potential repairs for a bile duct injury. Sharp, clean, and small injuries in a large CBD or common hepatic duct are more amenable to primary repair. Repair is generally performed over a T tube (A). It is important to bear in mind that the CBD is supplied via two main arteries running at the right and left border of the duct, entering at "3 o'clock" and "9 o'clock." As such, injuries that are less than 50% in circumference are less likely to have interrupted the blood supply on both sides and are therefore less likely to develop ischemic stricture with primary repair. If the duct is transected, nearly transected (>50% circumference), or very small, a Roux-en-Y hepaticojejunostomy is recommended (D). Injuries to the proximal CBD can be treated with a hepaticojejunostomy (D), while injuries to the distal CBD can be treated with a choledochoduodenostomy (E). If the bile duct injury is the result of thermal injury, a primary repair with a T tube placed through a separate choledochotomy is the preferred approach (C).

References: Oddsdottir, M, Hunter, JG. Gallbladder. In: Brunicardi FC, Andersen DK, Billiar TR, et al., eds. *Schwartz's principles of surgery.* 8th ed. New York: McGraw-Hill; 2005:1187–1200.

Garden JO, ed. *Hepatobiliary and pancreatic surgery.* 4th ed. New York: Elsevier; 2009:208.

18. E. The routine use of IOC to prevent bile duct injury is controversial, but most surgeons would say that routine use is unnecessary. Because the overall risk of bile duct injury is so small, to date there are no sufficiently large-scale randomized studies to answer this question. Most likely, the use of IOC will not prevent an injury to the CBD (A). However, IOC seems to allow earlier recognition of a CBD injury and prevent complete transection of the CBD. Although routine IOC will identify unsuspected CBD stones, in most instances, CBD stones are suspected preoperatively by abnormal liver function tests, a dilated CBD, or a history of gallstone pancreatitis. In a nationwide retrospective analysis, CBD injury was found in 0.39% of patients undergoing cholecystectomy with IOC and in 0.58% of patients without IOC (unadjusted relative risk, 1.49). After controlling for patient-level factors and surgeon-level factors, the risk of injury was increased when IOC was not used (adjusted relative risk, 1.71). Some surgeons prefer selective use of IOC and obtain what is known as the "critical view," whereby the cystic duct and artery are carefully identified and not clipped or cut until conclusive identification has been made. This is done by completely dissecting the Calot triangle free of all fat and fibrous tissue and dissecting the lower part of the gallbladder off the liver bed, such that only two skeletonized structures (the cystic duct and artery) are seen to be entering the gallbladder.

Reference: Saunders WB, Detry O, De Roover A, Detroz B. The role of intraoperative cholangiography in detecting and preventing bile duct injury during laparoscopic cholecystectomy. *Acta Chirurgica Belgica*. 2003;103(2):161–162.

19. C. Emphysematous cholecystitis occurs in less than 1% of acute cholecystitis cases. It is a disease that occurs predominantly in elderly diabetic men. The hallmark feature is characterized by gas within the gallbladder wall or lumen. This can be seen on plain radiograph, ultrasound, or computed tomography (CT) scan. Gangrene of the gallbladder is present in three-fourths of all cases, and perforation of the gallbladder occurs in more than 20% of cases (E). In one large series, the mortality rate was 25% and the morbidity rate was 50% despite aggressive treatment with broad-spectrum antibiotics and emergent surgery. In patients that are unstable, and not deemed suitable for general anesthesia (such as a patient on pressors or multiple medical problems), percutaneous drainage with cholecystostomy should be performed first. If the patient is more stable, cholecystectomy is preferred (B). Although prior studies suggested open cholecystectomy was preferred, laparoscopic cholecystectomy is an acceptable approach, provided a low threshold for conversion and standard principles are used. Antimicrobial coverage should include *Clostridia perfringens*, which is an anaerobic gram-positive rod and considered the most common cause of emphysematous cholecystitis (D). High-dose penicillin should be started immediately (A). Other common biliary pathogens associated with emphysematous cholecystitis include *Clostridia welchii*, *Escherichia coli*, *Enterococcus*, and *Klebsiella*.

References: Ahrendt SA, Pitt HA. Biliary tract. In: Townsend CM, Jr, Beauchamp RD, Evers BM, Mattox KL, eds. *Sabiston textbook of surgery: the biological basis of modern surgical practice*. 17th ed. Philadelphia: W.B. Saunders; 2004:1597–1642.

Tellez GS, Rodriguez-Montes L, Fernandez de Lis J. Acute emphysematous cholecystitis: report of twenty cases. *Hepatogastroenterology*. 1999;46(28):2144–2148.

20. B. Several studies have analyzed the role of preoperative biliary drainage via ERCP and stenting in patients with malignant obstructive jaundice who are to undergo a Whipple procedure. Theoretically, relief of jaundice might improve the operative risk of the subsequent Whipple procedure. However, a large meta-analysis and single-center studies failed to show improved morbidity and mortality rates with preoperative biliary drainage. In fact, the routine use of preoperative biliary drainage seems to increase the risk of infectious complications including wound infection (10% with drainage versus 4% without) and increases the risk of pancreatic fistula (10% with drainage versus 4% without). Thus, it should only be used selectively (e.g., presence of cholangitis or severe, intractable pruritus). It has not been demonstrated to decrease the risk of cholangitis (A), shorten hospital stay (D), or decrease the mortality rate (E). Additionally, obstructive jaundice provides the surgeon with a dilated

pancreatic duct at the time of surgery, making the pancreaticojejunostomy in a Whipple procedure easier to perform.

References: Ahrendt SA, Pitt HA. Biliary tract. In: Townsend CM, Jr, Beauchamp RD, Evers BM, Mattox KL, eds. *Sabiston textbook of surgery: the biological basis of modern surgical practice*. 17th ed. Philadelphia: W.B. Saunders; 2004:1597–1642.

Sewnath ME, Karsten TM, Prins MH, Rauws EJA, Obertop H, Gouma DJ. A meta-analysis on the efficacy of preoperative biliary drainage for tumors causing obstructive jaundice. *Ann Surg.* 2002;236(1):17–27.

Sohn TA, Yeo CJ, Cameron JL, Pitt HA, Lillemoe KD. Do preoperative biliary stents increase postpancreaticoduodenectomy complications? *J Gastrointest Surg.* 2000;4(3):258–267.

21. E. This patient presents with a history and findings consistent with cholangiohepatitis, also known as recurrent pyogenic cholangitis. It is endemic in Asia, although the incidence has been decreasing. Cholangiohepatitis affects both sexes equally (C). The etiology of cholangiohepatitis seems to be a combination of bacterial and parasitic (*Clonorchis sinensis*, *Opisthorchis viverrini*, and *Ascaris lumbricoides*) infections in the biliary tree. The bacteria deconjugate bilirubin, which has a greater propensity to precipitate as bile sludge. Brown pigment stones form as a consequence of the sludge and dead bacterial cells (B). In addition, the nucleus of the stone may harbor a parasite egg. The stones lead to recurrent episodes of cholangitis, liver abscesses, stricture formation, liver failure, and an increased risk of cholangiocarcinoma. Recurrence is high. Initial treatment is with ERCP and transhepatic cholangiography. Patients often require multiple interventions to clear the biliary tree. The patient may eventually require a biliary enteric bypass, but this would not be the initial procedure of choice. Metronidazole is the treatment of choice for amebic liver abscess (D). Hydatid liver disease is a liver cyst caused by *Echinococcus* and is associated with close contact with dogs and sheep (A).

22. D. Cancer of the gallbladder is predominantly adenocarcinoma. The majority of cases are discovered in an advanced state with distant metastases. Thus, the overall prognosis is very poor, with a 5-year survival rate of only 5%. The best chance of cure is if it is discovered incidentally at the time of cholecystectomy. It is 17 times more likely to be discovered in patients following open cholecystectomy as compared with laparoscopic cholecystectomy. Gallbladder cancer metastasizes first to the celiac axis lymph nodes. Recent studies indicate that those that are discovered incidentally and are superficial, such as carcinoma in situ and T1 lesions (do not extend into perimuscular connective tissue), and have negative margins, can be managed by cholecystectomy alone (B), with a 100% 5-year survival. Those that are more locally advanced, such as T2 through T4 lesions (those that invade the perimuscular connective tissue or directly invade the liver), are treated with a radical cholecystectomy, which includes subsegmental resection of segments IVb and V, plus hepatoduodenal ligament lymphadenectomy, which results in prolonged survival (C). The caveat is that there must be no evidence of distant metastases. In one series of 48 patients, the overall 5-year survival rate was 13%, but it was 60% for patients who underwent radical cholecystectomy. The radical cholecystectomy group had significantly longer survival than the simple cholecystectomy group for all stages except stage I (T1N0). Although port sites are associated with peritoneal disease and decreased survival, removing them does not improve survival and should not be done routinely in all patients with incidentally discovered gallbladder cancer (E). Radiation therapy with fluorouracil radiosensitization is the most commonly used postoperative treatment.

References: Oddsdottir, M, Hunter, J G. Gallbladder. In: Brunicardi FC, Andersen DK, Billiar TR, et al., eds. *Schwartz's principles of surgery*. 8th ed. New York: McGraw-Hill; 2005:1187–1200.

Reid KM, Ramos-De la Medina A, Donohue JH. Diagnosis and surgical management of gallbladder cancer: a review. *J Gastrointest Surg*. 2007;11(5):671–681.

Taner CB, Nagorney DM, Donohue JH. Surgical treatment of gallbladder cancer. *J Gastrointest Surg*. 2004;8(1):83–89.

Pitt SC, Jin LX, Hall BL, Strasberg SM, Pitt HA. Incidental gallbladder cancer at cholecystectomy: when should the surgeon be suspicious? *Ann Surg*. 2014;260(1):128–133.

23. B. Sclerosing cholangitis is characterized by the presence of multiple inflammatory fibrous thickenings resulting in irregular narrowing of the entire biliary tree (C). It is progressive and as such leads eventually to biliary obstruction, recurrent biliary infection, cirrhosis, and liver failure, as well as a significantly increased risk of cholangiocarcinoma (in 10%–20% of patients). All patients should be checked for an elevated level of CA 19-9. It is twice as common in men, and also tends to occur in younger patients (E). Risk factors for sclerosing cholangitis include inflammatory bowel disease, pancreatitis, and diabetes. The strongest association is with ulcerative colitis (A). Approximately two-thirds of patients have ulcerative colitis. In fact, it is usually discovered in these patients when an abnormal liver function test result is noted. Alkaline phosphatase is characteristically elevated out of proportion to an elevated bilirubin level. Patients may test positive for p-ANCA antibodies (in contrast to antimitochondrial antibodies for primary biliary cirrhosis). It is less commonly associated with Crohn disease. Other diseases associated with sclerosing cholangitis include Riedel thyroiditis and retroperitoneal fibrosis. Removing the colon in patients with ulcerative colitis does not affect the course of the sclerosing cholangitis. In addition, the severity of inflammation does not predict the onset of malignancy. All newly diagnosed patients with sclerosing cholangitis with or without an inflammatory bowel disease diagnosis should be scheduled for a screening colonoscopy. Patients can be managed initially with steroids, methotrexate, and cyclosporine, but the majority will ultimately require more invasive treatment including biliary stenting (D). Currently, the best option is liver transplantation in patients who progress to liver failure.

Reference: Oddsdottir, M, Hunter, JG. Gallbladder. In: Brunicardi FC, Andersen DK, Billiar TR, et al., eds. *Schwartz's principles of surgery*. 8th ed. New York: McGraw-Hill; 2005:1187–1200.

24. D. Gallbladder cancer is two to three times more common in females (C). It is also more common in Native Americans in both North and South America. Approximately 90% of patients with carcinoma also have gallstones. Large single stones have a much higher risk of cancer than multiple small stones, likely the result of creating more mucosal inflammation; large stones also are more likely to lead to cholecystoenteric fistulas. Other risk factors include choledochal cysts (which may be due to an abnormal pancreaticobiliary junction), sclerosing cholangitis, gallbladder polyps, and

exposure to carcinogens (nitrosamines, azotoluene). Obesity has recently been shown to be a risk factor for a wide range of cancers, including the gallbladder (E). Speckled cholesterol deposits on the gallbladder wall are a feature of cholesterolosis and are not associated with an increased risk of cancer (A). Selective mucosal calcium deposits (porcelain gallbladder) may have an increased risk of malignancy. Thickened nodules of mucosa and muscle in the gallbladder are a feature of adenomyomatosis (B). Tumor invading the lamina propria, but not yet invaded all the way through and to the underlying muscularis, is considered T1a disease and treated with simple cholecystectomy. Invasion to the underlying muscularis is T1b disease and requires resection of liver segments IVb and V and regional lymph node dissection.

References: Oddsdottir M, Hunter J. G. Gallbladder. In: Brunicardi FC, Andersen DK, Billiar TR, et al., eds. *Schwartz's principles of surgery*. 8th ed. New York: McGraw-Hill; 2005:1187–1200.

Stephen AE, Berger DL. Carcinoma in the porcelain gallbladder: a relationship revisited. *Surgery*. 2001;129(6):699–703.

Chen, G. L., Akmal, Y., DiFronzo, A. L., et al. (2015).

25. D. The exact etiology of choledochal cysts is unclear. The most likely explanation is that there is an anomalous pancreaticobiliary duct junction. Specifically, the pancreatic duct joins the common bile duct more than 1 cm proximal to the ampulla, resulting in a long common channel. The long channel leads to free reflux of pancreatic secretions into the biliary tract, resulting in increased biliary pressures and inflammatory changes in the biliary epithelium, which eventually lead to dilation and cyst formation. Although an abnormal pancreaticobiliary junction is present in the majority of patients with choledochal cysts, it is not uniformly seen. Choledochal cysts are more common in females and Asians. It classically presents in childhood with jaundice and an abdominal mass accompanied by abdominal pain. In infants, it may be confused with biliary atresia. However, less than 50% of patients present with all three features, and thus the diagnosis is often delayed. The most common presentation is nonspecific abdominal pain. The diagnosis is made by ultrasonography, which can sometimes detect the cyst antenatally. There are five types. Type I is the most common (90%) and consists of fusiform dilation of the bile duct. Type V, also known as Caroli disease, is characterized by multiple intrahepatic dilations. Because of the risk of malignant degeneration, treatment involves excising the cyst with a biliary enteric bypass (typically hepaticojejunostomy). The risk of malignancy increases with the more advanced age at which the cyst is detected. Type V (Caroli) will need a partial liver resection or liver transplant. Biliary smooth muscle (A), mucosa (E), ductal adventitia (C), and bile (B) are not thought to play a role in choledochal cyst disease.

References: Oddsdottir, M, Hunter, J. G. Gallbladder. In: Brunicardi FC, Andersen DK, Billiar TR, et al., eds. *Schwartz's principles of surgery*. 8th ed. New York: McGraw-Hill; 2005:1187–1200.

Todani T, Watanabe Y, Fujii T, Uemura S. Anomalous arrangement of the pancreatobiliary ductal system in patients with a choledochal cyst. *Am J Surg*. 1984;147(5):672–676.

26. C. Type I choledochal cysts are the most common type and are dilations of either the entire common hepatic duct and CBD or a segment of it. Management consists of excision of the entire cyst and a biliary enteric bypass. An exception is if the posterior wall of the cyst is stuck to the portal vein, which occasionally occurs due to ongoing inflammation. Roux-en-Y cyst jejunostomy alone would not be sufficient (E). Dissection of the posterior wall can sometimes be precarious because it may be stuck to the portal vein. In this case, the posterior wall should be left in situ and the mucosa fulgurated or curetted (Lilly procedure) because this will still theoretically remove the risk of malignancy. Type II choledochal cysts are diverticula that project from the CBD wall. Type III choledochal cysts are found in the intraduodenal portion of the CBD (also called a *choledochocele*). Type IVa cysts are characterized by multiple dilations of the intrahepatic and extrahepatic biliary tree. Most frequently, a large solitary cyst of the extrahepatic duct is accompanied by multiple cysts of the intrahepatic ducts. Type IVb choledochal cysts consist of multiple dilations that involve only the extrahepatic bile duct. Type V choledochal cysts (Caroli disease) consist of dilations of the intrahepatic biliary tree. Partial resection may be indicated for Type V choledochal cyst (A, B). There is no role for observation (D).

References: Ahrendt SA, Pitt HA. Biliary tract. In: Townsend CM, Jr, Beauchamp RD, Evers BM, Mattox KL, eds. *Sabiston textbook of surgery: the biological basis of modern surgical practice.* 17th ed. Philadelphia: W.B. Saunders; 2004:1597–1642.

Oddsdottir, M, Hunter, JG. Gallbladder. In: Brunicardi FC, Andersen DK, Billiar TR, et al., eds. *Schwartz's principles of surgery.* 8th ed. New York: McGraw-Hill; 2005:1187–1200.

Todani T, Watanabe Y, Fujii T, Uemura S. Anomalous arrangement of the pancreatobiliary ductal system in patients with a choledochal cyst. *Am J Surg.* 1984;147(5):672–676.

27. B. Perihilar cholangiocarcinomas are also known as Klatskin tumors. They are classified into four types based on whether they are limited to the common hepatic duct (type I), involve the bifurcation of the right and left hepatic ducts (type II), or enter into the secondary right (type IIIa) or left (type IIIb) intrahepatic ducts. Surgery is the only treatment that has shown potential for long-term survival, provided the tumor has no evidence of distant spread (D, E). Type I and II tumors involve resection of the entire extrahepatic biliary tree with portal lymphadenectomy and bilateral Roux-en-Y hepaticojejunostomies (C). More recently, an even more aggressive approach has been taken for type I and II tumors to include a hemihepatectomy to achieve negative margins. Using this approach, several authors have shown improved survival. For type III lesions, a similar aggressive approach using lobectomy is advocated. Adjuvant radiation therapy has also not been shown to improve either quality of life or survival in resected patients. Patients with unresectable disease are often offered treatment with 5-fluorouracil alone or in combination with mitomycin C and doxorubicin, but the response rates are low. A Whipple procedure would be appropriate for a distal CBD tumor (A).

References: Capussotti L, Muratore A, Polastri R, Ferrero A, Massucco P. Liver resection for hilar cholangiocarcinoma: in-hospital mortality and longterm survival. *J Am Coll Surg.* 2002;195(5):641–647.

Dinant S, Gerhards MF, Rauws EAJ, Busch ORC, Gouma DJ, van Gulik TM. Improved outcome of resection of hilar cholangiocarcinoma (Klatskin tumor). *Ann Surg Oncol.* 2006;13(6):872–880.

Lygidakis N, Sgourakis G, Dedemadi G. Long-term results following resectional surgery for Klatskin tumors: a twenty-year personal experience. *Hepatogastroenterology.* 2001;48(37):95–101.

Oddsdottir, M, Hunter, JG. Gallbladder. In: Brunicardi FC, Andersen DK, Billiar TR, et al., eds. *Schwartz's principles of surgery.* 8th ed. New York: McGraw-Hill; 2005:1187–1200.

28. E. Cholangiocarcinoma arises from bile duct epithelium (D). Although it can occur anywhere along the biliary tree, the majority occurs extrahepatically, while only 20% are intrahepatic (A). It is a locally aggressive cancer but can have direct spread to the liver and peritoneum. The Bismuth-Corlette classification system organizes cholangiocarcinoma by location: type I occurs below the confluence of the left and right hepatic ducts; type II occurs at the juncture of the left and right hepatic ducts; type III involves either the left or right hepatic duct; and type IV involves secondary extensions of either the left or right hepatic ducts (B). MRCP is an appropriate initial imaging study to define the anatomy and plan for surgical intervention. ERCP is the most valuable diagnostic tool and allows for biopsy brushings. Intrahepatic disease can be managed with hepatic wedge resection while extrahepatic disease needs resection with biliary-enteric bypass. However, this is only appropriate for patients that do not have extensive local disease (involvement of the portal vein trunk or hepatic arteries), nodal involvement, or distant metastases. Distal cholangiocarcinoma will need a pancreaticoduodenectomy. The National Comprehensive Cancer Network recommends consideration of chemoradiation in patients with positive margins or nodal disease, but it should not be done routinely (C).

Abdomen—Liver

4

NAVEEN BALAN, KATHRYN T. CHEN, AND DANIELLE M. HARI

ABSITE 99th Percentile High-Yields

I. Hepatocellular Carcinoma
   A. Etiology—arises in the setting of chronic inflammation or cirrhosis
      1. Hepatitis-C (most common), hepatitis-B, NAFLD (non-alcoholic fatty liver disease), EtOH, alpha-1-antitrypsin deficiency, hemochromatosis, Wilson disease, aflatoxin exposure
   B. Orthotopic liver transplant indications (MILAN criteria)
      1. One lesion <5 cm or 3 or less lesions each <3 cm, no vascular invasion or metastasis
   C. Liver resection indicated in good surgical candidates
   D. Options for patients who are poor surgical candidates: ablation (microwave/radiofrequency/cryoablation), TACE (transarterial chemoembolization)
   E. Future liver remnant (FLR): remaining liver following resection required to prevent liver failure
      1. Healthy patient: 20% to 25% needed; injured liver (e.g., post-chemo): 30% needed; cirrhotic patient: 40% needed
      2. Portal vein embolization of diseased segment to hypertrophy the contralateral (healthy) side offered to patients that fall below these thresholds
   F. Transjugular intrahepatic portosystemic shunt (TIPS)
      1. Emergent indication: massive esophageal variceal bleed refractory to medical and endoscopic therapy, needs decompression of the portal venous system; hepatic encephalopathy may develop

Mass	Background	Imaging	Management
Hemangioma	Most common benign tumor	CT—hypodense with peripheral nodular enhancement	Most are observed, surgery resection vs enucleation if symptomatic; can be associated with Kasabach-Merritt syndrome (consumptive coagulopathy from sequestration of platelets and congestive heart failure)
Focal nodular hyperplasia (FNH)	Benign, second most common	CT—hyperenhance on arterial phase with central scar, centrifugal filling on delayed	Tc-99m sulfur colloid test if unclear diagnosis (FNH will have normal/increased uptake), observation only, no intervention needed
Adenoma	Associated with oral contraceptive (OCP), steroid use	CT—hyperenhance on arterial phase, centripetal filling on delayed phase	Cessation of OCP with follow-up imaging, if persistent or enlarging then needs resection due to rupture/malignant degeneration risk; resection recommended for all males; will have decreased uptake on sulfur colloid scan

Mass	Background	Imaging	Management
Hydatid cyst	*Echinococcus granulosus* exposure	CT/US—cystic lesions with daughter cysts	Albendazole, if failure then proceed with PAIR (puncture, aspiration, injection, reaspiration)
Amebic abscess	Secondary to *Entamoeba histolytica*	CT—low-density mass with peripheral enhancing rim	Serologic testing; once diagnosis confirmed, then treat with metronidazole
Pyogenic abscess	Most due to biliary infections	CT—double target or cluster sign, air-fluid level	Percutaneous drain if >5 cm with antibiotics, if <5 cm in size, then antibiotics alone
Hepatocellular carcinoma (HCC)	Most common malignant tumor	CT—rapid arterial enhancement with rapid washout on portal venous phase	If imaging is consistent and AFP elevated, no need for biopsy; treat with resection, ablation, embolization, transplant
Fibrolamellar HCC	More common in women	CT—central scar that does not enhance	Surgery can be curative, otherwise need chemotherapy vs embolization

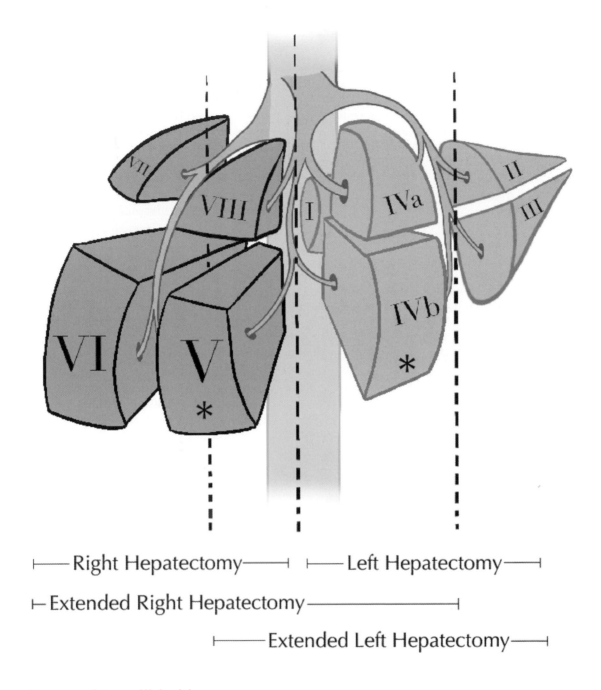

├────Right Hepatectomy────┤ ├────Left Hepatectomy────┤

├─Extended Right Hepatectomy────────────┤

├────Extended Left Hepatectomy────┤

*Resected in gallbladder cancer

The Couinaud classification describes functional liver anatomy as 8 independent segments based on independent vascular inflow, outflow, and biliary drainage. Cantlie line is a vertical plane dividing the liver into left and right lobes, extending from the inferior vena cava posteriorly to the middle of the gallbladder fossa anteriorly. A right hepatectomy resects segments V, VI, VII, and VIII. A left hepatectomy removes segments IVa, IVb, II, and III. An extended right includes the segments resected in a right hepatectomy plus IVa, IVb and sometimes the caudate lobe. An extended left hepatectomy resects the segments included in a left hepatectomy plus VIII and V. In all gallbladder cancers >T1a , V and IVb are resected. In T1a gallbladder, cholecystectomy alone is sufficient. The caudate lobe (segment I) is the only segment that drains directly into the inferior vena cava.

Fig. 4.1

Questions

1. A 48-year-old man with a history of Child-Pugh C cirrhosis secondary to nonalcoholic fatty liver disease is found to have multifocal hepatocellular carcinoma. Imaging shows a 2-cm lesion in segment VI, a 3-cm lesion in segment VII, and a 3-cm lesion in segment II. What is the appropriate management?
   A. Liver transplantation
   B. Right hepatectomy
   C. Chemotherapy
   D. Extended right hepatectomy
   E. Radiofrequency ablation of each lesion

2. An otherwise healthy 62-year-old woman is found to have anemia on her annual physical exam. After workup, she is found to have a sigmoid colonic adenocarcinoma and multiple hepatic lesions in the right hepatic lobe and several in the left hepatic lobe that are biopsy-proven metastatic adenocarcinoma. Her future liver remnant is estimated to be 15%. Which of the following is recommended?
   A. Chemotherapy alone
   B. Colectomy followed by chemotherapy
   C. Concomitant colectomy and right hepatectomy followed by chemotherapy
   D. Colectomy, postoperative chemotherapy, then transarterial chemoembolization (TACE) of liver lesions
   E. TACE of liver lesions

3. An 8-year-old girl presents with upper gastrointestinal (UGI) bleeding. The physical examination demonstrates splenomegaly. Her medical history is significant for a prolonged stay in the neonatal intensive care unit at birth due to prematurity, complicated by necrotizing enterocolitis. She has no history of travel outside the United States. Laboratory testing reveals a hematocrit of 20% and normal bilirubin, albumin, and international normalized ratio. After fluid resuscitation, an upper endoscopy is performed that reveals esophageal varices. The patient is given octreotide and undergoes sclerotherapy. Which of the following studies will most likely determine the cause of her UGI bleed?
   A. Duplex ultrasonography of the portal vein
   B. Duplex ultrasonography of the splenic vein
   C. CT scan of the abdomen
   D. MRI of the abdomen
   E. Liver biopsy

4. A 45-year-old man with a history of alcohol abuse presents with recurrent UGI bleeding. His history is significant for alcoholic pancreatitis. On upper endoscopy, he is found to have bleeding from isolated gastric varices. The bleeding is controlled medically. On CT imaging, the portal and superior mesenteric veins are patent, but the splenic vein is not visualized. Optimal management for this patient would be:
   A. Side-to-side portacaval shunt
   B. Mesocaval shunt
   C. Distal splenorenal shunt
   D. Long-term beta-blocker therapy
   E. Splenectomy

5. A 30-year-old Hispanic man with a history of alcohol abuse presents with a high fever, right upper quadrant pain, and leukocytosis. Ultrasonography reveals a 5-cm fluid collection in the right lobe of the liver. On the CT scan, the fluid collection shows a peripheral rim of edema. The cause of the fluid collection is most likely to be determined by:
   A. Blood cultures
   B. Stool cultures
   C. Percutaneous aspiration of liver
   D. Serologic tests
   E. Liver function tests

6. Definitive management of the patient in question 5 consists of:
   A. Oral metronidazole
   B. Broad-spectrum antibiotics and open surgical drainage
   C. Broad-spectrum antibiotics and early percutaneous aspiration of the abscess
   D. Broad-spectrum antibiotics and CT-guided catheter insertion to drain the abscess
   E. Broad-spectrum antibiotics and laparoscopic drainage

7. The most common benign tumor of the liver is:
   A. FNH
   B. Hepatic adenoma
   C. Hemangioma
   D. Mesenchymal hamartoma
   E. Inflammatory pseudotumor

8. Which of the following is true regarding liver cysts associated with polycystic liver disease?
   A. Laparoscopic fenestration is the preferred treatment option
   B. It has an autosomal recessive inheritance pattern
   C. They are typically symptomatic
   D. Oral estrogen therapy can be helpful
   E. Liver function tests are usually abnormal

9. Which of the following is the best method to prevent a first bleed in a patient with known large esophageal varices?
   A. Beta-blockade
   B. Transjugular intrahepatic portosystemic shunt (TIPS) placement
   C. Sclerotherapy
   D. Endoscopic ligation
   E. Selective portosystemic shunt placement

10. Which of the following is true regarding bile acids?
    A. Deoxycholic acid and lithocholic acid are primary bile acids
    B. Cholic and chenodeoxycholic acids are secondary bile acids
    C. Secondary bile acids are formed by intestinal bacteria
    D. After ingestion of food, bile acid concentration in the portal vein increases
    E. Ingestion of food leads to an inhibition of cholesterol 7-hydroxylase

11. Which of the following is true regarding the portal vein?
    A. It typically has one or two valves
    B. It supplies approximately one-third of the blood to the liver
    C. The normal pressure is 10 to 12 mm Hg
    D. It is formed by the confluence of the inferior mesenteric and splenic veins
    E. In the hepatoduodenal ligament, it is usually posterior to both the bile duct and hepatic artery

12. Focal nodular hyperplasia (FNH):
    A. Is typically symptomatic
    B. Is usually centrally located in the liver
    C. Is best confirmed with high-resolution computed tomography (CT)
    D. Poses a significant risk of rupture
    E. Is thought to be due to an embryonic disturbance in liver blood flow

13. The best screening approach for detecting early HCC in patients with chronic viral hepatitis is:
    A. Alpha-fetoprotein (AFP) level
    B. AFP level and ultrasonography
    C. Computed tomography
    D. Carcinoembryonic antigen (CEA) level
    E. Alkaline phosphatase level

14. A 36-year-old woman presents with right upper quadrant pain, jaundice, evidence of ascites, and an enlarged liver on physical examination. CT demonstrates marked hypertrophy of segment 1 of the liver, free fluid in the peritoneum, and inhomogeneous contrast enhancement of the remainder of the liver. This most likely indicates:
    A. Budd-Chiari syndrome
    B. Ruptured hepatic adenoma
    C. Ruptured hemangioma
    D. Acute hepatitis
    E. Schistosomiasis

15. Which of the following is true regarding hepatic adenomas?
    A. They do not occur in men
    B. They tend to appear "hot" on a sulfur colloid liver scan
    C. Rapid contrast enhancement on CT distinguishes them from FNH
    D. Rupture risk appears to be associated with tumor size
    E. They contain an abundance of nonparenchymal (Kupffer) cells

16. Which of the following treatments of a hydatid cyst located in the mid-right lobe of the liver is associated with the lowest recurrence rate, morbidity, and mortality?
    A. Long-term oral albendazole
    B. Laparoscopic cyst excision with omentoplasty
    C. Long-term oral mebendazole
    D. Surgical total pericystectomy with pre- and postoperative albendazole
    E. Percutaneous aspiration and injection of scolicidal agents

17. A 51-year-old male with liver cirrhosis presents with a moderately sized, reducible, umbilical hernia that occasionally causes pain. The skin is intact and there is no drainage. He has a significant amount of ascites. Serum bilirubin, albumin, and international normalized ratio are normal. He has no encephalopathy. He does not have any pain at the hernia site. Which of the following would be the most appropriate next step in management?
    A. TIPS placement
    B. Six-liter paracentesis followed by intravenous (IV) albumin replacement
    C. Proceed to surgical repair of the hernia
    D. Furosemide, spironolactone, and sodium restriction
    E. Observation

18. The most common identifiable source of a pyogenic liver abscess is:
    A. Seeding from the portal vein
    B. The biliary tree
    C. Hematogenous from endocarditis
    D. Direct extension of a nearby focus
    E. Inflammatory bowel disease

19. The principal mediators of fibrosis leading to cirrhosis in the liver are:
    A. Hepatocytes
    B. Ito (liver stellate) cells
    C. Endothelial cells
    D. Kupffer cells
    E. Clefts of Mall

20. Fibrolamellar carcinoma (FLC) of the liver:
    A. Is strongly associated with hepatitis B
    B. Most often occurs in elderly men
    C. Causes a marked elevation in AFP levels
    D. Often contains a central scar
    E. Has a worse prognosis than HCC

21. Which of the following is least likely to increase the risk of HCC?
    A. Toxins from Aspergillus
    B. Hydrocarbons
    C. Smoking
    D. Wilson disease
    E. Pesticides

22. The Model for End-Stage Liver Disease (MELD) score:
    A. Includes an assessment of the severity of ascites
    B. Includes the presence of encephalopathy
    C. Is similar to Child-Pugh in that they both use INR and serum creatinine
    D. Is not as useful as the Child-Pugh classification
    E. Predicts 3-month mortality in patients awaiting liver transplantation

23. Which of the following is true regarding the blood supply to the liver?
    A. The middle hepatic vein joins the right hepatic vein as it enters the inferior vena cava
    B. Veins from the caudate lobe drain primarily into the right hepatic vein
    C. The ligamentum venosum marks the location of the intrahepatic portal vein
    D. A replaced left hepatic artery most commonly arises from a branch of the celiac axis
    E. The proper hepatic artery gives rise to the gastroduodenal artery in most instances

24. Which of the following is not considered a poor predictor of survival after hepatic resection for a metastatic colorectal cancer?
    A. Hepatic metastasis measuring 4 cm
    B. Nodes positive in colon primary
    C. Hepatic metastasis developing 6 months after primary resection
    D. Four small hepatic metastases
    E. Very high CEA levels

25. The most common primary liver malignancy in children is:
    A. HCC
    B. FLC
    C. Intrahepatic cholangiocarcinoma
    D. Giant cell carcinoma
    E. Hepatoblastoma

26. The most accurate test for assessment of hepatic reserve before major hepatic resection is:
    A. Aminopyrine breath test
    B. Indocyanine green clearance
    C. Bromsulphthalein retention
    D. Sulfur colloid scan
    E. Bile acid tolerance

27. Which of the following is true regarding Budd-Chiari syndrome?
    A. It may benefit from percutaneous angioplasty and stenting
    B. Diagnosis is best made by portal venography
    C. The jaundice is caused by presinusoidal liver failure
    D. TIPS placement is contraindicated
    E. Liver function test is often normal

28. In patients with fulminant hepatic failure, the complication that most frequently leads to death is:
    A. Renal failure
    B. Pneumonia
    C. Hypoglycemia
    D. Intracranial hypertension
    E. Coagulopathy

29. A 30-year-old woman is found to have an incidental 3-cm mass in the liver on CT scan that intensely enhances in the arterial vascular phase. The lesion is "hot" on a technetium-99m–macroaggregated albumin liver scan. Which of the following is true about this lesion?
    A. It is usually centrally located
    B. It poses a significant risk of rupture
    C. It poses a significant risk of malignancy
    D. It is thought to be caused by an embryologic vascular injury
    E. It is composed of sheets of hepatocytes with no Kupffer cells

30. Which of the following is true regarding comparisons of amebic and pyogenic liver abscesses?
    A. Amebic abscesses have a much higher female preponderance
    B. Mortality rates are similar
    C. Both are more likely to occur in the left lobe
    D. Percutaneous aspiration is more likely to be needed with amebic abscesses
    E. Pyogenic abscesses are more likely to be multiple

31. A 30-year-old woman who is taking oral contraceptives is discovered to have a 4-cm asymptomatic solid mass in the right lobe of the liver on an ultrasound scan. CT demonstrates a central stellate scar within the mass that enhances on arterial phase. Management consists of:
    A. Observation
    B. Discontinuing oral contraceptives, repeating the CT scan in 6 months, and resection if the mass has not decreased in size
    C. Resection of the mass with a 1-cm margin
    D. Radiofrequency ablation
    E. Formal hepatic lobectomy

32. Which of the following is true regarding TIPS?
    A. It is contraindicated in patients with poorly controlled ascites
    B. It has a significant risk of causing encephalopathy
    C. It is considered to be a selective shunt
    D. It is best used for long-term portal decompression
    E. It has a low 1-year rate of shunt occlusion

33. A 30-year-old woman with symptoms and signs of symptomatic cholelithiasis is found to have gallstones and a 4-cm mass in the left lateral lobe of the liver on an ultrasound scan. The patient takes oral contraceptives but no other medications. Contrast-enhanced MRI reveals a lesion of low signal intensity with peripheral nodular enhancement, and T2-weighted images reveal high signal intensity. Management consists of:
    A. Laparoscopic cholecystectomy with a needle biopsy of the liver mass
    B. Laparoscopic cholecystectomy alone
    C. A trial of contraceptive cessation
    D. Open cholecystectomy with a wedge liver resection
    E. Open cholecystectomy with a left lateral segmentectomy

34. The most common cause of intrahepatic presinusoidal portal hypertension is:
    A. Alcohol
    B. Budd-Chiari syndrome
    C. Schistosomiasis
    D. Hemochromatosis
    E. PVT

35. During diagnostic laparoscopy preceding pancreaticoduodenectomy in a patient with pancreatic cancer, a 2-mm, firm, white lesion is noted on the periphery of the liver. Which of the following is true?
    A. The procedure should be aborted at this time
    B. The most likely etiology is a bile duct hamartoma
    C. Biopsy of the lesion should not be done at this time
    D. The patient likely has abnormal liver function tests (LFTs)
    E. Wedge resection of the liver should be performed

Answers

1. A. The most common indication for liver transplantation is end-stage liver disease (not cancer). However, the Milan criteria for liver transplantation arose in 1996 following a prospective cohort study that found orthotopic liver transplantation for select cirrhotic patients with hepatocellular carcinoma (HCC) to be efficacious. The specific criteria included patients with Child-Pugh B or C cirrhosis and HCC: either 1 lesion ≤5 cm or ≤3 lesions all ≤3 cm. Additionally, the cancer cannot involve major vascular structures or have evidence of extrahepatic spread. For Childs-Pugh A and early B cirrhotic pts with HCC that satisfy the Milan criteria, hepatic resection is an accepted option. A right hepatectomy would involve resection of segments V-VIII and an extended right hepatectomy would involve resection of segments IV-VI—neither option would treat segment II (B, D). Chemotherapy is reserved for patients with unresectable tumors, metastatic disease, or palliation (C). Radiofrequency ablation is useful in poor surgical candidates with multiple or small lesions but in this patient who has an indication for a surgical cure, it is not appropriate (E).

2. A. About 25% of patients with colorectal cancer present with synchronous liver metastases, and 30% will develop liver metastases during the course of their disease. Patients with colorectal cancer and hepatic metastasis may be appropriate surgical candidates with curative intent. Patients with liver metastases are considered candidates for hepatic resection based on the volume of liver remaining after resection and not the actual number of tumors. In patients with normal liver function, a 20% remnant is recommended but in a patient that has undergone neoadjuvant chemotherapy, a 30% to 35% remnant is recommended. Options include colon-first, liver-first, and concomitant resection. None of these three strategies demonstrates inferiority compared to the others. The surgery should be individualized to the patient based on concern for complications from the primary tumor, progression of liver disease, and difficulties in concomitant resection. However, the patient above has unresectable disease given the FLR of 15%. In this case, resection of the primary colon tumor is no longer advocated in the absence of complications such as obstruction, bleeding, or perforation (B, C). Chemotherapy alone is the appropriate choice (D). TACE is primarily reserved for patients with hepatocellular carcinoma. It involves injecting chemo followed by embolization of a major tumor artery which is often from hepatic artery (E).

3. A. Variceal bleeding in children is rare. The combination of esophageal varices and splenomegaly in the absence of evidence of cirrhosis (normal hepatic function) is highly suggestive of portal vein thrombosis (PVT). The diagnostic test of choice is a duplex ultrasound scan of the portal vein (B–E). PVT likely occurs because of a combination of factors that contributes to the Virchow triad (injury, stasis, and hypercoagulability). Many children with PVT have a history of neonatal umbilical vein catheterization (leading to portal venous injury), neonatal omphalitis (umbilical sepsis), or neonatal

intraabdominal sepsis (leading to infectious seeding of the portal vein). Some patients may have congenital webs in the portal vein (leading to stasis), and a smaller fraction have inherited hypercoagulable states. In one study of 100 neonates who underwent umbilical vein catheterization, portal vein ultrasonography demonstrated clinically silent PVT in 43%, and only 56% had complete or partial resolution. The etiology of PVT in adults is different. It is more likely associated with malignancy and cirrhosis. In most children, PVT is clinically silent until esophageal varices and UGI bleeding develop. Patients with PVT and without any bleeding should be started on anticoagulation. This also applies to asymptomatic patients because complete recanalization or partial resolution improves survival. Initial treatment of the bleeding varices is similar to that for adults and includes the use of sclerotherapy or banding as well as octreotide. Because PVT in children is not usually associated with cirrhosis, liver function is intact, and the overall prognosis for these children is reasonably good. Nevertheless, a portosystemic shunt should be considered in patients who are refractory to medical management.

References: Kim JH, Lee YS, Kim SH, Lee SK, Lim MK, Kim HS. Does umbilical vein catheterization lead to portal venous thrombosis? Prospective US evaluation in 100 neonates. *Radiology.* 2001;219(3):645–650.

Schettino GCM, Fagundes EDT, Roquete MLV, Ferreira AR, Penna FJ. Portal vein thrombosis in children and adolescents. *J Pediatr (Rio J).* 2006;82(3):171–178.

4. E. The finding of isolated gastric varices, without esophageal varices, is highly suggestive of splenic vein thrombosis. This condition leads to venous outflow obstruction of the spleen, resulting in massively dilated short gastric veins. The most common cause of splenic vein thrombosis is chronic pancreatitis, which leads to perivenous inflammation. It has been reported to occur in 4% to 8% of patients with chronic pancreatitis. Splenic vein thrombosis with gastric variceal formation is referred to as left-sided or sinistral portal hypertension. The mortality rate for gastric variceal bleeding exceeds 20%. Splenectomy is curative. Controversy exists as to whether prophylactic splenectomy is necessary when asymptomatic gastric varices are discovered in association with splenic vein thrombosis. A recent study suggests that gastric variceal bleeding from pancreatitis-induced splenic vein thrombosis occurs in only 4% of patients. Thus, prophylactic splenectomy is not recommended in asymptomatic patients, nor is it recommended concomitant with another planned abdominal operation. Bypass procedures carry a higher risk of morbidity and would not address the underlying problem (A–C). Long-term beta-blocker therapy is used as a prophylactic agent in patients with esophageal varices secondary to cirrhosis (D).

References: Agarwal AK, Raj Kumar K, Agarwal S, Singh S. Significance of splenic vein thrombosis in chronic pancreatitis. *Am J Surg.* 2008;196(2):149–154.

Heider TR, Azeem S, Galanko JA, Behrns KE. The natural history of pancreatitis-induced splenic vein thrombosis. *Ann Surg.* 2004;239(6):876–880.

Weber SM, Rikkers LF. Splenic vein thrombosis and gastrointestinal bleeding in chronic pancreatitis. *World J Surg*. 2003;27(11):1271–1274.

5. D. The diagnosis of an amebic liver abscess is made using a combination of the clinical presentation, ultrasound and CT scan features, and serologic testing. The causative organism is *Entamoeba histolytica*. Humans ingest the cysts through a fecal-oral route. The cyst becomes a trophozoite in the colon and invades the colonic mucosa, resulting in a diarrheal illness. The organism then reaches the liver via the portal vein. It leads to a liquefaction necrosis of the liver, leading to the description of an "anchovy paste" appearance of the fluid, which is a combination of blood and liquefied hepatic tissue. The infection is much more common in endemic areas such as Central and South America, India, and Africa, or in individuals who have had recent travel to those locations. Less than one-third of patients will have a history of a diarrheal illness. Amebic liver abscesses are much more common in patients with a history of heavy alcohol consumption, suggesting that alcohol increases susceptibility. CT scanning can help distinguish amebic liver abscesses from other entities, such as a pyogenic abscess and echinococcal cysts. The classic finding on CT is that of a single fluid collection in the right lobe with a rim of peripheral edema. It may be that the predilection for right lobe abscesses is due to receiving more drainage (and more bacteria) from the biliary and GI tract (via superior mesenteric and portal veins), as compared to the left lobe (via inferior mesenteric and splenic veins). So, it may be that the right lobe receives more bacteria and blood from GI and biliary infections. Culturing the liver abscess or stool does not usually yield ameba (B). The best test to establish the diagnosis is serologic testing using enzyme immunoassays. The test is typically not reliable until 7 to 10 days after the patient is infected. Conservative medical management of amebic liver abscess is safe. Percutaneous ultrasonography-guided aspiration is indicated only in patients who fail to improve clinically after 48 to 72 hours (C). Amebic liver abscesses may lead to mildly elevated transaminase and bilirubin levels, but these findings are nonspecific (E). Blood cultures are not indicated in the workup for amebic liver abscess (A).

References: Blessmann J, Binh HD, Hung DM, Tannich E, Burchard G. Treatment of amoebic liver abscess with metronidazole alone or in combination with ultrasound-guided needle aspiration: a comparative, prospective and randomized study: treatment of amoebic liver abscess. *Trop Med Int Health*. 2003;8(11):1030–1034.

McGarr PL, Madiba TE, Thomson SR. Amoebic liver abscess-results of a conservative management policy. *S Afr Med J*. 2003;93(2):132–136.

6. A. Amebic liver abscesses respond very well to oral metronidazole. Several studies have investigated whether percutaneous drainage is needed. Given the rapid response to oral metronidazole, aspiration or catheter-directed drainage is unnecessary in the majority of cases (B–E). Aspiration is only indicated if the diagnosis of amebic liver abscess is uncertain or if the patient does not respond appropriately to antibiotics within a few days. Metronidazole is administered for 7 to 10 days.

References: Akgun Y, Tacyildiz IH, Celik Y. Amebic liver abscess: changing trends over 20 years. *World J Surg*. 1999;23(1):102–106.

Blessmann J, Binh HD, Hung DM, Tannich E, Burchard G. Treatment of amoebic liver abscess with metronidazole alone or in combination with ultrasound-guided needle aspiration: a comparative, prospective and randomized study: treatment of amoebic liver abscess. *Trop Med Int Health*. 2003;8(11):1030–1034.

McGarr PL, Madiba TE, Thomson SR. Amoebic liver abscess-results of a conservative management policy. *S Afr Med J*. 2003;93(2):132–136.

7. C. Hemangiomas are the most common benign tumors of the liver. They are usually discovered incidentally and are typically asymptomatic. Diagnosis is generally made by characteristic features of CT and MRI. The main issues of which to be aware are that they can sometimes be difficult to distinguish from malignancy and that in children, in particular, giant hemangiomas (>5 cm) can lead to arteriovenous shunting with congestive heart failure and thrombocytopenia secondary to consumptive coagulopathy (Kasabach-Merritt syndrome). Hemangiomas can be removed by parenchymal sparing enucleation (not by formal resection). FNH is a benign asymptomatic liver lesion located on the periphery of the liver and typically discovered incidentally on CT scan (A). Hepatic adenomas present in young women and in association with oral contraceptive use (B). Mesenchymal hamartoma of the liver typically affects young males and is considered a benign lesion that may present with intraabdominal enlargement and respiratory distress particularly in the neonate (D). Inflammatory pseudotumor is a benign liver lesion that requires needle biopsy for correct diagnosis (E).

8. A. Polycystic liver disease is an autosomal dominant disorder that is seen in patients with polycystic kidney disease, or it can be seen with liver cysts alone (B). The majority of patients are asymptomatic from their liver, but on rare occasion, large cysts can produce severe abdominal pain requiring intervention (C). Various strategies have been used with varying degrees of success in symptomatic patients with liver cysts. Laparoscopic fenestration has emerged as the preferred treatment option and has a low risk of bleeding. Percutaneous aspiration, instillation of alcohol, and reaspiration (PAIR) is optimally suited for patients with single cysts but has been used in polycystic liver patients with a dominant cyst. Formal lobectomy is another option. When all other options have been exhausted, liver transplantation has been successful. To date, there is no successful medical management. However, patients are instructed to avoid factors that have been associated with increased cyst growth. Hormone replacement therapy with estrogens in particular has been linked to cyst growth and should therefore be avoided (D). Recently, octreotide has shown some preliminary promise in retarding cyst growth. Liver function tests are typically normal but can be elevated if there is gross displacement of liver parenchyma by massive liver cysts (E).

References: Abu-Wasel B, Walsh C, Keough V, Molinari M. Pathophysiology, epidemiology, classification and treatment options for polycystic liver diseases. *World J Gastroenterol*. 2013;19(35):5775–5786.

Que F, Nagorney DM, Gross JB Jr, Torres VE. Liver resection and cyst fenestration in the treatment of severe polycystic liver disease. *Gastroenterology*. 1995;108(2):487–494.

Sherstha R, McKinley C, Russ P, et al. Postmenopausal estrogen therapy selectively stimulates hepatic enlargement in women with autosomal dominant polycystic kidney disease. *Hepatology*. 1997;26(5):1282–1286.

9. D. Because of the high risk associated with esophageal varices, numerous studies have been undertaken to try to prevent first-time bleeds. The objective is to reduce portal venous pressure to less than 12 mm Hg without adding morbidity. Prophylaxis is important because the 1-year mortality rate is as high as 70% in cirrhotic patients. Prophylactic sclerotherapy, TIPS placement, and portosystemic shunting have not been shown to be effective (C). Conversely, both prophylactic β-adrenergic blockade and endoscopic ligation have been shown to be effective. Two large, randomized studies demonstrated that endoscopic ligation is even more effective than beta-blockade in bleed prevention (A). The former may be more appropriate in cases of medium to large esophageal varices. The combination of beta-blockade and endoscopic ligation is not recommended as it can increase the risk for adverse effects without an added benefit. In patients who are candidates for liver transplantation and have esophageal bleeding that is not controlled by medical management, TIPS is the best bridge while awaiting transplantation. TIPS can also be used as part of the acute management in patients with refractory variceal bleeding (B). Selective portosystemic shunt is reserved for patients that have failed all other management options because this carries a significant mortality rate and risk of hepatic encephalopathy (E). It is rarely performed today and only in an emergency setting.

References: Psilopoulos D, Galanis P, Goulas S, et al. Endoscopic variceal ligation vs. propranolol for prevention of first variceal bleeding: a randomized controlled trial. *Eur J Gastroenterol Hepatol.* 2005;17(10):1111–1117.

Sarin SK, Lamba GS, Kumar M, Misra A, Murthy NS. Comparison of endoscopic ligation and propranolol for the primary prevention of variceal bleeding. *N Engl J Med.* 1999;340(13):988–993.

10. C. Bile salts are made in the liver and then secreted to be used in the biliary tree and the intestine. Bile is composed of bile acids, pigments, phospholipids, cholesterol, proteins, and electrolytes. Bile salts are important for small intestinal absorption of fats and vitamins. Cholic acid and chenodeoxycholic acid are primary bile acids (A). They are made in the liver from cholesterol and then conjugated with glycine and taurine in the hepatocytes. The secondary bile acids are deoxycholic and lithocholic acids and are formed by intestinal bacterial modification of the primary bile acids (B). As a result of enterohepatic circulation, 95% of bile acids are returned to the liver via the portal circulation. They are reabsorbed passively in the jejunum and actively in the ileum. Bile salts are important in the absorption of dietary fats and fat-soluble vitamins. Major resection of the distal ileum results in fat malabsorption and deficiency in fat-soluble vitamins because it impairs the circulation of bile acids. It also lowers cholesterol levels because more cholesterol is used to make new bile salts. After ingestion of food, bile acid concentration in the liver decreases and the inhibition of cholesterol 7-hydroxylase decreases, resulting in an increase of bile acid secretion in the liver (D, E).

References: D'Angelica M, Fong Y. The liver. In: Townsend CM, Jr, Beauchamp RD, Evers BM, Mattox KL, eds. *Sabiston textbook of surgery: the biological basis of modern surgical practice.* 17th ed. Philadelphia: W.B. Saunders; 2004:1513–1574.

Siedelaff TD, Curley SA. Liver. In: Brunicardi FC, Andersen DK, Billiar TR, et al., eds. *Schwartz's principles of surgery.* 8th ed. New York: McGraw-Hill; 2005:1139–1186.

11. E. The portal vein has no valves (A). It supplies approximately 75% of the blood flow to the liver compared with 25% by the hepatic arteries (B). It is formed by the confluence of the superior mesenteric and splenic veins (D). The normal pressure in the portal vein is 3 to 5 mm Hg (C). The portal vein is most commonly located posterior (Portal is Posterior) to the common bile duct and hepatic artery in the hepatoduodenal ligament.

12. E. FNH is usually an incidental finding on a CT scan because most patients are asymptomatic (A), and it is not associated with a risk of rupture or subsequent malignancy (D). A hallmark feature of FNH is the presence of a hypodense central stellate scar on CT or magnetic resonance imaging (MRI) that enhances with contrast. MRI is the study of choice to confirm FNH and is often the test of choice to characterize liver lesions (C). FNH is usually located on the periphery of the liver (B). It may on occasion be difficult to distinguish from hepatic adenoma or fibrolamellar hepatocellular carcinoma. An early embryologic disturbance in liver blood flow is the postulated cause of FNH, which is supported by the findings of regenerative nodules. Resection is indicated when patients are symptomatic or if a definitive diagnosis cannot be made.

References: Gangahdar K, Deepa S, Chintapalli N. MRI evaluation of masses in the noncirrhotic liver. *Appl Radiol.* 2014;43(12):20–28.

Wanless IR, Mawdsley C, Adams R. On the pathogenesis of focal nodular hyperplasia of the liver. *J Hepatol.* 1985;5(6):1194–1200.

13. B. Screening for HCC is only of potential benefit in patients at high risk of developing HCC. The role and best test for screening for HCC in high-risk patients remain controversial. Studies in Asian patients with chronic viral hepatitis showed that a combination of ultrasonography and AFP is an effective screening tool. Recommendations are that AFP alone should not be used and that ultrasonography seems to be more efficient (A). The benefits of screening high-risk white patients are unclear, as is its cost-effectiveness. CT imaging can help establish the diagnosis of HCC by demonstrating a hyperintense lesion on arterial phase and rapid washout on venous phase (C). CEA can be used as a tool to measure response to treatment in patients with colorectal cancer (D). Alkaline phosphatase levels are not typically used for the diagnosis of HCC (E).

References: Daniele B, Bencivenga A, Megna AS, Tinessa V. Alpha-fetoprotein and ultrasonography screening for hepatocellular carcinoma. *Gastroenterology.* 2004;127(5 Suppl 1):S108–S112.

Tong MJ, Blatt LM, Kao VW. Surveillance for hepatocellular carcinoma in patients with chronic viral hepatitis in the United States of America. *J Gastroenterol Hepatol.* 2001;16(5):553–559.

14. A. The patient most likely has Budd-Chiari syndrome, a rare disorder caused by thrombosis of the hepatic inferior vena cava or the hepatic veins themselves that leads to hepatic venous outflow obstruction, postsinusoidal liver failure, and cirrhosis. The classic triad includes abdominal pain, ascites, and hepatomegaly. There are four forms: acute, chronic, asymptomatic, and fulminant. It is often associated with a hypercoagulable state that is either inherited (protein C, protein S, factor V Leiden, or antithrombin III deficiency) or acquired (myeloproliferative disorders, polycythemia vera, thrombocytosis, pregnancy). It is more common in women. The diagnosis can be made by duplex ultrasonography, which will show the thrombosed hepatic veins or inferior vena cava. The most prominent feature on a CT scan is caudate lobe (segment I) hypertrophy and inhomogeneous contrast enhancement. The treatment depends on the acuity of the presentation. Immediate treatment is with anticoagulation followed by percutaneous angioplasty with or without stenting. There are rare reports of successful thrombolysis. Subsequent treatment depends on whether the primary indication for an intervention is portal hypertension (TIPS or nonselective shunt) or liver failure (transplantation). The remaining answer choices do not present with the aforementioned findings (B–E).

References: Kim TK, Chung JW, Han JK, Kim AY, Park JH, Choi BI. Hepatic changes in benign obstruction of the hepatic inferior vena cava: CT findings. *AJR Am J Roentgenol.* 1999;173(5):1235–1242.

Slakey DP, Klein AS, Venbrux AC, Cameron JL. Budd-Chiari syndrome: current management options. *Ann Surg.* 2001;233(4):522–527.

Wu T, Wang L, Xiao Q, et al. Percutaneous balloon angioplasty of inferior vena cava in Budd-Chiari syndrome-R1. *Int J Cardiol.* 2002;83(2):175–178.

15. D. Distinguishing between FNH and a hepatic adenoma is important because the management of the former is observation, whereas the treatment of hepatic adenomas often requires surgical resection because of their known risk of malignant degeneration and risk of hemorrhage and spontaneous rupture. In a recent study, 70% of hepatic adenomas were symptomatic (abdominal pain), 29% of resected hepatic adenomas had evidence of hemorrhage, and 5% had malignancy present. Hepatic adenomas present in young women in association with oral contraceptive use. Though rare in men, they are associated with anabolic steroid use and glycogen storage diseases (A). Most authors recommend a selective approach to the resection of hepatic adenomas (only resect if symptomatic, >5 cm, or those that continue growing despite cessation of oral contraceptive use on repeat imaging), as rupture and malignant transformation risks are rare for those <5 cm. Resection is recommended in men regardless of size. Differentiating FNH and hepatic adenoma is not always straightforward. Both may show contrast enhancement in the arterial phase of a CT scan, so this does not help to differentiate them (C). FNH characteristically demonstrates a central scar. Adenomas may demonstrate increased fat signal on MRI compared with FNH. When CT and MRI are unable to distinguish adenoma from FNH, a sulfur colloid scan may be beneficial because adenomas will appear "cold" and FNHs "hot" because of the presence of Kupffer cells (B–E). Radiofrequency ablation is another potential option in managing hepatic adenomas, especially when multiple adenomas are present, or the patient is not a candidate for a major liver resection.

References: Cho SW, Marsh JW, Steel J, et al. Surgical management of hepatocellular adenoma: take it or leave it? *Ann Surg Oncol.* 2008;15(10):2795–2803.

Daniele B, Bencivenga A, Megna AS, Tinessa V. Alpha-fetoprotein and ultrasonography screening for hepatocellular carcinoma. *Gastroenterology.* 2004;127(5 Suppl 1):S108–S112.

Herman P, Pugliese V, Machado MA, et al. Hepatic adenoma and focal nodular hyperplasia: differential diagnosis and treatment. *World J Surg.* 2000;24(3):372–376.

Toso C, Majno P, Andres A, et al. Management of hepatocellular adenoma: solitary-uncomplicated, multiple and ruptured tumors. *World J Gastroenterol.* 2005;11(36):5691–5695.

16. D. Cystic hydatid disease of the liver is due to infection by the tapeworm *Echinococcus granulosus.* Another species, *Echinococcus multilocularis,* causes alveolar echinococcosis. Humans (and sheep) are intermediate hosts, whereas dogs are the definitive host. Diagnosis is established by an enzyme-linked immunosorbent assay test for *Echinococcus* antigen coupled with an ultrasound or CT scan. Characteristic features have led to four types described (Gharbi types): a simple cyst (type I), a cyst with free-floating hyperechogenic material called *hydatid sand* (type II), a cyst with a rosette appearance suggesting a daughter cyst (type III), and a cyst with a diffuse hyperechoic solid pattern (type IV). Treatment options for hydatid disease include oral anthelmintic agents (albendazole, mebendazole), laparoscopic or open cyst excision with omentoplasty (B), formal liver resection, total pericystectomy, and PAIR (E). Drug therapy alone is curative in only a small percentage of patients (A, C). The treatment of choice is a surgical total pericystectomy with pre- and postoperative albendazole. This has been demonstrated to have the lowest rates of recurrence, morbidity, and mortality. During aspiration or surgical treatment of hydatid cysts, extreme caution must be taken to avoid rupture of the cyst. Cyst rupture can result in release of protoscolices into the peritoneal cavity and can lead to anaphylaxis.

References: Etlik O, Arslan H, Bay A, et al. Abdominal hydatid disease: long-term results of percutaneous treatment. *Acta Radiol.* 2004;45(4):383–389.

Georgiou GK, Lianos GD, Lazaros A, et al. Surgical management of hydatid liver disease. *Int J Surg.* 2015;20:118–122.

Kabaalioğlu A, Ceken K, Alimoglu E, Apaydin A. Percutaneous imaging-guided treatment of hydatid liver cysts: do long-term results make it a first choice? *Eur J Radiol.* 2006;59(1):65–73.

Khuroo MS, Wani NA, Javid G, et al. Percutaneous drainage compared with surgery for hepatic hydatid cysts. *N Engl J Med.* 1997;337(13):881–887.

17. D. Patients with cirrhosis are at increased risk for umbilical herniation due to the increased intraabdominal pressure. The overlying skin can thin and eventually rupture, which is associated with high mortality. Child-Pugh A cirrhotics can proceed with elective surgery after medical optimization. Child-Pugh B cirrhotics have an increased risk during surgery, and the decision to operate should be individualized. Child-Pugh C is an absolute contraindication for elective surgery. Given that the patient above has poorly controlled ascites, he is a Child-Pugh B. Before surgical intervention in this patient, medical therapy needs to be initiated (C). Fixing the umbilical hernia without addressing the underlying ascites will increase the failure rate of the hernia repair. The initial treatment of ascites in a patient with cirrhosis includes a low-sodium diet and the use of the diuretics spironolactone and furosemide. In the majority of patients, this approach is successful. If the ascites is refractory to this management, the next step is large-volume (4–6 L) paracentesis. The paracentesis should be followed by an IV infusion of 25% salt-poor albumin (B). If the ascites is still not responsive, serial large-volume paracentesis can be used. TIPS is another option but should be reserved for patients with reasonably good liver function because those with advanced liver disease will have a high risk of the development of encephalopathy and hepatic decompensation (A). In the latter patient, the ideal option would be a liver transplantation. Peritoneovenous shunting is now rarely used because it has a high rate of shunt clotting and can induce disseminated intravascular coagulation. Observation would not be appropriate for a patient presenting with worsening ascites (E).

Reference: Choudhury J, Sanyal AJ. Treatment of ascites. *Curr Treat Options Gastroenterol.* 2003;6(6):481–491.

18. B. The classic triad associated with pyogenic liver abscess is the same as Charcot triad for cholangitis. It consists of right upper quadrant pain, fever, and jaundice, although only 10% of patients have all three features. Pyogenic liver abscess remains a highly lethal disease, with mortality rates, even in more recent large series, ranging from 10% to 20%. The most common etiology of pyogenic liver abscesses is the biliary tract. It is more likely to be associated with abnormal liver function tests compared with other infectious hepatic etiologies (e.g., amebic abscess, hydatid cyst) due to its proximity to the biliary tree. In most instances, management consists of IV antibiotics with percutaneous aspiration of the abscess with or without catheter drainage. Other etiologies include seeding of the portal vein from diverticular disease, appendicitis (D), inflammatory bowel disease (E), and systemic infections such as bacterial endocarditis (C). Amebic liver abscesses more commonly involve seeding from the portal vein (A). However, in a high percentage of pyogenic liver abscesses, the source is unclear.

Reference: Chu KM, Fan ST, Lai EC, Lo CM, Wong J. Pyogenic liver abscess. An audit of experience over the past decade. *Arch Surg.* 1996;131(2):148–152.

19. B. The Ito cells are also known as the hepatic stellate cells. They are located in the space of Disse and are characterized by the presence of lipid droplets because they store vitamin A. Ito cells play an important role in the liver's response to acute liver injury as well as in chronic liver injury. In these settings, the Ito cell differentiates into a myofibroblast-like cell that has a high capacity for fibrogenesis. The remaining answer choices do not play a role in mediating fibrosis (A, D, E).

Reference: Hautekeete ML, Geerts A. The hepatic stellate (Ito) cell: its role in human liver disease. *Virchows Arch.* 1997;430(3):195–207.

20. D. FLC has been considered to be a variant of HCC, but recent studies suggest that it is a distinct pathologic entity. FLC generally occurs in younger patients (median age 25 years) and HCC in older patients (median age 55 years) (B). Unlike HCC, the majority of patients with FLC do not have cirrhosis, are not hepatitis-B positive, and do not have an elevated AFP level (A–C). The tumor is usually well demarcated and may have a central fibrotic area. This can make it hard to distinguish from FNH. In the arterial phase of a CT scan, the central scar in FNH enhances because it actually represents a vascular entity, whereas the central scar in FLC does not enhance. Likewise, the central scar in FNH is hyperintense on gadolinium MRI. The prognosis overall tends to be better than that of HCC, mostly because of the absence of cirrhosis, but it still only carries a 5-year survival rate of 45% (E). It is associated with elevated neurotensin levels. Treatment is surgical resection.

References: Ichikawa T, Federle MP, Grazioli L, Madariaga J, Nalesnik M, Marsh W. Fibrolamellar hepatocellular carcinoma: imaging and pathologic findings in 31 recent cases. *Radiology.* 1999;213(2):352–361.

Kakar S, Burgart LJ, Batts KP, Garcia J, Jain D, Ferrell LD. Clinicopathologic features and survival in fibrolamellar carcinoma: comparison with conventional hepatocellular carcinoma with and without cirrhosis. *Mod Pathol.* 2005;18(11):1417–1423.

21. D. Both hepatitis B and C virus infections are factors for the development of HCC, whereas hepatitis A is not. Cirrhosis is not required for the development of HCC, and HCC is not an inevitable result of cirrhosis. Chronic alcohol abuse and smoking are also associated with an increased risk of HCC (C). Aflatoxin is linked to HCC (A). It is produced by *Aspergillus* species and can be found on contaminated peanuts and other grains. Other hepatic carcinogens include nitrites, hydrocarbons, solvents, pesticides, vinyl chloride, and Thorotrast (a contrast agent no longer used) (B, E). HCC has also been linked to metabolic liver diseases such as hereditary hemochromatosis. Wilson disease and primary biliary cirrhosis have not been consistently demonstrated to increase the risk of hepatocellular carcinoma.

Reference: van Meer S, de Man RA, van den Berg AP, et al. No increased risk of hepatocellular carcinoma in cirrhosis due to Wilson disease during long-term follow-up: liver cancer in Wilson disease. *J Gastroenterol Hepatol.* 2015;30(3):535–539.

22. E. The MELD score is used to prioritize patients awaiting liver transplantation and includes the serum total bilirubin and serum creatinine levels and the international normalized ratio (INR). The presence of encephalopathy or ascites does not factor into this score (A, B). MELD was originally designed to predict mortality after a TIPS procedure. The score ranges from 6 to 40. It has since been modified to add the serum sodium level because low serum sodium (<126 mEq/L) has been shown to be an independent risk of mortality in liver transplant recipients. The newly modified MELD score, in combination with American Society of Anesthesiologists class and patient age, has been shown to be predictive of perioperative mortality in patients with cirrhosis undergoing a wide variety of surgical procedures. The MELD score removes the subjectivity associated with other classification systems. In patients with end-stage liver disease awaiting transplantation, the 3-month mortality rate was 1.9% for those with a MELD score less than 9, whereas patients with a MELD score of 40 or more had a mortality rate of 71.3%. A MELD score >15 is required to be enlisted on the liver transplant list. Child-Pugh grade (based on bilirubin, albumin, INR, presence of ascites or encephalopathy) is another scoring system that can be used to measure hepatic reserve after hepatic resection (D). For each of the five criteria, a point (1–3) is assigned. Child-Pugh A includes 5 to 6 points (no mortality risk at 1 year), Child-Pugh B includes 7 to 9 points (20% 1-year mortality rate), and Child-Pugh C includes 10 to 15 points (55% 1-year mortality rate). INR and total bilirubin are the two variables the MELD and Child-Pugh score share in common (C).

Reference: Wiesner R, Edwards E, Freeman R, et al. Model for end-stage liver disease (MELD) and allocation of donor livers. *Gastroenterology.* 2003;124(1):91–96.

23. D. The right hepatic vein drains segments V, VI, VII and VIII and enters the vena cava. The caudate lobe, situated in the posterior right lobe, also drains directly into the inferior vena cava (B). The middle hepatic vein drains segments IVA, IVB, V, and VIII. The middle hepatic vein enters the inferior vena cava jointly with the left hepatic vein via a common orifice (A). The left hepatic vein drains segments II and III. The round ligament is a remnant of the umbilical vein and marks the location of the intrahepatic location of the left portal vein. The ligamentum venosum is a remnant of the ductus venosus and marks the border between the caudate lobe and the left lateral sector (C). In most instances, the common hepatic artery gives rise to the gastroduodenal artery and right gastric artery, after which the name changes to the proper hepatic artery (E). The proper hepatic artery becomes the right and left hepatic arteries. A replaced right hepatic artery arises from the superior mesenteric artery (most commonly) and is posterolateral to the portal vein. It is referred to as a replaced artery because it replaces the right hepatic artery coming off the proper hepatic artery. This is in contrast to an accessory right hepatic artery, which also comes off the superior mesenteric artery (most commonly) but is in *addition* to the right hepatic artery coming off the proper hepatic artery. A replaced left hepatic artery most commonly arises from the left gastric artery (branch of the celiac axis).

24. A. Several studies have analyzed predictors of poor long-term outcome after resection of hepatic metastasis from colorectal cancer. In one study, the factors were positive tumor margin, presence of extrahepatic disease, node-positive primary tumor, disease-free interval from primary tumor to metastases less than 12 months (C), more than one hepatic tumor, the largest hepatic tumor being larger than 5 cm, and a CEA level greater than 200 ng/mL. Using the last 5 factors, the authors recommended against hepatic resection for those with 3 or more points because the long-term outcome was poor. In another large study, the factors for adverse outcome were similar and included the number of hepatic metastases greater than three node-positive primary tumor (B), poorly differentiated primary tumor, extrahepatic disease (D), tumor diameter 5 cm or larger, CEA level greater than 60 ng/mL (E), and positive resection margin.

References: Fong Y, Fortner J, Sun RL, Brennan MF, Blumgart LH. Clinical score for predicting recurrence after hepatic resection for metastatic colorectal cancer: analysis of 1001 consecutive cases. *Ann Surg.* 1999;230(3):309–318.

Rees M, Tekkis PP, Welsh FKS, O'Rourke T, John TG. Evaluation of long-term survival after hepatic resection for metastatic colorectal cancer: a multifactorial model of 929 patients. *Ann Surg.* 2008;247(1):125–135.

25. E. Hepatoblastoma is the most common primary liver malignancy in children. It has been associated with familial polyposis syndrome. It presents typically with an asymptomatic abdominal mass, anemia, thrombocytosis, and elevated AFP levels. Patients may also first present with precocious puberty secondary to increased beta–human chorionic gonadotropin (β-hCG). Fetal histology has the best prognosis. Treatment is with chemotherapy first and then resection. Chemotherapy enables the subsequent hepatic resection to be less and may make tumors resectable that initially appear to be unresectable. FLC (B) has been considered to be a variant of HCC (A), but recent studies suggest that it is a distinct pathologic entity. Focal bile duct stenosis in older male patients without any biliary instrumentation is highly suggestive of intraductal cholangiocarcinoma (C). Giant cell (osteoclast-like) carcinoma of the liver is rare (D) but is more commonly seen in bone tumors.

Reference: Seo T, Ando H, Watanabe Y, et al. Treatment of hepatoblastoma: less extensive hepatectomy after effective preoperative chemotherapy with cisplatin and Adriamycin. *Surgery.* 1998;123(4):407–414.

26. B. In general, the Child-Pugh scoring system is useful in predicting hepatic reserve after hepatic resection. However, it loses its predictive value in Child-Pugh A patients. The indocyanine green clearance test is a study for measuring hepatic reserve before hepatic resection in combination with the Child-Pugh score. Indocyanine green binds to albumin and α_1-lipoproteins in liver parenchymal cells and thus rapidly clears from the plasma. It is then secreted in the bile. Hepatic reserve is measured by the amount of indocyanine green retained in the plasma after 15 minutes. If more than 15% remains in the plasma at 15 minutes, this is considered abnormal (retention rate 15% = clearance rate 85%). The remaining choices are less effective studies to assess for hepatic reserve (A, C–E).

Reference: Schneider PD. Preoperative assessment of liver function. *Surg Clin North Am.* 2004;84(2):355–373.

27. A. Budd-Chiari syndrome is due to thrombosis of the hepatic veins or intrahepatic vena cava. It is often due to an underlying hypercoagulable state. It leads to postsinusoidal portal hypertension because it is caused by hepatic venous outflow congestion (C). In contrast, presinusoidal portal hypertension develops secondary to congestion within the intrahepatic portal system. Liver function is oftentimes normal in presinusoidal portal hypertension while it is elevated in postsinusoidal portal hypertension (E). Diagnosis is made by CT scan and duplex ultrasound scan of the hepatic veins (B). Initial management is with heparinization followed by percutaneous angioplasty with or without stenting. Rare reports exist of successful thrombolysis. TIPS has also been used successfully (D). Those with decompensated liver function may require liver transplantation.

Reference: Slakey DP, Klein AS, Venbrux AC, Cameron JL. Budd-Chiari syndrome: current management options. *Ann Surg.* 2001;233(4):522–527.

28. D. Cerebral edema and intracranial hypertension (ICH) are the complications of fulminant hepatic failure most likely to result in adverse outcome and death (A–C, E). Liver failure is accompanied by high levels of ammonia, which can be detoxified in astrocytes leading to an accumulation of astrocyte glutamine. This is associated with increased intracellular osmolality and can lead to cerebral edema and eventually ICH. Thus, it is essential to monitor ICH as hepatic coma develops with intracranial pressure monitoring. This technology has been shown to be critical to the ongoing determination of a patient's candidacy for liver transplantation. Patients whose intracranial pressure increases to more than 20 mm Hg or whose cerebral perfusion pressure decreases to less than 60 mm Hg will have a high risk of irreversible brain injury. If the intracranial pressure is more than 50 mm Hg or the cerebral perfusion pressure is less than 40 mm Hg, transplantation is contraindicated. Coagulopathy in this patient population is not considered an absolute contraindication to invasive intracranial pressure monitoring.

Reference: Sass DA, Shakil A. Fulminant hepatic failure. *Liver Transpl.* 2005;11(6):594–605.

29. D. The patient has FNH. In contrast to hepatic adenomas, FNH typically is not associated with symptoms and does not pose any risks of rupture or malignant degeneration (B, C). These lesions intensely enhance in the arterial vascular phase of axial imaging studies. Characteristically, as many as two-thirds of lesions will demonstrate a central scar that enhances in the arterial phase (versus FLC, which remains hypodense). The lesions are often peripherally located (A). On a technetium-99m–macroaggregated albumin liver scan, FNH appears "hot" because of the presence of Kupffer cells, which take up sulfur colloid (E). The etiology is thought to be the result of an early embryologic vascular injury. FNH is rarely symptomatic. In patients with symptoms related to FNH, resection is indicated. Because the lesions are often peripheral, minimally invasive (laparoscopic) approaches to resection should be advocated. Resection of the lesion with a thin margin of normal liver parenchyma is curative, but formal segmental resection should be considered because such procedures are associated with lower morbidity.

30. E. The male-to-female ratio for amebic liver abscesses is approximately 10:1 versus 1.5:1 for pyogenic abscesses (A). Three-fourths of liver abscesses involve the right lobe of the liver (C). Pyogenic abscesses are more likely to be multiple. Amebic abscesses tend to occur in younger patients and in endemic areas. Heavy alcohol consumption is commonly reported for amebic infection and is also a risk factor for pyogenic abscesses. The majority of amebic abscesses are managed with antibiotics alone, whereas pyogenic abscesses often require aspiration or catheter-based drainage (D). The mortality for patients with amebic liver abscesses is 2% to 4%; however, the mortality for patients with pyogenic abscesses ranges from 10% to 20% (B).

31. A. The presence of a central stellate scar is considered diagnostic of FNH when the scar enhances in the arterial phase. FNH is thought to be the result of a response to an in utero disturbance in liver blood supply with a subsequent liver regeneration. There does not seem to be any link to oral contraceptive use and no risk of rupture or malignancy, so the management is observation (B). The size of the FNH lesion does not seem to be influenced by oral contraceptive use. The only indications for surgery would be if the diagnosis cannot be made preoperatively (particularly to distinguish FNH from FLC) with certainty or if the patient has symptoms (although the presence of symptoms suggests another pathology) (C–E). Change in the size of FNH on follow-up is rare.

Reference: Mathieu D, Kobeiter H, Maison P, et al. Oral contraceptive use and focal nodular hyperplasia of the liver. *Gastroenterology*. 2000;118(3):560–564.

32. B. TIPS has been shown to be useful in patients who do not respond to medical management of variceal bleeding. It is considered to be a nonselective shunt and is highly effective in the short term in preventing rebleeding (C, D). However, because it is nonselective, it has a significant risk of encephalopathy. Thus, it should be used with caution in patients who already have marginal hepatic reserve. TIPS is also useful in patients with refractory ascites (A). Recent studies suggest that it is also useful as a bridge to liver transplantation in patients with hepatorenal syndrome. It is not a good alternative to long-term portal decompression because the 1-year patency rate is only approximately 50% (E).

Absolute contraindications to TIPS placement are polycystic liver disease and right heart failure.

References: Colombato L. The role of TIPS in the management of portal hypertension. *J Clin Gastroenterol*. 2007;41:S344–S351.

Testino G, Ferro C, Sumberaz A, et al. Type-2 hepatorenal syndrome and refractory ascites: role of transjugular intrahepatic portosystemic stent-shunt in eighteen patients with advanced cirrhosis awaiting orthotopic liver transplantation. *Hepatogastroenterology*. 2003;50(54):1753–1755.

33. B. The MRI findings are characteristic of a hemangioma, given the peripheral nodular enhancement and the brightness on T2-weighted images. They have low-signal intensity on T1-weighted imaging. Hemangiomas are common benign liver lesions generally discovered incidentally on imaging studies. They may on occasion be difficult to distinguish from other lesions. MRI findings tend to be more specific than CT scan for hemangiomas. Rarely, hemangiomas are difficult to differentiate on MRI or CT scan. Hemangiomas can be definitively diagnosed by a technetium-99–labeled red cell scan with single-photon emission CT. Diagnostic findings include decreased activity on early images and subsequent delayed filling from the periphery. CT criteria that are specific for hemangioma include diminished attenuation on precontrast scan, peripheral contrast enhancement during the dynamic bolus phase of scanning, and complete isodense fill-in on delayed imaging. Given the vascular nature of hemangiomas, needle biopsy is contraindicated (A). Resection is also unnecessary (D, E). Hemangiomas are not associated with oral contraceptive use (C).

References: Freeny PC, Marks WM. Hepatic hemangioma: dynamic bolus CT. *AJR Am J Roentgenol*. 1986;147(4):711–719.

Reimer P, Rummeny EJ, Daldrup HE, et al. Enhancement characteristics of liver metastases, hepatocellular carcinomas, and hemangiomas with Gd-EOB-DTPA: preliminary results with dynamic MR imaging. *Eur Radiol*. 1997;7(2):275–280.

34. C. Portal hypertension is classified into three types: presinusoidal, sinusoidal, and postsinusoidal. Distinguishing between these causes is important because treatment may differ accordingly. Also, unlike the sinusoidal and postsinusoidal types, presinusoidal portal hypertension is more likely to be associated with a preserved liver function. Presinusoidal hypertension is further divided into intrahepatic and extrahepatic causes. Extrahepatic causes include portal and splenic vein thromboses (E). The most common intrahepatic etiology is schistosomiasis (*Schistosoma japonicum* and *Schistosoma mansoni*). The infection by a fluke leads to fibrosis and granulomatous reactions. In children, congenital hepatic fibrosis is another cause. Sinusoidal causes include alcoholism and other causes of cirrhosis (A). Other etiologies include hemochromatosis and Wilson disease (D). Postsinusoidal portal hypertension includes Budd-Chiari syndrome and congenital webs in the intrahepatic inferior vena cava (B).

35. B. Bile duct hamartomas are the most common lesions of the liver seen during laparotomy. They are often small (1–5 mm), firm, smooth, and white and occur in the periphery of the liver. It is important to differentiate these from metastatic lesions by taking intraoperative biopsies and sending them as frozen specimens (C). If it is found to be a metastatic lesion, the procedure should be aborted (A). Bile duct hamartomas do not typically distort hepatic parenchyma and do not lead to elevated LFTs. They do not need to be resected (E).

Abdomen—Pancreas

5

JOON Y. PARK AND DANIELLE M. HARI

ABSITE 99th Percentile High-Yields

I. Anatomic Variants of the Pancreas
   a. Annular pancreas
      i. Second portion of duodenum entrapped in pancreatic head from incomplete rotation of ventral pancreatic bud, associated with Down syndrome (trisomy 21)
      ii. Symptoms: duodenal obstruction (nausea and nonbilious emesis)
      iii. Treatment if symptomatic: nasogastric tube, duodenoduodenostomy
   b. Pancreatic divisum
      i. Failure of fusion of dorsal (Santorini) and ventral (Wirsung) ducts so that the duct of Santorini drains the majority of the pancreas via the minor papilla and the duct of Wirsung only drains the head and uncinate process via the major papilla
      ii. Symptoms: most are asymptomatic, some have recurrent pancreatitis
      iii. Treatment: endoscopic minor papilla sphincterotomy

II. Pancreatitis
   a. Most common cause of acute pancreatitis: gallstone (#2 EtOH)
   b. Most common cause of chronic pancreatitis: EtOH
   c. First step in workup is serum amylase/lipase and abdominal ultrasound; pancreatitis is a clinical diagnosis and does not require CT imaging unless there is suspicion for a complicated pancreatitis (e.g., necrotizing pancreatitis, hemorrhagic, pseudocyst)
   d. Distinction between necrotizing pancreatitis and infected necrotizing pancreatitis can be challenging to make; patients with progression to infection will often have a worsening clinical course and CT findings of extraluminal gas in the collection; FNA with culture should be performed to confirm the diagnosis but is not required to begin treatment
   e. Step-up approach to acute necrotizing pancreatitis (associated with improved mortality compared to open necrosectomy):
      i. NPO, fluid resuscitation; IV broad-spectrum antibiotics not routinely administered but should be given to patients in septic shock
      ii. Percutaneous versus endoscopic acute necrotic collection drainage
      iii. If no improvement in 72 hours, proceed to video-assisted retroperitoneal debridement (VARD)
   f. Peripancreatic fluid collections

	Interstitial pancreatitis	Necrotizing pancreatitis
<4 weeks	Acute peripancreatic fluid collection	Acute necrotic collection
>4 weeks	Pseudocyst	Walled off necrosis (WON)

      i. Conservative management for asymptomatic and small (<6 cm) pseudocysts for at least 6-weeks (most <6 cm resolve spontaneously, need mature wall for intervention)

      ii. Intervention indications: symptomatic, persistent and/or enlarging; managed with endoscopic cystogastrostomy for most

  g. Chronic pancreatitis surgical indications: intractable pain following maximal medical management

      i. Puestow: lateral pancreaticojejunostomy; decompressive procedure for obstruction; ideal for dilated main duct (≥6 mm) WITHOUT pancreatic head enlargement

      ii. Frey: lateral pancreatojejunostomy with duodenum-preserving coring out of the pancreatic head without division of the pancreas; ideal for dilated main duct (≥6 mm) AND enlarged pancreatic head

      iii. Beger: duodenum-sparing resection of most of the pancreatic head with division of the pancreatic body over the portal vein and reconstruction via a side-to-side and side-to-end pancreaticojejunostomy to drain the remaining head and tail of the pancreas; ideal for enlarged pancreatic head with normal sized main duct (<6 mm)

III. Pancreatic Cystic Lesions

  a. Best diagnostic test: MRCP; then confirm diagnosis with endoscopic ultrasound (EUS) and fine-needle aspiration (FNA)

Diagnosis	Notes	Pathology	Management
Mucinous cystic neoplasm	• Premalignant, 15% chance of malignancy • MUCH more common in women (>95% women), age 40s–50s • Usually in the body or head of the pancreas	Cyst walls with "ovarian-type" stroma Fluid: • Mucinous • Low amylase • High CEA	Resection

Intraductal papillary mucinous neoplasm (IPMN)	• Can be malignant (>60% risk of malignancy if any main duct component)
	• Nearly equal in men & women, age 60s–70s
	• Imaging: Diffuse or segmental pancreatic duct enlargement
		Fluid:
		• Mucinous
		• High amylase
		• High CEA
			Indications for resection:
			• Any main duct component (main-duct or mixed)
			• Branch-duct IPMN if ANY of the following:
			  ○ ≥3 cm
			  ○ Symptomatic (e.g., jaundice or pancreatitis)
			  ○ Enhancing mural nodule
			  ○ Main duct dilation >1 cm
			  ○ Intraductal mucin

Serous cystic neoplasm	• No malignant potential • Most commonly in the tail • Most have symptoms (epigastric pain, nausea, vomiting) • MUCH more common in women (90% women), age 70s • Imaging: honeycomb-like lesion with central scar and calcification	Uniform, cuboidal, glycogen-rich cells Fluid: • Serous • Low amylase • Low CEA	Resect if symptomatic, otherwise no treatment indicated as there is no malignant potential
Pseudocyst	• Suspect if recent episode of pancreatitis	Fluid: • Serous • High amylase • Low CEA	Surgery indicated if at least 6 weeks after episode of pancreatitis AND symptomatic OR >6 cm Most managed with endoscopic cystogastrostomy

IV. Pancreatic Neuroendocrine Tumors (PNETs)

  a. Types:

      i. Nonfunctional PNET: most common; usually present with large tumor because patients won't have symptoms until mass is large enough to cause mass effect

      ii. Insulinoma: most common functional PNET; low malignant potential (90% benign); most are sporadic, 5% associated with MEN1; presents with Whipple triad (hypoglycemia, symptoms of hypoglycemia, symptoms resolve with eating); diagnosis supported by the following labs (measured while hypoglycemic during a 72 hour fast)—insulin >10 mcU/mL with elevated C-peptide (≥2.5 ng/mL), fasting insulin to glucose ratio >0.4, no sulfonylurea or meglitinide detected; less likely to be detected with octreotide scan; if can't localize with CT, can try 18-F-DOPA PET scan

    1. Management:
- b. Manage symptoms with small, frequent meals
- c. If <2 cm AND >2 mm from the pancreatic duct: enucleate
- d. If >2 cm OR <2 mm from the pancreatic duct: formal resection
- e. If not a surgical candidate: give diazoxide (inhibits release of insulin from beta islet cells)

  iii. Gastrinoma: most common PNET in patients with MEN1 (20% associated with MEN1, 80% sporadic); second most common sporadic functional PNET; presents with refractory peptic ulcer disease (PUD), diarrhea; most have low-grade malignant behavior; when diagnosed, need to test calcium, PTH, prolactin (because associated with MEN1)
- 1. Diagnosis: confirmed if all 3 of the following are true: PUD, serum gastrin >1000 (while off PPI ×72 hours at least), gastric pH <2; if diagnosis is unclear, do secretin stimulation test: measure baseline gastrin, give 2 U/kg IV secretin, measure gastrin levels Q5min for 30 min; positive for gastrinoma if gastrin increases by ≥200
- 2. Management:
    - a. If <2 cm AND >2 mm from the pancreatic duct: enucleate
    - b. If >2 cm OR <2 mm from the pancreatic duct: formal resection

  iv. Glucagonoma: from alpha islet cells; presents with 4 Ds: dermatitis (necrolytic migratory erythema), diabetes, deep vein thrombosis, depression; most are malignant (75%); serum glucagon >1000; most in distal pancreas so present late without obstructive jaundice, management: formal resection (include splenectomy if doing distal pancreatectomy because of malignancy risk)

  v. VIpoma: presents with high-volume watery diarrhea, dehydration, muscle cramping, cutaneous flushing; most are malignant; labs that support the diagnosis: high VIP levels, hypokalemia, achlorhydria, metabolic acidosis, hypercalcemia, hyperglycemia; management: formal resection (include splenectomy if doing distal pancreatectomy)

  vi. Somatostatinoma: from delta cells; mostly malignant (90%); can be associated with neurofibromatosis 1; presents with steatorrhea, diabetes, gallstones, hypochlorhydria; diagnose with high fasting somatostatin levels; management: formal resection

V. Pancreatic adenocarcinoma
- a. Risk factors: increased age, smoking, obesity, new-onset diabetes in elderly
- b. Workup and staging: CT pancreas protocol, CA19-9, CT chest/abdomen/pelvis
- c. Consider diagnostic laparoscopy to assess for M1 disease prior to resection or neoadjuvant therapy
- d. Pancreatic adenocarcinomas with distant metastases (M1) are considered unresectable and treated with systemic therapy; those not associated with distant metastases are further classified below:

Classification	Arterial Contact	Venous Contact	Initial Management
Resectable	None	SMV/PV: ≤180° AND no contour irregularity IVC: no contact	Surgery*
Borderline Resectable	SMA/Celiac: ≤180°	SMV/PV: >180° and/or contour irregularity, appears reconstructable IVC: contact	Neoadjuvant therapy, restage, surgery if appropriate
Locally Advanced	SMA/Celiac: >180° (encasement)	Unreconstructable SMV/PV	Neoadjuvant therapy, restage, surgery if appropriate

SMV = superior mesenteric vein, PV = portal vein, IVC = inferior vena cava, SMA = superior mesenteric artery.
*Can also consider neoadjuvant therapy especially for high-risk masses, but most common ABSITE answer is still surgery for resectable disease.

e. If patient has biliary obstruction on presentation and cannot proceed directly to surgery, can have ERCP and stent placement; stent associated with increased risk of perioperative infection; should obtain a new CA19-9 level after biliary decompression

f. Generally, if a patient has a symptomatic pancreatic head mass, you can proceed with Whipple without a biopsy

g. If planning on neoadjuvant therapy, need EUS-guided biopsy prior to treatment; after completion of neoadjuvant therapy, restage with CT and CA19-9 and resect if appropriate

h. All pancreatic adenocarcinoma gets adjuvant therapy

i. Benefits of chemotherapy versus chemoradiation are not clear; either are appropriate

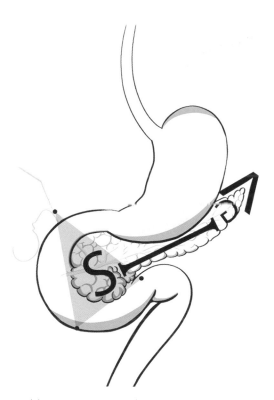

The apices of the "Gastrinoma Triangle," the most likely location of gastrinomas, are 1) where the cystic duct joins the common bile duct, 2) between the 2nd and 3rd parts of the duodenum, and 3) between the head and neck of the pancreas. Somatostatinomas are found in the head of the pancreas. Insulinomas can be found anywhere. VIPomas and Glucagonomas are typically found in the tail.

Fig. 5.1 Geography of Pancreatic Neuroendocrine Tumors.

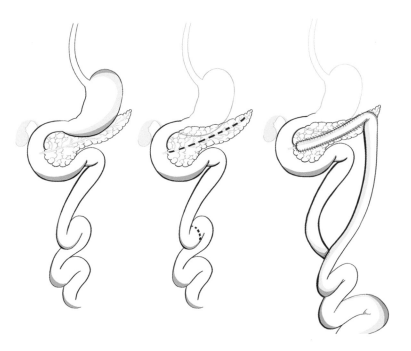

The Puestow procedure is the ideal surgery for patients with a normal sized pancreatic head and dilated pancreatic duct (>6 mm). The pancreatic duct is filleted open and a side-to-side pancreaticojejunostomy is created.

Fig. 5.2 The Puestow Procedure.

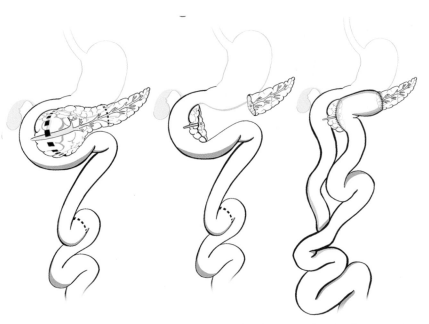

The Beger procedure is most suitable for patients with chronic pancreatitis who have an enlarged pancreatic head and small duct. The procedure preserves the bile duct and duodenum. Two anastomoses are created between the jejunum and the pancreas in a Roux-en-y configuration as shown above. Distal to the two pancreaticojejunostomies, a jejunojejunostomy is created.

Fig. 5.3 The Beger Procedure.

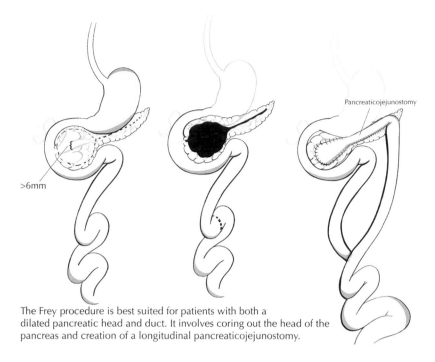

The Frey procedure is best suited for patients with both a dilated pancreatic head and duct. It involves coring out the head of the pancreas and creation of a longitudinal pancreaticojejunostomy.

Fig. 5.4 The Frey Procedure.

Questions

1. A 50-year-old man with a history of Roux-en-Y gastric bypass presents with epigastric pain and fullness two months after an episode of acute pancreatitis. CT scan reveals an 8-cm pancreatic pseudocyst that abuts the gastric fundus. What is the most appropriate management?
   A. Endoscopic cystogastrostomy via the gastric remnant
   B. Percutaneous drainage
   C. Surgical cystogastrostomy via the gastric remnant
   D. Surgical Roux-en-Y cyst-jejunostomy
   E. Repeat imaging in 4 weeks

2. A 55-year-old woman with a history of coronary artery disease is diagnosed with a resectable 3-cm insulinoma in the tail of the pancreas. She had a percutaneous angioplasty with drug-eluting stent placement three weeks ago and is on aspirin and clopidogrel. Despite eating small, frequent meals, she continues to have significant, intermittent light-headedness, palpitations, and diaphoresis daily. What is the most appropriate next step in management?
   A. Octreotide
   B. Diazoxide
   C. Neoadjuvant chemotherapy
   D. Continue aspirin and clopidogrel, proceed with enucleation
   E. Hold clopidogrel, continue aspirin, proceed with distal pancreatectomy

3. A 60-year-old man with chronic pancreatitis is presenting for follow-up. Despite alcohol and smoking cessation, oral analgesic medication, celiac axis nerve block, and ERCP with stent placement, he continues to have severe pain and foul-smelling diarrhea. Imaging reveals pancreatic calcification, an enlarged pancreatic head, and pancreatic duct diameter is 5 mm. What is the most appropriate management to help resolve his symptoms?
   A. Puestow procedure
   B. Frey procedure
   C. Beger procedure
   D. Minor papilla sphincterotomy
   E. Whipple

4. Which of the following is true regarding the role of endoscopic retrograde cholangiopancreatography (ERCP) and/or timing of surgery for acute biliary pancreatitis?
   A. In mild pancreatitis, laparoscopic cholecystectomy can be safely performed within 48 hours of admission
   B. ERCP with sphincterotomy should be used routinely before surgery
   C. If the total bilirubin fails to normalize, ERCP with sphincterotomy should be performed preoperatively
   D. In severe pancreatitis, early cholecystectomy reduces morbidity and mortality
   E. There is minimal risk of worsening the pancreatitis with the performance of ERCP

5. Which of the following is true regarding pancreatic cysts?
   A. Serous cystadenoma has malignant potential
   B. Asymptomatic patients with mixed-type intraductal papillary mucinous neoplasm (IPMN) should undergo conservative management
   C. Weight loss in patients with IPMN is mostly attributed to an elevated level of TNF-alpha
   D. Mucinous cystadenoma usually occurs in women and in the body or tail of the pancreas
   E. Asymptomatic mucinous cystadenoma can be managed with repeat imaging in 6 months

6. A 55-year-old man presents with a 12-hour history of epigastric pain, nausea, and vomiting. He has diffuse mild abdominal tenderness to palpation. Laboratory values are significant for serum amylase of 800 U/L, serum glucose of 130 mg/dL, chloride of 104 mEq/L, white blood cell count of 12,000 cells/μL, serum sodium of 125 mEq/L, and triglyceride levels of 1800 mg/dL. The most likely explanation for the hyponatremia is:
   A. Excessive fluid loss
   B. Inappropriate antidiuretic hormone response
   C. Excessive free water replacement
   D. Pseudohyponatremia
   E. Adrenal insufficiency

7. Management of pancreatic lymphoma is by:
   A. Pancreaticoduodenectomy
   B. Chemotherapy
   C. Pancreaticoduodenectomy with postoperative chemotherapy
   D. Radiation therapy
   E. Preoperative chemoradiation followed by pancreaticoduodenectomy

8. Which of the following is true regarding pancreas divisum?
   A. The duct of Santorini ends in a blind pouch
   B. The inferior portion of the pancreatic head drains through the duct of Santorini
   C. The majority of the pancreas drains through the duct of Santorini
   D. The duct of Wirsung drains through the minor papilla
   E. The ducts of Wirsung and Santorini fail to develop

9. The preferred definitive treatment for recurrent acute pancreatitis due to pancreas divisum is:
   A. Lateral pancreaticojejunostomy (Puestow procedure)
   B. Pancreaticoduodenectomy (Whipple procedure)
   C. Minor papilla sphincterotomy
   D. Major papilla sphincterotomy and pancreatic ductal septotomy
   E. Distal pancreatectomy

10. A 50-year-old male with chronic pancreatitis has failed medical management and is being considered for more invasive treatment. Which of the following is true regarding potential interventions?
    A. Pancreaticoduodenectomy (Whipple procedure) is inappropriate for chronic pancreatitis
    B. Endoscopic procedures have been shown to be superior to surgical treatment
    C. Lateral pancreaticojejunostomy (Puestow procedure) is appropriate if the pancreatic duct is larger than 6 mm
    D. The most common indication for invasive intervention in chronic pancreatitis is poor exocrine and endocrine function
    E. Long-term pain control is similar to either the Puestow, Beger, or Frey procedure

11. Adenocarcinoma of the pancreas arises most often from which anatomic site?
    A. Main pancreatic duct
    B. Branch pancreatic duct
    C. Pancreatic acinus
    D. Ampulla of Vater
    E. Pancreatic islet

12. A 60-year-old man presents with obstructive jaundice, acholic stools, and weight loss. An abdominal ultrasound scan demonstrates a dilated biliary tree and no gallstones. A dynamic contrast-enhanced CT scan demonstrates a solid mass localized to the head of the pancreas without evidence of distant metastasis, or adenopathy. Vascular involvement can't be excluded. The patient is otherwise in good health. Laboratory values are normal. Which of the following is the next step in the management?
    A. Exploratory laparotomy
    B. Diagnostic laparoscopy
    C. MRI
    D. Endoscopic ultrasound
    E. Positron emission tomography (PET) scan

13. Which of the following is true regarding alcohol and its relation to the pancreas and/or pancreatitis?
    A. It induces spasm of the sphincter of Oddi
    B. It decreases pancreatic secretion
    C. A single episode of binge drinking cannot lead to pancreatitis
    D. The type of alcohol consumed is an important risk determinant
    E. It inhibits chymotrypsin

14. A 48-year-old male presents with vague abdominal pain of 2 weeks duration. He was recently discharged for an episode of alcohol-related pancreatitis. Laboratory exam is remarkable for a mildly elevated serum amylase. A computed tomography (CT) scan demonstrates a 4-cm well-circumscribed peripancreatic fluid collection with homogenously low attenuation. The borders of the collection appear to be ill-defined. The patient is afebrile and hemodynamically stable. What is the most appropriate next step?
    A. Intravenous (IV) antibiotics and fluids
    B. Admit and place the patient on nothing by mouth (NPO)
    C. Percutaneous aspirate for carcinoembryonic antigen (CEA) level
    D. Exploratory laparotomy
    E. Observe

15. Which of the following is the *least* favorable management option for a chronic large pancreatic pseudocyst?
    A. Endoscopic transpapillary drainage using a stent
    B. Laparoscopic cystogastrostomy
    C. CT-guided drainage with a pigtail catheter
    D. Open Roux-en-Y cystojejunostomy
    E. Endoscopic transgastric cystogastrostomy

16. A 65-year-old man presents with a persistent skin rash of the lower abdomen and perineum, accompanied by intermittent vague left upper quadrant pain and recent weight loss. A chemistry panel reveals serum glucose to be 160 mg/dL, but results are otherwise unremarkable. CT reveals a large mass in the pancreas. Which of the following is true regarding the most likely condition?
    A. This patient is at higher risk for venous thromboembolic disease
    B. The mass is most commonly in the head of the pancreas
    C. The secretory peptide responsible for the symptoms also stimulates exocrine pancreatic flow
    D. Patients often have associated hypokalemia
    E. These are often benign lesions

17. The most common cause of chronic pancreatitis worldwide is:
    A. Gallstones
    B. Alcohol abuse
    C. Hereditary
    D. Hypertriglyceridemia
    E. Infectious

18. A 35-year-old cachectic woman presents with episodic severe watery diarrhea that has led to multiple hospital admissions for replacement of fluids and electrolytes over the course of several months. Stool cultures are repeatedly negative and she has no history of travel abroad. On examination, a mass is palpated in the epigastrium/right upper quadrant. CT reveals a large, bulky pancreatic mass with extension into the superior mesenteric vein and adjacent organs. The best palliative management option for this patient's symptoms is:
    A. Octreotide
    B. Streptozotocin
    C. Embolization
    D. Chemotherapy
    E. Radiation therapy

19. A 65-year-old male presents for evaluation of yellowing skin. Review of systems is significant for loose-fitting clothes, fatigue, and night sweats. Laboratory evaluation is remarkable for elevated total bilirubin. CT scan reveals a pancreatic mass. Which of the following is least likely to contribute to this condition?
    A. History of cholecystectomy
    B. Diabetes
    C. Smoking
    D. BRCA2
    E. Coffee consumption

20. A 41-year-old female presents with palpitations, trembling, diaphoresis, and confusion. Serum glucose is 48 mg/dL and C-peptide level is elevated. Her symptoms resolve with the administration of a carbohydrate load. Which of the following is true regarding the most likely condition?
    A. Elevated C-peptide and hypoglycemia rule out an exogenous source
    B. Patients will often have a mass in the neck of the pancreas
    C. The most sensitive study for localization is a high-resolution CT scan
    D. Recurrent lesions can be managed with streptozocin and 5-FU
    E. It is the least common functional pancreatic endocrine neoplasm

21. Octreotide scanning is most useful for localization of which of the following tumors?
    A. VIPoma
    B. Glucagonoma
    C. Pancreatic polypeptide-secreting tumor
    D. Gastrinoma
    E. Insulinoma

22. Which of the following is true regarding pancreatogenic (type 3) diabetes?
    A. Ketoacidosis is common
    B. The diabetes is easily controlled
    C. Peripheral insulin sensitivity is decreased
    D. Glucagon and pancreatic polypeptide (PP) levels are low
    E. Hyperglycemia is usually severe

23. A 30-year-old nurse presents with intermittent diaphoresis, trembling, and palpitations. Her fasting blood sugar is 50 mg/dL. Her insulin-to-C peptide ratio is greater than 1. Which of the following is the next step in management?
    A. CT scan of the abdomen
    B. Psychiatric counseling to discuss sulfonylurea abuse
    C. Psychiatric counseling to discuss exogenous insulin abuse
    D. Octreotide scan
    E. Magnetic resonance imaging

24. A 60-year-old alcoholic man presents with chronic, vague abdominal pain. He denies a history of pancreatitis and is otherwise in good health. CT reveals a 6-cm multiloculated, septated cyst at the tail of the pancreas. FNA of the cyst is nondiagnostic. Fluid amylase and CEA are in the high normal range. Management consists of:
    A. Distal pancreatectomy with possible splenectomy
    B. CT-guided drainage of the cyst
    C. Endoscopic cystogastrostomy
    D. Roux-en-Y cystojejunostomy
    E. Repeat imaging in 6 months

25. After a motor vehicle accident, persistent ascites develops in a 55-year-old man. Other than the ascites, CT findings are unremarkable. Paracentesis reveals clear fluid with an amylase level of 5000 U/L. The patient fails an attempt at bowel rest, parenteral nutrition, and paracentesis. Definitive management would consist of:
    A. Distal pancreatectomy
    B. Placement of pigtail catheter
    C. Roux-en-Y pancreaticojejunostomy
    D. Pancreaticoduodenectomy
    E. Placement of a transduodenal pancreatic duct stent

26. A 60-year-old man presents with chronic epigastric abdominal pain and jaundice. CT reveals diffuse swelling of the pancreas with compression of the intrapancreatic common duct. Needle biopsy of the pancreas reveals diffuse fibrosis and a plasma and lymphocytic infiltrate. Serum IgG levels are increased. Primary management consists of:
    A. Whipple procedure
    B. Steroids
    C. Chemotherapy
    D. Hepaticojejunostomy
    E. ERCP with stenting

27. A 61-year-old female undergoes a pancreaticoduodenectomy (Whipple) operation. On postoperative day five she becomes hypotensive, tachycardic, and has severe abdominal pain. Nasogastric tube demonstrates bilious output. She receives 2 L of fluids and BP improves to 110 mmHg. A CT scan reveals a significant amount of free (with HU [houndsfield units] of 25). The next step in her management is:
    A. Angiography with embolization
    B. Immediate take back to the OR
    C. IV octreotide drip
    D. Transfuse blood and transfer to ICU
    E. Upper endoscopy

28. Which of the following is true regarding anatomy or the embryologic development of the pancreas?
    A. The most commonly injured vessel during dissection behind the neck of the pancreas is the celiac vein
    B. The pancreas receives its arterial supply from only the celiac artery
    C. The ventral pancreas constitutes the head and part of the body of the pancreas
    D. Venous drainage of the pancreas is to the inferior vena cava
    E. The uncinate process is dorsal to the portal vein and superior mesenteric artery

29. A 35-year-old man presents with severe abdominal pain and diffuse abdominal tenderness. CT scan with IV contrast demonstrates areas of hypoattenuation in the pancreas. His vitals are stable. His temperature is 38.4°C. Which of the following is true regarding his condition?
    A. Fine-needle aspiration (FNA) for culture should be performed
    B. Early IV antibiotics have demonstrated improved survival
    C. Early necrosectomy decreases morbidity and mortality when compared with delayed intervention
    D. The patient should be observed with repeat imaging if he deteriorates clinically
    E. Percutaneous drainage should be performed

30. A 60-year-old woman presents with gallstone pancreatitis. Which of the following is the best predictor of a residual gallstone persisting in the common bile duct?
    A. Persistent elevation of the total bilirubin level
    B. A dilated common bile duct on admission
    C. Persistent elevation of the alkaline phosphatase level
    D. Persistent elevation of the serum amylase level
    E. Persistent abdominal pain

31. Which of the following pancreatic cystic lesions is almost exclusively found in a young female?
    A. Serous cystic adenoma
    B. Mucinous cystic neoplasm
    C. Side-duct IPMN
    D. Main-duct IPMN
    E. Solid pseudopapillary epithelial neoplasm

Answers

1. C. This patient has a symptomatic, large pancreatic pseudocyst. Since it has been at least 6 weeks after his episode of acute pancreatitis, and the pseudocyst is >6 cm, he should be offered definitive treatment (E). The majority of pancreatic pseudocysts are managed with endoscopic cystogastrostomy as it is minimally invasive and has a high success rate. In order to perform endoscopic cystogastrostomy, the pseudocyst must abut the gastric wall. However, the above patient has a history of Roux-en-Y gastric bypass. The gastric fundus is part of the remnant stomach and is not easily accessible endoscopically. As such, an endoscopic cystogastrostomy would not be routinely offered as this would require the expertise of a highly skilled endoscopist using double-push balloon endoscopy techniques (A). Percutaneous drainage is not an ideal option because there is a high rate of pancreaticocutaneous fistula formation and should be reserved for infected pancreatic pseudocysts in patients too unstable for endoscopy or surgery (B). Surgical options include cystogastrostomy or Roux-en-Y cyst-jejunostomy. In this case, the patient already has a Roux-en-Y bypass and cystogastrostomy is the more appropriate option to drain the pseudocyst without significantly altering the anatomy (D).

Reference: Nealon WH, Walser E. Surgical management of complications associated with percutaneous and/or endoscopic management of pseudocyst of the pancreas. *Ann Surg.* 2005;241(6):948–957.

2. B. This patient is experiencing symptoms of hypoglycemia secondary to her insulinoma despite adhering to eating frequent, small meals. The treatment of choice for insulinomas is surgical removal. If the insulinoma is small (<2 cm) and >2 mm away from the pancreatic duct, enucleation can be performed. Choice (D) is incorrect for two reasons: (1) it would be inappropriate to proceed with major pancreatic surgery while on dual antiplatelet therapy; and (2) because this patient's tumor is 3 cm, the treatment of choice is resection with distal pancreatectomy and not enucleation (D). However, because of her history of percutaneous coronary intervention with drug-eluting stent placement less than 1 month ago, she should continue dual antiplatelet therapy (E). After drug-eluting stent placement, dual antiplatelet therapy should ideally be continued for 6 months to minimize stent thrombosis. If urgent surgery is needed, clopidogrel can be temporarily held prior to the 6-month mark but should not be held within the first 4 to 6 weeks when stent thrombosis risk is the highest. Therefore, this patient's treatment should be focused on symptom management until she is ready for surgery. Diazoxide is the initial medication of choice to control symptoms in patients with insulinomas. It works by inhibiting the release of insulin from beta islet cells. While octreotide is a good option to control symptoms from VIPomas and glucagonomas, it does not work reliably for insulinomas as insulinomas do not always contain somatostatin receptors. Octreotide should only be considered as symptom management for insulinomas if octreotide scanning is positive (indicating that the tumor contains somatostatin receptors). Otherwise, octreotide will inhibit glucagon and actually worsen hypoglycemia (A). Chemotherapy is generally only considered for metastatic insulinomas and is inappropriate in this case as the majority of insulinomas are benign (C).

References: Valgimigli M, Bueno H, Byrne RA, et al. 2017 ESC focused update on dual antiplatelet therapy in coronary artery disease developed in collaboration with EACTS: The Task Force for dual antiplatelet therapy in coronary artery disease of the European Society of Cardiology (ESC) and of the European Association for Cardio-Thoracic Surgery (EACTS). *Eur Heart J.* 2018;39(3):213–260.

Gill GV, Rauf O, MacFarlane IA. Diazoxide treatment for insulinoma: a national UK survey. *Postgrad Med J.* 1997;73(864):640–641.

3. C. This patient has chronic pancreatitis with persistent pain despite medical management with celiac axis nerve block and is therefore a surgical candidate. When determining which procedure to perform, there are two main factors to consider: (1) if the pancreatic duct is dilated (≥6 mm), and (2) if the pancreatic head is involved. In the case of an enlarged pancreatic head and a normal-sized main pancreatic duct (<6 mm) (such as in this case), the most appropriate procedure is the Beger procedure, which involves duodenum-sparing resection of most of the pancreatic head with division of the pancreatic body over the portal vein and reconstruction via a side-to-side and side-to-end pancreaticojejunostomy to drain the remaining head and tail of the pancreas. When the pancreatic head is not involved and there is pancreatic ductal dilation of ≥6 mm, the Puestow procedure (lateral pancreaticojejunostomy) is most appropriate (A). When the pancreatic head is involved and the pancreatic duct is dilated, the most appropriate procedure is the Frey procedure, which involves coring out the pancreatic head and then performing lateral pancreaticojejunostomy (B). A Whipple includes a pancreaticoduodenectomy and is a highly morbid operation for benign disease (E). Minor papilla sphincterotomy is indicated for pancreatitis in the setting of pancreas divisum (D).

4. A. The presence of gallstones is the most common cause of acute pancreatitis worldwide, which is thought to be due to a gallstone causing transient obstruction at the ampulla of Vater. In most cases, the inflammation is mild to moderate, and the stone passes into the intestine spontaneously. In patients with severe pancreatitis, early cholecystectomy is associated with an increased morbidity and mortality, so cholecystectomy should be delayed until the pancreatitis is resolved (D). In mild to moderate pancreatitis, the timing of surgery is not critical, and early cholecystectomy (within 48 hours) can be performed safely. However, long delays result in as much as a 30% recurrence of pancreatitis. Routine ERCP to detect the presence of common duct stones is unnecessary because the probability of finding residual stones is low and the risk of ERCP-induced pancreatitis is significant (B, E). Preoperative ERCP should be reserved for patients with concomitant cholangitis or clear evidence of biliary obstruction (jaundice, persistent elevation of total bilirubin >4 mg/dL). Otherwise, an intraoperative cholangiogram should be performed, and if a common bile duct stone is detected, either a laparoscopic common duct exploration or a postoperative ERCP should be performed (C).

References: Chang L, Lo S, Stabile BE, Lewis RJ, Toosie K, de Virgilio C. Preoperative versus postoperative endoscopic retrograde cholangiopancreatography in mild to moderate gallstone pancreatitis: a prospective randomized trial. *Ann Surg.* 2000;231(1):82–87.

Kelly TR, Wagner DS. Gallstone pancreatitis: a prospective randomized trial of the timing of surgery. *Surgery.* 1988;104(4):600–605.

Rosing DK, de Virgilio C, Yaghoubian A, et al. Early cholecystectomy for mild to moderate gallstone pancreatitis shortens hospital stay. *J Am Coll Surg.* 2007;205(6):762–766.

5. D. Serous cystadenoma is a benign true cyst that most commonly occurs in women and in the pancreatic head. It is often asymptomatic, but large cysts (>4 cm) may cause vague abdominal pain. They do not need to be resected unless they are symptomatic (A). Mucinous cystadenoma is considered premalignant, has a female predominance, occurs commonly in the body or tail of the pancreas, and should always undergo resection (E). IPMN is divided into three types based on pancreatic duct involvement: main-duct, side-branch, and mixed-type. Main-duct IPMN carries up to a 50% risk of harboring malignant cells and should always be resected in surgically appropriate candidates. Mixed-type IPMN also has a higher risk and should be removed (B). Side-branch IPMN has a lower risk of malignancy and can be observed unless it is symptomatic, larger than 3 cm, or associated with mural nodules. The weight loss in patients with IPMN is mostly attributed to exocrine insufficiency from duct blockage and not TNF-alpha cachexia (C).

6. D. Severe hypertriglyceridemia leads to a falsely low sodium level. Water is displaced in the serum by lipids, resulting in an error in measurement. The danger is that the clinician who is unaware may try to correct the hyponatremia with hypertonic saline, leading to severe hypernatremia. Similarly, a significantly elevated level of serum glucose can also result in pseudohyponatremia. Excess volume loss secondary to emesis can lead to a hypovolemic hyponatremia but is accompanied by a hypochloremic metabolic alkalosis (A). Patients with gastrointestinal (GI) losses can have hyponatremia exacerbated by excessive free water replacement (C). Adrenal insufficiency may lead to hyponatremia secondary to the loss of action of aldosterone at the distal convoluted renal tubules but is accompanied by severe refractory hypotension and marked hyperkalemia (E).

Reference: Howard J, Reed J. Pseudohyponatremia in acute hyperlipemic pancreatitis: a potential pitfall in therapy. *Arch Surg.* 1985;120(9):1053–1055.

7. B. Primary pancreatic lymphoma is extremely rare. Thus, the management approach is based on case series and experience with lymphoma at other sites. Patients with pancreatic lymphoma may present with symptoms and CT findings suggestive of pancreatic adenocarcinoma, and as such, it may be difficult to diagnose preoperatively. However, suspicion of lymphoma should be raised in the presence of a large bulky pancreatic tumor or with more diffuse pancreatic involvement. This is one situation in which CT-guided needle biopsy of the mass is indicated because the majority of studies indicate that pancreatic lymphoma responds to chemotherapy as the primary modality. Surgery or radiation is not typically used in the management of pancreatic lymphoma (A, C–E).

References: Arcari A, Anselmi E, Bernuzzi P. Primary pancreatic lymphoma: a report of five cases. *Haematologica.* 2005;90(1), ECR09.

Bouvet M, Staerkel GA, Spitz FR, et al. Primary pancreatic lymphoma. *Surgery.* 1998;123(4):382–390.

Grimison P, Chin M, Harrison M. Primary pancreatic lymphoma-pancreatic tumors that are potentially curable without resection: a retrospective review of four cases. *BMC Cancer.* 2006;6.

8. C. In pancreatic divisum, the ducts of Wirsung and Santorini fail to fuse (E). The result is that the majority of the pancreas drains through the duct of Santorini and through the lesser papilla. The inferior portion of the pancreatic head and uncinate process drains through the duct of Wirsung and the major papilla (B, D). It is considered a normal anatomic variant and is seen in 10% of individuals. It is thought to lead to an increased risk of pancreatitis because the minor papilla sometimes cannot handle the higher flow of pancreatic juices. In another more common variant, the duct of Santorini ends in a blind pouch but still fuses with the Wirsung duct (A).

9. C. Pancreas divisum can lead to recurrent episodes of acute pancreatitis as well as chronic pancreatitis with intractable pain. Unlike other forms of chronic pancreatitis, however, marked dilation of the dorsal duct is unusual. As such, surgical decompressive procedures are not successful (A, B). For patients with recurrent attacks of acute pancreatitis, the best option is sphincterotomy of the minor papilla because the duct of Santorini is providing the primary drainage to the pancreas. A study from Marseille found a decreased rate of acute pancreatitis in 24 patients after minor papilla sphincterotomy and dorsal duct stenting. The complication rate was lower with sphincterotomy than with stent insertion. Major papilla sphincterotomy would not likely be helpful because it drains a minority of the pancreas in pancreatic divisum (D). Distal **pancreatectomy** is typically not needed (E).

Reference: Heyries L, Barthet M, Delvasto C, Zamora C, Bernard JP, Sahel J. Long-term results of endoscopic management of pancreas divisum with recurrent acute pancreatitis. *Gastrointest Endosc.* 2002;55(3):376–381.

10. C. The most common indication for surgical intervention in patients with chronic pancreatitis is chronic pain (D). Surgical drainage of a dilated pancreatic duct with distal obstruction is more effective than endoscopic approaches in patients with chronic pancreatitis (B). The Puestow procedure involves cutting open the length of the main pancreatic duct and anastomosing a Roux limb of jejunum to the duct but requires a dilated duct (>6 mm). Both the Whipple procedure (for inflammation limited to the pancreatic head) and total pancreatectomy are options for the treatment of intractable chronic pancreatitis, although they are associated with greater morbidity than a drainage procedure (A). The Beger procedure is another option, which resects the pancreatic head but spares the duodenum, stomach, and bile duct, but this is a technically challenging procedure. The Frey procedure is similar to Beger but easier to perform since it avoids the transection of the pancreatic neck over the superior mesenteric vessels. The best long-term pain control is achieved with longitudinal pancreaticojejunostomy with limited resection of the head of the pancreas, which Beger and Frey both satisfy, with Frey being the preferred option (E). However, Frey requires a dilated duct and pancreatic head.

References: Cahen DL, Gouma DJ, Nio Y, et al. Endoscopic versus surgical drainage of the pancreatic duct in chronic pancreatitis. *N Engl J Med.* 2007;356(7):676–684.

DiMagno MJ, DiMagno EP. Chronic pancreatitis. *Curr Opin Gastroenterol.* 2012;28(5):523–531.

Jawad ZAR, Kyriakides C, Pai M, et al. Surgery remains the best option for the management of pain in patients with chronic pancreatitis: a systematic review and meta-analysis. *Asian J Surg.* 2017;40(3):179–185.

Roch A, Teyssedou J, Mutter D, Marescaux J, Pessaux P. Chronic pancreatitis: a surgical disease? Role of the Frey procedure. *World J Gastrointest Surg.* 2014;6(7):129–135.

11. A. The majority of adenocarcinomas of the pancreas arise from the main pancreatic duct. Approximately 66% of pancreatic adenocarcinomas develop within the head or uncinate process of the pancreas. The remaining answer choices can lead to pancreatic adenocarcinoma, but it occurs less frequently (B, C, E). Carcinoma at the ampulla of Vater is most commonly duodenal adenocarcinoma (D).

Reference: Albores-Saavedra J, Schwartz AM, Batich K, Henson DE. Cancers of the ampulla of Vater: demographics, morphology, and survival based on 5,625 cases from the SEER program: Cancer of the Ampulla of Vater. *J Surg Oncol.* 2009;100(7):598–605.

12. D. In a patient with obstructive jaundice, the first study to perform is an abdominal ultrasound scan. In the absence of abdominal pain and in the presence of weight loss, it is highly likely that the diagnosis is malignancy. A dynamic, contrast-enhanced CT scan is highly effective in determining the resectability of the mass. In cases where vascular involvement is not clear, endoscopic ultrasonography has aided in determining resectability. Pancreatic cancer is considered unresectable if the tumor is encasing or occluding the superior mesenteric vein or portal vein and causing vein contour irregularity, as this is considered unreconstructable. Additionally, pancreatic cancer is considered unresectable if the tumor is abutting or encasing the superior mesenteric artery, hepatic artery, or celiac trunk by more than 180°. More frequently, endoscopic guided biopsy is being performed. The advantage of this approach is that there is no risk of tumor seeding because the area through which the needle is passed becomes part of the Whipple specimen. That being said, in the situation in which the mass appears to be resectable, percutaneous or endoscopic ultrasonography–guided biopsy is not considered necessary. Needle biopsy is prone to sampling error; therefore, a negative biopsy finding would not alter the plan to perform a Whipple procedure (A). Likewise, a positive biopsy finding would not alter the operative decision. Operative morbidity and mortality after the Whipple procedure are sufficiently low that one would accept the low likelihood (~5%) that the lesion is benign. Biopsy should be reserved for situations in which the lesion appears to be unresectable because it may guide chemotherapy. It is also indicated in situations in which the appearance of the mass suggests other less common pathologies such as pancreatic lymphoma. Diagnostic laparoscopy is often done before proceeding with a Whipple to confirm there are no obvious hepatic or peritoneal lesions (B). Suspected lesions are sent for a frozen sample. MRI may be a useful adjunct in patients with equivocal findings on CT or in cases where hepatic metastasis is suspected (C). The role of PET in cancer workup continues to develop but as of now it is unclear if PET adds

any additional information beyond what is provided with CT (E).

References: Small W, Hayes JP, Suh WW. ACR appropriateness criteria [r] borderline and unresectable pancreas cancer. *Oncology.* 2016;30(7):619–619.

Tummala P, Junaidi O, Agarwal B. Imaging of pancreatic cancer: an overview. *J Gastrointest Oncol.* 2011;2(3):168–174.

Wang WL, Ye S, Yan S, et al. Pancreaticoduodenectomy with portal vein/superior mesenteric vein resection for patients with pancreatic cancer with venous invasion. *Hepatobiliary Pancreat Dis Int.* 2015;14(4):429–435.

13. A. The exact mechanism by which alcohol induces pancreatitis is unclear. Ethanol induces spasm of the sphincter of Oddi, and this may lead to an increase in ductal pressure with a simultaneous brief stimulation of pancreatic secretion (B). It also increases pancreatic duct permeability, decreases pancreatic blood flow, and inappropriately activates chymotrypsin (E). Most patients with alcohol-related pancreatitis have a longstanding history of heavy drinking. The type of alcohol consumed is not important but rather the quantity and duration (D). The mean amount consumed in patients in whom pancreatitis develops is 100 to 175 g/day, although it can rarely develop after just one binge (C). Additionally, the risk of pancreatitis seems to be higher in patients who have a diet high in protein and fat.

14. E. The history of recent pancreatitis combined with the history of vague abdominal pain, elevated serum amylase, and CT scan demonstrating a peripancreatic fluid collection most likely represents pancreatic pseudocyst. Most patients with pseudocyst do not need admission and can continue to eat, although a low-fat diet is recommended. Admission and total parenteral nutrition (TPN) would only be recommended if they were unable to tolerate an oral diet (B). There is no reason to start IV antibiotics because he is not presenting with an infected pseudocyst (A). Initial management of pseudocysts is conservative via observation because most spontaneously resolve. Pancreatic cyst CEA level is considered the most accurate tumor marker for diagnosing a mucinous pancreatic cystic lesion. However, in the present setting, given the high suspicion for a pseudocyst, it would not be needed (C). Invasive interventions are inappropriate because most pseudocysts resolve spontaneously (D). Predictors of failure for conservative management include pancreatic pseudocysts larger than 6 cm or those that have persisted for more than 6 weeks. CT or ultrasound can be used to characterize interval changes in pancreatic pseudocysts.

15. C. Internal drainage is usually preferred to external drainage for a symptomatic pancreatic pseudocyst that has failed to resolve with conservative therapy. External drainage is associated with a higher rate of complications, including infection and pancreaticocutaneous fistula. The only indication for percutaneous drainage is in a patient with a documented or clinically apparent *infected* pancreatic pseudocyst that is unstable for a surgical or endoscopic procedure. Pseudocysts communicate with the pancreatic ductal system in 80% of cases. Internal drainage can be achieved endoscopically via a transmural approach or a transpapillary approach. This is gaining popularity making it the new first-line treatment for pancreatic pseudocyst. If there is portal hypertension (e.g., splenic vein thrombosis, underlying cirrhosis, esophageal or gastric varices), then surgical open internal drainage may be more appropriate. Options include a cystogastrostomy, a Roux-en-Y cystojejunostomy, and a cyst duodenostomy (A–B, D–E). Cystogastrostomy can be performed endoscopically, laparoscopically, or with a combined approach. Failure of the endoscopic approach can be predicted by the finding of major ductal disruption or stenosis on endoscopic retrograde cholangiopancreatography (ERCP) or magnetic resonance cholangiopancreatography. Regardless of the approach, biopsies of the cyst wall must be done to rule out malignancy.

References: Cantasdemir M, Kara B, Kantarci F, Mihmanli I, Numan F, Erguney S. Percutaneous drainage for treatment of infected pancreatic pseudocysts. *South Med J.* 2003;96(2):136–140.

Nealon WH, Walser E. Surgical management of complications associated with percutaneous and/or endoscopic management of pseudocyst of the pancreas. *Ann Surg.* 2005;241(6):948–957.

Yusuf TE, Baron TH. Endoscopic transmural drainage of pancreatic pseudocysts: results of a national and an international survey of ASGE members. *Gastrointest Endosc.* 2006;63(2):223–227.

16. A. Glucagonoma can be remembered by the 4 Ds: diabetes, dermatitis, deep vein thrombosis, and depression. The rash is termed *necrolytic migratory erythema* and tends to manifest on the lower abdomen or perineum. The mass characteristically appears in the tail of the pancreas along with VIPoma (a neuroendocrine tumor that secretes vasoactive intestinal polypeptide [VIP]). The responsible hormone, glucagon, inhibits exocrine pancreatic flow (C). The diagnosis of glucagonoma is confirmed by measuring fasting glucagon levels. Because the tumors are in the distal pancreas, the patient does not usually present with jaundice; as such, the diagnosis is often made late when the tumor is large. Because glucagonoma is most commonly malignant, it should be removed with enucleation (if <2 cm) or by distal pancreatectomy (E). Somatostatinoma can present with diabetes, gallstones, steatorrhea, and hypochlorhydria and most commonly occurs in the head of the pancreas along with pancreatic polypeptide-secreting tumor (B). Patients with VIPoma have large-volume secretory diarrhea and can lose enormous amounts of fluids and electrolytes including potassium (D).

References: Vinik A, Feliberti E, Perry RR. Glucagonoma syndrome. *Endotext.* 2014;27:89–107.

Schapiro H, Ludewig RM. The effect of glucagon on the exocrine pancreas. A review. *Am J Gastroenterol.* 1978;70(3):274–281.

17. B. For acute pancreatitis, gallstones and alcohol abuse are by far the two most common etiologies, with a slightly higher incidence of biliary pancreatitis. Biliary pancreatitis, however, leads to chronic pancreatitis far less often (A). Alcohol abuse is by far the most common cause of chronic pancreatitis. Although hypertriglyceridemia, infection (often viral), and hereditary syndromes can lead to acute pancreatitis, they occur less frequently than alcohol abuse and gallstones (C, D, E).

References: Fisher WE, Andersen DK, Bell RH, et al. Pancreas. In: Brunicardi FC, Andersen DK, Billiar TR, et al., eds. *Schwartz's principles of surgery.* 8th ed. New York: McGraw-Hill; 2005:1221–1296.

Steer ML. Exocrine pancreas. In: Townsend CM, Jr, Beauchamp RD, Evers BM, Mattox KL, eds. *Sabiston textbook of surgery: the biological basis of modern surgical practice.* 17th ed. Philadelphia: W.B. Saunders; 2004:1643–1678.

18. A. The patient most likely has a VIPoma. It has also been termed *WDHA* (watery diarrhea, hypokalemia, and achlorhydria) and Verner-Morrison syndrome. Patients have large-volume secretory diarrhea and can lose enormous amounts of fluids and electrolytes. Diagnosis is by CT scan, and most tumors have metastasized by the time of diagnosis. Another useful imaging tool is endoscopic ultrasonography. Even with distant metastasis, however, tumor debulking, hepatic artery embolization, and radiofrequency ablation of liver metastasis are useful in controlling symptoms (C, E). The best medical treatment of symptoms is achieved with octreotide, a somatostatin analogue. Chemotherapy has no role in the management of VIPoma (D). Streptozotocin is toxic to pancreatic beta cells and may be useful in the management of insulinoma (B).

Reference: Nguyen HN, Backes B, Lammert F, et al. Long-term survival after diagnosis of hepatic metastatic VIPoma: report of two cases with disparate courses and review of therapeutic options. *Dig Dis Sci.* 1999;44(6):1148–1155.

19. E. Coffee drinking has not been shown to be a risk factor for pancreatic cancer. Factors that are associated with a risk for pancreatic cancer include smoking (strongest and accounts for 25%–30% of all cases) (C), obesity, diabetes (B), atypical multiple mole melanoma, hereditary pancreatitis (A), familial adenomatous polyposis, hereditary nonpolyposis colon cancer, *BRCA2* (D), and Peutz-Jeghers syndrome. The role of alcohol in pancreatic cancer is debatable. More recently, a history of cholecystectomy and/or cholelithiasis has been demonstrated to be associated with an increased risk of pancreatic cancer (A).

References: Fan Y, Hu J, Feng B. Increased risk of pancreatic cancer related to gallstones and cholecystectomy: a systemic review and meta-analysis. *Pancreas.* 2016;45(4):503–509.

Lowenfels AB, Maisonneuve P. Epidemiology and prevention of pancreatic cancer. *Jpn J Clin Oncol.* 2004;34(5):238–244.

20. D. Insulinoma is the most common functional pancreatic endocrine neoplasm (E). The classic feature is the Whipple triad, which includes symptomatic fasting hypoglycemia, a documented serum glucose level of less than 50 mg/dL, and relief of symptoms with the administration of glucose. Patients will often present with recurrent episodes of syncope. They may also report palpitations, trembling, diaphoresis, confusion or disorientation, and seizures. The diagnosis is confirmed by demonstrating a low fasting blood sugar (insulin to glucose ratio of >0.3) and an elevated C peptide level. However, the advent of newer antidiabetic medications such as sulfonylureas can also present with a similar biochemical profile (A). Localization is achieved by CT scan and endoscopic ultrasonography. On occasion, they cannot be localized preoperatively, in which case, intraoperative ultrasonography is useful and is considered the most sensitive imaging study. In contrast to the other functional endocrine pancreatic neoplasms, an octreotide scan is poor at localizing insulinoma owing to the fact that these lesions may not express sufficient somatostatin receptors (C). They are evenly distributed throughout the head, body, and tail of the pancreas. There is no pancreatic tumor that characteristically appears in the neck of the pancreas (B). The majority of insulinomas are benign (90%). They can be treated with enucleation. Diazoxide inhibits insulin release and is occasionally used for preoperative control of symptoms related to hypoglycemia symptoms. For patients with recurrent or metastatic malignant insulinoma, tumor debulking may be beneficial as is the use of streptozocin and 5-FU.

References: Dewitt CR, Heard K, Waksman JC. Insulin and C-peptide levels in sulfonylurea-induced hypoglycemia: a systemic review. *J Med Toxicol.* 2007;3(3):107–118.

Halfdanarson TR, Rubin J, Farnell MB, Grant CS, Petersen GM. Pancreatic endocrine neoplasms: epidemiology and prognosis of pancreatic endocrine tumors. *Endocr Relat Cancer.* 2008;15(2):409–427.

21. D. Many pancreatic endocrine tumors have high concentrations of somatostatin receptors and can therefore be imaged with a radiolabeled form of the somatostatin analogue octreotide (indium-111 pentetreotide). Octreotide scanning has the advantage of whole-body scanning, which is useful in gastrinomas because they can present in a wide area. Used in combination with endoscopic ultrasonography, it detects more than 90% of gastrinomas. It is also useful for localizing carcinoid tumors. As many as 90% of gastrinomas are found in the Passaro triangle, an area defined by the junction of the cystic duct and common bile duct, the second and third portions of the duodenum, and the neck and body of the pancreas. Although a CT scan is also useful, an octreotide scan is particularly helpful in localizing gastrinomas smaller than 1 cm. Somatostatinoma and VIPoma tend to be large bulky tumors and are thus readily seen by CT (A). Glucagonoma may present with a mass seen in the pancreatic tail (B). Octreotide scanning will miss as many as 40% of insulinomas because they may not express sufficient somatostatin receptors (E). Pancreatic polypeptide (PP) seems to have an important role in glucose metabolism. PP regulates the expression of the hepatic insulin receptor gene. PP-secreting tumor is rare and often asymptomatic but can be established by the presence of an enhancing solitary pancreatic head tumor on CT imaging with elevated fasting PP level (C).

Reference: de Herder WW, Kwekkeboom DJ, Valkema R, et al. Neuroendocrine tumors and somatostatin: imaging techniques. *J Endocrinol Invest.* 2005;28(11 Suppl International):132–136.

22. D. Diabetes in the setting of chronic pancreatitis or after pancreatic resection is termed *type 3 diabetes.* It differs from type 1 and 2 diabetes in that it is associated with decreased glucagon and PP levels and insulin due to pancreatic loss or destruction. Because all three of these hormones regulate glucose levels, the ensuing diabetes is considered to be difficult to control (B). Furthermore, peripheral insulin sensitivity is increased, whereas hepatic insulin sensitivity is decreased (C). The result is that patients are prone to the development of hypoglycemia, but ketoacidosis and marked hyperglycemia are rare (A, E). For diabetes to develop as a result of pancreatitis, extensive destruction of the pancreas must occur. In fact, resections involving up to 80% of an otherwise normal gland can be done without endocrine insufficiency. This may help explain why not all post-Whipple patients develop poor glucose control.

23. C. Although the patient has symptomatic hypoglycemia, seemingly consistent with an insulinoma, her insulin-to-C peptide ratio is greater than 1. This combination, particularly in a health-care worker, is highly suggestive of factitious hypoglycemia with exogenous insulin abuse. The precursor

to insulin is proinsulin. Proinsulin is packaged in the pancreatic B cell, where it is cleaved to insulin and C peptide, which are then released into the circulation at an equal ratio. Insulin is cleared by the liver, whereas C peptide is cleared by the kidney and is cleared more slowly than insulin, such that the normal insulin-to-C peptide ratio is less than 1 during fasting. With a true insulinoma, both insulin and C peptide levels would be elevated; however, the ratio would still be less than 1. Factitious hypoglycemia will present with an insulin-to-C peptide ratio greater than 1 only if the patient is using exogenous insulin. In contrast, sulfonylurea abuse will have a ratio of less than 1 since it stimulates proinsulin release from the pancreas (B). Factitious hypoglycemia has been reported more frequently in health-care workers and is associated with a higher incidence of suicide, depression, and personality disorders. Thus, the patient should be referred for psychiatric counseling. Octreotide scan (D) is not useful in the workup for insulinoma but CT, MRI, or endoscopic ultrasound may demonstrate a pancreatic mass (A, E).

References: Lebowitz M, Blumenthal S. The molar ratio of insulin to C-peptide: an aid to the diagnosis of hypoglycemia due to surreptitious (or inadvertent) insulin administration. *Arch Intern Med.* 1993;153(5):650–655.

Waickus CM, de Bustros A, Shakil A. Recognizing factitious hypoglycemia in the family practice setting. *J Am Board Fam Pract.* 1999;12(2):133–136.

24. A. It is important to be aware that not all fluid-filled pancreatic abnormalities in a patient with a history of drinking represent pseudocysts (B–E). Some of these lesions may represent cystic neoplasms of the pancreas. Suspicion of a cystic neoplasm should be particularly increased in the absence of a history of pancreatitis, as in this patient. A cystic neoplasm should also be suspected when the CT scan demonstrates a solid component (septation) in the cystic lesion. The differential diagnosis includes serous cystadenoma, mucinous cystic neoplasm, intraductal papillary-mucinous adenoma, and solid pseudopapillary neoplasm. On a CT scan, a central scar is characteristic of a serous cystadenoma (although present in only 20%), whereas the finding of peripheral eggshell calcifications, although rare, is diagnostic of mucinous cystic neoplasm and highly suggestive of cancer. In the patient presented, the procedure of choice is surgical resection with distal pancreatectomy and splenectomy. This is based on several factors: the patient is having symptoms; he is a good candidate for surgery; the lesion is readily amenable to resection; and the lesion is large, has septations, and has multiple loculations. If, conversely, a patient has an incidentally discovered pancreatic cyst without symptoms, surgery is generally recommended if the risk of surgery is low. Before surgery, further studies are recommended to attempt to determine the malignant potential. The workup may include MRI, endoscopic ultrasonography to better delineate the mass, and CT-guided aspiration of the fluid for amylase level and tumor markers (carcinoembryonic antigen, CA 19–9, CA 125, CA 72–4, CA 15–3).

25. E. After surgery, trauma, or bouts of pancreatitis, persistent ascites or pleural effusions can develop. These are generally caused by a disruption of the pancreatic duct, with free extravasation of pancreatic fluid, leading to the development of an internal pancreatic fistula, which is rare.

More commonly, the extravasated fluid leads to the formation of a contained fluid collection known as a pseudocyst. Management of pancreatic ascites or effusion first requires establishing the diagnosis by obtaining a sample of the fluid and demonstrating a markedly elevated amylase level and a protein level greater than 25 g/L. Serum amylase may be elevated from reassertion across the peritoneal membrane. The recommended management is a stepwise progression, first with conservative management with bowel rest, parenteral nutrition, placing the patient NPO, and paracentesis to completely drain the fluid. If this fails to resolve the internal fistula, ERCP with pancreatic stenting is recommended. If this fails, surgery is indicated and should be tailored to the location of the ductal injury (B). For distal duct disruptions, a distal pancreatectomy is recommended (A), whereas for disruption of the body, a Roux-en-Y pancreaticojejunostomy is performed (C). Whipple procedure (pancreaticoduodenectomy) is not needed (D). Conservative therapy including somatostatin is successful in only approximately 50%, so nearly one-half will require an invasive procedure.

References: Gómez-Cerezo J, Barbado Cano A, Suárez I, Soto A, Rios JJ, Vazquez JJ. Pancreatic ascites: Study of therapeutic options by analysis of case reports and case series between the years 1975 and 2000. *Am J Gastroenterol.* 2003;98(3):568–577.

O'Toole D, Vullierme MP, Ponsot P, et al. Diagnosis and management of pancreatic fistulae resulting in pancreatic ascites or pleural effusions in the era of helical CT and magnetic resonance imaging. *Gastroenterol Clin Biol.* 2007;31(8–9 Pt 1):686–693.

26. B. Autoimmune pancreatitis is a form of chronic pancreatitis that is increasingly being recognized and can be confused with pancreatic lymphoma or pancreatic cancer. It presents most often as a diffusely enlarged hypoechoic pancreas. A CT scan often shows diffuse narrowing of the main pancreatic duct without the typical calcifications seen with chronic alcoholic pancreatitis. Pathology reveals a plasma cell and lymphocytic infiltrate. Laboratory values reveal increased levels of IgG and often diabetes. Antibodies against lactoferrin and carbonic anhydrase have been reported, but they are not a specific finding. The treatment of choice is steroid therapy, and the disease responds well to this management. Chemotherapy or invasive surgical/endoscopic procedures are not necessary (A, C–E).

References: Ketikoglou I, Moulakakis A. Autoimmune pancreatitis. Dig Liver Dis. 2005;37(3):211–215.

Okazaki K. Autoimmune-related pancreatitis. *Curr Treat Options Gastroenterol.* 2001;4(5):369–375.

27. A. This presentation is concerning for delayed bleeding following a pancreaticoduodenectomy (Whipple) procedure. This is most often due to a gastroduodenal artery stump leak. Fluid with HU >25 is most consistent with blood. CT may show a pseudoaneurysm, but this may not always be present. On hospital day 5, the tissue planes are often fragile, making it difficult to control bleeding in the operating room (B). After resuscitation with blood products, the most appropriate next step involves performing an angiography with embolization. A bleeding ulcer is also in the differential, but less likely in the absence of bloody nasogastric tube output and with CT findings, so upper endoscopy is not likely to be helpful (E). Esophagogastroduodenoscopy (EGD) needs to be selectively performed this early after surgery because the scope may compromise the freshly made

gastrojejunostomy anastomosis if the afferent/efferent limbs are to be evaluated. Transfusion of blood is appropriate but transport interventional suite should be next, as the patient may have a herald bleed followed by exsanguination (D). Octreotide has no role in the management of gastroduodenal artery stump bleeding (C). One study demonstrated that wrapping the gastroduodenal artery stump using the falciform ligament during surgery may decrease the risk of this complication.

References: Xu C, Yang X, Luo X. Wrapping the gastroduodenal artery stump during pancreatoduodenectomy reduced the stump hemorrhage incidence after operation. *Chin J Cancer.* 2014;26(3):299–308.

Han GJ, Kim S, Lee NK, et al. Prediction of late postoperative hemorrhage after Whipple procedure using computed tomography performed during early postoperative period. *Korean J Radiol.* 2018;19(2):284–291.

28. E. The ventral pancreas constitutes the uncinate process and inferior portion of the head of the pancreas, leaving the remainder the embryologic remnant of the dorsal pancreas (C). The uncinate process lies ventral to the aorta but dorsal to the portal vein and superior mesenteric artery. The most commonly injured vessel during dissection behind the neck of the pancreas is the superior mesenteric vein (A). The pancreas receives blood supply from two sources: the celiac axis (superior pancreaticoduodenal artery) and superior mesenteric artery (inferior pancreaticoduodenal artery) (B). Venous drainage of the pancreas is to the portal system (D).

29. D. CT scan with IV contrast demonstrating areas of hypoattenuation (nonperfused) in the pancreas in a patient with this presentation is concerning due to necrotizing pancreatitis. It is important to note that the necrotic pancreas is not usually infected initially. Thus, initial management of necrotizing pancreatitis is conservative with the avoidance of early invasive interventions. FNA with culture might be considered later (because infected necrosis typically develops weeks later) in the course of the hospitalization if the patient were to manifest evidence of sepsis such as leukocytosis, tachycardia, refractory abdominal pain, bacteremia, and/or persistent fevers (A). Prophylactic antibiotics for severe pancreatitis should not be routinely administered (B). In patients with proven (via needle aspiration) infected necrosis, minimally invasive percutaneous or endoscopic interventions (step-up approach) followed by video-assisted retroperitoneal debridement with the goal of postponing or obviating the need for open surgery is preferred (E). Furthermore, early necrosectomy has been shown to increase morbidity and mortality when compared with delayed intervention (C). In a patient that does not appear to have an infected necrotizing pancreatitis, it is appropriate to approach management conservatively with medical optimization and repeat CT scan if there is a deterioration in clinical status. It is best to allow the patient to manifest the severity of the disease before invasive interventions.

References: Bugiantella W, Rondelli F, Boni M, et al. Necrotizing pancreatitis: a review of the interventions. *Int J Surg.* 2016;28 Suppl 1:S163–S171.

Mier J, León EL, Castillo A, Robledo F, Blanco R. Early versus late necrosectomy in severe necrotizing pancreatitis. *Am J Surg.* 1997;173(2):71–75.

30. A. Although elevation of alkaline phosphatase can be seen with a residual common bile duct stone, the best predictor is a persistent elevation of the total bilirubin (C). Amylase is not typically elevated in this patient population (D). Because the pathophysiology of gallstone pancreatitis is transient obstruction of the ampulla of Vater by a gallstone, a significant number of patients will have some degree of common bile duct dilation on admission; as such, common bile duct dilation is not a specific finding (B). This differs from patients with symptomatic cholelithiasis, in which ductal dilation is frequently associated with common duct stones. Persistent abdominal pain can occur as a result of multiple etiologies and should be appropriately worked up with history and physical, laboratory studies, and/or imaging, if necessary (E).

References: Chan T, Yaghoubian A, Rosing D, et al. Total bilirubin is a useful predictor of persisting common bile duct stone in gallstone pancreatitis. *Am Surg*. 2008;74(10):977–980.

Chang L, Lo SK, Stabile BE, Lewis RJ, de Virgilio C. Gallstone pancreatitis: a prospective study on the incidence of cholangitis and clinical predictors of retained common bile duct stones. *Am J Gastroenterol*. 1998;93(4):527–531.

31. E. Solid pseudopapillary epithelial neoplasm is A rare tumor occurring almost exclusively in young women. It has low malignant potential and for the majority of patients, the tumor can be resected with curative intent regardless of the size. Metastasis and recurrence are uncommon. Serous cystic adenoma also occurs most commonly in women, but this has no malignant potential and does not need to be resected unless it is causing mass effect (A). Mucinous cystic neoplasm is considered a premalignant lesion, has a female predominance, occurs commonly in the body or tail of the pancreas, and should always undergo resection (B). Main-duct IPMN has a high risk of harboring malignant cells and should be resected (D). Side-duct IPMN can be managed conservatively unless it is symptomatic, larger than 3 cm, or associated with mural nodules (C).

Reference: Frost M, Krige JE, Bornman PC. Solid pseudopapillary epithelial neoplasm—A rare but curable pancreatic tumour in young women. *S Afr J Surg*. 2011;49(2):78–81.

Abdomen—Spleen

6

MARIA G. VALADEZ, BENJAMIN DIPARDO, AND ERIC R. SIMMS

ABSITE 99th Percentile High-Yields

I. Anatomy and Physiology
   A. White pulp contains macrophages and both B and T lymphocytes
   B. Red pulp is responsible for removing deformed or abnormal RBCs and nuclear remnants found in RBCs
   C. Splenocolic, gastrosplenic, splenorenal, and phrenicosplenic ligaments
      1. Short gastric arteries are found in the gastrosplenic ligament and can be a source of postoperative hemorrhage
      2. Splenic artery lies anterior and superior to the splenic vein
      3. Lack of normal peritoneal attachments results in a wandering spleen
   D. Accessory spleen
      1. Suspected if peripheral blood smear not consistent with asplenia after splenectomy or if recurrence of primary pathology; splenic hilum is the most common location followed by tail of pancreas

II. Splenic masses
   A. Most common benign splenic tumor: hemangioma
   B. Most common primary splenic tumor: non-Hodgkin lymphoma
   C. Parasitic cysts (most common worldwide but rare in the United States):
      1. Majority are hydatid cysts secondary to echinococcus; treated with partial or total splenectomy due to risk of rupture
   D. Nonparasitic cysts:
      1. Cysts can be true cysts or pseudocysts, but this differentiation is difficult to make preop; true cysts or primary cysts have epithelial lining and are congenital; pseudocysts or secondary cysts lack an epithelial lining and typically result from traumatic hematoma formation
      2. If asymptomatic, can be observed with serial imaging regardless of size; if symptomatic, treated with partial or total splenectomy
   E. Splenic abscesses
      1. Etiology: bacteremia, trauma, hemoglobinopathies, splenic artery embolization, following acute pancreatitis, immunosuppression, or trauma
      2. Most common organism: *Streptococcus pneumoniae*
      3. Treatment: IV antibiotics followed by splenectomy (gold standard)
      4. If poor surgical candidate with thick-walled unilocular abscess, treat with percutaneous drainage

III. Splenectomy
   A. Vaccinations
      1. Vaccinate against encapsulated organisms: *Streptococcus pneumoniae*, *Neisseria meningitidis*, and *Haemophilus influenzae*; ideally 2 weeks before surgery; 2 weeks after if emergent

2. Pneumococcal (PPSV23) vaccine should be given at least 8 weeks after the PCV13 vaccine with revaccination at 5 years; meningococcal (MenACWY) vaccination should be given 8 weeks after initial dose with revaccination every 5 years; also require yearly influenza and COVID vaccination
B. Postsplenectomy considerations
   1. Overwhelming postsplenectomy sepsis (OPSI) (<2% of patients due to loss of immunoglobulin M [IgM])
      a) Most cases occur early postsplenectomy, within first 2 years, and most common in younger patients undergoing splenectomy for hematologic disease; trauma splenectomy associated with lowest risk of OPSI
      b) Most common cause: *Streptococcus pneumoniae* infection
      c) Treatment: third-generation cephalosporins
   2. Peripheral smear findings:

Abnormality	Description
Howell-Jolly bodies	Nuclear remnants
Pappenheimer bodies	Iron deposits
Heinz bodies	Denatured hemoglobin
Target cells	Thickened RBC membrane

IV. Hematologic Diseases

	Condition	Pathophysiology	Management
Platelet disorders	Idiopathic thrombocytopenic purpura (ITP)	Antiplatelet IgG produced by spleen	Steroids first, followed by IVIG; splenectomy for refractory cases
	Thrombotic thrombocytopenic purpura (TTP)	Metalloproteinase deficiency causes defective vWF multimer cleaving	Plasmapheresis is first line; splenectomy for refractory cases
Hemolytic anemias	Hereditary spherocytosis	Spectrin, ankyrin band 3 protein, protein 4.2 abnormalities	Splenectomy is curative (if pigmented gallstones present, also need prophylactic cholecystectomy)
	Elliptocytosis	Membrane protein defect	Splenectomy rarely done
	Pyruvate kinase deficiency	Abnormal glucose metabolism	Splenectomy not indicated
	G6PD deficiency	X-linked recessive Crises precipitated by drugs, fava beans, etc.	Splenectomy not indicated
	Sickle cell anemia	Hemoglobin defect causes sickling	Splenectomy rarely indicated
	Thalassemia	Alpha or beta globulin defect interferes with RBC survival/ production	Splenectomy indicated for symptomatic splenomegaly, high transfusion requirements
	Autoimmune hemolytic anemias	Autoantibodies to RBC antigens Cold vs warm	Cold: no splenectomy Warm: splenectomy if refractory to steroid treatment

Questions

1. A 40-year-old female with ITP is about to undergo a splenectomy. Her preoperative platelet count is 40,000 cells/μL. Which of the following is true regarding perioperative platelet transfusions for ITP during splenectomy in this patient?
   A. Transfuse 2 units of platelets en route to OR
   B. Transfuse 2 units of platelets postoperatively even if no intraoperative bleeding
   C. Transfuse platelets upon clamping and ligating the splenic vein even if no intraoperative bleeding
   D. Transfuse platelets following splenic artery ligation even if no intraoperative bleeding
   E. Transfuse platelets following splenic artery ligation if patient continues to have intraoperative bleeding

2. A 29-year-old male who underwent emergent splenectomy for blunt abdominal trauma presents to the emergency department 3 weeks postoperatively complaining of progressive left upper quadrant abdominal pain and fever. On evaluation, he has a temperature of 38.5°C, a heart rate of 122 bpm, and a blood pressure of 112/68 mmHg. Labs demonstrate a white blood cell count of 21,000 cells/μL and a computed tomography (CT) scan shows a 7-cm fluid collection in the left upper quadrant. Which of the following is the most likely diagnosis?
   A. Iatrogenic colon perforation
   B. Pancreatic fistula
   C. Portal vein thrombosis
   D. OPSI
   E. Postoperative hemorrhage

3. A 12-year-old boy presents with ecchymosis and fever of 101.2°F. Laboratory exam is remarkable for platelet count of 30,000 cells/μL and hemoglobin of 8.2 mg/dL. Peripheral blood smear shows large and immature platelets. Review of systems is significant for an upper respiratory tract infection three weeks prior. His mother also notes that his urine has been pink. This is his second admission for this constellation of symptoms. Which of the following is true regarding this condition?
   A. Children are more likely to require splenectomy than adults
   B. In children, intravenous immunoglobulin is the initial approach to management
   C. The spleen is typically palpable on abdominal examination
   D. Children with platelet counts of 50,000 or fewer cells/μL should be hospitalized
   E. In children, this condition is often preceded by a viral illness

4. Which of the following is the best indication for splenectomy?
   A. Sarcoidosis
   B. Gaucher disease
   C. Myelofibrosis
   D. Hairy cell leukemia with neutropenia
   E. Secondary hypersplenism in a cirrhotic patient

5. A 30-year-old woman is found to have a signet ring calcification in the left upper quadrant on a plain abdominal radiograph. A CT scan confirms a 2-cm splenic artery aneurysm just beyond the take-off of the celiac axis. The pancreas appears normal. Which of the following is true regarding this condition?
   A. It is an uncommon visceral artery aneurysm
   B. In this patient, it is most likely a pseudoaneurysm
   C. It is associated with a double-rupture phenomenon
   D. The aneurysm typically arises in the proximal portion of the splenic artery
   E. Intervention is not needed

6. Two months after a splenectomy for ITP, the patient is noted to have petechiae and a decrease in platelet count. A peripheral blood smear is noteworthy for the absence of Howell-Jolly bodies. Which of the following is the best recommendation for a workup?
    A. CT scan of the abdomen
    B. Bone marrow biopsy
    C. No workup needed; administer steroids
    D. Radiolabeled RBC scan
    E. No workup needed; administer immunoglobulin

7. Which of the following is true regarding ITP?
    A. In adults, splenectomy should be performed once the diagnosis is established
    B. A chronic form is more likely to develop in adults than in children
    C. The diagnosis is effectively established by a peripheral blood smear
    D. Immunoglobulin is ineffective in increasing the platelet count
    E. In adults, splenectomy should be delayed until after the second relapse

8. Which of the following is true regarding TTP?
    A. It does not lead to hemolysis
    B. It is associated with liver failure
    C. Splenectomy is the first line of treatment in adults
    D. The Coombs test result is positive
    E. The most common cause of death is intracerebral hemorrhage

9. Which of the following is least likely to be seen in a postsplenectomy patient?
    A. Erythrocytes containing iron deposits
    B. Irregularly shaped and fragmented RBCs
    C. Persistent monocytosis
    D. Acanthocytes
    E. Erythrocytes containing nuclear fragments

10. A 50-year-old male has an incidentally discovered 8-cm nonparasitic splenic cyst. Which of the following is true about this condition?
    A. Splenectomy should be performed
    B. Most are symptomatic and present with left upper quadrant tenderness
    C. It may secrete CA 19-9
    D. The patient should undergo percutaneous aspiration
    E. It is a common incidental finding

11. A 7-year-old girl with hemolytic anemia who has failed conservative management is scheduled for an elective splenectomy. Which of the following is true regarding her condition?
    A. Preoperative right upper quadrant ultrasonography should be performed
    B. An intraoperative search for accessory splenic tissue is not necessary
    C. The most common intraoperative complication is injury to the pancreas
    D. Open splenectomy should be performed
    E. Surgery should be delayed until 10 years of age

12. A 35-year-old alcoholic male with human immunodeficiency virus (HIV) undergoes a splenectomy after being involved in a motor vehicle crash. Which of the following is true?
    A. The primary risk of OPSI is within the first year after splenectomy
    B. Suspected OPSI should initially be managed with a fluoroquinolone
    C. The majority of OPSI cases are due to *Haemophilus influenzae*
    D. Daily prophylactic antibiotic is recommended
    E. Loss of immunoglobulin G (IgG) is what predisposes postsplenectomy patients to OPSI

13. Which of the following indications for splenectomy poses the highest risk of postsplenectomy sepsis?
    A. Trauma
    B. ITP
    C. Hereditary spherocytosis
    D. Thalassemia major
    E. Hereditary elliptocytosis

14. A 32-year-old female with rheumatoid arthritis presents for evaluation of recurrent infections. Physical exam is significant for splenomegaly. Laboratory exam demonstrates marked neutropenia. Which of the following is true concerning this condition?
    A. Splenectomy is the initial treatment of choice
    B. There is a tendency for upper extremity ulcers to form in this patient population
    C. The neutrophil count does not improve with surgical intervention
    D. Patients have antibodies against neutrophil nuclei
    E. Corticosteroids are contraindicated

15. Which of the following is true regarding hereditary spherocytosis?
    A. It is transmitted as an autosomal recessive trait
    B. The spleen is typically smaller than normal
    C. Spherocytosis on blood smear improves following splenectomy
    D. It is associated with leg ulcers
    E. A positive direct Coombs test result confirms the diagnosis

16. After splenectomy for a myeloproliferative disorder, a 40-year-old woman presents with anorexia, abdominal pain, and a low-grade fever. Her white blood cell (WBC) count is 14,000 cells/μL and her platelet count is 500,000 cells/μL. A noncontrast CT scan reveals diffuse small bowel edema and mild ascites. The most likely diagnosis is:
    A. OPSI
    B. Portal vein thrombosis
    C. Primary peritonitis
    D. Ischemic colitis
    E. Perforated duodenal ulcer

17. The most common cause of spontaneous splenic rupture worldwide is:
    A. Leukemia
    B. Malaria
    C. Hemophilia
    D. Hemolytic anemia
    E. Hodgkin lymphoma

18. The most common indication for elective splenectomy is:
    A. Staging for Hodgkin lymphoma
    B. Hereditary spherocytosis
    C. ITP
    D. TTP
    E. Autoimmune hemolytic anemia

19. In comparing laparoscopic with open splenectomy for hematologic disorders, which of the following is true?
    A. Open splenectomy has better long-term results with respect to response rates
    B. The length of hospital stay is the same
    C. The operative mortality rate is lower with laparoscopic splenectomy
    D. Laparoscopic splenectomy has emerged as the standard of care
    E. Laparoscopic splenectomy is frequently associated with increased cost to the patient

Answers

1. E. Splenectomy for ITP can be safely performed in most patients without the need for platelet transfusions. Transfusing platelets preoperatively does not reduce transfusion requirements intraoperatively (A). Platelet transfusion is most effective after the splenic artery is ligated because the newly transfused platelets are not at risk for sequestration (B, C). Splenic vein ligation would not prevent platelet sequestration (C). Transfusions can be avoided if there is no intraoperative bleeding (D).

Reference: Goel R, Ness PM, Takemoto CM, Krishnamurti L, King KE, Tobian AAR. Platelet transfusions in platelet consumptive disorders are associated with arterial thrombosis and in-hospital mortality. *Blood*. 2015;125(9):1470–1476.

2. B. This patient presenting with fever, tachycardia, leukocytosis, and a left upper quadrant fluid collection after emergent splenectomy likely has a pancreatic fistula from iatrogenic injury to the tail of the pancreas, which lies in the splenorenal ligament (B). Portal vein thrombosis (PVT) should be considered in a patient with fever and abdominal pain after splenectomy. Although PVT might cause a fever, it would not be associated with a left upper quadrant fluid collection (C). The diagnosis of PVT can be made with CT imaging demonstrating portal vein dilation and a filling defect or with Duplex scan. OPSI is a life-threatening condition caused by absent IgM, which requires prompt treatment with broad-spectrum antibiotics. While a high index of suspicion for OPSI should be maintained in this patient with fever after splenectomy, the left upper quadrant fluid collection and gradually progressive course make pancreatic fistula a more likely diagnosis (D). Iatrogenic colon perforation would present in the immediate postoperative period with systemic signs of infection and worsening diffuse abdominal pain (A). Similarly, postoperative hemorrhage will present in the immediate postoperative period with tachycardia and hypotension requiring blood products and possibly angioembolization or surgical exploration (E). The most common source of bleeding after splenectomy is the short gastric arteries.

3. E. ITP is an autoimmune disorder caused by the formation of antiplatelet IgG autoantibodies produced in the spleen. Platelets are opsonized by the antiplatelet antibodies and are then removed prematurely, leading to the low platelet count. In adults, it is two to three times more common in women, whereas it occurs with equal frequency in boys and girls. Patients typically present with ecchymoses or petechiae. Others may exhibit minor bleeding from the gums or nose, excessive menstruation, or blood in the stool or urine. Life-threatening bleeding as an initial presentation is uncommon. In children, the presentation is often preceded by a viral illness. The spleen is usually not enlarged (C). The diagnosis is one of exclusion and is based on the history, physical examination, complete blood count, and examination of the peripheral smear, which should exclude other causes of thrombocytopenia. The peripheral blood smear frequently shows large, immature platelets. Bone marrow aspiration is not routinely used but is appropriate in patients over the age of 60 and in patients considering splenectomy. The bone marrow aspirate shows normal or increased megakaryocytes. The management depends on the age of the patient, the platelet count, and the severity of symptoms. In children, the majority present with mild cases that are self-limited and do not need any medical therapy (A–B). In fact, children with platelet counts greater than 30,000 cells/μL should not be hospitalized and do not routinely require treatment if they are asymptomatic or have only minor purpura (D). In adults, that threshold is greater than 20,000/μL. The first line of therapy is oral prednisone at a dose of 1 to 1.5 mg/kg/day. Another effective therapy is intravenous (IV) immunoglobulin, which is used if corticosteroids are ineffective. Splenectomy is indicated for failure of medical therapy, for prolonged use of steroids with side effects, and for most cases of a first relapse, particularly if there is preoperative bleeding. Patients with low platelet counts of less than 10,000/μL should have platelets available for surgery but should not receive them preoperatively because they will be consumed. Platelets should be given for those who continue to bleed after ligation of the splenic pedicle. The one exception is if there is preoperative bleeding; platelets can be given before or at the time of incision during splenectomy. Urgent splenectomy plays a role in severe, life-threatening bleeding, in conjunction with medical therapy in both adults and children. Splenectomy provides a permanent response in 75% to 85% of patients.

Reference: George JN, Woolf SH, Raskob GE, et al. Idiopathic thrombocytopenic purpura: a practice guideline by explicit methods for the American Society of Hematology. *Blood.* 1996;88(1):3–40.

4. D. General indications for splenectomy include symptomatic splenomegaly, hypersplenism, hemolytic anemia, thrombocytopenia, or other cytopenia. Splenectomy is not indicated for sarcoidosis, Gaucher disease, or myelofibrosis, unless they have hypersplenism (A–C). Splenectomy is not indicated for patients with portal hypertension (E). Hairy cell leukemia gets its name from hair-like cytoplasmic projections in lymphocytes that are seen on a peripheral smear. Treatment is with chemotherapy, but splenectomy is useful in increasing cell counts, improving pain, and early satiety. With newer chemotherapeutic agents, the role of splenectomy is decreasing.

5. C. Splenic artery aneurysms are the most common visceral artery aneurysms (A). Women are four times more likely to be affected than men. The aneurysm usually arises in the middle to distal portion of the splenic artery (D). The risk of rupture is very low and is likely dependent on size and hormonal influences. Once rupture occurs, the mortality rate ranges from 35% to 50%. Splenic artery aneurysm is particularly problematic in pregnancy because rupture imparts a risk of mortality to both mother and fetus. Most patients are asymptomatic and seek medical attention based on an incidental radiographic finding (a ring-like calcification on a plain abdominal radiograph located in the left upper quadrant). Indications for treatment of true aneurysms include the presence of symptoms, pregnancy, and women of childbearing age who intend to become pregnant. Pseudoaneurysms are usually associated with inflammatory processes, are inherently unstable, and thus should be treated. For asymptomatic patients, size greater than 2 cm is an indication for surgery. Most splenic artery aneurysms can be observed; however, because this woman is of childbearing age, treatment would be indicated (E). The majority of splenic artery aneurysms are true aneurysms (B). Pseudoaneurysms occur most commonly in association with an episode of severe pancreatitis with erosion into the vessel. The patient presented has no evidence of pancreatitis. Splenic artery aneurysms are associated with a double-rupture phenomenon in which there is an initial herald bleed into the lesser sac and then rupture into the peritoneal cavity.

6. D. When a recurrence of a platelet count decrease after splenectomy for ITP develops in a patient, one must consider the possibility of an accessory spleen that was missed. The presence of an accessory spleen is suggested by the absence of Howell-Jolly bodies on a peripheral blood smear. This patient needs to be appropriately worked up starting with radionuclide imaging to determine if an accessory spleen is present (C, E). The sensitivity of CT scan in identifying an accessory spleen is 60% (A). Bone marrow biopsy has no role (B). Identification of an accessory spleen in a patient who remains severely thrombocytopenic warrants surgical excision of the accessory spleen. Rituximab may also be considered in this patient population.

References: Quah C, Ayiomamitis GD, Shah A, Ammori BJ. Computed tomography to detect accessory spleens before laparoscopic splenectomy: is it necessary? *Surg Endosc.* 2011;25(1):261–265.

Ghanima W, Khelif A, Waage A, et al. Rituximab as second-line treatment for adult immune thrombocytopenia (the RITP trial): a multicentre, randomised, double-blind, placebo-controlled trial. *Lancet.* 2015;385(9978):1653–1661.

7. B. Adults are more likely to get a chronic, more insidious form of ITP than children. In adults, women are affected two to three times more often than men, whereas, in children, it is equally common in boys and girls. The diagnosis of ITP is one of exclusion. The peripheral blood smear shows a low platelet count as well as large, immature platelets but does not establish the diagnosis (C). IV immunoglobulin therapy is effective in both children and adults in increasing the platelet count (D). In adults, splenectomy is indicated for failure of medical therapy (steroids, immunoglobulin), for prolonged use of steroids beyond 3 to 6 months, and for most cases of a first relapse (A, E).

8. E. The first line of treatment for TTP is plasma exchange by removing the patient's plasma and exchanging it with fresh-frozen plasma (C). Splenectomy is not very effective in TTP and should be used as salvage therapy in refractory cases. Features of TTP include thrombocytopenia, microangiopathic hemolytic anemia, and neurologic complications. The pathophysiology involves abnormal platelet clumping, likely due to large multimers of von Willebrand factor, which results in thrombotic episodes in the microvascular circulation. The narrowed lumens in the microvascular circulation lead to increased shear stress on red blood cells (RBCs), causing them to lyse (A). Symptoms and signs include petechiae; fever; neurologic symptoms such as headaches, seizures, and even coma; and renal failure (B). The peripheral blood smear shows schistocytes, nucleated RBCs, and basophilic stippling. The most common cause of death is intracerebral hemorrhage. TTP can be distinguished from autoimmune hemolytic anemia, in that the result of the Coombs test is negative in TTP (D).

Reference: Coppo P, Froissart A, French Reference Center for Thrombotic Microangiopathies. Treatment of thrombotic thrombocytopenic purpura beyond therapeutic plasma exchange. *Hematology Am Soc Hematol Educ Program.* 2015;(1):637–643.

9. B. After splenectomy, target cells, Howell-Jolly bodies (erythrocytes containing nuclear fragments), Heinz bodies, Pappenheimer bodies (erythrocytes containing iron deposits), and spur cells (acanthocytes) are seen (A, D–E). These inclusions (bodies) are normally pitted by the spleen. Leukocytosis, persistent monocytosis, and increased platelet counts commonly occur after splenectomy as well (C). The increase in WBC count is primarily mature neutrophils. The white blood cell (WBC) count typically increases within 1 day after splenectomy but may remain elevated for as long as several months. Asplenic patients have been found to have subnormal IgM levels. The spleen is a major site of production for the opsonins properdin and tuftsin, and splenectomy results in decreased serum levels of these proteins. Schistocytes (irregularly shaped and fragmented RBCs) are pathologic and indicate either disseminated intravascular coagulation or traumatic hemolytic anemia (such as TTP).

10. C. Nonparasitic splenic cysts are rare (E). They are most commonly asymptomatic, but when patients have symptoms, they frequently complain of left upper quadrant tenderness with referred pain to the left shoulder (B). Asymptomatic cysts can safely be observed regardless of size (A). Additionally, percutaneous aspiration is met with high recurrence rates (D). Patients should be managed with observation and serial ultrasound imaging to assess for interval growth. It has been shown that splenic cysts may secrete tumor markers such as CA 19-9, but they do not have malignant potential.

References: Boybeyi O, Karnak I, Tanyel FC, Ciftçi AO, Senocak ME. The management of primary nonparasitic splenic cysts. *Turk J Pediatr.* 2010;52(5):500–504.

Bresadola V, Pravisani R, Terrosu G, Risaliti A. Elevated serum CA 19-9 level associated with a splenic cyst: which is the actual clinical management? Review of the literature. *Ann Ital Chir.* 2015;86(1):22–29.

11. A. In the pediatric population, preoperative workup for hemolytic anemia should include a right upper quadrant ultrasound to look for cholelithiasis because these patients are susceptible to developing pigment stones. If these are present, concomitant splenectomy and cholecystectomy would

be considered. Laparoscopic splenectomy has emerged as the gold standard for most children (D). Intraoperatively, before removal of the spleen, there should always be a search for an accessory spleen, particularly in a patient with a hematologic indication for splenectomy (B). There is no need to delay surgery until 10 years of age (E). Most surgeons agree that the minimum accepted age is 5 years, but there have been reports of splenectomy in patients as young as 2 years old. Although the pancreatic tail is at risk of injury, the most common intraoperative complication is hemorrhage that can occur during hilar dissection (C).

References: Sheng J, Wu Y. A report of two cases of splenectomy in children younger than two years old with hereditary spherocytosis. *J Pediatr Surg Case Rep.* 2015;3(2):84–86.

Vecchio R, Intagliata E, Marchese S, La Corte F, Cacciola RR, Cacciola E. Laparoscopic splenectomy coupled with laparoscopic cholecystectomy. *JSLS.* 2014;18(2):252–257.

12. D. OPSI is a significant concern in the asplenic patient and can occur in 0.05% to 2% of postsplenectomy patients. It is due to loss of IgM (E). These patients continue to be at an increased risk many years after splenectomy (A). Management of OPSI requires prompt identification and initiation of supportive care with a third-generation cephalosporin (B). The majority of OPSI cases are due to *Streptococcus pneumoniae* (C), followed by *H. influenzae* type B, *Neisseria meningitides*, and group A *streptococcus*. Daily prophylactic antibiotic use is indicated for children younger than 5 and for immunocompromised patients because they may not be able to mount an appropriate response to pneumococcal vaccination. Asplenic patients may also have mild degrees of thrombocytosis and leukocytosis, Howell-Jolly bodies in RBCs, and an increased number of target cells. Howell-Jolly bodies are nuclear remnants in circulating erythrocytes that appear basophilic (blue). Normally, erythrocytes expel their DNA before exiting the bone marrow.

References: Fishman D, Isenberg DA. Splenic involvement in rheumatic diseases. *Semin Arthritis Rheum.* 1997;27(3):141–155.

Piliero P, Furie R. Functional asplenia in systemic lupus erythematosus. *Semin Arthritis Rheum.* 1990;20(3):185–189.

Theilacker C, Ludewig K, Serr A, et al. Overwhelming postsplenectomy infection: A prospective multicenter cohort study. *Clin Infect Dis.* 2016;62(7):871–878.

13. D. All of the answer choices can lead to postsplenectomy sepsis (A–C, E). The incidence and mortality rate for postsplenectomy sepsis are highest in patients with underlying hematologic conditions, particularly thalassemia major and sickle cell disease. Children have a higher risk than adults. In a large review, the incidence of infection after splenectomy in children (younger than 16 years old) was 4.4%, compared with 0.9% in adults. Severe infection after splenectomy for benign disease was very uncommon, except in infants and children younger than 5 years of age. Patients are also more susceptible to malaria.

References: Davidson RN, Wall RA. Prevention and management of infections in patients without a spleen. *Clin Microbiol Infect.* 2001;7(12):657–660.

Holdsworth RJ, Irving AD, Cuschieri A. Postsplenectomy sepsis and its mortality rate: actual versus perceived risks. *Br J Surg.* 1991;78(9):1031–1038.

Leonard AS, Giebink GS, Baesl TJ, Krivit W. The overwhelming postsplenectomy sepsis problem. *World J Surg.* 1980;4(4):423–432.

14. D. The triad of rheumatoid arthritis, splenomegaly, and neutropenia is called Felty syndrome. It is present in 3% of patients with rheumatoid arthritis. The pathophysiology involves the coating of the white blood cell surface with immune complexes, leading to their sequestration and clearance in the spleen. An increased risk of infections due to neutropenia ensues. The size of the spleen can vary from nonpalpable to massively enlarged. Initial treatment with corticosteroids typically improves the neutrophil count, but the effects are not always permanent (A, E). Hematopoietic growth factors and methotrexate have also been used. There is a tendency for leg ulcers to form in these patients (B). Other indications for splenectomy include transfusion-dependent anemia and profound thrombocytopenia. Responses to splenectomy are excellent, with more than 80% of patients showing a durable increase in white blood cell count. The neutrophil count typically improves immediately, although the relative number of neutrophils may remain subnormal (C). However, neutrophil function improves.

15. D. Hereditary spherocytosis (HS) is an RBC membrane disorder that leads to hemolytic anemia. It is autosomal dominant and the most common hemolytic anemia requiring splenectomy (A). It is due to an inherited dysfunction or deficiency in one of the RBC membrane proteins (spectrin, ankyrin, band 3 protein, or protein 4.2), which causes the membrane lipid bilayers to destabilize, leading to a lack of membrane deformability. The spleen sequesters and destroys these nondeformable RBCs. Most patients are asymptomatic, but they may have mild jaundice from hemolysis and splenomegaly on physical examination (B). Laboratory features include a mild to moderate anemia, a low mean corpuscular volume, an elevated mean corpuscular hemoglobin concentration, and an elevated red cell distribution width. Laboratory values also reflect the hemolysis and rapid cell turnover with an elevated reticulocyte count, lactate dehydrogenase, and unconjugated bilirubin. Unlike autoimmune hemolytic anemia, the direct Coombs test result is negative in HS (E). In HS, RBCs tend to lyse at lower concentrations of salt than normal. Splenectomy is curative for HS and serves as the sole mode of therapy, but patients continue to have spherocytosis on blood smear (C). Due to ongoing red cell lysis, gallstones are common. When gallstones are found, prophylactic cholecystectomy is recommended, particularly in children. Another feature of HS is leg ulceration, which is another indication for early splenectomy. These ulcers heal after splenectomy. The cause of the ulceration is unclear but may be a result of increased blood viscosity that reduces oxygen levels in the leg tissues. Alternatively, recent studies suggest that hemolysis leads to nitric oxide resistance, endothelial dysfunction, and end-organ vasculopathy, as is seen in sickle cell disease.

Reference: Kato GJ, McGowan V, Machado RF, et al. Lactate dehydrogenase as a biomarker of hemolysis-associated nitric oxide resistance, priapism, leg ulceration, pulmonary hypertension, and death in patients with sickle cell disease. *Blood.* 2006;107(6):2279–2285.

16. B. This patient most likely has PVT; it should be suspected in patients with fever and abdominal pain after splenectomy. This patient is predisposed to PVT formation because of her hypercoagulability from a combination of thrombocytosis after splenectomy and the setting of a myeloproliferative disorder. PVT is uncommon (occurrence rate ranging from 2% to 8%) but not rare, and the greatest risk is in cases involving splenomegaly with a myeloproliferative disorder. Postsplenectomy PVT typically presents with anorexia, abdominal pain, leukocytosis, and thrombocytosis, as demonstrated in this patient. A high index of suspicion, early diagnosis with contrast-enhanced CT, and immediate anticoagulation are keys to successful treatment of PVT. Patients undergoing splenectomy should be treated with deep venous thrombosis prophylaxis, including pneumatic compression devices, and with subcutaneous or low-molecular-weight heparin. OPSI is an uncommon complication in postsplenectomy patients and may present with nonspecific flu-like symptoms that rapidly progress to fulminant sepsis (A). Primary peritonitis is often a monobacterial infection occurring in cirrhotic patients with ascites (C). Ischemic colitis presents with left-sided abdominal pain and bloody diarrhea in elderly patients with low-flow states, such as those with severe dehydration, heart failure, shock, and trauma (D). Perforated duodenal ulcer initially presents with epigastric pain, followed by diffuse tenderness, abdominal rigidity, and rebound tenderness (E).

References: an't Riet M, Burger JW, van Muiswinkel JM, Kazemier G, Schipperus MR, Bonjer HJ. Diagnosis and treatment of portal vein thrombosis following splenectomy: portal vein thrombosis following splenectomy. *Br J Surg.* 2000;87(9):1229–1233.

Winslow ER, Brunt LM, Drebin JA, Soper NJ, Klingensmith ME. Portal vein thrombosis after splenectomy. *Am J Surg.* 2002;184(6):631–636.

17. B. Spontaneous rupture of the spleen is an uncommon dramatic abdominal emergency that requires immediate diagnosis and prompt treatment to ensure the patient's survival. Spontaneous rupture rarely occurs in a histologically proven normal spleen and in such cases is called a *true spontaneous rupture.* Spontaneous rupture usually occurs in a diseased spleen and is called *pathologic spontaneous rupture.* Infectious diseases have been cited in most cases involving splenic rupture but are rare in hematologic malignancies despite frequent involvement of the spleen (A, E). Malaria is the number one cause worldwide and infectious mononucleosis is the number one cause in the United States. With malaria, changes in splenic structure can result in hematoma formation, rupture, hypersplenism, torsion, or cyst formation. An abnormal immunologic response may result in massive splenic enlargement. Spontaneous rupture of the spleen is an important and life-threatening complication of *Plasmodium vivax* infection but is rarely seen in *Plasmodium falciparum* malaria. Other less frequent causes of spontaneous splenic rupture include hemolytic anemia, hemophilia, myelodysplastic disorders, lupus, dialysis, and multiple myeloma (C, D).

Reference: Hamel CT, Blum J, Harder F, Kocher T. Nonoperative treatment of splenic rupture in malaria tropica: review of literature and case report. *Acta Trop.* 2002;82(1):1–5.

18. C. The most common indication for splenectomy is trauma to the spleen, whether iatrogenic or accidental. In the past, staging for Hodgkin disease was the most common indication for elective splenectomy (A). ITP is now the most frequent indication for splenectomy in the elective setting, followed by HS, autoimmune hemolytic anemia, and TTP (B, D–E).

Reference: Schwartz SI. Role of splenectomy in hematologic disorders. *World J Surg.* 1996;20(9):1156–1159.

19. D. The laparoscopic approach typically results in longer operative times, shorter hospital stays, and lower morbidity rates (B, E). It has similar blood loss and mortality rates compared with open splenectomy (A, C). Cost analysis reveals that higher operating room charges are seen with laparoscopic splenectomy. However, several studies have found that the total cost to the patient is less with the laparoscopic procedure due to the shortened hospital stay (E). The laparoscopic approach has emerged as the standard for nontraumatic elective splenectomy.

References: Beauchamp RD, Holzman MD, Fabian TC. Spleen. In: Townsend CM, Jr, Beauchamp RD, Evers BM, Mattox KL, eds. *Sabiston textbook of surgery: the biological basis of modern surgical practice.* 17th ed. Philadelphia: W.B. Saunders; 2004:1679–1710.

Parks AE, McKinlay, R. Spleen. In: Brunicardi FC, Andersen DK, Billiar TR, et al., eds. Schwartz's principles of surgery. 8th ed. New York: McGraw-Hill; 2005:1297–1318.

Alimentary Tract— Esophagus

AMANDA C. PURDY AND ERIC R. SIMMS

7

ABSITE 99th Percentile High-Yields

I. Anatomy and Surgical Approaches
  A. Blood supply:
   1. Cervical esophagus → inferior thyroid artery
   2. Thoracic esophagus → direct branches off thoracic aorta
   3. Abdominal esophagus → branches from the left gastric and inferior phrenic arteries
  B. Surgical approaches:
   1. Cervical esophagus: left cervical incision
   2. Proximal and mid-thoracic esophagus: right posterolateral thoracotomy
   3. Distal thoracic esophagus: left posterolateral thoracotomy

II. Hiatal Hernias

Types of Hiatal Hernias

Type	Description	Management
I	Sliding hiatal hernia GE junction slides above the diaphragm	• If asymptomatic, no treatment indicated • If patient has GERD, can treat medically and consider fundoplication and hiatal hernia repair if medical management fails
II	Paraesophageal hernia The fundus herniates through the hiatus	• Elective hiatal hernia repair and fundoplication recommended to reduce risk of future complications (gastric volvulus, incarceration/strangulation)
III	Sliding + paraesophageal hernia Combination of types 1 and 2 *More common than type 2*	
IV	Paraesophageal hernia that includes organs besides the stomach	

  A. Gastric Volvulus
   1. Gastric volvulus is a complication of large hiatal hernias, where the stomach herniates into the chest and volvulizes; can lead to gastric ischemia and necrosis
   2. Borchardt triad is present in 70% of acute gastric volvulus: severe epigastric pain, inability to vomit, inability to pass nasogastric tube
   3. First steps of management are NG tube decompression and IV fluid resuscitation; NG decompression may resolve volvulus; if NG tube cannot be placed, patients need emergent surgery

III. Barrett Esophagus (BE)
  A. Intestinal metaplasia (stratified squamous epithelium → columnar epithelium with goblet cells) of the distal esophagus secondary to acid reflux; increased risk of esophageal adenocarcinoma
  B. During the initial endoscopy:

1. If NO mucosal irregularities or nodules are seen, proceed with 4-quadrant biopsies every 2 cm within the segment of BE
2. If any mucosal irregularities or nodules ARE seen, endoscopically resect the irregular area(s) and obtain 4-quadrant biopsies every 1 cm within the segment of BE

C. Medical management of GERD (PPI) & one of the following (based on endoscopy findings):

Pathology Finding	Management
No dysplasia	• Consider surveillance endoscopy with 4-quadrant biopsies every 2 cm within the segment of Barrett esophagus every 3–5 years
Low-grade dysplasia	• Endoscopic eradication (radiofrequency ablation, photodynamic therapy, or cryotherapy) OR • Surveillance endoscopy in 3–6 months with 4-quadrant biopsies every 1 cm within the segment of Barrett esophagus
High-grade dysphasia	• Endoscopic mucosal resection*Classically, high-grade dysplasia was treated with esophagectomy; however, endoscopic resection is a much less invasive acceptable alternative

IV. Motility Disorders
   A. Achalasia (classic triad: dysphagia [most common], regurgitation, weight loss)
      1. Due to the progressive degeneration of ganglion cells in the myenteric plexus in the esophageal wall
      2. Esophagram: may see "bird's beak" appearance
      3. Manometry: no peristalsis in the esophageal body and a hypertonic lower esophageal sphincter that fails to completely relax during swallowing
      4. Management:
         a) Heller myotomy: best option (to resolve the obstruction at the LES); myotomy of the inner circular and outer longitudinal muscles, extending 6 cm up the esophagus and 2 cm onto the stomach with partial fundoplication (to prevent subsequent reflux) (incomplete myotomy may occur due to inadequate mobilization of GE junction)
         b) Pneumatic endoscopic dilation: appropriate in patients who are not surgical candidates; will likely need repeated dilations over time
         c) POEM (per oral endoscopic myotomy)
   B. Divides ONLY circular muscle fibers (cricopharyngeus), longer myotomy
   C. Advantages: less invasive with similar symptom relief as Heller myotomy
   D. Disadvantages: technically demanding with long learning curve; up to 50% of patients can have acid reflux following the procedure
      a) Nonoperative options (for poor operative risk patients, lose efficacy over time): calcium channel blockers, nitrates, and botulism toxin injections; botulism toxin injections only work for a few months, and should be avoided in patients who are surgical candidates as they may disrupt surgical planes
   E. Zenker diverticulum (dysphagia, coughing, spontaneous regurgitation and halitosis)
      1. A false (pulsion) diverticulum through Killian triangle due to a failure of the cricopharyngeus muscle to relax during swallowing
      2. Management options:
         a) Open surgery: cricopharyngeal myotomy +/− diverticulectomy or diverticulopexy; the most important aspect is the myotomy, which fixes the underlying problem; if the diverticulum is large (>5 cm) and causing mass effect, resection recommended
         b) Endoscopic esophagodiverticulostomy: uses stapler or energy devices to divide the cricopharyngeus endoscopically; ONLY for large diverticula >3 cm (if diverticulum too small, the cricopharyngeal myotomy will be incomplete)
         c) Open surgery has lower recurrence rates and slightly higher complication rates than endoscopic management

V. Esophageal Tumors
   A. Leiomyoma (hypoechoic mass on endoscopic ultrasound, more common in males)
      1. Most common benign tumor of the esophagus, arise from the smooth muscle cells (mesenchymal); if <5 cm, resect endoscopically
      2. If >5 cm, surgically enucleate (via VATS or laparoscopy)

B. Esophageal cancer
   1. Adenocarcinoma and squamous; adenocarcinoma more common in the United States
   2. Use endoscopic ultrasound to determine T stage, CT for N stage
   3. Localized: limited to the mucosa or invading lamina propria (and N0, M0)
      a) Endoscopic resection for T1a = within the mucosa (to the lamina propria or muscularis mucosa)
      b) Esophagectomy for T1b = within the submucosa
      c) Neoadjuvant chemoradiation first if >T2 = to the muscularis propria
   4. Regional: (nodal disease but M0)
      a) Neoadjuvant chemoradiation first, followed by esophagectomy
      b) Need 15 nodes for proper oncologic staging
   5. Distant (palliative care)
   6. Esophagectomy, transhiatal approach (left cervical and abdominal incisions) or transthoracic approach (right thoracotomy and abdominal incision); similar outcomes, transhiatal may be associated with shorter length of hospital stay
   7. Conduit choices after esophagectomy include the stomach (most common, need to preserve the right gastroepiploic artery for perfusion), the colon, and the jejunum
   8. Special circumstances
      a) Upper esophageal cancer (within 5 cm of the upper esophageal sphincter); chemoradiation as primary treatment modality
      b) Distal esophageal cancer (within 5 cm of GE junction)
         (1) Some may originate in esophagus and others in stomach
         (2) Depending on location, may spread to mediastinal or abdominal nodes
         (3) Most receive neoadjuvant or perioperative chemoradiation prior to surgery

VI. Esophageal Perforation
   A. Etiologies: iatrogenic by instrumentation (most common at cricopharyngeus), spontaneous (Boerhaave, occurs 5 cm above GE junction on left), trauma, caustic ingestion
   B. Workup: CXR (may see left-sided effusion), esophagram with gastrografin → if negative or inconclusive: esophagram with thin barium
      1. *Gastrografin major side effect: pneumonitis if aspirated*
      2. *Barium major side effect: severe peritonitis/mediastinitis*
   C. Management: start with NPO, IV fluid resuscitation, broad-spectrum antibiotics including antifungals
   D. Nonoperative management: if patient hemodynamically stable, not septic, with mild symptoms, and a contained perforation (minimal mediastinal contamination)
   E. Surgical approach: right posterolateral thoracotomy for proximal or middle one-third, left posterolateral thoracotomy for lower one-third
   F. Management depends on etiology of perforation
      1. Malignant obstruction
         a) Early cancer: perform esophagectomy
         b) Advanced cancer: esophageal stenting
      2. Benign obstruction
         a) If due to achalasia, perform myotomy on contralateral side
      3. Normal esophagus
   G. Repair of perforation
      a) Extend myotomy to expose full length of mucosal injury (musical injury often longer than muscle injury)
      b) Debride all nonviable tissue
      c) Two-layer closure (mucosa with absorbable suture and muscle with nonabsorbable suture)
      d) Reinforce repair with intercostal flap

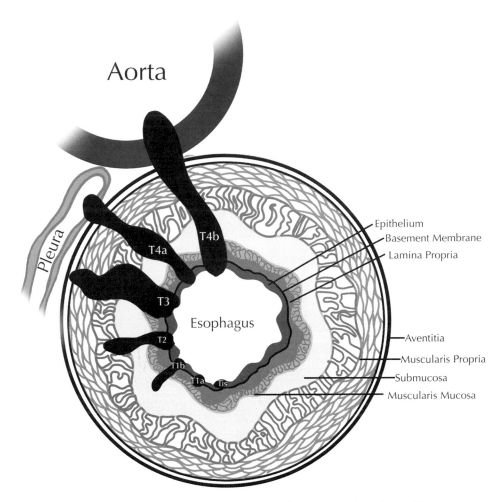

T staging is the same for both esophageal adenocarcinoma and squamous cell carcinoma. T1a tumors invade the lamina propria or muscularis mucosa. These tumors can be resected endoscopically. T1b tumors invade the submucosa and must be treated with esophagectomy. T2 tumors and above must be managed with neoadjuvant therapy and they invade the muscularis propria. T3 invade the aventitia. T4 tumors invade adjacent structures and are divided into resectible and unresectible tumors. T4a tumors invade the pleura, pericardium, or diaphragm and are resectible. T4b are unresectible tumors and invade the aorta, vertebral body, or trachea.

Fig. 7.1

Questions

1. A 40-year-old woman with a history of Raynaud disease presents for evaluation of dysphagia. Barium esophagram shows reflux but no structural abnormalities, and upper endoscopy shows reflux esophagitis. Manometry shows absent peristalsis of the distal esophagus and decreased tone of the lower esophageal sphincter. Initial management consists of:
   A. Laparoscopic Heller myotomy with partial fundoplication
   B. Proton pump inhibitor and metoclopramide
   C. Pneumatic dilation
   D. Calcium channel blocker
   E. Nissen fundoplication

2. A 63-year-old man with a history of GERD presents for progressive dysphagia over the past 4 months. Esophagram shows an irregular lesion in the distal esophagus. Endoscopy with biopsy and endoscopic ultrasound confirms a 2 cm irregular mass with invasion into the submucosa. Imaging does not show any distant masses or abnormal lymph nodes. What is the first step in treatment?
   A. Chemotherapy
   B. Chemoradiation
   C. Endoscopic resection
   D. Enucleation
   E. Esophagectomy

3. A 20-year-old man presents to your office after being hospitalized for lye ingestion. Esophagoscopy revealed a high-grade esophageal caustic injury, and the patient was treated with supportive care. The patient asks about the long-term complications after caustic injury to the esophagus. Which of the following is true?
   A. He is at increased risk for esophageal adenocarcinoma
   B. He should undergo endoscopic surveillance beginning 6 weeks after ingestion
   C. The most common complication is an esophageal stricture
   D. Adult caustic ingestion is less severe than pediatric ingestion
   E. Early use of a neutralizing agent decreases the risk of subsequent stricture formation

4. A 35-year-old woman is in the recovery room after endoscopic dilation of a peptic stricture in the mid-thoracic esophagus. She begins to complain of chest pain and odynophagia. She is hemodynamically stable and chest radiograph does not show any free air or pleural effusion. Esophagram with water-soluble contrast is normal. What is the most appropriate next step in management?
   A. CT scan of the chest, abdomen, and pelvis with IV and oral contrast
   B. Esophagram with thin barium
   C. Nasogastric tube placement
   D. Left posterolateral thoracotomy
   E. Right posterolateral thoracotomy

5. Which of the following is true regarding the surgical approach, anatomy, or blood supply to the esophagus?
   A. Outer longitudinal muscle is an extension of the cricopharyngeus muscle
   B. Cervical esophagus is supplied by the inferior thyroid artery
   C. The narrowest point in the esophagus is at the aortic arch
   D. Branches off the intercostal arteries are the major blood supply to the thoracic esophagus
   E. The standard surgical approach to the midesophagus is a left thoracotomy

6. Which of the following statements is true about Mallory-Weiss syndrome?
   A. The chief pathologic finding is spontaneous perforation of the esophagus
   B. It typically occurs on the right side
   C. It is usually associated with air in the mediastinum
   D. Endoscopy should be performed to confirm the diagnosis
   E. Esophageal balloon tamponade is an appropriate option in cases of persistent bleeding

7. A 40-year-old female has been using a proton pump inhibitor (PPI) to control gastroesophageal reflux disease (GERD) for the past 7 years. She is otherwise healthy. She was seen in clinic and deemed a suitable candidate for definitive surgical intervention. During the operation, after the phrenoesophageal ligament is mobilized, her distal esophagus is inspected, and it appears shortened. Preoperative upper gastrointestinal study did not identify a hiatal hernia. Which of the following will most likely need to be done?
   A. Proceed with a standard Nissen fundoplication
   B. Proceed with a Dor fundoplication
   C. Perform Collis gastroplasty
   D. Abort the operation and initiate management with steroids
   E. Take several biopsies before aborting the operation

8. A 51-year-old male has been undergoing yearly endoscopy with biopsy for Barrett esophagus (BE). His most recent biopsy demonstrates high-grade dysplasia without nodules. Which of the following is the best next step in management?
   A. Esophagectomy with reconstruction
   B. Repeat endoscopy with biopsy in 3 months
   C. Endoscopic radiofrequency ablation
   D. Antireflux operation
   E. Oncology referral for consideration of neoadjuvant chemotherapy

9. Barrett esophagus:
   A. Is a congenital abnormality
   B. Occurs more frequently in women
   C. When diagnosed, should be treated with an antireflux procedure to prevent cancer
   D. Diagnosis requires replacement of a 3-cm segment of the squamous cells by columnar epithelium
   E. Features the presence of goblet cells

10. Which of the following is true regarding Barrett esophagus?
   A. PPIs are considered a more effective treatment option than H2 blockers
   B. Dietary restrictions such as those used for patients with GERD are not useful
   C. Patients with short- and long-segment Barrett esophagus have a similar risk of high-grade dysplasia
   D. Use of high-dose PPIs with aspirin is contraindicated
   E. Photofrin is a useful treatment modality

11. Esophageal manometry performed in a patient with a true paraesophageal hernia will demonstrate that the LES is:
   A. Above the normal position
   B. At the normal position
   C. Hypertensive
   D. Hypotensive
   E. Short

12. Which of the following statements about a paraesophageal hernia is true?
   A. It is associated with anemia
   B. It does not pose a risk for incarceration and strangulation
   C. Diagnosis is not readily made with upper endoscopy
   D. It is usually caused by a traumatic injury
   E. It rarely requires operative repair

13. Which of the following will predispose a patient to the development of esophageal disease?
   A. LES length of 3 cm
   B. Resting LES pressure of 8 mm Hg
   C. Resting upper esophageal sphincter (UES) pressure of 70 mm Hg
   D. Abdominal length less than 1 cm
   E. Relaxation of LES with swallowing

14. A 52-year-old male with cirrhosis and known esophageal varices presents with a large amount of hematemesis. Which of the following statements is true?
   A. Beta blockade is ineffective for preventing rebleeding
   B. The most important next step is endoscopy for both diagnostic and therapeutic interventions
   C. Prophylactic antibiotics do not improve survival
   D. Early administration of vasoactive drugs does not improve outcomes
   E. Endoscopic band ligation has been demonstrated to be superior to endoscopic sclerotherapy

15. A 59-year-old diabetic male with a history of chronic obstructive pulmonary disease (COPD) and prior congestive heart failure presents with a 2-year history of progressively difficult swallowing. Esophagram demonstrates a dilated proximal esophagus with abrupt tapering distally. Manometry shows high pressure in the lower esophageal sphincter (LES) at rest and failure of the LES to relax after swallowing. Upper endoscopy is negative. Which of the following is true regarding this patient?
    A. The underlying condition is characterized by high-amplitude peristaltic waves of the esophagus
    B. Laparoscopic esophagomyotomy with complete fundoplication is the treatment of choice
    C. A trial of calcium channel blockers should be started
    D. Esophageal pneumatic dilation is the next step in management
    E. Peroral endoscopic myotomy (POEM) is the treatment of choice

16. During the course of an upper endoscopy for manometry confirmed achalasia, the endoscopist thinks he may have caused an inadvertent perforation of the left lower distal esophagus. The patient is stable and shows no signs of sepsis. Esophagogram confirms a markedly dilated esophagus with a distal-free perforation. Management consists of:
    A. Intravenous (IV) antibiotics, placing patient NPO (nothing by mouth), and close observation
    B. Left thoracotomy, primary repair, longitudinal myotomy on the contralateral side
    C. Laparoscopic primary repair and longitudinal myotomy on the ipsilateral side
    D. Esophagectomy with immediate reconstruction
    E. Esophageal stent placement

17. A 36-year-old male presents for consultation regarding an incidental esophageal mass seen on computed tomography (CT) scan. This was performed after he was involved in a motor vehicle collision (MVC). He had no serious injuries and was discharged the same day. Barium swallow demonstrates a smooth, crescent-shaped filling defect. Which of the following is true regarding this mass?
    A. Resection with a 1-cm margin is the treatment of choice
    B. They most commonly present with satellite tumors
    C. They have no risk of malignant degeneration
    D. Esophageal ultrasonography may be useful
    E. A preoperative endoscopic biopsy should be performed

18. Which of the following statements is true about Zenker diverticulum?
    A. It is a true diverticulum
    B. It is best diagnosed with esophagoscopy
    C. It is unlikely to cause aspiration
    D. It is a pulsion diverticulum
    E. Small diverticula (<3 cm) are best managed endoscopically

19. Over the past 2 years, a 50-year-old man repeatedly reported difficulty swallowing, which he described as a lump in his throat. He has noticed expectoration of excess saliva, dysphagia, intermittent hoarseness, regurgitation of undigested food hours later, and some weight loss. Which of the following is true of the most likely diagnosis?
    A. Swallowing is easiest immediately after waking up in the morning and gets increasingly difficult throughout the course of the day
    B. It is best managed with diverticulectomy alone through a left cervical incision
    C. It involves an outpouching of the muscularis propria
    D. Esophagectomy will improve survival
    E. The patient should likely be started on chemoradiation

20. A 39-year-old male presents in clinic to discuss his care before starting neoadjuvant chemoradiation for esophageal cancer. His albumin is 2.4 mg/dL. Which of the following is true regarding nutritional optimization for this patient?
    A. He should begin parenteral nutrition
    B. Percutaneous gastrostomy tube should not be offered
    C. Esophageal stent placement has been consistently demonstrated to improve nutritional status
    D. Nasogastric tube insertion has been shown to improve nutritional status
    E. Stent migration and chest discomfort are uncommonly reported in patients with esophageal stents

21. Which of the following is true regarding surgical intervention for esophageal cancer?
    A. Ivor Lewis esophagectomy involves an upper midline laparotomy and a left thoracotomy
    B. Transthoracic esophagectomy (TTE) is associated with a shorter total hospital length of stay when compared to a transhiatal esophagectomy (THE)
    C. There is no difference in mortality between the use of TTE or THE in the surgical treatment of esophageal cancer
    D. TTE is associated with fewer complications when compared with THE
    E. THE is performed with a right cervical incision and midline laparotomy

Answers

1. B. This patient has dysphagia in the setting of scleroderma, an autoimmune connective tissue disease most common in women between the ages of 30 and 50. Raynaud occurs in 90% of scleroderma patients and presents with the classic triad of color change, including an initial pallor secondary to vasospasm, followed by cyanosis and rubor. Approximately 90% of patients have gastrointestinal involvement, and the esophagus is the most common site. Patients with scleroderma develop fibrous replacement of the smooth muscle layer of the esophagus, resulting in decreased peristalsis of the lower portion of the esophagus and hypotonicity of the lower esophageal sphincter which may present with dysphagia, reflux, and peptic strictures. The most appropriate initial management is a PPI and a promotility agent. Antireflux procedures (Nissen) are relatively contraindicated in patients with scleroderma, as up to 70% of patients suffer from dysphagia postoperatively (E). Laparoscopic Heller myotomy and pneumatic dilation are both acceptable first-line treatments for achalasia in patients who are good surgical candidates; however, they are not indicated for esophageal dysmotility due to scleroderma (A, C). Patients with achalasia will have absent peristalsis of the esophageal body and *hypertonicity* of the lower esophageal sphincter. Calcium channel blockers, which may be indicated in achalasia, diffuse esophageal spasm, and nutcracker esophagus, can actually worsen dysmotility in scleroderma (D).

Reference: Carlson DA, Hinchcliff M, Pandolfino JE. Advances in the evaluation and management of esophageal disease of systemic sclerosis. *Curr Rheumatol Rep.* 2015;17(1):475.

2. E. This patient has esophageal adenocarcinoma, the most common esophageal malignancy in the United States. This patient has a T1b lesion with no evidence of nodal disease or distant metastasis and is a candidate for esophagectomy. Important T stages to remember for esophageal adenocarcinoma are T1a (invasion into the lamina propria or muscularis mucosa), T1b (invasion into the submucosa), and T2 (invasion into the muscularis propria). Patients with T1a lesions with no abnormal lymph nodes are candidates for endoscopic resection (C). Patients with T1b lesions with no abnormal lymph nodes should proceed with esophagectomy. Lymph node involvement is directly proportional to esophageal tumor depth or T stage. The incidence of positive lymph nodes is 20% for T1a and 50% for T1b tumors. Patients with T2 lesions or any lymph node involvement should proceed with neoadjuvant chemoradiation (A, B). Enucleation is not an appropriate treatment for esophageal adenocarcinoma, as a formal resection with lymph node dissection is warranted (D). Enucleation is a treatment option for esophageal leiomyomas.

Reference: National Comprehensive Cancer Network. Esophageal and Esophagogastric Junction Cancers (Version 5.2020). https://www.nccn.org/professionals/physician_gls/PDF/esophageal.pdf. Accessed December 30, 2020.

3. C. The most common complication after caustic injury to the esophagus is stricture formation; the likelihood of developing a stricture is directly correlated with the severity of injury. Most strictures occur within 2 months of ingestion. A less common long-term risk after caustic injury to the esophagus is the development of *squamous cell* esophageal carcinoma (A). Because of this risk, the American Society for Gastrointestinal Endoscopy recommends routine endoscopic screenings every 2 to 3 years, beginning 10 to 20 years after caustic esophageal injury (B). Adult caustic ingestion tends to be more severe than pediatric cases (D). Neutralizing agents are never indicated in caustic ingestions and do not prevent subsequent complications (E). Neutralizing reactions between acidic and alkaline substances create exothermic reactions that cause further thermal injury. Patients with focal necrosis (grade III caustic injury) should be started on broad-spectrum IV antibiotics.

References: Cheng HT, Cheng CL, Lin CH, et al. Caustic ingestion in adults: the role of endoscopic classification in predicting outcome. *BMC Gastroenterol.* 2008;8(1):31.

ASGE Standards of Practice Committee, Evans JA, Early DS, et al. The role of endoscopy in Barrett's esophagus and other premalignant conditions of the esophagus. *Gastrointest Endosc.* 2012;76(6):1087–1094.

4. B. This patient with chest pain and odynophagia after dilation of an esophageal stricture should be evaluated for iatrogenic esophageal perforation. Iatrogenic injuries are the most common cause of esophageal perforations and occur at anatomic areas of narrowing, including the cricopharyngeus and GE junction. When an esophageal perforation is suspected, initial workup includes plain radiographs of the neck, chest, and/or abdomen depending on the suspected location of the perforation. The next step is esophagram with water-soluble contrast. If normal, the next step is a thin barium esophagram, which is more sensitive. CT with contrast is less sensitive than esophagram (A). Blind nasogastric tube placement is not appropriate in the setting of a suspected esophageal injury and may cause further injury (C). Surgical management prior to confirming the diagnosis is premature (D, E). If the patient is found to have a free perforation of the mid-thoracic esophagus, repair via a right posterolateral thoracotomy would be appropriate. Injuries to the distal thoracic esophagus are approached via a left posterolateral thoracotomy.

Reference: Bladergroen MR, Lowe JE, Postlethwait RW. Diagnosis and recommended management of esophageal perforation and rupture. *Ann Thorac Surg.* 1986;42(3):235–239.

5. B. The esophagus is a 2-layered muscular conduit connecting the oropharynx to the stomach. The outer muscular layer is longitudinal while the inner layer is circular and considered an extension of the cricopharyngeus muscle (A). Several anatomic areas of narrowing exist in the esophagus with the cricopharyngeus muscle contributing to the narrowest portion of the esophagus. Other anatomic areas of narrowing occur at the aortic arch and the diaphragm (C). The cervical esophagus is supplied by the thyrocervical trunk off the subclavian artery. The major branches of the thyrocervical trunk can be remembered by the mnemonic "STAT" (suprascapular artery, transverse cervical artery, ascending cervical artery, and inferior thyroid artery). The thoracic esophagus is primarily supplied by branches directly off the aorta. The surgical approach to the esophagus can be divided into thirds. The distal third of the esophagus is approached by a left thoracotomy, while the proximal and midesophagus are approached with a right thoracotomy, as the aorta is in the way during a left thoracotomy (E).

6. D. The mechanism of a Mallory-Weiss tear is similar to that of an esophageal perforation (Boerhaave syndrome) but differs in that the injury is not full thickness (A). It is the result of forceful vomiting or coughing, such as after an alcohol drinking binge. The classic description is retching followed by vomiting of blood. The presence of a hiatal hernia is a predisposing factor and is found in a majority of patients. This situation exposes the LES to high pressures, which results in a partial-thickness mucosal tear and bleeding most commonly 3 to 5 cm above the gastroesophageal junction on the left side (B). Boerhaave syndrome results in a full-thickness tear causing esophageal perforation (A). These patients often present in sepsis with air in the mediastinum and a pleural effusion. Severe sepsis in the setting of esophageal perforation mandates surgical intervention (C). Most bleeding from Mallory-Weiss tears stops spontaneously with nonsurgical management (E). Patients should undergo endoscopy to confirm the diagnosis. Recent studies suggest that the area of bleeding is best managed by injecting sclerosing agents or epinephrine to prevent rebleeding. Esophageal balloon tamponade is contraindicated as it can convert a partial thickness tear into a full-thickness esophageal laceration. Additionally, it will not stop the bleeding as it is usually arterial and not venous. In cases not amenable to endoscopic therapy, operative management consists of oversewing the laceration through an anterior longitudinal gastrotomy in the middle third of the stomach.

Reference: Llach J, Elizalde JI, Guevara MC, et al. Endoscopic injection therapy in bleeding Mallory-Weiss syndrome: a randomized controlled trial. *Gastrointest Endosc.* 2001;54(6):679–681.

7. C. Roughly 15% of the adult population in the United States have GERD. Most patients can initially be managed conservatively with the use of PPI. Indications for surgical intervention include failure of conservative management, patient preference for definitive intervention despite successful medical management (e.g., patient would like to avoid lifelong need for medication), and complications associated with GERD including Barrett esophagus or extra-esophageal manifestations (asthma, cough, hoarseness). The standard surgical intervention involves a Nissen fundoplication. If a shortened esophagus is encountered during surgery (abdominal length <1 cm), then a Collis gastroplasty will need to be performed to lengthen it and minimize tension during antireflux repair (A). In most patients, about 3 cm of intraabdominal esophagus can be mobilized and thereby avoid the need to lengthen the esophagus. An anterior (Dor) fundoplication may be considered in patients with underlying esophageal dysmotility (B). Although scleroderma can present with a shortened or fibrotic esophagus, this is a diffuse process and will involve the entire esophagus. In addition, most patients will have

extra esophageal disease (D). In the above patient, a biopsy should be considered. However, the long duration of GERD and absence of any systemic symptoms (fevers, night sweats, weight loss) make carcinoma unlikely, and thus the surgery should proceed (E).

Reference: Kunio NR, Dolan JP, Hunter JG. Short esophagus. *Surg Clin North Am.* 2015;95(3):641–652.

8. C. The management of BE with carcinoma has evolved considerably in recent years. Esophagectomy with reconstruction was once considered the standard of care for high-grade dysplasia, but this has been largely replaced by minimally invasive endoscopic techniques such as radiofrequency ablation (RFA) (A). A large meta analysis published in the *New England Journal of Medicine* demonstrates that RFA is associated with a high rate of disease eradication and reduced risk of the development of carcinoma. Although no randomized control trial currently exists to support this recommendation, endoscopic therapy is now the favored approach for high-grade dysplasia in BE without suspicious nodules. Endoscopic ablation or repeat endoscopy in 3 to 6 months with 4-quadrant biopsies every 1 cm within the segment of BE are appropriate options in patients with low-grade dysplasia (B). These patients should also be offered an antireflux procedure such as a Nissen procedure or medical management with PPI, even if asymptomatic. (D). Oncology referral is premature because there is not yet a cancer diagnosis established for the above patient (E).

References: Bennett C, Green S, Decaestecker J, et al. Surgery versus radical endotherapies for early cancer and high-grade dysplasia in Barrett's oesophagus. *Cochrane Database Syst Rev.* 2012;11:CD007334.

Almond M, Barr L. Management controversies in Barrett's oesophagus. *Gastroenterology.* 2014;49(2):195–205.

Shaheen NJ, Sharma P, Overholt BF, et al. Radiofrequency ablation in Barrett's esophagus with dysplasia. *N Engl J Med.* 2009;360(22):2277–2288.

9. E. BE occurs in 5% to 7% of patients with GERD. It is an acquired pathology (A). The hallmark feature is the presence of intestinal goblet cells, which signifies intestinal metaplasia, on endoscopic biopsy. It occurs more commonly in males with a 3:1 ratio (B). Once BE develops, the risk of adenocarcinoma is approximately 0.5% per year. In one large study, the prevalence of cancer was 4%. Management of BE is initially medical, provided there is no evidence of severe dysplasia. However, surveillance for dysplasia is recommended in patients with BE. If severe dysplasia is present, endoscopic radioactive ablation or esophagectomy are recommended (D). In patients with BE without dysplasia, a randomized study comparing medical management with antireflux surgery showed that there were no differences between the two treatments with regard to preventing progression to dysplasia and adenocarcinoma, although antireflux surgery was more efficient than medical treatment (C).

References: Drewitz DJ, Sampliner RE, Garewal HS. The incidence of adenocarcinoma in Barrett's esophagus: a prospective study of 170 patients followed 4.8 years. *Am J Gastroenterol.* 1997;92(2):212–215.

Parrilla P, Martínez de Haro LF, Ortiz A, et al. Long-term results of a randomized prospective study comparing medical and surgical treatment of Barrett's esophagus. *Ann Surg.* 2003;237(3):291–298.

Peters, J. H, DeMeester, T. R. Esophagus and diaphragmatic hernia.

10. A. Although pharmacologic treatment for BE should be similar to that for GERD, most authorities agree that the use of PPIs is more effective in treating patients with BE. The ASPECT trial demonstrated that high-dose PPI and aspirin chemoprevention therapy, especially in combination, significantly and safely reduces the rate of cancer progression in patients with BE (D). Interestingly, in vivo studies have shown that nonsteroidal antiinflammatory drugs (NSAIDs) and statins can reduce the progression of cancer in patients with Barrett esophagus. The ASPECT trial may provide more powerful evidence to suggest the use of NSAIDs in patients with Barrett esophagus for chemoprophylaxis. Long-segment Barrett esophagus has a higher risk for high-grade dysplasia (C). Photofrin has not been demonstrated to be a useful modality (E). Dietary restrictions are helpful in Barrett esophagus and include the avoidance of fatty foods, chocolate, peppermint, alcohol, coffee, ketchup, mustard, or vinegar (B).

References: Cameron JL, Cameron AM. The management of Barrett's esophagus. In: Cameron JL, Cameron AM, eds. *Current surgical therapy*. 11th ed. Philadelphia: W.B. Saunders; 2014.

Shapiro J, van Lanschot JJB, Hulshof MCCM, et al. Neoadjuvant chemoradiotherapy plus surgery versus surgery alone for oesophageal or junctional cancer (CROSS): long-term results of a randomised controlled trial. *Lancet Oncol*. 2015;16(9):1090–1098.

Jankowski JAZ, de Caestecker J, Love SB, et al. Esomeprazole and aspirin in Barrett's oesophagus (AspECT): a randomised factorial trial. *Lancet*. 2018;392(10145):400–408.

11. B. Hiatal hernias are divided into three types. Type I, or a sliding hiatal hernia, is the most common. In this hernia, the gastroesophageal junction moves upward into the posterior mediastinum along with part of the stomach, such that the LES is above its normal position (A). The majority of these hernias are asymptomatic. Those who do have symptoms typically experience heartburn and regurgitation. In type II, or paraesophageal hernias, the gastroesophageal junction and therefore the LES are in their normal positions, as is the cardia. However, the gastric fundus is dislocated upward. The LES is neither hypertensive nor hypotensive (C, D). A type III hernia is a combination of types I and II. A hypertensive LES is characteristic of achalasia. In GERD, the LES pressure is low. GERD seems to begin from gastric distention. The distention leads to a shortening of the LES (E). As the sphincter shortens, its resting pressure decreases. The location of the LES (in the normal abdominal position or in the mediastinum) is important in GERD. Loss of abdominal length of the LES causes a decrease in LES pressure because it is no longer subjected to the positive pressure of the abdomen.

12. A. A paraesophageal hernia, or type II hiatal hernia, is also called a *rolling-type hiatal hernia*. The widened hiatus permits the fundus of the stomach to protrude into the chest, anterior and lateral to the body of the esophagus. The gastroesophageal junction remains below the diaphragm. The herniated gastric fundus rotates in a counterclockwise direction and is prone to becoming incarcerated and strangulated. This herniated portion of the stomach develops mucosal erosions (Cameron ulcers) that can lead to chronic blood loss and anemia in up to one-third of patients. Patients can also have dysphagia, heartburn, and abdominal pain. Diagnosis can be made by a barium swallow. Upper endoscopy can readily make the diagnosis on a retroflex view (C). Although incarceration is rare, most surgeons recommend elective repair of paraesophageal hernias because of the potential risk of strangulation (B, E). It is not typically preceded by trauma (D).

13. D. Manometry is an important diagnostic tool to identify predisposing conditions for esophageal disease. Characteristics of an abnormal LES include resting pressure less than 6 mmHg (normal range is 6–26 mmHg), overall length of less than 2 cm, and abdominal length less than 1 cm (A, B). Relaxation of LES with swallowing is a function of the normal swallowing mechanism and dysfunction will increase the risk for the development of achalasia (E). The resting UES is 60 to 80 mmHg (C). High UES pressures will predispose patients to pulsion diverticulum and difficulty with swallowing.

14. E. Acute variceal bleeding (AVB) is the leading cause of upper GI bleeding in patients with cirrhosis, and the management can be challenging. Early recognition and intervention are important because the progression to sepsis and multiorgan failure confers a dismal prognosis with over 90% mortality. The most important next steps in a cirrhotic presenting with AVB involve the airway, breathing, and circulation (ABCs). Airway management should take precedence over controlling AVB (B). After the ABCs, the recommended approach involves a combination of vasoactive drugs (octreotide) and endoscopic intervention. Medical management should be initiated as soon as possible because it can reduce the rate of active bleeding and improve the yield of endoscopic intervention (D). Several randomized controlled trials have been performed comparing endoscopic band ligation versus endoscopic sclerotherapy and have demonstrated the superiority of the former in both controlling bleeding and safety profile. Infection has been demonstrated to be an important predictor of mortality in AVB. Patients that receive prophylactic fluoroquinolones have been shown to have a reduced incidence of AVB and improved survival (C). In patients with chronic esophageal varices, beta-blockers can be used to prevent episodes of rebleeding (A).

References: Calès P, Masliah C, Bernard B, et al. Early administration of vapreotide for variceal bleeding in patients with cirrhosis. *N Engl J Med*. 2001;344(1):23–28.

Hou MC, Lin HC, Liu TT, et al. Antibiotic prophylaxis after endoscopic therapy prevents rebleeding in acute variceal hemorrhage: a randomized trial. *Hepatology*. 2004;39(3):746–753.

Jensen DM, Kovacs T, Randall G. Emergency sclerotherapy vs rubber band ligation for actively bleeding esophageal varices in a randomized prospective study. *Gastrointest Endosc*. 1994;40:241.

Lo GH, Lai KH, Cheng JS, et al. Emergency banding ligation versus sclerotherapy for the control of active bleeding from esophageal varices. *Hepatology*. 1997;25(5):1101–1104.

15. D. This patient has achalasia, a primary motility disorder of the esophagus, specifically of the LES. The pathogenesis is presumed to be neurogenic degeneration of ganglion cells, which can be idiopathic or infectious (i.e., Chagas disease from *Trypanosoma cruzi*). The degeneration results in a failure of the LES to relax on swallowing, leading to an increase in intraluminal esophageal pressure, marked esophageal dilation (with an air–fluid level on radiograph), and loss of progressive peristalsis in the body of the esophagus. The classic triad of symptoms is dysphagia, regurgitation, and weight loss. There are four basic treatment options, all of which are considered palliative procedures as there is no cure. According to recent American College of Gastroenterology Clinical Guidelines, initial therapy should be *either* graded pneumatic dilation or laparoscopic surgical myotomy with a *partial* fundoplication in patients fit to undergo surgery. Esophageal pneumatic dilation is a better option in patients with higher operative risk and is safer than previously thought, but patients will often require multiple dilations over time. For low-risk patients or those who have failed balloon dilation, a laparoscopic esophagomyotomy with an anterior fundoplication (Dor) or partial, 270-degree posterior fundoplication (Toupet) should be performed. A recent multicenter, randomized controlled trial found that although a lower percentage of patients with a Toupet fundoplication had an abnormal 24-hour pH test when compared with a Dor fundoplication, the differences were not statistically significant, and either approach would be appropriate. A complete fundoplication, or a Nissen, has a high chance of causing recurrent dysphagia in this patient population (B). Medical management with calcium channel blockers and nitroglycerin can help relax the LES, but this treatment only relieves symptoms in less than 10% of patients. These medications are only considered in patients who are not appropriate surgical candidates (C). In high-risk elderly patients, injection of the LES with botulinum toxin can provide short-term relief. Botulinum toxin should be avoided in patients who would otherwise be appropriate surgical candidates because it can ruin the anatomic planes required for surgery. Nutcracker esophagus is characterized by high-amplitude peristaltic waves of the esophagus (A). Esophageal diverticula can be associated with a hypertrophic upper esophageal sphincter. POEM is an emerging option but requires a long learning curve. Up to 50% of patients can have acid reflux following the procedure (E).

References: Campos GM, Vittinghoff E, Rabl C. Endoscopic and surgical treatments for achalasia: a systemic review and meta-analysis. *Ann Surg.* 2009;249(1):45–57.

Hoogerwerf WA, Pasricha PJ. Achalasia: treatment options revisited. *Can J Gastroenterol.* 2000;14(5):406–409.

Rawlings A, Soper NJ, Oelschlager B, et al. Laparoscopic Dor versus Toupet fundoplication following Heller myotomy for achalasia: results of a multicenter, prospective, randomized-controlled trial. *Surg Endosc.* 2012;26(1):18–26.

Vaezi M, Richter J, Wilcox C. Botulinum toxin versus pneumatic dilatation in the treatment of achalasia: a randomized trial. *Gut.* 1999;44(2):231–239.

16. B. The decision of how to proceed in an iatrogenic esophageal perforation depends on five factors: whether it is a free or contained perforation, the duration of time that the perforation has been present, the underlying pathology in the esophagus, whether severe inflammation is present at surgery, and the patient's condition. As a general rule, if the perforation is contained, as shown on an esophagogram, management can be conservative (A). If it is a small free perforation, surgery is indicated with primary repair with or without an intercostal muscle flap. Resection of an injured esophagus with cervical esophagostomy (spit fistula), gastrostomy, and feeding jejunostomy is reserved for situations in which there has been a long delay in diagnosis (>72 hours), severe inflammation is present, or the patient is extremely ill or disabled (B). If the underlying disease

requires an esophagectomy (e.g., cancer, severe burn), immediate esophagectomy with reconstruction is recommended if feasible (limited inflammation and minimal delay) (D). Stenting is generally reserved for unresectable cancer (E). An iatrogenic perforation in a patient with achalasia will need to have the perforation addressed as discussed above and will also need definitive management of the underlying disease provided the person is not extremely ill. The treatment of choice is a left thoracotomy, primary repair, and longitudinal myotomy on the contralateral side with or without fundoplication. Laparoscopic repair is increasing in popularity but will still need a myotomy on the contralateral side of the perforation (C).

References: Fernandez FF, Richter A, Freudenberg S, Wendl K, Manegold BC. Treatment of endoscopic esophageal perforation. *Surg Endosc.* 1999;13(10):962–966.

Hunt DR, Wills VL, Weis B, Jorgensen JO, DeCarle DJ, Coo IJ. Management of esophageal perforation after pneumatic dilation for achalasia. *J Gastrointest Surg.* 2000;4(4):411–415.

17. D. Leiomyomas are the most common benign tumor in the esophagus, accounting for more than 50% of benign tumors. However, benign masses constitute only 10% of esophageal tumors. They have a small risk of malignant degeneration (C). Leiomyomas only become symptomatic when they are very large (>5 cm). Otherwise, they are incidentally discovered during the course of other studies. They have a characteristic appearance on barium swallow of a smooth, crescent-shaped filling defect that encroaches on the lumen. On endoscopy, the mucosa is usually intact, and the tumor moves up and down with swallowing. If it has the characteristic appearance, the tumor should not undergo biopsy because of an increased risk of mucosal perforation. This can create scarring that may affect later efforts at resection (E). Esophageal ultrasonography is very useful in the diagnosis of leiomyomas because it will demonstrate a homogeneous region of hypoechogenicity. Treatment is to enucleate the mass, which can be done via a videoscopic approach with intraoperative esophagoscopy (A). The cell of origin of these tumors is mesenchymal. The average age at presentation is 38 years, and they are twice as common in males and most commonly located in the lower two-thirds of the esophagus. Leiomyomas are usually solitary, but multiple tumors are seen in as many as 10% of patients (B).

Reference: Aurea P, Grazia M, Petrella F, Bazzocchi R. Giant leiomyoma of the esophagus. *Eur J Cardiothorac Surg.* 2002;22(6):1008–1010.

18. D. A Zenker diverticulum is a false esophageal diverticulum that does not contain all layers of the esophagus; it is also a type of pulsion diverticulum (A). A pulsion diverticulum forms at a point of weakness and is due to alterations in luminal pressure. Conversely, a traction diverticulum is from external pulling on the esophageal wall, such as from inflamed lymph nodes with tuberculosis. Zenker diverticulum is the most common type of esophageal diverticulum. It usually presents in older patients (>60 years). It characteristically arises at a point of weakness, most commonly at the Killian triangle, which is formed by the inferior fibers of the inferior constrictor muscle and the superior border of the cricopharyngeus muscle. Patients typically present with dysphagia, regurgitation of undigested food, halitosis, episodes of aspiration, and salivation (C). With the characteristic history, the first diagnostic study is a barium swallow. In the absence of other pathology (such as an irregular mucosa), endoscopy is not needed (B). Treatment is surgical by either open or endoscopic techniques. The open technique involves cervical esophagomyotomy with stapling and amputation of the diverticulum. The endoscopic technique involves division of the common wall between the diverticulum and the esophagus. Studies have shown that results with the endoscopic technique are better with larger diverticula (E). Diverticula smaller than 3 cm are too short to accommodate one cartridge of staples and to allow complete division of the sphincter; therefore, this size is considered a contraindication to this technique.

References: Bonavina L, Bona D, Abraham M, Saino G, Abate E. Long-term results of endosurgical and open surgical approach for Zenker diverticulum. *World J Gastroenterol.* 2007;13(18):2586–2589.

Collard JM, Otte JB, Kestens PJ. Endoscopic stapling technique of esophagodiverticulostomy for Zenker's diverticulum. *Ann Thorac Surg.* 1993;56(3):573–576.

Narne S, Cutrone C, Bonavina L, Chella B, Peracchia A. Endoscopic diverticulotomy for the treatment of Zenker's diverticulum: results in 102 patients with staple-assisted endoscopy. *Ann Otol Rhinol Laryngol.* 1999;108(8):810–815.

19. A. Cricopharyngeal dysfunction has multiple causes, including such neurogenic and myogenic etiologies as stroke, multiple sclerosis, peripheral neuropathy, Parkinson disease, and dermatomyositis. The exact cause is unknown, but the primary theory is that the cricopharyngeus muscle, which is normally in a state of tonic contraction, fails to relax and allow the passage of food into the cervical esophagus. This produces a Zenker diverticulum, which is considered a false diverticulum (only involves an outpouching of the mucosa and submucosa) and can be confirmed with a barium swallow (C). Endoscopic evaluation of a suspected Zenker diverticulum is discouraged as it can lead to an iatrogenic perforation. Patients describe difficulty swallowing food, which worsens throughout the day as the diverticulum increasingly gets filled with food. Another key element of the diagnosis is the classic history of an inability to handle saliva secretion, such that the patient describes expectoration of saliva. Patients also report hoarseness. Diverticulectomy is often performed during surgery for a Zenker diverticulum. However, the most important aspect of management is cricopharyngeal myotomy, which is necessary to correct the underlying pathology (B). Weight loss results from a decreased caloric intake. Although one should always be suspicious of carcinoma in a patient with difficulty swallowing and weight loss, the long duration of symptoms makes carcinoma unlikely (D, E).

References: Cameron JL, Cameron AM. The management of Barrett's esophagus. In: Cameron JL, Cameron AM, eds. Current surgical therapy. 11th ed. Philadelphia: W.B. Saunders; 2014.

Cameron JL, Cameron AM. The management of pharyngeal esophageal (Zenker) diverticula. 11th ed. Philadelphia, PA: W.B. Saunders; 2014.

20. B. Patients with newly diagnosed esophageal cancer frequently present with poor nutritional status, which only worsens after starting neoadjuvant therapy. As such, although nutritional optimization is an important component in the management of esophageal cancer, the optimal approach remains undefined. Percutaneous gastrostomy, however, should be discouraged because it may compromise the gastric conduit needed during esophageal reconstruction and will delay chemotherapy for an additional 2 to 4 weeks. The role for parenteral nutrition is limited because of its high cost and high rate of complications (A). Nasogastric tube insertion can lead to migration of the tube and aspiration (D). Esophageal stents are frequently offered because they can significantly improve the dysphagia associated with esophageal cancer. Unfortunately, its role in improving nutritional status has had inconsistent results in the literature (C). Stent migration and chest discomfort are common and lead to the frequent removal of the stents (E). Additional studies are needed to determine the best approach for nutritional optimization in this patient population.

References: Jones CM, Griffiths EA. Should oesophageal stents be placed before neo-adjuvant therapy to treat dysphagia in patients awaiting oesophagectomy? Best evidence topic (BET). *Int J Surg.* 2014;12(11):1172–1180.

Mão-de-Ferro S, Serrano M, Ferreira S, et al. Stents in patients with esophageal cancer before chemoradiotherapy: high risk of complications and no impact on the nutritional status. *Eur J Clin Nutr.* 2016;70(3):409–410.

Naharaja V, Cox MR, Eslick GD. Safety and efficacy of esophageal stents preceding or during neoadjuvant chemotherapy for esophageal cancer: a systemic review and meta-analysis. *J Gastrointest Oncol.* 2014;5(2):119–126.

21. C. Surgical intervention in esophageal cancer is an area of active research. The three standard approaches include TTE, THE, and a combination of the two using a three-incision esophagectomy. TTH was initially described as a two-stage procedure by Dr. Ivor Lewis in which he performed mobilization of the stomach using an upper midline laparotomy incision followed by resection of the esophagus using a right thoracotomy incision several days later (A). A large multicenter prospective study comparing THE and TTE failed to demonstrate any difference in overall mortality and morbidity between the two approaches (D). However, THE has been shown in several studies to be associated with a lower total hospital length of stay (B). THE is performed with a left cervical incision and midline laparotomy (E). It is often performed for patients with distal esophageal cancer.

References: D'Amico TA. Outcomes after surgery for esophageal cancer. *Gastrointest Cancer Res.* 2007;1(5):188–196.

Hulscher JB, Tijssen JG, Obertop H, van Lanschot JJ. Transthoracic versus transhiatal resection for carcinoma of the esophagus: a meta-analysis. *Ann Thorac Surg.* 2001;72(1):306–313.

Litle VR, Buenaventura PO, Luketich JD. Minimally invasive resection for esophageal cancer. *Surg Clin North Am.* 2002;82(4):711–728.

Rentz J, Bull D, Harpole D, et al. Transthoracic versus transhiatal esophagectomy: a prospective study of 945 patients. *J Thorac Cardiovasc Surg.* 2003;125(5):1114–1120.

Alimentary Tract—Stomach

NAVEEN BALAN, AMY KIM YETASOOK, AND KATHRYN T. CHEN

8

ABSITE 99th Percentile High-Yields

I. Ulcers
   A. Peptic ulcer disease (PUD): imbalance of pepsin/acid and mucosal protection
      1. Almost always caused by *Helicobacter pylori* (gram-negative spirochete) and NSAID overuse
      2. Triple therapy: PPI, clarithromycin, amoxicillin, or metronidazole ×14 days
      3. Daintree Johnson classification for types of gastric ulcers
         a) Type I: along lesser curvature in the antrum, solitary, not acid associated
         b) Type II: prepyloric, solitary, acid associated
         c) Type III: prepyloric and duodenal, one in each location, acid associated
         d) Type IV: proximal stomach/cardia, solitary, not acid associated
         e) Type V: anywhere in the stomach, usually multiple, NSAID associated
      4. Biopsy all gastric ulcers: higher risk of cancer

Operation	Procedure	Result	Complication
Antrectomy	Resection of distal stomach (need reconstruction with Billroth I or II)	Removal of antral G cells	Incomplete antrectomy can lead to continued ulcer disease
Truncal vagotomy (TV)	Ligation of anterior and posterior vagal trunks 4 cm proximal to GEJ	Removal of vagal stimulation to gastric body parietal cells, decreasing acid secretion	Loss of parasympathetic innervation to pylorus which prevents gastric emptying (primarily to solid foods)
Selective vagotomy (SV)	Ligation of anterior and posterior vagal trunks distal to hepatic/celiac branches		Lower rate of delayed gastric emptying but higher risk of recurrent ulcer disease
Highly selective vagotomy (HSV)	Similar to SV except preserves crow's foot fibers innervating pylorus and antrum		Lowest rate of delayed gastric emptying but highest risk of recurrent ulcer disease
Pyloroplasty	Widen the pyloric channel, multiple approaches	Improved gastric emptying (usually with TV/SV)	Can lead to rapid gastric emptying

   B. Surgical indications: surgery for bleeding PUD entails oversewing of the ulcer (to ligate the bleeding artery) with consideration for truncal vagotomy (to decrease acid secretion); more time-consuming procedures (selective vagotomy) reserved for elective ulcer surgery, as are antrectomy and Billroth II (when obstruction complicates PUD)

1. Truncal vagotomy and selective vagotomy always need drainage procedure (e.g., pyloroplasty) whereas highly selective vagotomy does not

Duodenal Ulcer*	
Problem	*Treatment*
Bleeding	Oversew bleeder
Perforation	Graham patch

*For gastric ulcer, first-line treatment is same; however, first biopsy ulcer to rule out malignancy.

II. Upper Gastrointestinal Bleed
   A. Medical management: hydration, PPI bid (noninferior to continuous PPI) ×72 hours
   B. Procedural interventions: endoscopic hemostasis attempts ×2, angioembolization (usually GDA); 2nd look EGD only for high-risk lesion (visible vessel or adherent clot)
   C. Surgery indications: multiple failed endoscopies, hemodynamic instability, associated perforation

III. Bariatric Surgery
   A. Indications:
      1. BMI >40 (morbid obesity) or BMI 35 to 40 with ≥1 weight-related comorbidity (diabetes, hypertension, hyperlipidemia, GERD, obstructive sleep apnea, pseudotumor cerebri, severe life-limiting arthritis)
   B. Sleeve gastrectomy: most commonly performed, lower excess body weight (EBW) loss and incidence of vitamin deficiency; postoperative complications include staple line leak, bleeding, de novo reflux, incisura stricture, twisting/kinking of sleeve, weight regain
   C. Roux-en-Y gastric bypass: higher EBW loss and incidence of vitamin deficiency; postoperative complications include anastomotic leak, internal hernia, marginal ulcer, perforated marginal ulcer, bile reflux, jejunojejunostomy, intussusception, roux stasis syndrome, gastrogastric fistula, dumping syndrome, and weight regain
   D. Pulmonary embolus is leading cause of death, occurring within a few weeks after discharge
   E. Common postoperative complications:

Complication	Symptoms	Etiology	Management
Alkaline reflux (requires surgery more than any other postgastrectomy syndrome)	Bilious emesis does NOT relieve epigastric pain	Bile reflux into the stomach usually with Billroth II anatomy	Workup with EGD (pathology: foveolar hyperplasia with mucosal congestion and edema); confirm with HIDA demonstrating biliary secretion into stomach/esophagus; treatment: convert to Roux-en-Y
Small intestinal bacterial overgrowth (SIBO)	Bloating, chronic watery diarrhea	Bacterial overgrowth in blind loop due to immotility	Labs for B12 deficiency, macrocytic anemia, confirm with lactulose breath test and treat with antibiotics (rifaximin)
Early dumping syndrome	Nausea, vomiting, diarrhea 15–30 min postprandially	Hyperosmolar load and release of serotonin, neurotensin, bradykinins, and enteroglucagon	Eat smaller, more frequent meals with low carbs, high protein, and fat throughout the day, separate solids from liquids, octreotide is most effective
Late dumping syndrome	Dizziness, fatigue, diaphoresis 1–3 h postprandially	High carbohydrate load causing hyperinsulinemia leading to reactive hypoglycemia	Similar to above; if refractory, convert to Roux-en-Y
Marginal ulcer	Nausea, pain, and perforation/bleeding at anastomosis	NSAIDs, smoking, *H. pylori* infection, acid exposure to small bowel	Discontinue NSAIDs, treat *H. pylori*, give acid suppression therapy, bleeding or perforation may need surgery

IV. Gastric Cancer
  A. Adenocarcinoma: risk factors include *H. pylori* infection, diet (high salt, nitrosamine-containing foods), obesity, smoking, ETOH, hereditary diffuse gastric cancer (*CDH1* mutations)
    1. Staging: EGD for biopsy, EUS for T/N stage, CT chest/abdomen/pelvis, +/− PET-CT, diagnostic laparoscopy to evaluate for peritoneal disease
    2. Early gastric cancer: cTis or T1a-endoscopic or surgical resection; T1b-surgical resection with 5 cm gross margins to achieve R0 resection
    3. Locoregional disease: T2+ or nodal involvement need neoadjuvant chemotherapy followed by surgical resection and adjuvant chemotherapy
    4. Surgical options: distal versus subtotal versus total gastrectomy with R0 goal, need 16 lymph nodes; *CDH1* needs total gastrectomy, also acceptable option for palliation in stage IV disease
    5. Siewert-Stein classification:
       a) Type I: epicenter within 1 to 5 cm above GE junction, treat as esophageal cancer
       b) Type II: epicenter within 1 cm above and 2 cm below GE junction, treat as esophageal cancer
       c) Type III: epicenter within 2 to 5 cm below GE junction, treat as stomach cancer
    6. Incidence of PROXIMAL gastric cancer has been rising the fastest (due to obesity and reflux); proximal gastric cancer is two times more common in men and white race
    7. *H. pylori* is PROTECTIVE against proximal gastric cancer but associated with increased risk of distal gastric cancer
  B. Gastrointestinal stromal tumor (GIST)
    1. Endoscopy: submucosal mass with central umbilication and ulceration
    2. Essential features: majority due to mutations in protooncogene *KIT* (most common) or *PDGFRA*; spindle cell histology; can occur anywhere along GI tract, but stomach is most common (60%) followed by jejunum/ileum
    3. High-risk features for recurrence: tumor size >5 cm or >5 mitoses/hpf
    4. Imatinib: tyrosine kinase inhibitor, highest response rate with exon 11 *KIT* mutation
       a) Neoadjuvant therapy: use when surgical resection will result in significant morbidity
       b) Adjuvant therapy: high-risk features for recurrence and tumor rupture during surgery
  C. MALT lymphoma: B-cell lymphoma, arises in the setting of chronic *H. pylori* infection
    1. Histology: lymphoepithelial lesions are pathognomonic
    2. Treatment: triple or quadruple antibiotic therapy will eradicate cancer in majority of early cases

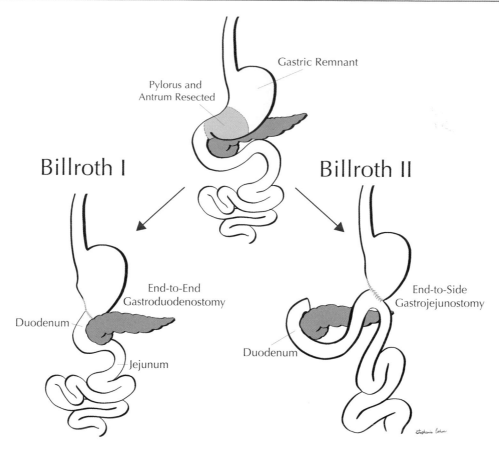

In the **Billroth I** operation, the distal stomach is resected and an anastamosis is created between the gastric remnant and the duodenum in an end-to-end fashion. There is no duodenal stump, and there is only one suture line. Although a Billroth I is more physiologic, it is associated with higher rates of gastric outlet obstruction.

In a **Billroth II** reconstruction, an anastamosis is created between the gastric remnant and the jejunum in a side-to-side or end-to-side fashion. There are two suture lines, one to close the duodenal stump and the other at the gastrojejunostomy.

Fig. 8.1

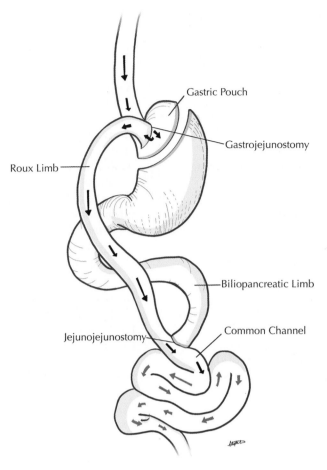

Fig. 8.2

Questions

1. A 56-year-old male with fatigue undergoes upper endoscopy after initial workup shows a microcytic anemia. He is found to have an ulcer with irregular borders with biopsy showing a dense lymphoid infiltrate with prominent lymphoepithelial lesions. Which of the following is true for this malignancy?
   A. Tumors with chromosomal translocation t(11;18) respond poorly to antibiotics
   B. After successful treatment, yearly endoscopy is used for surveillance
   C. It is most commonly a result of a gram-positive rod
   D. There is no role for surgical resection
   E. Early-stage disease requires chemoradiation as first-line treatment

2. A 46-year-old female was incidentally found to have a pedunculated mass along the greater curvature of the stomach on CT imaging following a motor vehicle collision. Further workup with endoscopy shows a submucosal mass with central umbilication and ulceration that is found to be CD117-positive after biopsy. Which of the following is true regarding the management of this lesion?
   A. It is considered a radiosensitive tumor
   B. The highest response rate to therapy involves mutations in the KIT proto-oncogene at exon 11
   C. It arises from an endodermal-derived component
   D. Most patients become symptomatic early in the course of their disease
   E. Early tumors can be treated with endoscopic mucosal resection

3. A 41-year-old female presents to the emergency department with acute severe abdominal pain and nausea but no vomiting. She reports a history of uncomplicated Roux-en-Y gastric bypass years ago but denies other abdominal surgeries. Abdominal exam reveals mild tenderness without guarding or rebound tenderness. A CT scan shows dilated proximal small bowel but no intraabdominal free air or fluid. What is the next best step in the management of this patient?
   A. Advise the patient to eat smaller, more frequent meals
   B. Exploratory laparotomy
   C. Nasogastric tube decompression followed by 24-hour water-soluble contrast challenge
   D. Antibiotic therapy
   E. Upper endoscopy

4. A 40-year-old male with severe epigastric pain is found to have multiple duodenal ulcers on EGD. What is the normal location of the cells that secrete the majority of the hormone that is being overproduced in this patient?
   A. Stomach body
   B. Stomach antrum
   C. Pancreas
   D. Duodenum
   E. Jejunum

5. Three years after a laparoscopic Roux-en-Y gastric bypass (LRYGB), a 45-year-old male presents with symptoms and signs of a small bowel obstruction (SBO). He reports a 150-lb weight loss. Which of the following is the most likely etiology?
   A. An internal hernia
   B. Adhesions
   C. Roux compression due to mesocolon scarring
   D. Kinking of the jejunojejunostomy
   E. Incarcerated abdominal wall hernia

6. A 79-year-old male with chronic back pain and chronic obstructive pulmonary disease (COPD) requiring supplemental oxygen presents to the emergency department (ED) with epigastric abdominal pain that started suddenly 2 days ago. His abdominal examination is significant for epigastric tenderness but is otherwise unremarkable. A computed tomography (CT) scan demonstrates a small amount of free air under the right hemidiaphragm but no contrast extravasation. An upper gastrointestinal (GI) water-soluble contrast study demonstrates a duodenal ulcer but no extravasation. Which of the following is the best management?
   A. Nasogastric tube decompression, intravenous (IV) antibiotics, and proton pump inhibitor (PPI)
   B. Exploratory laparotomy
   C. Diagnostic laparoscopy
   D. Oral antibiotics, clear liquid diet for 2 weeks, and follow-up in clinic
   E. Serial abdominal exam in the ED for 6 to 8 hours and, if improving, he may be discharged with oral antibiotics

7. Which of the following is true regarding the management of obesity?
   A. Indications for bariatric surgery include a body mass index (BMI) greater than 30 with weight-related comorbidities or BMI greater than 35
   B. Sibutramine acts by inhibiting pancreatic lipase
   C. Roux-en-Y gastric bypass (RYGB) does not have a restrictive component
   D. RYGB has a lower 30-day mortality compared with biliopancreatic diversion (BPD)
   E. Patients with obesity-related comorbidities do not need to attempt nonoperative management before obesity surgery

8. Which of the following is the gold standard for the diagnosis of gastroparesis?
   A. Upper endoscopy
   B. Plain abdominal x-rays
   C. Nuclear medicine scan
   D. CT
   E. It is considered a clinical diagnosis.

9. Which of the following is true regarding gallstone disease after weight loss surgery?
   A. The rate of postoperative cholecystectomy is the same regardless of the type of weight loss surgery
   B. Prophylactic cholecystectomy should be performed at the time of surgery in most patients
   C. Ursodiol is recommended for 6 months after gastric bypass surgery
   D. Decreased secretion of calcium and mucin contributes to gallstone formation after weight loss surgery
   E. Acute cholecystitis after weight loss surgery is uncommon

10. Which of the following is the first manifestation of gastric leak following Roux-en-Y gastric bypass?
    A. Abdominal pain
    B. Tachycardia
    C. Nausea
    D. Increased serum glucose
    E. Tachypnea

11. A 45-year-old male with a history of laparoscopic gastric banding 5 years ago presents to the ED with complaints of pain at his port site. He first noticed it several days ago after he got his gastric band adjusted in clinic. On exam, the port site appears erythematous, warm, and is tender to palpation. He is afebrile and normotensive. Which of the following is the best next step?
    A. CT of the abdomen
    B. Admit to the hospital, start IV antibiotics and fluid resuscitation
    C. EGD
    D. Incision and drainage
    E. Discharge with oral antibiotics

12. A 60-year-old man presents with a 12-hour history of worsening epigastric pain. He has a history of duodenal ulcer, and the results of a recent biopsy 2 weeks earlier were negative for *Helicobacter pylori*. Upright chest radiograph demonstrates free air under the diaphragm. The patient is hemodynamically stable. At surgery, a perforated duodenal ulcer is found with mild peritoneal contamination. Which of the following is the best management option?
    A. Graham patch of duodenal ulcer
    B. Graham patch of duodenal ulcer with truncal vagotomy and pyloroplasty
    C. Truncal vagotomy and antrectomy with Billroth I reconstruction
    D. Truncal vagotomy and antrectomy with Billroth II reconstruction
    E. Graham patch of duodenal ulcer with a highly selective vagotomy

13. Which of the following is true regarding postvagotomy diarrhea?
    A. It is effectively treated with octreotide
    B. It does not improve with oral cholestyramine
    C. Cardiovascular manifestations are common
    D. Most patients require the creation of a reversed jejunal segment
    E. Diarrhea may improve with the administration of codeine

14. A 45-year-old woman is undergoing an exploratory laparotomy for Zollinger-Ellison syndrome (ZES). Preoperative localization studies failed to demonstrate the location of the tumor. At surgery, no obvious tumor is seen despite an extensive Kocher maneuver and careful inspection. An intraoperative ultrasound scan is negative. The next step in the management would be:
    A. Closing the abdomen
    B. Distal pancreatectomy and splenectomy
    C. Proximal pancreaticoduodenectomy
    D. Blind proximal duodenotomy
    E. Blind distal duodenotomy

15. Which of the following is true regarding TNM (tumor, nodes, and metastases) staging for gastric adenocarcinoma?
    A. Computed tomography scan is the most accurate means of determining T and N staging
    B. The accuracy of endoscopic ultrasound (EUS) is higher for N stage than T stage
    C. Fifteen lymph nodes are required for an oncologic resection to appropriately stage the patient
    D. Magnetic resonance imaging (MRI) with gadolinium should be routinely performed
    E. T3 invades the subserosa

16. Which of the following is associated with hypergastrinemia?
    A. Diabetes
    B. Hypothyroidism
    C. Hyperparathyroidism
    D. Chronic gastritis
    E. D-cell hyperplasia

17. A 46-year-old male undergoes a distal gastrectomy for a tumor in the gastric antrum that was biopsy proven to be adenocarcinoma. The specimen is sent for pathology. Pathology reveals microscopic evidence of tumor at the margins. Which of the following most accurately describes this resection?
    A. D1 resection
    B. D2 resection
    C. R0 resection
    D. R1 resection
    E. R2 resection

18. Which of the following is considered to be a risk factor for gastric cancer?
    A. Pernicious anemia
    B. Blood group O
    C. Carbonated acidic soda
    D. Female sex
    E. Diabetes

19. Which of the following is true regarding the types of gastric ulcers?
    A. Type II ulcers are the most common
    B. Type IV ulcers occur near the gastroesophageal junction
    C. Type I ulcers usually have increased acid secretion
    D. Type III ulcers are associated with decreased acid secretion
    E. Type I gastric ulcers are prepyloric

20. Which of the following is true regarding gastrointestinal stromal tumor (GIST)?
    A. The extent of the tumor is best determined preoperatively by endoscopy
    B. They arise from smooth muscle cells
    C. Malignant potential is readily determined by histologic features
    D. They can be managed by laparoscopic wedge resection
    E. They rarely present with GI bleeding

21. Which of the following is true regarding postgastrectomy bile reflux?
    A. It is more likely to occur after a Billroth I than a Billroth II reconstruction
    B. Symptoms usually correlate with the amount of bile entering the stomach
    C. In symptomatic patients, medical management is generally effective
    D. Creation of a Roux-en-Y gastrojejunostomy is an effective surgical option
    E. Most patients with bile reflux into the stomach will develop symptoms

22. The best test for localization of a gastrinoma is:
    A. MRI
    B. CT
    C. Abdominal ultrasound
    D. Octreotide scan
    E. Selective angiography

23. The best test to confirm eradication of *H. pylori* after treatment is:
    A. *H. pylori* serology
    B. Urea breath test
    C. Rapid urease test
    D. Histologic biopsy
    E. Antral mucosal biopsy with culture

24. Which of the following is true regarding a highly selective vagotomy (HSV)?
    A. The anterior and posterior vagal trunks are divided
    B. The nerve of Grassi is spared
    C. The anterior Latarjet nerve is divided
    D. The crow's feet to the antrum are spared
    E. The celiac branch is divided

25. The most common metabolic disorder after gastric resection is a deficiency of:
    A. Iron
    B. Vitamin B12
    C. Folate
    D. Calcium
    E. Vitamin D

26. Which of the following is true regarding ZES?
    A. Symptoms decrease with fasting
    B. Ulcers are most often located in the distal duodenum
    C. It is most commonly familial
    D. It is the most common functional neuroendocrine tumor
    E. Treatment with proton pump inhibitors (PPIs) can control symptoms in the majority of patients

27. A 70-year-old man presents with an 8-hour history of acute abdominal pain and a history of melena. On examination, the patient is febrile to 101°F, with a blood pressure of 105/70 mmHg and a heart rate of 130 beats per minute and has diffuse abdominal tenderness with rebound and guarding. The rectal examination is guaiac positive. Laboratory values are significant for a white blood cell count of 16,000 cells/μL and a hematocrit of 26%. CT demonstrates extravasation of oral contrast in the proximal duodenum. After resuscitation, management consists of:
    A. Closure of the perforation with omental patch plus an HSV
    B. Closure of the perforation and omental patch via the open approach
    C. Perform duodenotomy over perforation, oversew posterior ulcer, close duodenotomy, and place omental patch
    D. Vagotomy and antrectomy with oversewing of the posterior ulcer and omental patch
    E. Closure of the perforation and omental patch via laparoscopic approach

28. A 50-year-old woman with a history of diabetes presents with symptoms of early satiety, nausea, vomiting, and epigastric pain. Upper endoscopy reveals a large mass of undigested food particles in the stomach that is partially obstructing the pylorus. Which of the following is true regarding this condition?
    A. Most patients require surgery
    B. It can be treated with oral administration of cellulase
    C. Psychiatric treatment is critical in long-term management
    D. The patient likely has patchy areas of alopecia
    E. Peptic ulcer disease is a risk factor

29. A 70-year-old man presents to the ED with sudden onset of severe epigastric pain associated with retching but with little vomitus. His blood pressure is 140/90 mmHg and his heart rate is 90 beats per minute. Attempts by the ED physician to place a nasogastric tube are unsuccessful. An upright chest radiograph reveals a large gas bubble just above the left diaphragm. Which of the following is true regarding this condition?
    A. The stomach is likely twisted along the axis, transecting the lesser and greater curvature
    B. In children it is largely due to a paraesophageal hernia
    C. It is associated with Bergman's triad
    D. Percutaneous gastrostomy tube for definitive management is acceptable in select patients
    E. It is initially managed conservatively for the majority of patients

30. Which of the following describes the association between Sister Mary Joseph nodule and gastric cancer?
    A. A metastatic left axillary lymph node
    B. A metastatic left supraclavicular lymph node
    C. An ovarian mass from gastric metastasis
    D. Umbilical metastasis suggesting carcinomatosis
    E. An anterior nodule palpable on rectal examination suggesting drop metastasis

31. A 68-year-old woman presents with an upper GI hemorrhage. She has a history of ulcer disease and has recently completed a treatment for *H. pylori*. Upper endoscopy reveals brisk arterial bleeding from a duodenal ulcer located on the posterior wall. Despite numerous attempts to control the bleeding endoscopically, the ulcer continues to bleed. The patient has received 4 units of blood. Her hematocrit is 25%, her blood pressure is 110/60 mmHg, and her heart rate is 120 beats per minute. Which of the following is the best management option?
    A. Duodenotomy, oversewing the ulcer, truncal vagotomy, and pyloroplasty
    B. Duodenotomy and oversewing the ulcer
    C. Truncal vagotomy and antrectomy with Billroth I reconstruction
    D. Truncal vagotomy and antrectomy with Billroth II reconstruction
    E. Highly selective vagotomy

32. A 42-year-old alcoholic male with recurrent episodes of pancreatitis presents to the ED with one episode of hematemesis in the morning. He does not appear to have any active bleeding currently. CT scan demonstrates splenic artery thrombosis. Lipase and liver function tests are normal. EGD demonstrates isolated gastric varices that are not currently bleeding and one 2-cm ulcer at the angularis. Which of the following endoscopic features confers the lowest risk of rebleeding?
    A. Oozing ulcer
    B. Nonbleeding ulcer with overlying clot
    C. Nonbleeding visible vessel
    D. Visible ulcer base
    E. Flat pigmented spot

33. Which of the following is true regarding gastric polyps?
    A. Fundic gastric polyps have the highest risk of harboring malignant cells
    B. Adenomatous gastric polyps are the most common type
    C. Hamartomatous polyps are associated with *H. pylori* infection
    D. Heterotopic polyps most commonly present with gastrointestinal bleeding
    E. Inflammatory polyps do not have a risk of malignancy

34. Bleeding from a Dieulafoy gastric lesion is due to:
    A. Antral vascular ectasia
    B. Abnormal gastric rugal folds
    C. Ingested foreign material
    D. An abnormal submucosal vessel
    E. A premalignant lesion

35. The most sensitive and specific diagnostic test for gastrinoma is:
    A. Basal and stimulated gastric acid outputs
    B. Octreotide scan
    C. Fasting serum gastrin
    D. Calcium stimulation test
    E. Secretin stimulation test

Answers

1. A. Lymphoepithelial tissue on biopsy is virtually pathognomonic for gastric MALT lymphoma, an indolent malignancy primarily thought to arise from chronic *H. pylori* infection (gram-negative spirochete) (C). Treatment with triple therapy or quadruple therapy antibiotics to eradicate *H. pylori* is the first-line treatment for patients with early-stage 1 or 2 disease. Most cases take 1 year to achieve remission; however, although rare, it can take up to 3 years. Refractory cases, as well as stage 3 and 4 disease, require chemoradiation using CHOP (cyclophosphamide, doxorubicin, vincristine, and prednisone) (E). Surgical resection is reserved for cases complicated by perforation, bleeding, or obstruction (D). Tumor biology affects the response to antibiotics, namely the t(11;18) chromosomal translocation that has a <5% response to antibiotics alone and requires additional treatment with radiation therapy or rituximab. After successful treatment with antibiotics, surveillance endoscopy is needed 3 months after treatment to check for eradication of *H. pylori* and to evaluate for recurrence (B).

Reference: Liu H, Ye H, Ruskone-Fourmestraux A, et al. T(11;18) is a marker for all stage gastric MALT lymphomas that will not respond to H. pylori eradication. *Gastroenterology.* 2002;122(5):1286–1294.

2. B. Gastric GIST can be diagnosed on upper endoscopy, classically as a submucosal mass with central umbilication and ulceration. On pathologic evaluation, the majority express CD117 (c-kit), as well as CD-34. It arises from mesodermal-derived components and grows intraluminal (C). Patients thus present late with obstruction or they outgrow the blood supply, presenting with necrosis and hemorrhage into the gastric lumen (D). GISTs are not radiosensitive or responsive to traditional chemotherapy (A). However, the KIT proto-oncogene encodes for a receptor tyrosine kinase that, when mutated, becomes constitutively active and leads to mitogenic activity and tumorigenesis. Imatinib, a tyrosine kinase inhibitor (TKI), has emerged as an important adjunct in the management of gastric GISTs, with high response rates: 90% for exon 11 mutations and 50% for exon 9 mutations in KIT. Neoadjuvant therapy with imatinib can be used to downsize tumors when upfront surgical resection would result in significant morbidity. Adjuvant imatinib is indicated in patients with high-risk features for recurrence: extragastric tumors >5 cm or >5 mitoses/50 hpf or gastric tumors >10 cm or >5 mitoses/50 hpf, or patients with tumor rupture. The most common adverse effect of imatinib is edema. While small Tis or T1a gastric adenocarcinomas can be treated with endoscopic resection, complete resection of gastric GISTs typically requires at least a wedge resection (E).

3. B. One of the more feared postoperative complications following Roux-en-Y gastric bypass is acute afferent loop syndrome with small bowel obstruction (SBO) of the biliopancreatic limb. A high index of suspicion is needed to diagnose this complication, usually based on patient symptoms and evidence of proximal SBO on imaging. Unlike most adhesive SBOs, which can be decompressed with vomiting, obstruction of the afferent loop via an internal hernia causes a closed loop obstruction with a high risk of perforation with urgent surgical exploration indicated to relieve the obstruction. Eating smaller, more frequent meals is the first-line treatment of early dumping syndrome postgastrectomy (A). Nasogastric tube decompression with water-soluble contrast challenge is the conservative management for adhesive SBO and is not appropriate in this patient (C). Antibiotic therapy is a treatment for small intestine bacterial overgrowth (SIBO) but not for bowel obstruction (D). While upper endoscopy would be useful in the diagnosis of reflux gastritis or marginal ulcer, it would be of low utility in this patient (E).

4. B. This patient with multiple duodenal ulcers likely has Zollinger-Ellison syndrome secondary to hypersecretion of gastrin from a gastrinoma. Gastrin is usually produced by antral G cells and acts on parietal cells to produce hydrochloric acid and chief cells to produce pepsinogen, both cell types of which are most predominant in the stomach body (A). The pancreas is the site of the secretion of many hormones including somatostatin from D cells, insulin from beta cells, and glucagon from alpha cells (C). The duodenum and jejunum are the sites of the secretion of cholecystokinin (CCK) from I cells and secretin from K cells (D, E). The duodenum is the most common site for gastrinomas (50%–88%), followed by the pancreas (25%).

5. A. The most common etiology of small bowel obstruction in the United States is adhesions from previous abdominal surgery. However, this does not hold true for patients that have previously had an LRYGB. In this procedure, a potential hernia site (Petersen space hernia) is created, increasing the risk for the development of an internal hernia, which is the most common cause of SBO in this patient population with an incidence of 1% to 5%. This potential space results from herniation of intestinal loops through a defect in the mesentery and between small bowel limbs, transverse mesocolon, and the retroperitoneum. Additionally, when compared to its open counterpart, the laparoscopic approach further facilitates a Petersen hernia because of the decreased frequency of postoperative adhesions, which seemingly have a physiologic role of preventing bowel mobility, and thus, internal herniation. Risk of SBO is significantly higher with a retrocolic versus an antecolic approach. Roux compression due to mesocolon scarring is the second most common etiology for SBO in patients with LRYGB followed by adhesions (B, C). Kinking of the jejunojejunostomy and incarcerated abdominal wall hernia occur less frequently (D, E).

Reference: Champion JK, Williams M, Husain S, Johnson AR. Small-bowel obstruction after laparoscopic Roux-en-Y gastric bypass: etiology, diagnosis, and management. *Arch Surg.* 2003;13(4):988–993.

6. A. Nonoperative management for perforated peptic ulcer disease is gaining popularity and is now accepted as an appropriate first-line management for poor surgical candidates (e.g., COPD using home oxygen) who are stable, have no evidence of peritonitis, and have no contrast extravasation. Conservative management is also more favorable if the duration of symptoms has lasted more than 24 hours. By this time the perforation has typically been sealed. Self-sealing of the perforation is achieved by either adhesion formation to the caudate lobe, the greater omentum, the gallbladder, or the falciform ligament. In one study, only 3 out of 109 patients managed nonoperatively developed an intraabdominal abscess (which can be managed with antibiotics and percutaneous drainage). This may speak to the intrinsic immune function of the omentum and the fact that the upper GI tract has a low bacterial load. Eighty percent of nonoperative cases respond favorably, and morbidity is not significantly increased. Patients deemed appropriate candidates for nonoperative management should be admitted, placed NPO (nothing by mouth), and given IV fluid resuscitation, IV antibiotics covering gram-negative and anaerobic organisms, and PPIs. Nasogastric tube insertion is critical to help decompress the stomach and allow the perforation to heal. CT scan may be considered for patients who fail to improve or those who deteriorate clinically. Surgery is the next step for patients who fail conservative management (B, C). Outpatient follow-up is not appropriate because nonoperative management should be performed in a monitored setting with frequent abdominal exams and follow-up esophagogastroduodenoscopy (EGD) to ensure that the perforation has sealed (D, E).

References: Nusree R. Conservative management of perforated peptic ulcer. *Thai J Surg.* 2005;26:5–8.

Hanumanthappa MB, Gopinathan S, Guruprasad R. A nonoperative treatment of perforated peptic ulcer: a prospective study with 50 cases. *J Clin Diagnostic Res.* 2012;41:4161.

7. D. Obesity has been linked to multiple comorbidities, including hypertension and diabetes, and is on the rise. As such, many clinicians have turned to medical management and/or bariatric surgery to help fight this epidemic in cases where diet and exercise fail. Two FDA-approved medications to help treat obesity include sibutramine and orlistat. Sibutramine blocks the presynaptic uptake of serotonin, thereby potentiating its anorexic effects in the CNS. Orlistat inhibits pancreatic lipase, which decreases dietary fat absorption and results in weight loss (B). A significant complication limiting its use for most patients is severe flatulence. Indications for weight loss surgery include BMI >35 with associated obesity-related comorbidities (e.g., hypertension, diabetes) or BMI >40 (A). Additionally, all patients will need to demonstrate that they have successfully attempted and failed nonoperative weight loss management such as diet and exercise programs (E). Patients will also need to be evaluated by a physiatrist and deemed suitable for the procedure. The four standard approaches in the United States include laparoscopic gastric banding, sleeve gastrectomy, BPD, and RYGB. Laparoscopic gastric banding and sleeve gastrectomy are considered restrictive procedures as they physically limit the intake of food. BPD is considered a malabsorptive procedure as it involves constructing an alimentary channel distally to the GI tract and thereby preventing the absorption of caloric intake. RYGB is considered a combined approach and involves creating a small restricted gastric remnant (restrictive component) and a roux-limb from the stomach to the distal jejunum (malabsorptive component) (C). These procedures result in up to 50% resolution of weight-related comorbidities and up to 50% excess weight loss. Compared to BPD, RYGB has a lower 30-day mortality and is slightly favored by surgeons as it is technically easier to perform. RYGB has a slightly higher mean excess weight loss at 2 years compared to sleeve gastrectomy, but sleeve gastrectomy has a higher perioperative leak rate. Both procedures are equally effective in eliminating type 2 diabetes mellitus.

References: Duarte MIX de T, Bassitt DP, Azevedo OC de, Waisberg J, Yamaguchi N, Pinto Junior PE. Impact on quality of life, weight loss and comorbidities: a study comparing the biliopancreatic diversion with duodenal switch and the banded Roux-en-Y gastric bypass. *Arq Gastroenterol.* 2014;51(4):320–327.

Santry HP, Gillen DL, Lauderdale DS. Trends in bariatric surgical procedures. *JAMA.* 2005;294(15):1909–1917.

O'Brien P. Surgical treatment of obesity. *Endotext.* 2016;19:29–46.

Zingmond DS, McGory ML, Ko CY. Hospitalization before and after gastric bypass surgery. *JAMA.* 2005;294(15):1918–1924.

8. C. Gastroparesis is defined as delayed gastric emptying without a mechanical cause for obstruction. Although diabetes is the most common known cause of gastroparesis (29%), idiopathic gastroparesis occurs more frequently (36%). The most common symptoms are nausea, early satiety, and abdominal bloating. Most patients do not have abdominal pain. Although symptoms alone can be suggestive of this condition, it needs to be confirmed by imaging (E). Gastric emptying scintigraphy (delayed gastric emptying study) is the gold standard in diagnosing gastroparesis. This involves asking the patient to eat a small meal along with a radioactive tracer. The rate of emptying is measured 1, 2, 3, and 4 hours after the meal is ingested. If more than 10% of the meal remains in the stomach after 4 hours, the study is considered consistent with gastroparesis (A, B, D).

9. E. Gallstone formation occurs in 30% to 52% of patients undergoing weight loss surgery, but only 7% to 15% are symptomatic. Among those 7% to 15% who do become symptomatic, acute cholecystitis is uncommon. Rapid weight loss is a known risk factor for cholelithiasis. In fact, excess weight loss greater than 25% is considered the strongest predictor of postoperative cholecystectomy and occurs more commonly in patients who have had a gastric bypass versus laparoscopic banding or sleeve gastrectomy (A). Several mechanisms have been shown to contribute to gallstone formation during weight loss including increased secretion of calcium and mucin into bile, increased concentrations of arachidonic acid derivatives, and bile stasis secondary to stringent dietary restrictions postoperatively (D). Prophylactic cholecystectomy at the time of weight loss surgery has been a point of debate in the surgical community. Proponents argue that it helps prevent the morbidity of symptomatic biliary disease and avoids the need for treatments such as endoscopic retrograde cholangiopancreatography (ERCP), which can be particularly challenging in this patient population (e.g., RYGB). However, it has been shown in several large studies that the rate of postoperative cholecystectomy remains under 15%; therefore, the routine removal of the gallbladder during weight loss surgery is not currently supported by the American Society of Metabolic and Bariatric Surgery (B). In contrast, symptomatic patients may undergo concomitant cholecystectomy safely. Ursodiol after gastric bypass can significantly decrease the rate of gallstone formation, but because it has not been shown to be cost effective and lead to improved outcomes, it is not routinely recommended (C).

References: D'Hondt M, Sergeant G, Deylgat B, Devriendt D, Van Rooy F, Vansteenkiste F. Prophylactic cholecystectomy, a mandatory step in morbidly obese patients undergoing laparoscopic Roux-en-Y gastric bypass? *J Gastrointest Surg.* 2011;15(9):1532–1536.

Shiffman ML, Shamburek RD, Schwartz CC, Sugerman HJ, Kellum JM, Moore EW. Gallbladder mucin, arachidonic acid, and bile lipids in patients who develop gallstones during weight reduction. *Gastroenterology.* 1993;105(4):1200–1208.

Sugerman HJ, Brewer WH, Shiffman ML, et al. A multicenter, placebo-controlled, randomized, double-blind, prospective trial of prophylactic ursodiol for the prevention of gallstone formation following gastric-bypass-induced rapid weight loss. *Am J Surg.* 1995;169(1):91–96.

Tucker ON, Fajnwaks P, Szomstein S, Rosenthal RJ. Is concomitant cholecystectomy necessary in obese patients undergoing laparoscopic gastric bypass surgery? *Surg Endosc.* 2008;22(11):2450–2454.

Villegas L, Schneider B, Provost D, et al. Is routine cholecystectomy required during laparoscopic gastric bypass? *Obes Surg.* 2004;14(2):206–211.

10. B. The rate of obesity is rising in the United States and an increasing number of patients are undergoing weight loss surgery. Gastric leak in the early postoperative period may be an indication to go back to the operating room, so early recognition of this complication is important. The first manifestations of a gastric leak are tachycardia and fever (A, C–E). This may also be accompanied by tachypnea, abdominal pain, chest pain, oliguria, and/or hypotension.

Reference: Bekehit M, Katri K, Nabil W. Earliest signs and management of leakage after bariatric surgeries: single institute experience. *Alexandria J Med.* 2013;49(1):29–33.

11. A. Laparoscopic gastric banding involves placing an inflatable balloon around the proximal stomach at the angle of His. A properly placed lap band will have an approximately 45° upward angle from the horizontal plane on a plain film of the abdomen. The procedure was very popular when it first appeared but lost traction after subsequent studies demonstrated that it was far inferior to gastric bypass. Additionally, patients with laparoscopic bands were more likely to require revisions for complications associated with the gastric band. One such complication is band erosion (BE) into the stomach and/or adjacent organs. This may present as port site erythema (inflammation tracking down the tube), fooling the clinician into thinking the patient may only have an overlying skin infection. In fact, most patients with BE presenting with port site erythema do not have a subfascial port infection. BE can occur many years after surgery, and one proposed mechanism involves overtightening of the band (e.g., after clinic visit). CT of the abdomen should be performed in patients suspected of having BE and, if found, the port site should be completely deflated and the patient should be scheduled for laparoscopic removal of the band. EGD may demonstrate BE if it has completely eroded into the gastric lumen but may miss partial BE (C). Incision and drainage are not indicated because there is no abscess (D). The patient should be monitored for the development of a subsequent port site infection, but the first step is to get a CT scan (B–E).

References: Dilorenzo N, Lorenzo M, Furbetta F. Intragastric gastric band migration and erosion: an analysis of multicenter experience on 177 patients. *Surg Endosc.* 2013;27(4):1151–1157.

Naef M, Naef U, Mouton WG, Wagner HE. Outcome and complications after laparoscopic Swedish adjustable gastric banding: 5-year results of a prospective clinical trial. *Obes Surg.* 2007;17(2):195–201.

Stroh C, Hohmann U, Will U, et al. (2008).

12. E. In the majority of patients with a perforated duodenal ulcer, simple closure of the ulcer with an omental (Graham) patch is all that is necessary (A). This is then followed by treatment of *H. pylori.* In addition, a Graham patch alone should be used if the patient is unstable, if there is extensive exudative peritonitis, or if the perforation is long standing (>24 hours). However, in the setting of a patient with a known ulcer diathesis who has either already been treated for *H. pylori* or is *H. pylori* negative, an ulcer surgery should be added to the operation, provided the patient is a good operative risk, is hemodynamically stable, and does not have extensive peritonitis. The options are either to perform a highly selective vagotomy (HSV) or a vagotomy and pyloroplasty (B). An HSV is the preferred approach in the stable good-risk patient, provided the surgeon is comfortable with the procedure. Pyloroplasty is typically performed along with a vagotomy because the widened outlet from the stomach to the duodenum helps circumvent any unwanted effects of the decreased gastric peristalsis and overall change in gastric emptying patterns that occur following vagotomy. The entire procedure can be performed laparoscopically in select patients. Truncal vagotomy and antrectomy (C, D) is generally not recommended in the setting of perforation because of the high associated morbidity and mortality rates.

References: Cadiere GB, Bruyns J, Himpens J, Van Alphen P, Verturyen M. Laparoscopic highly selective vagotomy. *Hepatogastroenterology.* 1999;46(27):1500–1506.

Jordan PH Jr, Thornby J. Perforated pyloroduodenal ulcers: long-term results with omental patch closure and parietal cell vagotomy. *Ann Surg.* 1995;221(5):486–488.

Siu WT, Leong HT, Law BKB, et al. Laparoscopic repair for perforated peptic ulcer: a randomized controlled trial. *Ann Surg.* 2002;235(3):313–319.

13. E. Postvagotomy syndromes include diarrhea, gastric atony, and incomplete vagotomy (leading to recurrent ulceration). Diarrhea follows truncal vagotomy and may be confused with dumping syndrome. The diarrhea associated with vagotomy occurs more frequently and is not associated with the other cardiovascular manifestations seen with dumping syndrome (C). The initial treatment is similar to that for dumping syndrome, with dietary modifications such as frequent small meals with decreased fluid intake and an increase in fiber. A proposed mechanism of the diarrhea is an increase in stool bile salts. Oral cholestyramine is often helpful because it binds bile salts (B). Loperamide and codeine have also been shown to delay intestinal transit time and improve symptoms. In the very rare patient who does not respond to medical management, reversal of a segment of jejunum is effective in slowing transit time and improving diarrhea (D). Octreotide is not effective for postvagotomy diarrhea and may make the situation worse by decreasing pancreatic secretions and thus increasing steatorrhea (A).

References: Duncombe V, Bolin T, Davis A. Double-blind trial of cholestyramine in post-vagotomy diarrhea. *Gut.* 1977;18(7):531–535.

O'Brien JG, Thompson DG, Mcintyre A. Effect of codeine and loperamide on upper intestinal transit and absorption in normal subjects and patients with postvagotomy diarrhea. *Gut.* 1988;29(3):312–318.

14. D. More than 80% of gastrinomas are localized preoperatively. For those that cannot be localized, surgical exploration is still indicated because excision of the primary tumor leads to a decreased rate of liver metastasis. When exploring, it is important to be aware that 80% of gastrinomas are found within the gastrinoma (Passaro) triangle, an area defined by the junction of the cystic duct and common bile duct, the second and third portions of the duodenum, and the neck and body of the pancreas. As many as 60% of gastrinomas are within the wall of the duodenum, primarily in the first and second portions and can be very small. Thus, the next maneuver would be to perform a blind proximal duodenotomy to manually palpate the duodenal wall for tumors. Closing the abdomen (A) would be inappropriate. Blind distal pancreatectomy and splenectomy (these share blood supply) (B) or distal duodenotomy (E) would have very low yields. A pancreaticoduodenectomy (Whipple procedure) (C) would not be indicated in this setting. It is potentially indicated for multiple duodenal or proximal pancreatic head tumors that could not be enucleated.

15. C. Achieving an adequate lymphadenectomy with a ≥15 lymph node harvest during an oncologic resection of gastric cancer is important in accurately staging the patient and reducing the nodal false negative rate. Staging of gastric cancer involves depth of invasion (T1 invades lamina propria; T2, muscularis propria or subserosa; T3, serosa; T4, adjacent structures), nodes, and distant metastasis (E). EUS is the best modality for assessing tumor depth of invasion and nodal status. It is approximately 80% accurate in determining whether the tumor is transmural (invading serosa, T3) but only 50% accurate in assessing whether pathologically enlarged lymph nodes are present (B). EUS seems to be more accurate with advanced disease than early disease. CT scanning is the preferred method for determining distant metastases, but it is not as useful for T and N staging (A). The routine use of MRI and positron emission tomography scanning for staging of gastric cancer has not as yet been established (D). N1 disease includes 1 to 6 regional nodes; N2, 7 to 15 regional nodes; and N3, more than 15 regional nodes.

References: Puli SR, Batapati Krishna Reddy J, Bechtold ML, Antillon MR, Ibdah JA. How good is endoscopic ultrasound for TNM staging of gastric cancers? A meta-analysis and systematic review. *World J Gastroenterol.* 2008;14(25):4011–4019.

Willis S, Truong S, Gribnitz S, Fass J, Schumpelick V. Endoscopic ultrasonography in the preoperative staging of gastric cancer: accuracy and impact on surgical therapy. *Surg Endosc.* 2000;14(10):951–954.

Xi W, Zhao C, Ren G. Endoscopic ultrasonography in preoperative staging of gastric cancer: determination of tumor invasion depth, nodal involvement and surgical respectability. *World J Gastroenterol.* 2003;9(2):254–257.

16. D. When considering gastrinoma, it is important to be aware of the differential diagnosis of an elevated gastrin level. Causes of hypergastrinemia with increased acid production include gastrinoma, G-cell hyperplasia (not D-cell) (E), retained antrum after distal gastrectomy, renal failure, and gastric outlet obstruction. Hypergastrinemia with normal or low acid production includes pernicious anemia, postvagotomy states, use of acid-suppressive medication, and chronic gastritis. Hypothyroidism is associated with a low gastrin level, whereas hyperthyroidism increases gastrin levels (B). Diabetes (A) and hyperparathyroidism (C) do not affect gastrin levels.

References: Seino Y, Matsukura S, Inoue Y, Kadowaki S, Mori K, Imura H. Hypogastrinemia in hypothyroidism. *Am J Dig Dis.* 1978;23(2):189–191.

Korman MG, Laver MC, Hansky J. Hypergastrinemia in chronic renal failure. *BMJ.* 1972;1(5794):209–210.

17. D. R0 resection is resection of all gross and microscopic tumors (C). R1 indicates removal of all macroscopic disease but microscopic margins are positive for disease. An R2 resection indicates that gross residual disease is left behind (E). A D1 resection (A) refers to removal of perigastric lymph nodes; D2 (B) refers to the additional resection of lymph nodes along the named vessels around the stomach. A D3 resection is a D2 resection plus removal of para-aortic lymph nodes.

18. A. Risk factors for gastric cancer include dietary factors such as a large consumption of smoked meats, pickled foods, high nitrates, and high salt, whereas a diet high in fruits and vegetables may be protective (D, E). Other risk factors include smoking, low socioeconomic status, Black race, *H. pylori* infection, chronic atrophic gastritis, blood type A, previous partial gastrectomy, achlorhydria, pernicious anemia, polyps (adenomatous and hyperplastic), male sex, and certain familial syndromes such as hereditary nonpolyposis colorectal cancer, Li-Fraumeni syndrome, familial adenomatous polyposis, and Peutz-Jeghers syndrome (B, D). Peutz-Jeghers syndrome is associated with a markedly increased risk of cancer in the esophagus, stomach, small bowel, colon, pancreas, breast, lung, uterus, and ovary, with a cumulative 93% risk of cancer. Carbonated acidic soda has not been shown to increase the risk for cancer (C). Gastric cancer has been categorized by Lauren into intestinal and diffuse types based on histology. The intestinal type is thought to be more related to environmental factors, is associated with chronic gastritis, and is well differentiated. The diffuse type is usually poorly differentiated and associated with signet rings and occurs in younger patients and in association with familial disorders and with type A blood. The diffuse type has a worse prognosis.

References: Berndt H, Wildner GP, Klein K. Regional and social differences in cancer incidence of the digestive tract in the German Democratic Republic. *Neoplasma.* 1968;15(5):501–515.

Giardiello FM, Brensinger JD, Tersmette AC, et al. Very high risk of cancer in familial Peutz-Jeghers syndrome. *Gastroenterology.* 2000;119(6):1447–1453.

Wynder EL, Kmet J, Dungal N, Segi M. An epidemiological investigation of gastric cancer. *Cancer.* 1963;16(11):1461–1496.

19. B. Gastric ulcers have been categorized into five types. The most common is the type I lesion (≈60%) (A), which is located near the angularis incisura at the border between the antrum and the fundus, usually along the lesser curve. These patients usually have normal or decreased acid secretion. Type II gastric ulcers are located in the fundus and are associated with a concomitant duodenal ulcer. Type III gastric ulcers are prepyloric. Both types II and III gastric ulcers are usually associated with increased gastric acid secretion. Type III ulcers are thought to behave like duodenal ulcers. Type IV gastric ulcers are located near the gastroesophageal junction. Like type I ulcers, type IV gastric ulcers have normal or low acid production and are associated with impaired mucosal defense. Type V gastric ulcers are considered a diffuse process and are associated with NSAID use.

20. D. GISTs were previously called *leiomyomas* or *leiomyosarcomas* because they were thought to arise from smooth muscle cells, but they in fact originate from mesenchymal components (from Cajal cells) (B). They stain positive for CD117 (c-kit). They are most commonly found in the stomach and, although rare, they are the most common mesenchymal tumors of the intestinal tract. Because they are not epithelial tumors and grow in the wall of the stomach, they tend to be large at the time of presentation. They cause mucosal ulceration and frequently present with GI bleeding (E). Large tumors may also produce symptoms of weight loss, abdominal pain, and fullness and early satiety. An abdominal mass may be palpable. An endoscopic biopsy specimen may be negative in as many as one-half of cases due to sampling error because most of the tumor is submucosal (A). A CT scan provides a better assessment of the extent of the tumor. Determining whether a GIST is malignant is not straightforward because there are no discriminating cellular features (C). The malignant potential is determined by mitotic activity (>5 mitoses/50 high power field) with 1 cm. Lymph node dissection is not necessary because tumors spread hematogenously and lymph node metastasis is extremely rare. Wedge resection with 1 cm margins is adequate treatment in most cases. This can be performed laparoscopically. However, microscopically positive margins have not been demonstrated to affect survival.

References: Dempsey DT. Stomach. In: Brunicardi FC, Andersen DK, Billiar TR, et al., eds. *Schwartz's principles of surgery.* 8th ed. New York: McGraw-Hill; 2005:933–996.

Mercer DW, Robinson EK. Stomach. In: Townsend CM, Jr, Beauchamp RD, Evers BM, Mattox KL, eds. *Sabiston textbook of surgery: the biological basis of modern surgical practice.* 17th ed. Philadelphia: W.B. Saunders; 2004:1265–1322.

Novitsky YW, Kercher KW, Sing RF, Heniford BT. Long-term outcomes of laparoscopic resection of gastric gastrointestinal stromal tumors. *Ann Surg.* 2006;243(6):738–745.

Sexton JA, Pierce RA, Halpin VJ, et al. Laparoscopic gastric resection for gastrointestinal stromal tumors. *Surg Endosc.* 2008;22(12):2583–2587.

Malangoni MA, et al. Stomach. In: Cameron JL, ed. *Current surgical therapy.* 8th ed. Philadelphia: Mosby; 2004:67–100.

21. D. Bile reflux into the stomach can occur without previous surgery, but in most instances it follows ablation of the pylorus, such as after gastric resection or pyloroplasty. After such procedures, most patients will have bile in the stomach on endoscopic examination, along with some degree of gross or microscopic gastric inflammation. However, only a small fraction of patients will have a significant degree of symptoms such as nausea, epigastric pain, and bilious vomiting consistent with alkaline (bile) reflux gastritis (B, E). Symptoms often develop months or years after the index operation. The differential diagnosis includes afferent or efferent loop obstruction, gastric stasis, and small bowel obstruction. These other diagnoses can be ruled out using a combination of abdominal radiographs, upper endoscopy, and abdominal CT scan. A hepatoiminodiacetic acid (HIDA) scan is particularly helpful for demonstrating bile reflux. Bile reflux and gastritis are more likely to occur after Billroth II reconstruction (A) than after Billroth I and least likely after vagotomy and pyloroplasty. Medical management of symptomatic patients is not particularly effective (C). The surgical procedure of choice is to convert the Billroth II into a Roux-en-Y gastrojejunostomy with a lengthened jejunal limb (at least 45 cm).

22. D. More than 90% of gastrinomas have receptors for somatostatin. Octreotide scanning (somatostatin receptor scintigraphy) has been shown to be the most sensitive test for localization of gastrinomas. However, successful localization depends on size and location. Somatostatin receptor scintigraphy is poor for very small tumors (<1.1 cm) and for small primary duodenal tumors. Duodenal gastrinomas are best localized by endoscopic ultrasonography. Abdominal ultrasound is not helpful (C). Failure to detect the tumor preoperatively should not preempt surgical exploration because an additional 33% will be found at surgery. CT and angiography may also be useful adjuncts in detecting gastrinoma (B, E). Aside from MRI's utility in detecting liver metastasis, it is not often employed in the workup for a presumed gastrinoma (A).

Reference: Alexander HR, Fraker DL, Norton JA, et al. Prospective study of somatostatin receptor scintigraphy and its effect on operative outcome in patients with Zollinger-Ellison syndrome. *Ann Surg.* 1998;228(2):228–238.

23. B. A urea breath test is the best way to confirm eradication of *H. pylori*. The test relies on the fact that the bacteria hydrolyze urea. The patient is given radiolabeled urea to ingest orally. If *H. pylori* is present, the urea will be converted to ammonia and radiolabeled bicarbonate, which is then exhaled as carbon dioxide. The amount of exhaled carbon dioxide is quantified. Positive *H. pylori* serology (A) provides evidence of current infection if the patient has never been treated for it but will remain positive even after successful treatment; thus, it is not useful in this setting. Antral mucosa biopsy (E) with histologic examination (D) for the organism is the gold standard test. It is useful in the initial evaluation of patients with upper GI symptoms because it permits evaluation of the stomach via endoscopy at the time of biopsy. However, given its invasive nature and increased cost, it is not routinely recommended to confirm eradication. Cultures of the gastric mucosa are not routinely available at every laboratory, and a repeat endoscopy is required. The rapid urease test, also known as the campylobacter-like organism (CLO) test (C), is ideally used if another endoscopy and biopsy are being performed. The study requires placing a sample of gastric mucosa in a urea solution and then using a pH indicator to demonstrate the production of ammonia.

24. D. HSV is also known as a parietal cell vagotomy or proximal gastric vagotomy. The goal of the operation is to divide the vagal nerves of the proximal two-thirds of the stomach where the parietal cells are located and preserve the distal third to maintain antral function and thus not require a drainage procedure (such as a pyloroplasty). This results in fewer complications than the classic truncal vagotomy. The operation spares the main anterior and posterior vagal trunks (A) but divides the branches of the anterior and posterior Latarjet nerves that directly innervate the proximal stomach (C). The distal 7 cm (approximately) of nerves, known as the crow's feet, are spared. Likewise, the celiac and hepatic branches are spared (E). Proximally, it is important to divide the nerve of Grassi, which is a branch off the posterior trunk of the vagus (B). It is often referred to as the criminal nerve of Grassi because failure to divide this branch leads to a higher ulcer recurrence rate. With the recognition of *H. pylori* as the main etiology of peptic ulcer, the role of surgery has greatly diminished. HSV is still indicated in certain rare situations, such as patients who do not respond to medical management, patients who are bleeding who do not respond to endoscopic management, or with perforation in patients with a longstanding ulcer diathesis.

25. A. Gastric resection leads to numerous disturbances in metabolism. These include deficiencies of iron, vitamin B12 (B), folate (C), fat-soluble vitamins (E), and calcium (D). Of these, iron deficiency is the most common. Iron is absorbed in the duodenum and is facilitated by an acidic environment. After gastric resection, overall iron intake is decreased, and the reduced acidity impairs absorption. Reduction in the parietal cell mass from gastric resection leads to a decrease in intrinsic factor, which is necessary for the enteric absorption of vitamin B12, occurring in the terminal ileum. This leads to a megaloblastic anemia. Furthermore, an acidic environment facilitates the bioavailability of vitamin B12. Vitamin B12 deficiency usually only develops when at least one-half of the stomach is resected. Fat malabsorption can occur after gastrectomy (particularly with a Billroth II reconstruction) because of inadequate mixing of food with bile and digestive enzymes. This leads to a decreased absorption of fat-soluble vitamins. Calcium is absorbed in the duodenum and small bowel and is also facilitated by an acid environment. Long-term deficiencies manifest as osteoporosis. Folate deficiency is rare.

26. E. ZES (gastrinoma) is caused by uncontrolled secretion of gastrin by a pancreatic or a duodenal neuroendocrine tumor. Most cases are sporadic, but 20% are inherited (C). The inherited or familial form of gastrinoma is associated with multiple endocrine neoplasia type 1. Gastrinoma is the most common functional neuroendocrine tumor in multiple endocrine neoplasia type 1 but insulinoma is the most common overall (D). The most common symptoms are epigastric pain, gastroesophageal reflux, and diarrhea. The massive acid hypersecretion leads to a secretory diarrhea that persists even with fasting (A). The majority will have demonstrable peptic ulceration that is most commonly located in the proximal duodenum (B). Unlike typical ulcers, those associated with gastrinoma on occasion will be found in the distal duodenum or jejunum. Ulcers in these locations should raise suspicion for gastrinoma, as should recurrent or refractory peptic ulcers, ulcers in association with secretory diarrhea, finding gastric rugal hypertrophy or esophagitis-related stricture on endoscopy, bleeding or perforated ulcer, family history of ulcer, and ulcers in the setting of hypercalcemia or kidney stones. PPIs are highly effective in relieving the symptoms of ZES, although definitive treatment consists of localizing and resecting the tumor.

Reference: Meijer JL, Jansen JB, Lamers CB. Omeprazole in the treatment of Zollinger-Ellison syndrome and histamine H2-antagonist refractory ulcers. *Digestion*. 1989;44 Suppl 1:31–39.

27. C. The presentation of oral contrast extravasation in the proximal duodenum (or free air under the diaphragm) combined with melena, anemia, and guaiac-positive stool is highly suggestive of a "kissing" duodenal ulcer. This represents a rare combination of an anterior duodenal ulcer that perforates into the peritoneum and a synchronous posterior ulcer that erodes into the gastroduodenal artery and bleeds.

The majority of anterior perforated ulcers can be managed by simple ulcer closure with an omental (Graham) patch. This can be achieved via an open or laparoscopic approach. In this patient, one must rule out a bleeding posterior ulcer. This would best be achieved via an anterior duodenotomy across the pylorus. If a posterior ulcer is identified, it should be oversewn.

References: Dasmahapatra KS, Suval W, Machiedo GW. Unsuspected perforation in bleeding duodenal ulcers. *Am Surg*. 1988;54(1):19–21.

Hunt PS, Clarke G. Perforation in patients with bleeding ulcer. *ANZ J Surg*. 1991;61(3):183–185.

Stabile BE, Hardy HJ, Passaro E. "Kissing" duodenal ulcers. *Arch Surg*. 1979;114(10):1153–1156.

28. B. Bezoars are accumulations of indigestible material in the stomach. Bezoars often produce nonspecific symptoms and are usually found incidentally in patients undergoing upper gastrointestinal endoscopy or imaging. There are two types. Phytobezoars are composed of undigested vegetable matter (as in this patient). Risk factors for phytobezoars include previous gastric surgery and gastroparesis such as from diabetes. Peptic ulcer disease is not a risk factor (E). Bezoars produce obstructive symptoms but can also cause ulceration and bleeding. Diagnosis is suggested by an upper GI series and confirmed by endoscopy. Treatment generally consists of a combination of enzymatic degradation, endoscopic disruption, irrigation, and removal. Enzyme therapy can be performed with papain (present in meat tenderizers) or with cellulase. However, the use of papain has been associated with hypernatremia, gastric ulceration, and esophageal perforation, such that cellulase is preferred. More recently, nasogastric Coca-Cola lavage has been successfully used. The mechanism responsible is believed to be a combination of the mucolytic effect of sodium bicarbonate ($NaHCO_3$) and digestion of the bezoar by CO_2 bubbles, all of which is exaggerated by the cola's acidity. Trichobezoars are composed of hair. It occurs most commonly in girls and young women who swallow their hair (trichophagia). Interestingly, most have long hair with patchy areas of alopecia (D), and many have an underlying psychiatric disorder; thus psychiatric care is important in prevention (unlike phytobezoars) (C). The hair creates a cast of the stomach and strands of hair can extend into the small bowel (the so-called Rapunzel syndrome). Large trichobezoars are likely to require surgical removal because they are less likely to respond to enzymatic degradation (A).

References: Bonilla F, Mirete J, Cuesta A, Sillero C, González M. Treatment of gastric phytobezoars with cellulase. *Rev Esp Enferm Dig*. 1999;91(12):809–814.

Ladas SD, Triantafyllou K, Tzathas C, Tassios P, Rokkas T, Raptis SA. Gastric phytobezoars may be treated by nasogastric Coca-Cola lavage. *Eur J Gastroenterol Hepatol*. 2002;14(7):801–803.

Walker-Renard P. Update on the medicinal management of phytobezoars. *Am J Gastroenterol*. 1993;88(10):1663–1666.

29. D. Gastric volvulus is associated with Borchardt triad (sudden onset of severe upper abdominal pain, recurrent retching without vomitus, and an inability to pass a nasogastric tube). Etiology is either primary (due to congenital changes in the gastric ligaments) or secondary to anatomic abnormalities, usually paraesophageal or diaphragmatic hernias. Even if gastric volvulus is associated with anatomic abnormalities, these do not always need to be addressed for definitive management. In elderly patients or poor surgical candidates who cannot tolerate a long operation, once the stomach is detorsed (either endoscopically or surgically), definitive therapy can consist of as little as a gastropexy usually via percutaneous gastrostomy tube. Bergman triad (mental status changes, petechiae, and dyspnea) is seen with fat emboli syndrome (C). The volvulus can be either organoaxial (twisting around the axis between the gastroesophageal junction and pylorus), which is twice as common, or mesenteroaxial (twisting along the axis between the lesser and greater curvature) (A). Gastric volvulus most commonly occurs in association with a diaphragmatic defect. The stomach becomes trapped in the defect and twists. In children, the defect is congenital (such as a Bochdalek hernia), whereas in adults, it is more often traumatic or secondary to paraesophageal hernias (B). Gastric volvulus can also occur in the absence of a diaphragmatic defect. In such situations, there is typically a congenital absence of intraperitoneal visceral attachments. It is seen in association with a wandering spleen, a condition in which the spleen also lacks peritoneal attachments and is prone to torsion. Gastric volvulus is a surgical emergency because there is a high risk of gastric necrosis if it is unrecognized (E). If the stomach is compromised, a gastric resection may be needed. If a volvulus is found without necrosis and without a diaphragmatic defect, then detorsion and gastropexy are performed.

References: Carter R, Brewer LA 3rd, Hinshaw DB. Acute gastric volvulus. A study of 25 cases. *Am J Surg.* 1980;140(1):99–106.

Uc A, Kao SC, Sanders KD, Lawrence J. Gastric volvulus and wandering spleen. *Am J Gastroenterol.* 1998;93(7):1146–1148.

Wasselle JA, Norman J. Acute gastric volvulus: pathogenesis, diagnosis, and treatment. *Am J Gastroenterol.* 1993;88(10):1780–1784.

30. D. A metastatic left supraclavicular lymph node is called the *Virchow node* (Troisier sign) (B). Intraabdominal cancers tend to metastasize to the left secondary to lymph drainage into the left subclavian vein via the thoracic duct. A metastatic left axillary lymph node from gastric cancer is called an *Irish node* (A). A Blumer shelf is a palpable nodule on rectal examination suggesting a drop metastasis (E). An ovarian mass from a gastric metastasis is also known as Krukenberg tumor. (C) An umbilical nodule (Sister Mary Joseph node) suggests carcinomatosis. Although associated with gastric cancer, it may represent any metastatic lesion, most commonly from an intraabdominal cancer. It was named after Dr. William Mayo's surgical assistant, who made the observation while scrubbing patients for gastric surgery that those with umbilical nodules had widely metastatic and unresectable gastric cancer. Current recommendations are that if such nodules are found on physical examination, the patient should undergo fine-needle aspiration because such umbilical nodules may sometimes represent benign disease.

References: Fleming MV, Oertel YC. Eight cases of Sister Mary Joseph's nodule diagnosed by fine-needle aspiration. *Diagn Cytopathol.* 1993;9(1):32–36.

Giner Galvañ V. Sister Mary Joseph's nodule. Its clinical significance and management. *An Med Interna.* 1999;16(7):365–370.

31. A. Bleeding from duodenal ulcers can be controlled endoscopically in the majority of patients; thus surgery is rarely indicated. Predictors of failure of endoscopic management include the presence of shock or a large ulcer (>2 cm). Even when bleeding recurs after having been controlled endoscopically, endoscopic treatment can again be attempted with a high rate of success, thus avoiding surgery. The bleeding is usually from a posterior ulcer that has eroded into the gastroduodenal artery (remember anterior ulcers cause a free perforation and peritonitis, posterior ulcers penetrate and bleed). Surgical management decisions should be based on the hemodynamic stability of the patient, the patient's overall medical condition, and whether the patient has a history of ulcer disease that has been treated for *H. pylori*. In the patient who is actively bleeding, the duodenum should be opened across the pylorus as is used in a pyloroplasty. The ulcer bed should be oversewn with multiple figure-of-eight sutures. If the patient has a history of ulcers that have been treated for *H. pylori* and is stable in the operating room, an ulcer operation should be performed. The best option in this type of emergent setting is to perform a truncal vagotomy and to close the longitudinal duodenotomy in a transverse fashion as with a pyloroplasty. If the patient is a high surgical risk and unstable, another option would be to simply perform a smaller duodenotomy, oversew the ulcer, simply close the duodenotomy, and treat postoperatively for *H. pylori* (B). Although vagotomy and antrectomy are another option, they would seldom be used in the emergent setting because of the higher associated morbidity rate (D, E). An HSV (C) would not address the actively bleeding ulcer.

References: Brullet E, Calvet X, Campo R, Rue M, Catot L, Donoso L. Factors predicting failure of endoscopic injection therapy in bleeding duodenal ulcer. *Gastrointest Endosc.* 1996;43(2):111–116.

Lau JY, Sung JJ, Lam YH, et al. Endoscopic retreatment compared with surgery in patients with recurrent bleeding after initial endoscopic control of bleeding ulcers. *N Engl J Med.* 1999;340(10):751–756.

32. D. Recurrent episodes of acute pancreatitis predispose patients to developing splenic vein thrombosis, which can result in isolated gastric varices. Historically, patients were offered a splenectomy as a prophylactic measure to prevent severe upper GI bleeding. However, with improved imaging we are better able to identify splenic vein thrombosis, and we now know that only 4% of patients will have clinically significant gastric variceal bleeding, so routine splenectomy has fallen out of favor. This patient also has a concomitant ulcer, which could have been contributing to hematemesis. The Forrest classification grades peptic ulcers based on endoscopic features and allows the clinician to determine risk of rebleeding. The risk decreases in the following order: active spurting bleeding (17%–100%), active oozing bleeding (17%–100%), nonbleeding visible vessel (0%–81%), adherent clot (14%–36%), flat pigment spot (0%–13%), and clean visible ulcer base (0%–10%) (A–C, E). Although patients with high-risk peptic ulcers (active bleeding/oozing, nonbleeding visible vessel) may benefit from a second-look endoscopy, current guidelines recommend against routine second-look endoscopy.

References: Forrest JH, Finlayson NDC, Shearman DJC. Endoscopy in gastrointestinal bleeding. *Lancet.* 1974;304(7877):394–397.

Heider TR, Azeem S, Galanko JA, Behrns KE. The natural history of pancreatitis-induced splenic vein thrombosis. *Ann Surg.* 2004;239(6):876–882.

Laine L, Jensen DM. Management of patients with ulcer bleeding. *Am J Gastroenterol.* 2012;107(3):345–360.

33. E. Hyperplastic polyps are by far the most common gastric polyps (70%–90%) (B). Other types include adenomatous, hamartomatous, inflammatory (pseudopolyps), fundic gland, and heterotopic. Hyperplastic polyps are seen in association with chronic atrophic gastritis, which is due to *H. pylori* infection (C). Hyperplastic polyps are further classified into polypoid foveolar hyperplasia and typical hyperplastic polyps. Polypoid foveolar hyperplasia does not seem to have malignant potential, whereas the typical hyperplastic polyp has an approximately 2% chance of developing malignancy. Adenomatous polyps have the highest risk of malignancy (10%–20%), and the risk of malignancy seems to be related to size and histology (greater risk for villous than tubular) (A). Fundic gastric polyps are associated with long-term PPI use, and the risk of cancer is negligible. Additionally, hamartomatous, inflammatory, and heterotopic polyps do not seem to have a risk of malignancy. Heterotopic polyps are usually the result of ectopic pancreatic tissue and are typically benign lesions without clinical significance (D). However, large heterotopic polyps can lead to obstruction and intussusception. Treatment for most polyps is simply endoscopic polypectomy. Additional surgical resection is recommended for polyps that are sessile and larger than 2 cm, those with areas of invasive tumor, and those that cause symptoms (bleeding or pain).

References: Orlowska J, Jarosz D, Pachlewski J, Butruk E. Malignant transformation of benign epithelial gastric polyps. *Am J Gastroenterol.* 1995;90(12):2152–2159.

Jalving M, Koornstra JJ, Wesseling J, Boezen HM, DE Jong S, Kleibeuker JH. Increased risk of fundic gland polyps during long-term proton pump inhibitor therapy. *Aliment Pharmacol Ther.* 2006;24(9):1341–1348.

34. D. A Dieulafoy lesion is a congenital malformation in the stomach (typically on the lesser curvature) characterized by a submucosal artery that is abnormally large and tortuous. As a result of its relatively superficial location, it may erode through the mucosa and become exposed to gastric secretions, leading to massive upper GI hemorrhage. On endoscopy, the mucosa of the stomach appears normal, and the only finding is a pinpoint area of mucosal defect with brisk arterial bleeding. The lesion may easily be missed if the bleeding is not active. Dieulafoy lesion is not premalignant (E) and is not associated with the ingestion of foreign material (C). Treatment is endoscopic, via electrocautery, heater probe, or injection with a sclerosing agent. Surgery, which consists of a wedge resection, is reserved for the rare patient who is not controlled endoscopically. Antral vascular ectasia (A) is seen in a condition known as watermelon stomach and can lead to significant acute or chronic GI blood loss. Dilated mucosal blood vessels containing thrombus, mucosal fibromuscular dysplasia, and hyalinization are prominent features. It derives its name from the mucosal vessels that create parallel lines in the mucosal folds (B). The stomach is typically not enlarged. It is seen predominantly in elderly women with autoimmune disease or elderly males with cirrhosis.

Reference: Selinger CP, Ang YS. Gastric antral vascular ectasia (GAVE): an update on clinical presentation, pathophysiology, and treatment. *Digestion.* 2008;77(2):131–137.

35. E. The most sensitive and specific test for gastrinoma (ZES) is the secretin stimulation test. An IV bolus of secretin is administered, and gastrin levels are checked before and after injection. An increase in serum gastrin of 120 pg/mL or greater has the highest sensitivity and specificity for gastrinoma. There are numerous other causes of hypergastrinemia. They can be divided into those associated with an increased acid production and those with a decreased acid production (A). In the latter situation, the hypergastrinemia is reactive due to hypo- or achlorhydria. In addition to ZES, G-cell hyperplasia, gastric outlet obstruction, and retained antrum after Billroth II reconstruction are associated with increased acid production. Reactive hypergastrinemia is seen with atrophic gastritis, pernicious anemia, and gastric cancer; in patients receiving H_2-receptor antagonists and PPIs; and after vagotomy. Hypergastrinemia is also seen in chronic renal failure due to decreased catabolism. Given this broad differential, fasting serum gastrin levels (C) are not sufficiently specific to establish the diagnosis of ZES in the majority of patients unless gastrin levels are extremely high (>1000 pg/mL). The secretin stimulation test has higher sensitivity and specificity than the calcium stimulation test (D). The calcium stimulation test is used if the secretin test result is negative and there is a high suspicion for ZES in the presence of hypergastrinemia. Once the diagnosis of ZES is established, a nuclear octreotide scan (B) seems to be the most sensitive test to localize the tumor.

Reference: Berna M, Hoffmann K, Long S. Serum gastrin in Zollinger-Ellison syndrome: II. Prospective study of gastrin provocative testing in 293 patients from the National Institutes of Health and comparison with 537 cases from the literature: evaluation of diagnostic criteria, proposal of new criteria, and correlations with clinical and tumoral features. *Medicine.* 2006;(6):331–364.

Alimentary Tract— Small Bowel

9

ZACHARY N. WEITZNER, FORMOSA CHEN,
AND BEVERLEY A. PETRIE

ABSITE 99th Percentile High-Yields

I. Duodenum
   A. Releases alkaline mucus from Brunner glands to neutralize gastric acid
   B. S cells release secretin (inhibits gastric acid, stimulates pancreatic bicarb, increases bile production in liver) and I cells release cholecystokinin (CCK) (inhibits gastric emptying, stimulates pancreatic enzyme production, increases bile, gallbladder contraction, satiety)
   C. Leafy appearing villi, absorb iron, eroded in celiac disease
   D. Bulb: 1st segment; ulcerations due to *Helicobacter pylori*, Zollinger–Ellison syndrome
   E. Descending: 2nd segment; pancreatic and common bile duct empty
   F. Transverse: 3rd segment; anterior to inferior vena cava, aorta, vertebral column
   G. Ascending: 4th segment; joins jejunum; ends at ligament of Treitz
   H. Blood supply: celiac axis via gastroduodenal artery and SMA axis via pancreaticoduodenal arteries

II. Jejunum
   A. Does not have Brunner glands; thus marginal ulcers are more likely with Billroth II than with Billroth I
   B. Begins at ligament of Treitz
   C. Identifiable by long vasa recta from SMA and plicae circularis
   D. Dense villi for absorption of water, lipids, NaCl, glucose, amino acids

III. Ileum
   A. Three meters long, short vasa recta from SMA, flatter mucosa with Peyer patches lymphoid tissue
   B. Terminal ileum (TI) is chief site of absorption of B12, folate, and bile salts (conjugated in TI, unconjugated elsewhere in ileum)

IV. Absorptive Defects
   A. Diagnostic tests
      1. Sudan red stain: detects presence of fat in stool
      2. Schilling test: detects B12 deficiency; oral labeled B12 given with unlabeled IM B12 to force urinary excretion; if radiolabeled B12 in urine, able to absorb B12; if none, repeated with PO intrinsic factor; if labeled B12 in urine → pernicious anemia; if not, primary small bowel (SB) malabsorption
      3. D-xylose test: PO D-xylose given, if not excreted in urine, then primary SB absorption deficit
   B. Short Gut Syndrome (SGS)
      1. Defined by malabsorption due to loss of intestinal length; diagnosis based on symptoms
      2. Due to both loss of absorption and decreased transit time
      3. Risk of SGS with less than 180 cm of small bowel; lower risk with competent ileocecal valve
         a) Having 50% to 100% of functional large intestine is equivalent to 50 cm small bowel
         b) Ileum can adapt after resection by dilating, elongating, increasing size of villi to increase absorption, more important than jejunum in SGS

4. Complications: total parenteral nutrition (TPN) associated liver disease, cholelithiasis, calcium oxalate nephrolithiasis, coagulopathy, bacterial overgrowth, sepsis
5. Tx: prevention of sepsis, slow transit (loperamide, etc.), reduce GI secretion with octreotide and PPI, restrict oxalate in diet
6. Teduglutide: GLP-2 agonist to promote intestinal absorption and health
7. Surgical tx: slow transit by interposing colon, reversing intestinal segments, lengthening procedures (STEP), intestinal transplantation

V. Structural Disease
   A. Duodenal diverticula
   1. Most common small bowel diverticula; most are asymptomatic
   2. Operate only if symptomatic with small bowel obstruction (SBO), biliary obstruction, concern for malignancy

VI. Mechanical Disease
   A. Small bowel obstruction
   1. Most commonly due to adhesions in first world; hernia elsewhere
   2. Early small bowel follow-through (SBFT) to determine likelihood of resolution with conservative management
   3. Closed-loop obstruction may have normal lactate
   4. Avoid nitrous oxide during anesthesia as gas third spaces
   5. Law of LaPlace: $P = 2T/r$
   6. Malignancy is suspected for SBO in a virgin abdomen; always check for a hernia
   B. Stricture
   1. Heineke-Mikulicz: stricture <7 cm, longitudinal incision on antimesenteric bowel closed in transverse fashion
   2. Finney: stricture 7 to 15 cm, longitudinal enterotomy on antimesenteric bowel sutured in side-to-side isoperistaltic enteroenterostomy
   3. Jaboulay: stricture 10 to 20 cm, 2 enterotomies anastomosed in side-to-side fashion bypassing strictured segment
   4. Michelassi: stricture >15 cm or multiple consecutive strictures, bowel divided at midpoint of stricture, stenotic areas overlapped, longitudinal enterotomies along stricture, then anastomosed in side-to-side isoperistaltic fashion

VII. Small Bowel Neoplasms
   A. Carcinoid: most common SB neoplasm
   1. Slow-growing tumors of Kulchitsky enterochromaffin cells, usually nonfunctional, carcinoid syndrome when functional
   2. Most commonly located in ileum followed by rectum
   3. Strong desmoplastic reaction and mesenteric fibrosis surrounding can obstruct
   4. Carcinoid syndrome: secretes serotonin, histamine, VIP, bradykinin, prostaglandins which cause flushing, diarrhea, bronchoconstriction, and right-sided valvular heart disease (most commonly tricuspid insufficiency); tx=octreotide
   5. Elevated chromogranin-A, pancreatic polypeptide, NSE, 5-HIAA
   6. Resect if possible; can debulk liver mets
   7. Gastric carcinoid (types I and II have hypergastrinemia; type III does not)
      a) Type I: autoimmune etiology associated with atrophic gastritis; associated with hypergastrinemia and in setting of chronic atrophic gastritis or pernicious anemia, rarely malignant, usually women, small and multicentric; if less than 1 cm without concerning risk factors, can remove endoscopically
      b) Type II: associated with the Zollinger-Ellison syndrome (hypergastrinemia) and MEN-1; grows slowly but more likely to metastasize to lymph nodes and distant sites; somatostatin analogs may be initiated and result in tumor regression; needs gastric resection
      c) Type III: usually poorly differentiated neuroendocrine cell, normal gastrin level, high rate of cancer, and usually needs partial gastrectomy and lymph node dissection

8. Appendiceal carcinoid:
   a) <2 cm at tip: appendectomy
   b) >2 cm or at base of appendix: right hemicolectomy
9. Bronchial carcinoid:
   a) Carcinoid tumors may be diagnosed by bronchoscopy, appearing as pink or purple friable endobronchial masses covered by intact epithelium
   b) Tx: Complete surgical resection with mediastinal lymph node sampling or dissection, regardless of the presence of nodal involvement
10. Diagnosis
    a) Octreotide scan: best for localizing; indium 111-labeled somatostatin scintigraphy
    b) Ga-68 DOTATATE PET/CT: better than octreotide scan for localizing NETs
    c) Chromogranin A level most sensitive for detection

B. Adenocarcinoma
   1. Second most common primary SB tumor
   2. Risk factors: smoking, EtOH, peptic ulcer disease, celiac disease, Crohn disease, FAP, HNPCC, PJS
   3. Goal is R0 resection with 10 mesenteric lymph nodes, may need Whipple

C. Lymphoma
   1. From lymphoid tissues such as Peyer patches, thus more common in jejunum and ileum
   2. B-cell NHL most common, better prognosis than T-cell lymphomas
   3. Enteropathy-associated T-cell lymphoma has poor prognosis, associated with celiac
   4. Tx is surgical resection with adjuvant CHOP or R-CHOP chemotherapy

D. Metastases
   1. Melanoma most common; colon, breast, lung, kidney also seen

VIII. Fistulas and Ileostomies

A. High output fistula >500 cc/day, unlikely to spontaneously resolve
B. Check for *FRIENDS*: foreign bodies, radiation, inflammation/inflammatory bowel disease, neoplasm, distal obstruction, steroids/sepsis
C. High ileostomy output considered >1200 cc/day and managed with antimotility agents, maintain hydration
D. Loss of bicarb leads to uric acid nephrolithiasis in high output fistulae and ostomies

IX. Crohn Disease

A. Abdominal pain, diarrhea +/− hematochezia, ileitis, obstruction, perianal disease, lateral fissures
B. Aphthous ulcers, anemia, vitamin deficiencies, malnutrition, cholesterol gallstones, oxalate kidney stones, blind loop syndrome, fistulae, megaloblastic anemia (decreased B12)
C. Extraintestinal sx that resolve with resection: uveitis, erythema nodosum
D. Extraintestinal sx that do not resolve with resection: ankylosing spondylitis, pyoderma gangrenosum
E. Tx: induction therapy with steroids (sometimes infliximab), maintenance therapy with biologics and mesalamine/sulfasalazine
F. Skip lesions, rare rectal involvement but common perianal involvement, fat creeping, deep transmural ulcers that are serpiginous, common stenotic lesions, noncaseating granulomas on histology
G. Surgery to treat obstruction, maintain intestinal length; do not perform fistulotomies

Heineke-Mikulicz Stricturoplasty

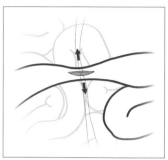
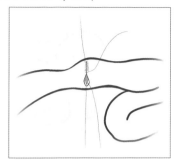

Finney Stricturoplasty

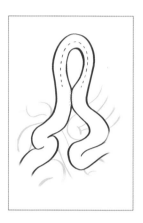
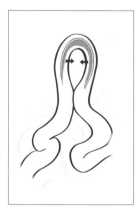
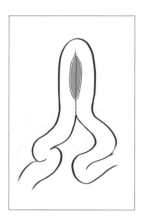
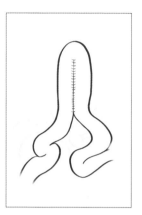

The Heineke-Mickulicz stricturoplasty is best suited for short strictures (≤7 cm). The technique is performed by making a longitudinal incision on the antimesenteric side of the bowel, extending from 2 cm proximal to 2 cm distal to the stricture, and then closing in a transverse fashion.

The Finney Stricturoplasty is used for longer strictures up to 15 cm. An enterotomy is created in a longitudinal fashion, and a loop is folded over itself at its midpoint section to create a U shape. The edges of the bowel are sutured together to create a short side-to-side enteroenterostomy.

Fig. 9.1 Heineke-Mikulicz Stricturoplasty and Finney Stricturoplasty.

Questions

1. A 55-year-old woman with a history of total abdominal colectomy with end ileostomy for refractory Crohn disease presents with a bulge adjacent to her ileostomy. The bulge has been present for months and has always been easily reducible. However, she frequently develops bloating, obstipation, and low ostomy output requiring manual reduction of the bulge. What is the best treatment option for this patient?
   A. Primary parastomal hernia repair
   B. Relocation of her ileostomy with mesh closure of the previous defect
   C. Parastomal hernia repair with mesh
   D. Ileal pouch-anal anastomosis
   E. Observation

2. A 62-year-old female presents to clinic for her 2-week follow-up appointment after undergoing a low anterior resection with diverting loop ileostomy for rectal cancer. Her incisions are healing well. She states her ostomy has put out 1.9 L per day and she has doubled her daily fluid intake due to increased thirst. Her serum creatinine remains normal and she has no electrolyte abnormalities. What is the best treatment option for this patient?
   A. Admission to the hospital for IV hydration
   B. Oral loperamide and close outpatient monitoring
   C. Revision to a more distal ostomy
   D. Methylnaltrexone and close outpatient monitoring
   E. Observation

3. A 55-year-old man with a history of heavy nonsteroidal antiinflammatory drugs (NSAID) use is admitted with a perforated antral ulcer. He undergoes a Billroth II reconstruction. On postoperative day 4, he develops acute abdominal pain and hemodynamic instability. Which of the following complications is most likely causing this presentation?
   A. Anastomotic leak of gastrojejunostomy
   B. Efferent limb syndrome
   C. Duodenal stump blowout
   D. Marginal ulcer
   E. Internal hernia

4. Two weeks after an open aortic aneurysm repair, the patient presents with marked abdominal distention without nausea or vomiting. There is no tenderness on abdominal examination. Plain films are unremarkable. CT scan reveals a large amount of ascites but is otherwise unremarkable. Paracentesis reveals turbid fluid that is culture negative. Fluid analysis reveals a triglyceride level of 400 mg/dL. The white blood cell count is 600 cells/μL with a predominance of lymphocytes. Which of the following is true about this condition?
   A. The patient should be placed on total parental nutrition (TPN) and NPO
   B. Octreotide is not useful
   C. The patient should immediately be reexplored
   D. Interventional radiology (IR) embolization is first-line treatment
   E. Most patients respond to a high-protein, low-fat diet with medium-chain triglycerides

5. Which of the following is true regarding short bowel syndrome in adults?
   A. The presence of an intact ileocecal valve reduces malabsorption
   B. It is defined as less than 300 cm of the residual small bowel
   C. Resection of the ileum is better tolerated than resection of the jejunum
   D. The presence of an intact colon does not alter the severity
   E. It is most commonly caused by multiple operations requiring small bowel resection

6. Which of the following is true regarding the management of short bowel syndrome?
   A. Glutamine should be avoided
   B. Octreotide is the cornerstone of management
   C. Codeine is contraindicated
   D. Early enteral feeding is indicated
   E. Patients who require TPN after 6 months will require permanent TPN

7. A 6-year-old boy has short bowel syndrome caused by midgut volvulus that developed during infancy and has since been dependent on TPN, which he has tolerated well. He has approximately 28 cm of small bowel remaining with an intact colon. The small bowel is markedly dilated without evidence of small bowel obstruction. Which of the following is the best option?

   A. Serial transverse enteroplasty procedure (STEP)
   B. Continue with TPN
   C. Small bowel transplantation
   D. Small bowel tapering procedure
   E. Tapering and lengthening procedure (Bianchi)

8. Which of the following is true regarding small bowel neoplasms?

   A. Adenocarcinoma is the most common type
   B. Small bowel lymphoma most commonly occurs in the duodenum
   C. The incidence of primary small intestinal cancers is increasing
   D. Five-year survival is higher for adenocarcinoma compared with carcinoid tumors
   E. Small bowel lymphoma is primarily treated by chemotherapy

9. A 68-year-old woman presents with an exacerbation of congestive heart failure and acute abdominal pain. Physical examination of the abdomen is significant for mild diffuse abdominal tenderness but no rebound or guarding. CT arteriography of the abdomen demonstrates diffuse narrowing of the superior mesenteric artery (SMA) and its branches but no vascular occlusion, pneumatosis, free air, or portal venous gas. Which of the following is an appropriate management option?

   A. IV heparin drip
   B. Exploratory laparotomy
   C. Aggressive fluid resuscitation
   D. Intraarterial papaverine
   E. Increase cardiac output

10. Which of the following is true regarding carcinoid?

   A. The majority of carcinoid syndrome is from appendiceal tumors that have metastasized
   B. The most common symptom of carcinoid syndrome is diarrhea
   C. Chromogranin A will not be elevated in nonfunctioning tumors
   D. Patients are at an increased risk for glossitis
   E. Urinary 5-hydroxyindoleacetic acid (5-HIAA) is not sensitive for detecting metastatic carcinoid

11. Which of the following is the best test for prognosis and monitoring treatment response in carcinoid tumors?

   A. Platelet serotonin levels
   B. 24-hour urinary 5-HIAA test
   C. Serum chromogranin A levels
   D. Serum serotonin levels
   E. Neuron-specific enolase

12. Which of the following is true regarding small bowel obstruction?

   A. The most common worldwide etiology is adhesions from prior surgery
   B. It is more frequent with upper intestinal than lower intestinal surgery
   C. In a complete closed-loop obstruction, serum lactate can be normal
   D. Partial obstruction symptoms typically improve within 24 hours with conservative management
   E. Abdominal pain disproportionate to exam findings occurs early in the setting of obstruction

13. Which of the following is true regarding duodenal diverticula?

   A. They tend to occur on the antimesenteric side of the bowel
   B. Most are identified in young patients
   C. Treatment with endoscopic interventions is contraindicated
   D. Malabsorption due to bacterial overgrowth within the diverticula mandates surgery
   E. When discovered incidentally at surgery, they should be left alone

14. Which of the following is the most common cause of obscure GI bleeding in adults?

   A. Small intestine angiodysplasia
   B. Meckel diverticulum
   C. Crohn disease
   D. Infectious enteritis
   E. Vasculitis

15. Which of the following is true regarding GISTs of the small bowel?

   A. Most patients are symptomatic with GI bleeding
   B. They stain positive for CD134
   C. Patients deemed candidates for chemotherapy should receive it for 1 year
   D. A patient with a 6-cm tumor should receive adjuvant chemotherapy
   E. Malignancy is primarily determined by evidence of local invasion

16. A hernia sac containing a Meckel diverticulum is known as:
    A. Petit hernia
    B. Littre hernia
    C. Spigelian hernia
    D. Richter hernia
    E. Grynfeltt hernia

17. Superior mesenteric artery (SMA) (Wilkie) syndrome:
    A. Involves the second portion of the duodenum
    B. Causes venous outflow obstruction from the left kidney
    C. Is best diagnosed with arteriography
    D. Should initially be managed with a high caloric intake diet
    E. Is best managed by gastrojejunostomy

18. A 45-year-old woman with a history of laparotomy and 5000 cGy of abdominal and pelvic irradiation for ovarian cancer 10 years ago presents with symptoms and signs of an acute bowel obstruction. CT scan shows a complete small bowel obstruction at the level of the mid jejunum with no evidence of any masses. Which of the following is true about this condition?
    A. If a stricture is present, it is best managed by strictureplasty
    B. Steroids should be administered
    C. Acute radiation enteritis is due to an obliterative arteritis
    D. The risk of this complication increases in the setting of diabetes
    E. The degree of radiation damage is not affected by whether the patient received chemotherapy

19. A 75-year-old male with a history of chronic obstructive pulmonary disease (COPD) presents to the ED with a 1-day history of abdominal distention and nausea. He denies abdominal pain. Abdominal examination is benign. Laboratory values are normal. CT scan demonstrates free air under the diaphragm and thin-walled, air-filled cysts within the bowel wall. Which of the following is true regarding this condition?
    A. Laparotomy is indicated
    B. The primary form occurs more commonly than the secondary form
    C. It is unlikely to be related to the patient's COPD
    D. It is most commonly seen in the ileum
    E. It is associated with steroid use

20. Which of the following is true regarding Peutz-Jeghers syndrome?
    A. Patients should begin breast and cervical cancer screening at age 25
    B. It is autosomal recessive
    C. Small bowel obstruction is uncommon
    D. Prophylactic colectomy is recommended to most patients starting at age 20
    E. These patients are not at increased risk for small bowel cancer

21. Which of the following is correct with regards to Crohn disease?
    A. Mesenteric fat wrapping is considered pathognomonic
    B. Symptoms of ankylosing spondylitis improve with resection of diseased bowel
    C. The majority of patients with an initial presentation of terminal ileitis progress to Crohn disease on long-term follow-up
    D. Exaggerated skin injury after minor trauma (pathergy) is a commonly associated condition
    E. Pyoderma gangrenosum is commonly found on the initial presentation of Crohn disease

22. Which intestinal cells have been implicated in the formation of gastrointestinal stromal tumors (GISTs)?
    A. Goblet cells
    B. Interstitial cells of Cajal
    C. Enteroendocrine cells
    D. Paneth cells
    E. Absorptive enterocytes

23. A 46-year-old woman is about to undergo hepatic resection for a metastatic carcinoid tumor. During anesthesia induction, her blood pressure decreases to 80 mmHg systolic and her heart rate increases to 110 beats per minute. Her entire body appears flushed. Her temperature is normal, as is end-tidal CO2. Management consists of:
    A. Corticosteroids
    B. Antihistamine
    C. Octreotide
    D. Abort operation
    E. Dantrolene

24. A 70-year-old woman presents with vague abdominal pain, diarrhea, steatorrhea, and anemia with an elevated mean corpuscular volume. Her medical and surgical history is unremarkable. A CT scan of the abdomen and pelvis is negative. An upper GI series and small bowel follow-through are significant only for a large jejunal diverticulum. Which of the following is true regarding this patient?

    A. It is typically caused by an autoimmune etiology
    B. A long-chain triglyceride diet may be helpful
    C. The diverticulum should be resected
    D. Broad-spectrum antibiotics are indicated only if the patient presents with a fever and leukocytosis
    E. Vitamin B12 is indicated

25. A 57-year-old male with no past surgical history presents with 2 days of abdominal pain, nausea, and vomiting. On exam he is distended and tympanic and is mildly tender to palpation without rebound or guarding. He has no groin hernias. Computed tomography (CT) scan demonstrates multiple dilated loops of small bowel with a transition point in the distal small bowel, with some adjacent mesenteric fat stranding. He has a mild leukocytosis. His last bowel movement was 1 day ago. He has not passed flatus for over a day. He has not had any similar symptoms previously. A nasogastric (NG) tube is placed, intravenous (IV) fluids are administered, and the patient is placed NPO (nothing by mouth). Which of the following is the best next step in management?

    A. A 24-hour trial of NG tube suction, then exploratory laparotomy if high output continues
    B. Exploratory laparotomy
    C. Water-soluble oral contrast challenge
    D. Water-soluble oral and rectal contrast challenge
    E. Diagnostic laparoscopy

26. Which of the following has been shown to be the most efficacious means of reducing postoperative ileus in patients undergoing bowel resection?

    A. Early ambulation
    B. Gum chewing
    C. Alvimopan
    D. Ketorolac combined with reduction in opioid use
    E. Nasogastric intubation

27. Which of the following is true regarding Crohn disease?

    A. It is more common in individuals of high socioeconomic status
    B. The most common indication for surgery is perforation
    C. It has a unimodal distribution
    D. It is more prevalent in females
    E. The most common initial presentation is an acute onset of abdominal pain and diarrhea

28. The earliest lesion characteristic of Crohn disease is:

    A. Aphthous ulcer
    B. Caseating granuloma
    C. Noncaseating granuloma
    D. Cobblestone mucosa
    E. Serosal thickening

29. Which of the following is the best therapeutic option for mild active Crohn disease?

    A. Sulfasalazine
    B. Prednisone
    C. Budesonide
    D. Metronidazole
    E. Infliximab

30. Which of the following is true regarding the principles of operative management of the small bowel in Crohn disease?

    A. The optimal margin is at least 4 cm beyond grossly visible disease
    B. Frozen section should be obtained to confirm the absence of active disease in at least one margin
    C. A 3-cm strictured segment of duodenum is best managed by resection
    D. A 10-cm strictured segment of jejunum can be managed by a Heineke-Mikulicz strictureplasty rather than by resection
    E. Strictures longer than 10 cm are best managed by resection

Answers

1. C. This patient presents with a chronic, reducible parastomal hernia. The definitive treatment for parastomal hernia repair is ostomy reversal; however, given this patient's Crohn disease, ostomy takedown with ileoanal anastomosis or ileal pouch-anal anastomosis is contraindicated (D). Given the recurrent discomfort and intermittent obstruction from her hernia, simple observation would not be appropriate (E). Once taught as the surgical treatment of choice for parastomal hernia repair, ostomy relocation is no longer advised as it creates the potential for a new parastomal hernia and for hernias from prior ostomy site and laparotomy incisions. SAGES now recommends against ostomy relocation as the treatment of parastomal hernias (B). Primary parastomal hernia repair results in high tension with a high rate of hernia recurrence (A). The most effective treatment for parastomal hernias adjacent to ostomies that are unable to be reversed is mesh repairs (C). Standard approaches include the Sugarbaker repair, in which an underlay mesh is placed on the defect with the stoma exiting the peritoneum at the side of the mesh, and the keyhole approach, when the stoma is brought through a hole created in the mesh.

Reference: Gillern S, Bleier JIS. Parastomal hernia repair and reinforcement: the role of biologic and synthetic materials. *Clin Colon Rectal Surg.* 2014;27(4):162–171.

2. B. This patient presents with high ostomy output, usually defined as over 1.2 L per day. High ostomy output can result in dehydration, loss of bicarbonate resulting in uric acid nephrolithiasis, and skin breakdown. In the absence of dehydration or electrolyte abnormalities requiring inpatient admission, high ostomy output can be managed as an outpatient with close follow-up and titration of oral loperamide or Lomotil. When high ostomy output results in symptomatic dehydration or electrolyte disturbances, admission for inpatient hydration and monitoring is recommended (A). Ostomy revision is not typically required for high ostomy output and diverting loop ileostomies are usually distal enough to adequately absorb fluid (C). Methylnaltrexone is an opioid antagonist used to treat opioid-induced ileus and is not absorbed enterally (D). Observation is not appropriate for high ileostomy output (E).

3. C. The most serious complication after a Billroth II reconstruction is a duodenal stump blowout. In a Billroth II, the pylorus and antrum are resected, and the first portion of the duodenum is oversewn. The biliary system drains into the duodenum, which then rejoins path of food at a surgically constructed gastrojejunostomy. The inflammation caused by a perforated ulcer results in inflammation of the duodenum, which may leak after oversewing. Additional causes of duodenal stump blowout include afferent limb obstruction and pancreatitis. Efferent limb syndrome is the result of obstruction of the efferent limb distal to the gastrojejunostomy, resulting in bile reflux and bilious emesis (B). Anastomotic leak of the gastrojejunostomy is possible but less common and catastrophic than duodenal stump blowout. A marginal ulcer is more likely to occur after a Billroth II reconstruction,

as compared to after a Billroth I, because the alkaline environment secreted by Brunner glands in the duodenum is not present in the jejunum. However, marginal ulcers, which are present on the jejunal side of the anastomosis, present with abdominal pain and possible upper GI bleeding (D). Any procedure that can result in adhesions has the potential to cause an internal hernia, though the highest chance is after a gastric bypass. The presentation of internal hernia is typically indolent with vague abdominal pain, nausea, and vomiting and can be confused for gastroenteritis or peptic ulcer disease. A high index of suspicion is required, and the diagnosis often requires diagnostic laparoscopy for confirmation (E).

4. E. The patient has chylous ascites. In Western countries, chylous ascites is most often due to malignancy and cirrhosis, whereas infectious etiologies such as tuberculosis and filariasis predominate in Eastern and developing countries. Other causes include postlaparotomy inflammatory disorders, trauma, radiation therapy, congenital lymphatic abnormalities, and pancreatitis. The operations most associated with this complication include aortic aneurysm repair, retroperitoneal lymph node dissection, inferior vena cava surgery, and liver transplantation, because these are operations in which retroperitoneal lymphatics are most likely to be interrupted. The mechanisms thought to lead to the development of chylous ascites include exudation of chyle due to obstruction of the cisterna chyli, direct leakage of chyle through a lymphoperitoneal fistula, and exudation through dilated retroperitoneal vessels. The diagnosis of chylous ascites is best established by analysis of the fluid. Chyle typically has a turbid appearance; however, it may be clear in fasting patients. Elevated triglyceride levels in the fluid are considered diagnostic, usually above 200 mg/dL, although some use a threshold above 110 mg/dL. In addition, the white blood cell count is greater than 500, with a predominance of lymphocytes. The total protein level is between 2.5 and 7.0 g/dL. Cultures are negative, except for cases of tuberculosis, in which adenosine deaminase is also positive in the fluid. The initial treatment of chylous ascites is to administer a high-protein, low-fat diet with medium-chain triglycerides. This diet minimizes chyle production and flow. Medium-chain triglycerides are absorbed by the intestinal epithelium and are transported to the liver through the portal vein and do not contribute to chylomicron formation. Conversely, long-chain triglycerides are converted to monoglycerides and free fatty acids, which are then transported to the intestinal lymph vessels as chylomicrons. If this diet regimen fails, placing the patient NPO and on TPN with octreotide has been shown to be useful in patients with postoperative chylous ascites (A, B). If these medical approaches fail, then lymphoscintigraphy is often useful to localize lymph leaks and the site of obstruction. In some instances, IR can percutaneously inject glue to stop leak. Surgical reexploration with localization and closure of the lymphatic leak should be performed if leak persists beyond 2 weeks (C). Alternatively, in facilities with capabilities to perform percutaneous lymphangiography, embolization of lymphatics may be attempted after failed dietary management (D). This latter complication may be due to a high plasminogen concentration in the ascitic fluid.

Reference: Cárdenas A, Chopra S. Chylous ascites. *Am J Gastroenterol.* 2002;97(8):1896–1900.

5. A. The total length of small bowel is approximately 20 feet (each foot is equal to ≈30 cm), or approximately 600 cm (6 m). Short bowel syndrome is defined as the presence of less than 180 cm of residual and functional small bowel in adult patients (B). Thus, resection of less than 50% of the small intestine is generally well tolerated. In approximately 75% of cases, short bowel syndrome results from one massive small bowel resection, as opposed to multiple sequential resections (E). In adults, the most common etiologies include acute mesenteric ischemia, malignancy, and Crohn disease. In pediatric patients, the most common etiologies include intestinal atresia, midgut volvulus, and necrotizing enterocolitis. Resection of the jejunum is better tolerated than resection of the ileum because the absorption of bile salts and vitamin B12 occurs in the ileum (C). An intact ileocecal valve is thought to reduce malabsorption because it increases the residence time of the chyme in the small intestine. Likewise, an intact colon is important because it has a tremendous water-reabsorbing capacity and electrolytes and can also absorb fatty acids (D). With an intact colon, a shorter small bowel remnant is tolerated. The key to preventing short bowel syndrome is avoidance of excessive small bowel resection. In Crohn patients, the use of strictureplasty as opposed to resection is recommended when possible. Also, one should resect only obviously dead bowel in acute mesenteric ischemia, leaving marginal bowel in situ and performing a second-look procedure.

6. D. In the early phase of short bowel syndrome, treatment is directed at slowing intestinal transit; reducing GI secretions; and maintaining nutrition, fluid, and electrolyte balance. Transit time is slowed by the administration of narcotics such as codeine and diphenoxylate, as well as with the antimotility agents Lomotil (diphenoxylate and atropine) and loperamide (C). Massive small bowel resection is associated with hypergastrinemia and acid hypersecretion. The increased acidity in the small bowel results in the inhibition of digestive enzymes. This can be controlled with H2 receptor antagonists or proton pump inhibitors such as omeprazole and thus should be started in all patients with short gut syndrome (B). Nutrition is achieved with the institution of TPN. In addition, enteral feeding should be instituted as soon as postoperative ileus has resolved. Enteral feeding assists in the process of intestinal adaptation and prevents the development of villous atrophy associated with being NPO for a prolonged period of time. Glutamine is helpful because it serves as a trophic factor for the gut and is considered the principal fuel of the small intestine (A). Cholestyramine is also useful in controlling diarrhea due to unabsorbed bile salts. The role of octreotide is controversial. Short-term use leads to a reduction in diarrhea, but long-term use may lead to steatorrhea, gallstones, and an inhibition of intestinal adaptation. More recently, a high-carbohydrate, low-fat enteral diet rich in glutamine combined with growth hormone administration has shown promise in improving intestinal absorptive capacity.

Intestinal adaptation occurs over a period of 1 to 2 years in most adults. Thus, the final determination of whether permanent TPN will be necessary is not determined until after this period (E).

7. A. Many patients with short bowel syndrome can eventually discontinue TPN, particularly if the bowel length is more than 120 cm in adults or more than 60 cm in children. Treatment options for short bowel syndrome depend on the length of small bowel remaining, whether the remnant small bowel is markedly dilated, whether the patient remains TPN dependent, and whether multiple complications of TPN have developed such as catheter-related infections, vena cava thrombosis, and liver damage (B). A short remnant (<90 cm in adults, <30 cm in children) of small bowel poses a challenging dilemma. If the remnant of small bowel is short and markedly dilated without evidence of obstruction, the best option would be an intestinal lengthening procedure. The dilated bowel lends itself to lengthening by applying a series of transverse linear staples on the mesenteric border and then on the antimesenteric border. The procedure is known as the serial transverse enteroplasty procedure. The Bianchi procedure is another option. However, it is technically much more demanding and associated with a risk of creating ischemia and anastomotic leaks and thus has a higher complication rate and an increased need for reoperation (E). Tapering of the small bowel alone would be indicated for patients with a longer small bowel remnant (>60 cm in children) who have marked bowel distention with evidence of stasis and bacterial overgrowth (D). Tapering alone would not be appropriate in someone with such a short segment of small bowel. Small bowel transplantation is also an option but is reserved for the patient with a short segment and who is TPN dependent (such as this patient) in whom, in addition, complications have developed from the TPN, as mentioned (C). If liver failure has developed in the patient, small bowel transplantation can be combined with liver transplantation.

References: Kim HB, Lee PW, Garza J, Duggan C, Fauza D, Jaksic T. Serial transverse enteroplasty for short bowel syndrome: a case report. *J Pediatr Surg.* 2003;38(6):881–885.

Sudan D, Thompson J, Botha J, et al. Comparison of intestinal lengthening procedures for patients with short bowel syndrome. *Ann Surg.* 2007;246(4):593–601.

8. C. Malignant tumors of the small bowel are rare. However, the incidence has nearly doubled since the 1970s. The most common tumor is carcinoid (37.4%), followed by adenocarcinoma (36.9%), lymphoma (17%), and GISTs (8%) (A). Small bowel lymphomas most commonly involve the ileum (as do carcinoids), whereas adenocarcinomas are most common in the duodenum (periampullary), and GISTs are evenly distributed throughout the small bowel (although most common in the stomach) (B). Small bowel lymphomas are predominantly the non-Hodgkin type. In children younger than age 10, they are the most common intestinal neoplasm. The propensity for involvement of the ileum is due to its high concentration of lymphoid tissue (C). The primary treatment of small bowel lymphoma (as well as all other small bowel malignancies) is surgical resection including the affected mesentery (E). There is no clear, well-defined role for radiation therapy or chemotherapy for the majority of small bowel malignancies. The exception is the use of Gleevec (imatinib mesylate) for GISTs. The 5-year survival rate is higher for carcinoid compared with adenocarcinoma (64.6% versus 32.5%) (D).

References: Balthazar EJ, Noordhoorn M, Megibow AJ, Gordon RB. CT of small-bowel lymphoma in immunocompetent patients and patients with AIDS: comparison of findings. *AJR Am J Roentgenol.* 1997;168(3):675–680.

Bilimoria KY, Bentrem DJ, Wayne JD, Ko CY, Bennett CL, Talamonti MS. Small bowel cancer in the United States: changes in epidemiology, treatment, and survival over the last 20 years. *Ann Surg.* 2009;249(1):63–71.

9. E. The presentation is most consistent with nonocclusive mesenteric ischemia, which accounts for approximately 20% to 30% of acute mesenteric ischemia cases. This condition typically affects elderly patients and presents in the setting of a decrease in cardiac output, such as after an acute myocardial infarction, exacerbation of congestive heart failure, or after cardiac surgery. There are no laboratory tests to establish the diagnosis of bowel ischemia with certainty, although the presence of lactic acidosis is considered ominous. The initial diagnostic test of choice for suspected acute mesenteric ischemia is CT angiography. It is helpful in identifying the etiology, which includes an embolus that would be visualized as an occlusion just distal to the origin of the SMA; acute thrombosis of the SMA, which would appear as an occlusion in association with diffuse calcifications within the vessel; mesenteric venous thrombosis, which would demonstrate a lack of contrast filling of either the portal or superior mesenteric vein; and nonocclusive mesenteric ischemia, which would simply show diffuse spasm. The standard treatment for SMA embolus is operative embolectomy with resection of ischemic or infarcted bowel, although there are some reports of the use of thrombolytic therapy in the absence of signs of bowel compromise (B). The treatment for acute thrombosis is surgical bypass from either the aorta or the iliac artery to the more distal SMA. For mesenteric venous thrombosis, the treatment is heparin alone, provided there is no suggestion of infarcted bowel (A). For nonocclusive mesenteric ischemia, the goal of treatment is to restore intestinal blood flow, which is most successfully done by correcting the underlying cause to improve cardiac output. This may be accomplished with inotropes in the setting of cardiogenic shock. In addition to supportive care, selective intraarterial infusion of a vasodilator, such as papaverine hydrochloride into the SMA to reverse splanchnic vasoconstriction, can be helpful but is not first-line therapy when medical management of cardiac dysfunction may be successful (D). Aggressive fluid resuscitation should be used with caution as nonocclusive mesenteric ischemia often occurs in the setting of decompensated congestive heart failure (as in the above patient), which may worsen with multiple fluid boluses (C). The mortality rate for nonocclusive mesenteric ischemia is approximately 50%.

References: Bassiouny HS. Nonocclusive mesenteric ischemia. *Surg Clin North Am.* 1997;77(2):319–326.

Kozuch P, Brandt L. Review article: diagnosis and management of mesenteric ischemia with an emphasis on pharmacotherapy. *Aliment Pharma Ther.* 2005;21(3):201–215.

Trompeter M, Brazda T, Remy CT, Vestring T, Reimer P. Nonocclusive mesenteric ischemia: etiology, diagnosis, and interventional therapy. *Eur Radiol.* 2002;12(5):1179–1187.

10. D. While it was long believed that the appendix was the most common source of carcinoid tumor, a large SEER database study found that the small intestine accounted for 55% of cases, followed by the rectum (20%), and then the appendix (17%). The most common location in the small bowel is the ileum (A). Carcinoid syndrome most commonly presents with flushing followed by diarrhea and bronchospasms (B). Most gut carcinoid tumors do not cause the syndrome because vasoactive substances (serotonin, histamine, dopamine, substance P, prostaglandins) from these tumors enter the portal vein and are metabolized by the liver before reaching the systemic circulation. For carcinoid syndrome to develop, these substances need to be released directly into the systemic circulation. Thus, the syndrome develops in the setting of bronchial carcinoids (which do not drain into the liver), retroperitoneal invasion (where retroperitoneal veins drain directly into the systemic circulation), or in the presence of liver metastasis. A 24-hour urinary 5-HIAA test is highly sensitive and specific for detecting metastatic carcinoid and is considered the gold-standard test to establish the diagnosis (E). However, it is not as sensitive for detecting nonfunctional carcinoid tumors. Screening for a carcinoid tumor (as opposed to establishing the diagnosis of carcinoid syndrome) is probably best achieved with serum chromogranin A because it will be elevated in both functioning and nonfunctioning tumors (C). Normally, most dietary tryptophan is converted into nicotinic acid (niacin, vitamin B3). In the presence of carcinoid tumors, there is a shift toward conversion to 5-hydroxytryptophan, which is then converted to serotonin. Serotonin is then metabolized to 5-HIAA. The shift away from conversion to tryptophan to nicotinic acid can result in pellagra, which can present with diarrhea, dermatitis (rough scaly skin, glossitis, angular stomatitis), dementia, and/or hypoalbuminemia.

References: Swain CP, Tavill AS, Neale G. Studies of tryptophan and albumin metabolism in a patient with carcinoid syndrome, pellagra, and hypoproteinemia. *Gastroenterology.* 1976;71(3):484–489.

Nobels FR, Kwekkeboom DJ, Coopmans W, et al. Chromogranin A as serum marker for neuroendocrine neoplasia: comparison with neuron-specific enolase and the alpha-subunit of glycoprotein hormones. *J Clin Endocrinol Metab.* 1997;82(8):2622–2628.

Zuetenhorst JM, Taal BG. Metastatic carcinoid tumors: a clinical review. *Oncologist.* 2005;10(2):123–131.

Maggard MA, O'Connell JB, Ko CY. Updated population-based review of carcinoid tumors. *Ann Surg.* 2004;240(1):117–122.

11. C. Serum chromogranin A is the most sensitive marker for detecting neuroendocrine tumors in general. It has also been shown to be the most useful marker for detecting recurrence and response to treatment. Because the level of chromogranin A correlates with tumor burden, it is a useful marker for treatment response. A high level correlates with a worse prognosis. Platelet serotonin level is also useful in detecting carcinoid tumors (A). However, platelets become rapidly saturated with serotonin; thus, it is not a useful tool for monitoring treatment response (D). 5-HIAA is also thought to be useful; however, several studies indicate that chromogranin A is more sensitive for recurrence and a better prognosticator (B). Neuron-specific enolase has a high specificity but a low sensitivity for the detection of carcinoid tumor (E).

References: Bajetta E, Ferrari L, Martinetti A, et al. Chromogranin A, neuron specific enolase, carcinoembryonic antigen, and hydroxyindole acetic acid evaluation in patients with neuroendocrine tumors. *Cancer*. 1999;86(5):858–865.

Eriksson B, Oberg K, Stridsberg M. Tumor markers in neuroendocrine tumors. *Digestion*. 2000;62 Suppl 1(1):33–38.

Janson ET, Holmberg L, Stridsberg M, et al. Carcinoid tumors: analysis of prognostic factors and survival in 301 patients from a referral center. *Ann Oncol*. 1997;8(7):685–690.

Nikou GC, Lygidakis NJ, Toubanakis C, et al. Current diagnosis and treatment of gastrointestinal carcinoids in a series of 101 patients: the significance of serum chromogranin-A, somatostatin receptor scintigraphy and somatostatin analogues. *Hepatogastroenterology*. 2005;52(63):731–741.

12. C. Mechanical SBO is the most frequently encountered surgical disorder of the small intestine and, in the United States, is most commonly due to intraabdominal adhesions related to previous abdominal surgery. However, worldwide it is most commonly due to a hernia (A). The risk of readmission for adhesions is greatest for patients undergoing lower abdominal surgery and seems to be in the 9% range long term (B). Diagnosis of obstruction can be made with CT scan, small bowel series, or enteroclysis (fluoroscopic examination of the small bowel using liquid contrast). The majority of patients can be managed nonoperatively with nasogastric decompression and nutritional support. This is successful in 65% to 81% of patients, and resolution of symptoms most commonly occurs within 48 hours (D). However, any signs and symptoms suggestive of ischemic bowel are an indication for urgent operative intervention. The incidence of strangulation is no greater than with SBO that presents later. Features of strangulated obstruction such as abdominal pain disproportionate to abdominal findings are suggestive of intestinal ischemia and are not usually an early finding (E). Serum lactate levels are 90% sensitive and 87% specific for the presence of bowel ischemia. However, it is possible that patients with a complete closed-loop obstruction (more commonly with volvulus) can have a normal lactate level. This is because obstruction of venous drainage prevents lactic acid produced by enterocytes from reaching systemic circulation. If nasogastric decompression fails to resolve the obstruction, surgery is indicated. The timing of surgery is debatable. In one large series, surgery was recommended for failure of nasogastric decompression after 6 days and in another study after 10 to 14 days. The morbidity and mortality rates of early small bowel obstruction are very low.

References: Ellozy SH, Harris MT, Bauer JJ, Gorfine SR, Kreel I. Early postoperative small-bowel obstruction: a prospective evaluation in 242 consecutive abdominal operations. *Dis Colon Rectum*. 2002;45(9):1214–1217.

Matter I, Khalemsky L, Abrahamson J, Nash E, Sabo E, Eldar S. Does the index operation influence the course and outcome of adhesive intestinal obstruction? *Eur J Surg*. 1997;163(10):767–772.

Parker MC, Ellis H, Moran BJ, et al. Postoperative adhesions: ten-year follow-up of 12,584 patients undergoing lower abdominal surgery. *Dis Colon Rectum*. 2001;44(6):822–829.

Stewart R, Page C, Brender J. The incidence and risk of early postoperative small bowel obstruction: a cohort study. *Am J Surg*. 1987;154(6):643–647.

Tavakkoli A, Ashley SW, Zinner MJ. Small Intestine. In: Brunicardi F, Andersen DK, Billiar TR, Dunn DL, Hunter JG, Matthews JB, Pollock RE, eds. *Schwartz's principles of surgery*. 10th ed. New York: McGraw-Hill Education; 2015:1146–1151.

Atluri P, Karakousis GC, Porrett PM, Kaiser LR, eds. *Surgical review: an integrated basic and clinical science study guide*. 2nd ed. Philadelphia: Lippincott Williams and Wilkins; 2005.

13. E. Acquired diverticula consist of mucosa and submucosa but lack a complete muscularis and are thus considered false diverticula. They are most commonly located in the second portion of the duodenum near the ampulla of Vater and are referred to as periampullary diverticula. They arise on the mesenteric border in areas of weakness in the bowel wall where blood vessels penetrate (A). Periampullary diverticula are associated with cholangitis, pancreatitis, and sphincter of Oddi dysfunction. Duodenal diverticula are also associated with choledocholithiasis. These latter complications are thought to be due to the location of the periampullary diverticulum, which may lead to obstruction and stasis of the common duct. The majority of patients presenting with biliary complications who are discovered to have a duodenal diverticulum can be safely treated endoscopically (C). If this is not successful, surgical diverticulectomy is recommended. Care must be taken during diverticulectomy to identify and preserve the sphincter, which may require cannulation of the common bile duct. These false diverticula are also found in the jejunum and ileum. They are distinguished from a Meckel diverticulum, which is a true diverticulum present at birth. Duodenal diverticula are most often discovered between ages 56 and 76 years during upper endoscopy, endoscopic retrograde cholangiopancreatography, or abdominal imaging in as many as 6% of patients (B). They are asymptomatic in the majority of patients, and thus surgery is not recommended if they are discovered incidentally either on imaging or intraoperatively. Complications are estimated to occur in 6% to 10% of patients. They may cause symptoms of malabsorption due to bacterial overgrowth within the diverticula. This can be treated with antibiotics (D). Less commonly, bleeding can arise within the diverticulum, or diverticulitis can develop, leading to perforation, which usually occurs into the retroperitoneum. Perforation requires laparotomy, and closure of the duodenal defect can be challenging and may require placing a loop of jejunum over the defect as a serosal patch.

References: Kennedy RH, Thompson MH. Are duodenal diverticula associated with choledocholithiasis? *Gut*. 1988;29(7):1003–1006.

Tham TCK, Kelly M. Association of periampullary duodenal diverticula with bile duct stones and with technical success of endoscopic retrograde cholangiopancreatography. *Endoscopy*. 2004;36(12):1050–1053.

Vaira D, Dowsett JF, Hatfield AR, et al. Is duodenal diverticulum a risk factor for sphincterotomy? *Gut*. 1989;30(7):939–942.

14. A. The majority of lesions responsible for GI bleeding are seen with upper endoscopy or colonoscopy. Obscure GI bleeding refers to persistent or recurrent bleeding for which no source has been identified by these modalities. Obscure bleeding can be either occult (meaning not visible to the eye) or overt (such as melena and hematochezia). In most instances, the source of obscure bleeding is the small bowel. Small intestine angiodysplasias account for 75% of cases of obscure bleeding in adults (B–E). Other causes include Crohn disease, infectious enteritis, neoplasms, and vasculitis. A Meckel diverticulum is the most common cause of obscure GI bleeding in children. Localization of small bowel lesions is difficult with standard studies. Options include push enteroscopy and small bowel barium studies, capsule endoscopy, radiolabeled red blood cell scanning, and angiography (although these latter two are only useful in the setting of active bleeding).

Reference: Pennazio M, Santucci R, Rondonotti E, et al. Outcome of patients with obscure gastrointestinal bleeding after capsule endoscopy: report of 100 consecutive cases. *Gastroenterology.* 2004;126(3):643–653.

15. D. GISTs were previously termed *leiomyomas* or *leiomyosarcomas.* It now seems that they are mesenchymal tumors. GISTs are classified into three types: spindle cell (70%), epithelioid type (20%), and mixed spindle and epithelioid cell type (10%). GISTs stain positive for CD34, the human progenitor cell antigen, as well as for CD177, the c-kit proto-oncogene protein (B). The stomach is the most common site in the GI tract. Small bowel GISTs may be incidental discoveries at surgery for other disorders. The majority of patients are asymptomatic (A). However, those that do present with symptoms tend to be very large and bulky at presentation. In one large study, the median size of a symptomatic GIST was 11 cm. They tend to present with evidence of obstruction or GI bleeding. The standard treatment is surgical resection with 1 cm margins. However, microscopically positive margins have not been demonstrated to affect survival. GISTs of the small intestine carry a high mortality rate, likely due to the late presentation. Only 28% of patients were alive at a median follow-up of 20 months in one study. Determining whether a GIST is benign or malignant is difficult because seemingly benign tumors may behave in a malignant fashion with local recurrence. The risk of malignancy can be remembered by "the rule of 5s": tumors >5 cm or >5 mitoses per 50 high-power field (E). The adjuvant treatment of GISTs includes chemotherapy with imatinib (Gleevec), a tyrosine kinase inhibitor. In one study, imatinib controlled tumor growth in as many as 85% of advanced GISTs. Currently, imatinib is recommended for unresectable, metastatic, or recurrent lesions. Adjuvant therapy should continue for a total of 3 years (C). Patients that harbor an exon 9 KIT mutation will require a higher dose of imatinib (800 mg daily versus 400 mg). The most useful indicators of survival and the risk of metastasis include the size of the tumor at presentation, the mitotic index, location within the GI tract, and the absence of tumor rupture.

References: Blay JY, Bonvalot S, Casali P, et al. Consensus meeting for the management of gastrointestinal stromal tumors. Report of the GIST Consensus Conference of 20-21 March 2004, under the auspices of ESMO. *Ann Oncol.* 2005;16(4):566–578.

Crosby JA, Catton CN, Davis A, et al. Malignant gastrointestinal stromal tumors of the small intestine: a review of 50 cases from a prospective database. *Ann Surg Oncol.* 2001;8(1):50–59.

Dematteo RP, Ballman KV, Antonescu CR, et al. Adjuvant imatinib mesylate after resection of localised, primary gastrointestinal stromal tumour: a randomised, double-blind, placebo-controlled trial. *Lancet.* 2009;373(9669):1097–1104.

Joensuu H, Eriksson M, Sundby Hall K, et al. One vs three years of adjuvant imatinib for operable gastrointestinal stromal tumor: a randomized trial: A randomized trial. *JAMA.* 2012;307(12):1265–1272.

16. B. A hernia sac containing a Meckel diverticulum is called a *Littre hernia.* Lumbar hernias can be either congenital or acquired and occur in the lumbar region of the posterior abdominal wall. Hernias through the superior lumbar triangle (Grynfeltt triangle) (E) are more common than those through the inferior lumbar triangle (the Petit triangle) (A). The Petit triangle is bounded by the external oblique muscle, latissimus dorsi muscle, and iliac crest. The Grynfeltt triangle is bounded by the quadratus lumborum muscle, the 12th rib, and the internal oblique muscle. A spigelian hernia occurs through the spigelian fascia, which is composed of the aponeurotic layer between the rectus muscle medially and the semilunar line laterally (C). Nearly all spigelian hernias occur in the spigelian belt located below the umbilicus but above the epigastric vessels. The absence of posterior rectus fascia may contribute to an inherent weakness in this area. A Richter hernia occurs when only the antimesenteric border of the bowel herniates through the fascial defect (D). It involves only a portion of the circumference of the bowel. As such, incarceration and strangulation may occur in the absence of any evidence of bowel obstruction.

Reference: Skandalakis PN, Zoras O, Skandalakis JE, Mirilas P. Spigelian hernia: surgical anatomy, embryology, and technique of repair. *Am Surg.* 2006;72(1):42–48.

17. D. The SMA leaves the aorta at a downward and acute angle. SMA syndrome or Wilkie syndrome is a rare condition characterized by compression of the third portion of the duodenum by the SMA as it passes over this portion of the duodenum (A). It occurs most often in the setting of profound weight loss. Factors that predispose to the condition include supine immobilization, scoliosis, placement of a body cast, and eating disorders. Symptoms include profound nausea and vomiting, abdominal distention, weight loss, and postprandial epigastric pain, which varies from intermittent to constant, depending on the severity of the duodenal obstruction. Weight loss usually occurs before the onset of symptoms. It is believed to occur more commonly in women, likely secondary to the increased prevalence of anorexia. However, a recent study of SMA syndrome among intellectually disabled children showed that it predominantly affects males. The diagnosis can be made by a CT scan, which demonstrates a decreased aortomesenteric angle and a decreased distance between the aorta and the SMA, as well as evidence of obstruction of the duodenum (C). It can also be diagnosed by a barium upper GI series or hypotonic duodenography, demonstrating abrupt or near-total cessation of flow of barium from the duodenum to the jejunum. Conservative measures that are tried initially are primarily focused on weight gain to increase the mesenteric root fat pad. The operative treatment is duodenojejunostomy (E). Nutcracker syndrome is characterized by compression of the left renal vein by the aorta, superior to the duodenum (B).

References: Adson DE, Mitchell JE, Trenkner SW. The superior mesenteric artery syndrome and acute gastric dilatation in eating disorders: a report of two cases and a review of the literature. *Int J Eat Disord.* 1997;21(2):103–114.

Agrawal GA, Johnson PT, Fishman EK. Multidetector row CT of superior mesenteric artery syndrome. *J Clin Gastroenterol.* 2007;41(1):62–65.

Geskey JM, Erdman HJ, Bramley HP, Williams RJ, Shaffer ML. Superior mesenteric artery syndrome in intellectually disabled children. *Pediatr Emerg Care.* 2012;28(4):351–353.

18. D. The small-intestinal epithelium is acutely susceptible to radiation injury because radiation has its greatest impact on rapidly proliferating cells. Radiation-induced injury to the bowel can present with acute or chronic enteritis. Approximately 75% of patients undergoing radiation therapy for abdominal and pelvic cancers develop acute radiation enteritis transiently. Chronic radiation enteritis results from an obliterative arteritis in the submucosal vessels, while acute radiation enteritis is a transient period of nausea, vomiting, diarrhea, and abdominal pain that occurs around 3 weeks after treatment (C). This leads to progressive submucosal fibrosis and stricture formation. Not infrequently, patients with radiation-induced injury may develop a small bowel obstruction. The risk of radiation enteritis correlates with the amount of radiation received. It is uncommon if the total radiation dose is less than 4000 cGy. The risk of radiation damage increases if the patient received chemotherapy or has underlying vascular disease or diabetes (E). Early symptoms of radiation damage include diarrhea, abdominal pain, and malabsorption and are usually self-limited. The treatment of acute radiation enteritis includes antispasmodic agents, analgesic agents, and antidiarrheal agents. Steroids are not used in the management of radiation enteritis (B). Only a small group of patients with chronic radiation enteritis will require surgery for either SBO from stricture formation or fistulas. Unlike Crohn disease, for which strictureplasty is used, it is not recommended for radiation enteritis because there is a high risk of tissue breakdown (A). The extent of macroscopic radiation injury is difficult to determine on gross inspection. Extensive lysis of adhesions should be avoided because this creates a risk of an enterotomy and subsequent fistula formation as well. The two main surgical procedures are primary resection with reanastomosis or bypass. If the source of obstruction is a loop of bowel stuck in the pelvis, it is best treated with a bypass rather than an attempt to take down the adhesions and risk injury.

References: Galland RB, Spencer J. Natural history and surgical management of radiation enteritis. *Br J Surg.* 1987;74(8):742–747.

Tavakkoli A, Ashley SW, Zinner MJ. Small Intestine. In: Brunicardi F, Andersen DK, Billiar TR, Dunn DL, Hunter JG, Matthews JB, Pollock RE, eds. *Schwartz's principles of surgery.* 10th ed. New York: McGraw-Hill Education; 2015:1146–1151.

19. E. Pneumatosis intestinalis is a radiographic finding and not a disease unto itself. Its discovery on imaging is vexing because it can be a completely benign finding, or it can be associated with life-threatening bowel ischemia. It has been divided into primary and secondary pneumatosis intestinalis. The primary form is less common and is termed *pneumatosis cystoides intestinalis* (B). It consists of thin-walled, air-filled cysts within the bowel wall, usually in the colon, but it can occur anywhere in the GI tract (D). It is an incidental finding, and the diagnosis is readily made on plain radiograph or CT scan. The gas can appear as linear, curvilinear, bubbly, or cystic. There is no specific treatment (A). Secondary pneumatosis intestinalis occurs when there is an underlying disease process. The exact cause of pneumatosis intestinalis is unclear, but there seem to be several pathways that allow gas to enter the bowel wall. Immunodeficient and inflammatory bowel states lead to a loss of mucosal barrier function that may permit air to enter the bowel wall. Bowel obstruction leads to gas formation under pressure. Alterations in bacteria flora, with invasion of the bowel wall, likewise lead to gas formation. In adults, secondary pneumatosis intestinalis is most often associated with COPD (C). It is also

seen with collagen vascular disease, celiac sprue, Crohn disease, use of steroids, and in immunodeficient states. More ominously, it is also associated with ischemic bowel. Thus, it is important to recognize that not all cases of pneumatosis are benign. In neonates, it is most commonly associated with necrotizing enterocolitis. The finding of pneumatosis intestinalis in association with necrotizing enterocolitis does not mandate surgical exploration. It is also seen with pyloric stenosis, Hirschsprung disease, and other causes of bowel obstruction. Pneumoperitoneum can rarely be the result of a benign case of pneumatosis intestinalis because the air-filled cysts are thin-walled and can burst.

References: Mularski RA, Ciccolo ML, Rappaport WD. Nonsurgical causes of pneumoperitoneum. *West J Med.* 1999;170(1):41–46.

Peter S, Abbas M, Kelly K. The spectrum of pneumatosis intestinalis. *Arch Surg.* 2003;138(1):68–75.

Hsueh KC, Tsou SS, Tan KT. Pneumatosis intestinalis and pneumoperitoneum on computed tomography: beware of non-therapeutic laparotomy. *World J Gastrointest Surg.* 2011;3(6):86–88.

20. A. Peutz-Jeghers syndrome features mucocutaneous melanotic pigmentation and hamartomatous polyps (not adenomatous) of the small intestine. It is an autosomal dominant inherited syndrome (B). The skin lesions are found in the circumoral region of the face, buccal mucosa, forearms, palms, soles, digits, and perianal area, whereas the hamartomas are usually in the jejunum and ileum. The most common symptom is recurrent colicky abdominal pain (C). Symptoms of a bowel obstruction develop in as many as 50% of patients, which is usually due to intussusception or obstruction by the polyp itself. Hemorrhage or chronic anemia can also occur as a result of the polyps. The polyps can also undergo adenomatous change. Patients are at significantly increased risk of developing cancer in the GI tract (esophagus, stomach, small intestine, colon, and pancreas) and extraintestinal cancer (testis, breast, uterus, ovary). Female patients should begin breast and cervical cancer screening starting at age 25. Over the long term, cancer develops in as many as 90% of patients. Compared with the general population, they are at 500 times increased risk of the development of small intestine cancer (E). Operative intervention is only indicated in the presence of symptoms (D).

References: Boardman LA, Pittelkow MR, Couch FJ, et al. Association of Peutz-Jeghers-like mucocutaneous pigmentation with breast and gynecologic carcinomas in women. *Medicine (Baltimore).* 2000;79(5):293–298.

Giardiello FM, Brensinger JD, Tersmette AC, et al. Very high risk of cancer in familial Peutz-Jeghers syndrome. *Gastroenterology.* 2000;119(6):1447–1453.

Wu YK, Tsai CH, Yang JC. Gastroduodenal intussusception due to Peutz-Jeghers syndrome: a case report. *Hepatogastroenterology.* 1994;41(2):134–136.

van Lier MGF, Wagner A, Mathus-Vliegen EMH, Kuipers EJ, Steyerberg EW, van Leerdam ME. High cancer risk in Peutz-Jeghers syndrome: a systematic review and surveillance recommendations. *Am J Gastroenterol.* 2010;105(6):1258–1264.

21. A. The finding of "creeping fat" or mesenteric fat wrapping is a gross feature of Crohn disease that is considered pathognomonic. It indicates the encroachment of mesenteric fat onto the serosal surface of the bowel. The presence of fat wrapping correlates well with the presence of underlying acute and chronic inflammation. A recent study suggests that adiponectin, an adipocyte-specific protein with antiinflammatory properties found in mesenteric adipose tissue, may play an important role in the inflammation seen in Crohn disease. Terminal ileitis refers to any acute inflammation of the distal ileum adjacent to the ileocecal valve and is therefore not pathognomonic. Terminal ileitis is associated with numerous infectious causes including *Yersinia enterocolitica* and pseudotuberculosis, *Mycobacterium*, cytomegalovirus (in acquired immunodeficiency syndrome), *Salmonella*, *Campylobacter*, and *Shigella*, among others. The finding of terminal ileitis does not warrant bowel resection. Overall, a minority of patients (10% in one study) who present with terminal ileitis progress to Crohn disease on long-term follow-up (C). The majority of extraintestinal manifestations in inflammatory bowel disease improve with bowel resection but ankylosing spondylitis and primary sclerosing cholangitis do not (B). Pyoderma gangrenosum is rarely the initial presentation of Crohn disease (E). These patients present with small papules often on the lower extremities that resemble a "cat's paw" appearance and can progress to larger ulcerations with necrotic centers. Rarely, patients develop pathergy, a condition in which minor trauma leads to the development of large and difficult-to-heal ulcers (D). Debridement of these lesions should be avoided because this worsens the lesion. Infliximab or another tumor necrosis factor-alpha inhibitor should be used.

References: Menachem Y, Gotsman I. Clinical manifestations of pyoderma gangrenosum associated with inflammatory bowel disease. *Isr Med Assoc J.* 2004;6(2):88–90.

Yamamoto K, Kiyohara T, Murayama Y, et al. Production of adiponectin, an anti-inflammatory protein, in mesenteric adipose tissue in Crohn's disease. *Gut.* 2005;54(6):789–796.

Hatemi I, Hatemi G, Celik AF, et al. Frequency of pathergy phenomenon and other features of Behçet's syndrome among patients with inflammatory bowel disease. *Clin Exp Rheumatol.* 2008;26(4 Suppl 50):S91–S95.

22. B. There are four main cell types in the small intestine: absorptive enterocytes (E), which make up 95% of intestinal cells; goblet cells (A); Paneth cells (D); and enteroendocrine cells (C). Goblet cells secrete mucus. Paneth cells secrete several substances including lysozyme, tumor necrosis factor, and cryptidins, which assist in host mucosal defense. There are more than 10 distinct types of enteroendocrine cells that secrete various gut hormones. The interstitial Cajal cell is a specialized cell of mesodermal origin that seems to regulate peristalsis. It is referred to as an intestinal pacemaker cell. The cells normally express KIT, a tyrosine kinase receptor. These cells have been implicated as the cells of origin of GISTs.

References: Miettinen M, Majidi M, Lasota J. Pathology and diagnostic criteria of gastrointestinal stromal tumors (GISTs): a review. *Eur J Cancer.* 2002;38:S39–S51.

Sircar K, Hewlett BR, Huizinga JD, Chorneyko K, Berezin I, Riddell RH. Interstitial cells of Cajal as precursors of gastrointestinal stromal tumors. *Am J Surg Pathol.* 1999;23(4):377–389.

23. C. The patient has a carcinoid crisis. This has been described after anesthetic induction as well as after other stressful situations such as biopsies or invasive procedures. Carcinoid crisis is characterized by hypotension, bronchospasms, flushing, and tachycardia. The primary treatment is IV octreotide administered as a bolus of 50 to 100 µg. Even

more rarely, a carcinoid crisis can manifest with hypertension. Octreotide is effective for a hypertensive crisis as well. Adjunctive treatment with antihistamines may also be of benefit due to frequent histamine release from carcinoid tumors (B). If the above measures do not resolve the crisis, then aborting the procedure may be necessary (D). Dantrolene is the preferred choice of management for malignant hyperthermia (E). This diagnosis is supported by an increase in end-tidal CO_2. Corticosteroids are not used in the management of carcinoid crisis (A).

References: Bax NDS, Woods HF, Batchelor A, Jennings M. Octreotide therapy in carcinoid disease. *Anticancer Drugs.* 1996;7(Suppl 1):17–22.

Warner RR, Mani S, Profeta J, Grunstein E. Octreotide treatment of carcinoid hypertensive crisis. *Mt Sinai J Med.* 1994;61(4):349–355.

24. E. The patient has a blind loop syndrome, which is due to bacterial overgrowth (A). Symptoms include diarrhea, steatorrhea, megaloblastic anemia, weight loss, abdominal pain, and deficiencies of fat-soluble vitamins. The megaloblastic anemia is due to the utilization of vitamin B12 by the bacteria. The underlying cause may be an intestinal abnormality such as a diverticulum, fistula, and intestinal stricture, or it may follow a Billroth II procedure. In the patient presented, the large jejunal diverticulum is likely the etiology. The diagnosis can be confirmed by various means. A barium study is useful to define the anatomic abnormality. The D-xylose test involves ingesting xylose, which is metabolized by the bacteria. Excessive CO_2 in the breath confirms the diagnosis. Cultures of the small intestine can be obtained; however, passing an intestinal tube distal enough to obtain an adequate culture can be challenging. Another useful study is the Schilling test. Oral radiolabeled vitamin B12 is administered along with parenteral unlabeled vitamin B12. The unlabeled vitamin B12 saturates liver receptors. Thus, if the oral radiolabeled vitamin B12 is properly absorbed and liver receptors are saturated, the radiolabeled vitamin B12 will be excreted in high concentrations in the urine. With pernicious anemia and blind loop syndrome, oral absorption will be low, and thus urinary excretion of radiolabeled vitamin B12 will be low. When the test is repeated after the addition of intrinsic factor, vitamin B12 excretion will increase, whereas with blind loop syndrome, vitamin B12 excretion will remain low. The initial treatment of blind loop syndrome consists of broad-spectrum antibiotics including metronidazole with tetracycline as well as vitamin B12 supplementation given parenterally. This should be given to all patients presenting with blind loop syndrome (D). Prokinetic agents do not seem to help. In addition, dietary modifications such as a lactose-free diet are useful because patients with blind loop syndrome often become lactose intolerant. Medium-chain triglyceride diets are more readily absorbed than long-chain triglycerides because they do not require digestive enzymes (B). Resection of the diverticulum is not recommended initially (C). Surgery should be reserved for patients who fail repeated medical management attempts.

References: Ross CB, Richards WO, Sharp KW, Bertram PD, Schaper PW. Diverticular disease of the jejunum and its complications. *Am Surg.* 1990;56(5):319–324.

Woods K, Williams E, Melvin W, Sharp K. Acquired jejunoileal diverticulosis and its complications: a review of the literature. *Am Surg.* 2008;74(9):849–854.

25. C. Surgical dogma has stated that a small bowel obstruction (SBO), in the absence of prior surgery or visible external hernia, requires surgical intervention, as the differential invariably are all surgical diseases, such as internal hernia, appendicitis, intussusception, inflammatory bowel disease, malignancy, or obstructed Meckel diverticulum. However, in a recent study, as many as 40% of SBO in patients without prior history of surgery resolved nonoperatively. Of those that required surgical intervention, the majority were found to have adhesions despite no prior operations (A). Most centers have transitioned to a water-soluble oral contrast challenge to help decide which patients with adhesive SBOs will require surgical intervention. This is being performed even in patients without prior abdominal surgery. This entails performing nasogastric decompression for two hours followed by administration of a water-soluble contrast either by mouth or via NG tube. This is followed by plain films 8 hours later. Patients with plain films demonstrating contrast in the colon after 8 hours are unlikely to require surgical intervention while those without contrast in the colon after 8 hours are more likely to fail nonoperative management (C). Rectal contrast is not typically used in the workup nor in management of adhesive SBO (D).

Reference: Ng YYR, Ngu JCY, Wong ASY. Small bowel obstruction in the virgin abdomen: time to challenge surgical dogma with evidence: Small bowel obstruction in the virgin abdomen. *ANZ J Surg.* 2018;88(1–2):91–94.

26. C. Postoperative ileus remains a major source of prolonged hospitalization in patients undergoing abdominal surgery. The use of early ambulation, early postoperative feeding protocols, and routine nasogastric intubation have not been shown to be associated with earlier resolution of postoperative ileus (A, E). Reducing opioid use in combination with the use of nonsteroidal antiinflammatory drugs such as ketorolac has been shown to reduce the duration of ileus in most studies. The mechanism may be a combination of the reduction in opioids and the antiinflammatory properties of ketorolac. However, ketorolac has been associated with an increased risk of operative site and gastrointestinal (GI) bleeding as well as fluid retention (D). Recently, ketorolac has been also shown to increase the risk of readmission and reinterventions after GI surgery. Another drug that has been investigated is erythromycin, which is useful for gastroparesis because it works by its agonistic effect on the motilin receptor. However, it does not seem to be useful for ileus and should be avoided in cases of obstruction, as would all promotility agents (B). Metoclopramide is a dopaminergic antagonist with antiemetic and prokinetic properties, but it has also not been shown to be useful for ileus. Gum chewing has had conflicting results in the literature, but a recent randomized controlled trial from New Zealand demonstrated a significant reduction in postoperative ileus in patients with colorectal cancer undergoing bowel resection (27% versus 48%). The most efficacious agent, however, is alvimopan (Entereg), which has been demonstrated in randomized studies to improve postoperative ileus in patients undergoing bowel resection. Alvimopan is an opioid receptor antagonist. It binds μ-opioid receptors in the GI tract and selectively inhibits the opioid effects on GI function and motility while not affecting opioid analgesia. It is the first US Food and Drug Administration–approved drug for postoperative ileus. It is approved for short-term (maximum 15 doses over 5 days) in-hospital use only. Patients on long-term narcotics (e.g., for chronic pain) should not use Alvimopan because this population has an increased risk of myocardial infarction.

References: Ludwig K, Enker WE, Delaney CP, et al. Gastrointestinal tract recovery in patients undergoing bowel resection: results of a randomized trial of alvimopan and placebo with a standardized accelerated postoperative care pathway. *Arch Surg.* 2008;143(11):1098–1105.

Wolff BG, Weese JL, Ludwig KA, et al. Postoperative ileus-related morbidity profile in patients treated with alvimopan after bowel resection. *J Am Coll Surg.* 2007;204(4):609–616.

Su'a BU, Hill AG. Perioperative use of chewing gum affects the inflammatory response and reduces postoperative ileus following major colorectal surgery. *Evid Based Med.* 2015;20(5):185–186.

Kotagal M, Hakkarainen TW, Simianu VV, Beck SJ, Alfonso-Cristancho R, Flum DR. Ketorolac use and postoperative complications in gastrointestinal surgery. *Ann Surg.* 2016;263(1):71–75.

27. A. Crohn disease is the most common primary surgical disease of the small bowel. Acute onset of abdominal pain and diarrhea is not the most common presentation for Crohn disease; the majority of patients first present with an insidious onset of vague abdominal discomfort (E). It has a bimodal distribution, with one large peak in the second and third decades of life and a second smaller peak in the sixth decade (C). Several risk factors for Crohn disease have been identified, including living in northern latitudes, Ashkenazi Jewish descent, smoking, and a familial inheritance. The relative risk among first-degree relatives of patients with Crohn disease is as high as 14 to 15 times greater than in the general population. It is also more common in urban areas and in patients with a high socioeconomic status. Most studies suggest that Crohn disease is approximately of equal prevalence in females and males (D). Breastfeeding may also be protective against the development of Crohn disease. Although medical management is the first-line treatment for Crohn disease, about 75% of patients will ultimately need surgery. The most common reasons for surgery include fistula, abscess, and obstruction; perforation is quite rare (B).

References: Passier JLM, Srivastava N, van Puijenbroek EP. Isotretinoin-induced inflammatory bowel disease. *Neth J Med.* 2006;64(2):52–54.

Strong SA. Surgical management of Crohn's disease. In: Holzheimer RG, Mannick JA, eds. *Surgical treatment: evidence-based and problem oriented.* Munich: Zuckschwerdt; 2001:714–725.

28. A. In the early stages of Crohn disease, patients demonstrate small superficial ulcers in the mucosa known as aphthous ulcers. These superficial ulcers are often surrounded by a halo of erythema. The ulcers form as a result of submucosal lymphoid follicle expansion. As the disease progresses, the ulcers coalesce to form larger ulcers, which are stellate shaped, as well as deep linear ulcers. Further coalescence of the ulcers leads to a cobblestone appearance (D), which is a hallmark of Crohn disease. Other hallmarks of Crohn disease include noncaseating granulomas (C), transmural inflammation, serosal thickening (E), and "skip lesions," meaning that the areas of intestinal inflammation are discontinuous. The noncaseating granulomas are found in both areas of active disease, and grossly normal-appearing intestine is seen in all layers of the bowel wall and in mesenteric lymph nodes (B). Because the inflammation is transmural, inflamed loops of bowel become adhered to one another, thereby leading to fibrosis, stricture formation, intraabdominal abscess, fistulas, and, rarely, free perforation.

Reference: Levine MS. Crohn's disease of the upper gastrointestinal tract. *Radiol Clin North Am.* 1987;25(1):79–91.

29. A. Numerous pharmacologic agents are used to treat Crohn disease. Treatment options should be divided into those used for maintenance therapy for mild active disease, those used to treat an acute exacerbation, and drugs for maintaining remission. In patients with mild active disease, the most commonly used drug is sulfasalazine, an aminosalicylate that acts as an antiinflammatory agent. This is particularly useful in patients with colitis and ileocolitis. Mesalamine is another antiinflammatory agent in the same family as sulfasalazine. It seems to have fewer side effects owing to the fact that it is activated by colonic bacteria, thus limiting its action to the colon. For acute flare-ups, the treatment of choice remains corticosteroids, prednisone in particular. Prednisone is highly effective in inducing remission (in approximately three-fourths of patients); however, due to the side effects of long-term use, it is not recommended for long-term prevention of remission (B). Budesonide (C), a synthetic glucocorticoid, is another option. It has an advantage over prednisone in that it has a markedly reduced systemic absorption and thus fewer long-term side effects. Nevertheless, it can also suppress the adrenal gland. If corticosteroids are ineffective in inducing remission, the next step would be to administer infliximab (E), a monoclonal antibody that targets tumor necrosis factor-alpha. Care must be used in administering infliximab. Because it targets tumor necrosis factor-alpha, a cytokine that regulates inflammatory reactions, patients who receive infliximab are at increased risk of acquiring opportunistic infections such as tuberculosis and aspergillosis. It is also associated with activation of latent multiple sclerosis, demyelinating central nervous system disorders, and worsening congestive heart failure. Infliximab has also been shown to be effective in healing complex fistulas associated with Crohn disease. Rarely, it has been associated with T-cell lymphoma and almost exclusively in young teenage males. Antibiotics have an adjunctive role in the treatment of infectious complications associated with Crohn disease (D). They are used to treat patients with perianal disease, enterocutaneous fistulas, and active colon disease and aid in situations in which bacterial overgrowth has occurred. Once remission has been achieved after an acute flare-up, it is important to maintain remission. Although corticosteroids would theoretically be useful, the side effects preclude long-term administration. Infliximab is used to maintain remission, as are azathioprine and 6-mercaptopurine. These latter drugs act by inhibiting DNA synthesis and thus suppressing the function of T cells and natural killer cells. A second-line agent for maintenance of remission is methotrexate.

30. D. Approximately three-fourths of patients with Crohn disease will eventually require surgery. Indications for surgery include failure of medical management, intestinal obstruction, fistula, abscess, bleeding, and perforation. In children, growth retardation is another indication. Because patients with Crohn disease will often require repeat operations, it is important to avoid unnecessary resection of small bowel because this puts the patient at risk of short bowel syndrome. As such, several principles of surgical management should be followed. Surgical resection should be limited to the segment of bowel that is causing the complication. Other areas of active disease should be left alone, provided they are not causing obvious complications. Resection margins of 2 cm beyond grossly visible disease are recommended (A). Resection margins have not been shown to affect recurrence. The presence of microscopic disease in the resection margin also does not adversely affect outcome or recurrence. Thus, frozen section is unnecessary (B). When the indication for surgery is SBO, strictureplasty has been shown to be equally effective as resection for jejunal and ileal disease while sparing bowel length. Two types of strictureplasty are recommended: the Heineke-Mikulicz pyloroplasty (for strictures <12 cm in length) and the Finney pyloroplasty (for strictures ≤25 cm in length) (E). A potential drawback of these techniques is that they may potentially leave an undetected malignancy behind. Thus, during the course of a strictureplasty, biopsy specimens of any intraluminal ulcerations should be taken. Duodenal Crohn disease is much less common, and thus guidelines are less clear. However, current recommendations are to perform a bypass of duodenal strictures, such as with a gastrojejunostomy and duodenojejunostomy, depending on the location. Duodenal resection is not recommended (C). Duodenal strictureplasty has been rarely reported. For colon disease, resection is recommended, again limiting resection to the diseased segment causing symptoms. In a metaanalysis, 90% of recurrences occurred at nonstrictureplasty sites.

References: Fazio V, Marchetti F, Church M. Effect of resection margins on the recurrence of Crohn's disease in the small bowel: a randomized controlled trial. *Ann Surg.* 1996;224(4):563–571.

Tichansky D, Cagir B, Yoo E, Marcus SM, Fry RD. Strictureplasty for Crohn's disease: meta-analysis. *Dis Colon Rectum.* 2000;43(7):911–919.

Yamamoto T, Fazio VW, Tekkis PP. Safety and efficacy of strictureplasty for Crohn's disease: a systematic review and meta-analysis: W. Donald Buie, M.d., editor. *Dis Colon Rectum.* 2007;50(11):1968–1986.

Alimentary Tract— Large Intestine 10

JOSEPH HADAYA, FORMOSA CHEN, AND BEVERLEY A. PETRIE

ABSITE 99th Percentile High-Yields

I. Adequate Colonoscopy Metrics
   A. Should be able to intubate the cecum in ≥90% of all cases and in ≥95% of cases when the indication is screening in a healthy adult
   B. Adenoma detection rates of at least 25% in patients >50 years old who are undergoing screening colonoscopy
   C. The mean withdrawal time is ≥6 minutes in colonoscopies with normal results that are performed in patients with intact anatomy
   D. Mucosally based pedunculated polyps and sessile polyps <2 cm in size are resected or documentation of unresectability is made
   E. Perforation rates should not exceed 1 in 500 colonoscopies overall, and 1 in 1000 screening colonoscopies
   F. Incidence of polypectomy bleeding should be <1%
   G. Postpolypectomy bleeding is managed nonoperatively in ≥90% of cases

II. Initial Colonoscopy Screening Guidelines

Risk factor	Screening
Normal risk	Start at age 50 and continue every 10 years; alternatives to colonoscopy include annual fecal occult blood test (FOBT) or flexible sigmoidoscopy every 5 years or annual FOBT plus flexible sigmoidoscopy every 5 years
First-degree family member with colorectal cancer prior to age 60	Start at age 40 or 10 years prior to first-degree members diagnosis age; continue screening every 5 years
Two first-degree family members with colorectal cancer diagnosis at any age	Start at age 40 or 10 years prior to first-degree members diagnosis age; continue screening every 5 years
Ulcerative colitis (UC)	Colonoscopy every 1–2 years starting 8 years after onset of disease or at same time of primary sclerosing cholangitis (PSC) diagnosis
Familial adenomatous polyposis (FAP)	Annual sigmoidoscopy starting at age 10–12
Lynch syndrome	Colonoscopy every 1–2 years starting at age 20, or 10 years prior to age of diagnosis of youngest affected family member
Personal cancer history	Colonoscopy at 1 year following resection, or 6 months if no preoperative completion colonoscopy was performed; then every 3 years

III. Postcolonoscopy Frequency Guidelines Based on Findings

Finding	Recommended interval for surveillance colonoscopy
No abnormalities	10 years
1–2 tubular adenomas <10 mm	7–10 years
3–4 tubular adenomas <10 mm	3–5 years
5–10 tubular adenomas <10 mm	3 years
Adenoma >10 mm	3 years
Adenoma with tubulovillous or villous histology	3 years
Adenoma with high-grade dysplasia	3 years
>10 adenomas	1 year
Piecemeal resection of adenoma ≥20 mm	6 months

   A. Surgically resect polyps that are unable to be endoscopically removed
      1. If T1 lesion present, polypectomy is sufficient if all the following are true: (1) margins are clear of dysplasia and cancer by 1 to 2 mm (pedunculated), or submucosal invasion <1 to 2 mm (nonpedunculated), (2) no lymphovascular or perineural invasion is present, (3) moderate-well differentiated lesion, (4) en bloc endoscopic resection; all others require a formal oncologic resection with adequate lymphadenectomy

IV. Staging of Colon Cancer and Management

Stage	TNM staging	Management
Stage I	T1-2, N0, M0	Colectomy
Stage II	T3-4, N0, M0	Colectomy (with en bloc resection of adjacent organs, if needed); high-risk features (obstruction, T4, <12 LN harvested, high-grade tumor, perineural or lymphovascular invasion) should get adjuvant chemotherapy
Stage III	Any T, N1 or N2, M0	Colectomy with adjuvant chemotherapy
Stage IV	Any T, Any N, M1	Diffuse metastatic disease: systemic chemotherapy Oligometastatic liver/lung disease: neoadjuvant vs adjuvant chemotherapy, staged vs simultaneous colectomy and metastatectomy

V. Familial Adenomatous Polyposis (FAP)
   A. Autosomal dominant, mutations in *APC* gene (tumor suppressor); up to 25% are *de novo* mutations; mean age for polyp development is 16 to 18 years, with diffuse polyposis at age 20 to 40, colon cancer in approximately 100%, left-sided
   B. Increased risk of cancer is due to substantial number of adenomas at early age rather than intrinsic malignant potential of each adenoma (versus hereditary nonpolyposis colorectal cancer)
   C. Surgery: generally, by age 20, or for high-grade dysplasia, suspected colorectal cancer, gastrointestinal bleeding, rapid increase in polyp number or inability to survey; surgical options: proctocolectomy with ileal–pouch anal anastomosis (IPAA), total colectomy with ileorectal anastomosis (IRA) or end ileostomy
   D. Postcolectomy surveillance necessary (risk for malignancy at rectal cuff or within ileal pouch)

VI. Hereditary Nonpolyposis Colon Cancer (HNPCC/Lynch Syndrome)
   A. Autosomal dominant, mutations in DNA mismatch repair (MMR) genes (*MLH1, MSH2, MSH6, PMS2*)
   B. Risk of colorectal cancer 12% to 90%, occurs at younger age than average risk; adenomacarcinoma sequence progresses faster in HNPCC than sporadic disease, synchronous lesions common (7%) as well as metachronous
   C. Amsterdam II criteria (family history-based screening): at least 3 relatives with colorectal or Lynch-associated cancer, involving at least 2 generations, at least 1 diagnosed before age 50, at least 1 is a first-degree relative of the other two, and familial adenomatous polyposis excluded ("3-2-1-1-0 rule")

VII. Ulcerative Colitis and Crohn's Disease
   A. Ulcerative colitis
      1. Contiguous inflammation from rectum extending proximally, spares anus, mucosal disease only, crypt abscesses are common
      2. Extraintestinal manifestations include ankylosing spondylitis, primary sclerosing cholangitis, uveitis, pyoderma gangrenosum (ankylosing spondylitis and primary sclerosing cholangitis do not improve after proctocolectomy)
      3. Management: mesalamine or infliximab for maintenance therapy; steroids for acute flares
      4. Indications for elective surgery include growth failure in children, intractable disease despite escalating medical therapy, chronic steroid dependence, dysplasia, or malignancy
      5. Elective surgical options: total proctocolectomy with ileal pouch–anal anastomosis (IPAA), total abdominal colectomy with ileorectal anastomosis (in rare cases where rectum is spared, although rectum must be screened for malignancy), total abdominal colectomy with end ileostomy
      6. Pouchitis: inflammation/infection of pouch, treat with ciprofloxacin or metronidazole
      7. Emergent surgery: severe colitis with toxic megacolon, perforation, or bleeding; perform total abdominal colectomy with end ileostomy (possible pouch formation later)
   B. Crohn's disease
      1. Transmural inflammation with skip lesions, any segment affected (terminal ileum most common) but generally spares rectum; strictures, fistula, granulomas and creeping fat common
      2. Extraintestinal manifestations include arthralgias, megaloblastic anemia, erythema nodosum
      3. Maintenance therapy for mild disease includes mesalamine or immunomodulator (azathioprine, 6-mercaptopurine, methotrexate); for moderate to severe disease, infliximab (or other anti-TNF therapy) monotherapy or infliximab plus azathioprine
      4. Acute disease managed with steroids, anti-TNF agents, or immunomodulators
      5. Surgery reserved for complications (strictures, perforation, obstruction, malignancy, fistula); most commonly strictures

VIII. Sigmoid and Cecal Volvulus
   A. If no evidence of peritonitis, ischemia, or perforation, sigmoid volvulus can be managed with flexible sigmoidoscopy to detorse and reduce bowel, place rectal tube (decompression), and allow for bowel preparation; high risk of recurrence, so sigmoidectomy with primary anastomosis should be performed within 1 to 3 days
   B. For peritonitis, ischemia, or inability to detorse: emergency resection (with end colostomy)
   C. Cecal volvulus is not amenable to endoscopic therapy and should be managed surgically with right colectomy due to high risk of recurrence

IX. *Clostridium difficile* Colitis
   A. Anaerobic, gram-positive rod; healthcare acquired infection, can present up to 3 to 4 weeks after antibiotic administration (even single dose); updated 2021 guidelines below

Clinical	Treatment
Initial episode	Preferred: fidaxomicin 200 mg BID for 10 days Alternative: oral vancomycin 125 mg 4× daily for 10 days OR If above unavailable, oral metronidazole 500 mg ×3 daily for 10 days
1st recurrence	Preferred: fidaxomicin 200 mg BID for 10 days, OR BID for 5 days followed by once every other day for 20 days Alternative: vancomycin 125 mg 4× daily for 10 days
2nd and 3rd recurrence	Preferred: fidaxomicin 200 mg BID for 10 days, OR BID for 5 days followed by once every other day for 20 days Alternative: vancomycin 125 mg 4× daily for 10 days followed by rifaximin 400 mg 3× daily for 20 days
4th recurrence	Fecal microbiota transplantation
Fulminant infection (hypotension, ileus, megacolon*)	Vancomycin 500 mg 4× daily; if ileus, consider adding rectal instillation of vancomycin; IV metronidazole (500 mg every 8 hours) should be administered with oral or rectal vancomycin, particularly if ileus is present

*Should consider total abdominal colectomy as well

X. Diverticulitis

  A. Mild uncomplicated diverticulitis, minimal to no comorbidities, no systemic signs of infection, minimal pain, and able to tolerate oral intake) can be treated without antibiotics; for abscesses >3 cm in size, percutaneous drainage recommended

  B. After resolution of complicated diverticulitis, the patients should undergo colonoscopy if none recently (higher risk of associated malignancy)

  C. For patients with complicated diverticulitis (fistula, obstruction, stricture or abscess requiring drainage), elective colectomy typically recommended

  D. For patients with uncomplicated diverticulitis, decision for elective colectomy may be considered for those with multiple, recurrent admissions for uncomplicated diverticulitis that decrease quality of life; young age should not be a determinant to recommend surgery

  E. For patients presenting with diffuse peritonitis or failure of nonoperative management, urgent sigmoidectomy should be offered and if expertise is present, minimally invasive surgery should be employed

  F. Primary anastomosis is preferable to Hartmann procedure in hemodynamically stable, immunocompetent patients younger than 85 years, even in Hinchey III or Hinchey IV disease (LADIES trial); however, this decision should be individualized

  G. Hartmann procedure preferred in hemodynamically unstable patients, immunocompromised, those on pressors

Category	Findings/symptoms	Management
Emergent Conditions		
Hinchey I	Pericolonic abscess	Antibiotics, bowel rest, and percutaneous drainage if abscess >3 cm
Hinchey II	Pelvic abscess	
Hinchey III	Purulent peritonitis	Surgery: Hartmann procedure vs resection with primary anastomosis, diverting ileostomy (controversial)
Hinchey IV	Feculent peritonitis	
Elective		
Smoldering diverticulitis	Chronic abdominal pain	Sigmoidectomy if disease is debilitating
Stricture	Thin stools, constipation	
Colovesical fistula	Pneumaturia, fecaluria, recurrent UTI	Sigmoidectomy, fistula takedown (postoperative Foley catheter to decompress bladder)

XI. Lower GI Bleeding

  A. Initial evaluation: colonoscopy is preferred in stable patients, allows for diagnosis, localization, potential intervention, and proctoscopy

   1. Should be performed as soon as patient is resuscitated and has completed adequate bowel preparation, which may only include a Fleet enema prior to scope; limited utility without preparation, with low cecal intubation rates and obstructed views; nasogastric tube can be placed for administrating bowel preparation and to rule out upper GI bleed; if bleeding briskly, consider simultaneous upper endoscopy

  B. If bleeding briskly, and source not visualized with colonoscopy, consider angiography (therapeutic, accurate localization) or tagged RBC scan (most sensitive, detects bleed <0.5 cc/min)

  C. If hemodynamically unstable, upper GI bleeding ruled out with EGD, hemorrhoids ruled out with proctoscopy, and bleeding source still not found, but high suspicion for distal to ileocecal valve, proceed with total abdominal colectomy (segmental resection discouraged)

XII. Ischemic Colitis: bloody diarrhea and left-sided abdominal pain in elderly with volume depletion, risk factors include cardiovascular disease and a short interval of volume depletion/hypotension; watershed areas (splenic flexure) most commonly affected

  A. Cross-sectional imaging generally shows nonspecific segmental colon thickening; best study is endoscopy, which demonstrates clearly demarcated patchy areas of erythema and ulceration

   1. Conservative management with fluid resuscitation typically effective; antibiotics to prevent bacterial translocation

Questions

1. A 42-year-old man with no past medical history presents with a 5-day history of left lower quadrant abdominal pain. He is found to have sigmoid diverticula with associated pericolonic stranding and mesenteric lymphadenopathy on CT imaging. He is treated with IV antibiotics, his pain resolves, a diet is restarted, and he is transitioned to oral antibiotics and discharged. Which of the following is most appropriate?
   A. Add probiotics
   B. Schedule elective sigmoid colectomy
   C. Schedule colonoscopy
   D. No further recommendations
   E. Schedule repeat CT scan of the abdomen and pelvis with IV contrast

2. A 68-year-old female presents to the emergency department (ED) with obstipation, nausea, and gradually worsening abdominal distention. She is afebrile with normal vital signs and has moderate distention on examination with mild abdominal tenderness. A CT scan of the abdomen and pelvis suggests a large bowel obstruction with a transition point in the left (descending) colon and multiple hypoattenuating masses in the liver and base of the lungs. There is also evidence of small bowel dilation. He is afebrile and hemodynamically stable. A nasogastric tube is placed. What is the next best step in the management of this patient?
   A. Colonoscopy and uncovered stent placement
   B. Colonoscopy and covered stent placement
   C. Left colectomy
   D. Diverting loop ileostomy
   E. Initiate inpatient chemotherapy

3. Which of the following is true about colonic physiology?
   A. The colon absorbs the majority of water in the gastrointestinal tract
   B. Sodium is absorbed actively via Na^+,K^+-ATPase
   C. Ammonia reabsorption is unaffected by luminal pH
   D. Chloride is secreted
   E. It produces no nutrients

4. A 55-year-old woman undergoes laparoscopy for presumed appendicitis. At surgery, she is found to have perforated appendicitis with what appears to be peritoneal studding. The patient undergoes appendectomy and biopsy of the peritoneum. Final pathology reveals appendiceal adenocarcinoma. Subsequent workup reveals no evidence of additional metastatic spread to the liver or lungs. Further treatment would consist of:
   A. No further treatment
   B. Systemic chemotherapy
   C. Intraperitoneal chemotherapy
   D. Cytoreductive surgery and hyperthermic intraperitoneal chemotherapy
   E. Cytoreductive surgery and systemic chemotherapy

5. A 73-year-old female with no significant medical problems is found to have a 3-cm hepatic flexure mass on screening colonoscopy. A biopsy demonstrates moderately differentiated adenocarcinoma. Her laboratory tests are notable for microcytic anemia and normal liver function tests. Which of the following is the most appropriate preoperative staging strategy?
   A. CT scan of the chest, abdomen, and pelvis, and transrectal endoscopic ultrasound
   B. CT scan of the chest, abdomen, and pelvis, and carcinoembryonic antigen
   C. CT scan of the chest, abdomen, and pelvis, MRI of the brain, and carcinoembryonic antigen
   D. PET/CT of the chest, abdomen, and pelvis, MRI of the brain, and carcinoembryonic antigen
   E. PET/CT of the chest, abdomen, and pelvis, MRI of the brain

6. A 45-year-old woman with a 15-year history of pancolitis from UC undergoes surveillance colonoscopy. No polyps are detected. Random biopsy samples are taken, and final pathology findings reveal high-grade dysplasia from the sigmoid colon region. Recommended management would be:
   A. Repeat colonoscopy in 6 months with additional random biopsies
   B. Sigmoid colectomy
   C. Total colectomy with ileorectal anastomosis
   D. Total proctocolectomy with ileostomy
   E. Restorative proctocolectomy with ileal pouch–anal anastomosis

7. The earliest manifestation of ulcerative colitis is:
   A. Mucosal ulcerations
   B. Mucosal edema
   C. Plasmacytosis
   D. Pseudopolyps
   E. Crypt abscesses

8. With appendicitis during pregnancy, the factor most strongly associated with fetal mortality is:
   A. Fetal gestational age
   B. Open appendectomy instead of laparoscopy
   C. Maternal comorbidities
   D. Appendiceal rupture
   E. Delay in antibiotic administration

9. Which of the following is true about hereditary nonpolyposis colon cancer (HNPCC) (Lynch syndrome)?
   A. It is not associated with a higher risk of upper genitourinary tract cancer.
   B. It is considered an autosomal recessive syndrome.
   C. Screening colonoscopy should begin at age 12.
   D. Colonic malignancy has the same prognosis as sporadic cancer.
   E. Modified Amsterdam criteria requires one family member to be diagnosed before age 40.

10. Which of the following is true regarding familial juvenile polyposis?
    A. It is autosomal recessive
    B. The polyps are hamartomas
    C. The risk of colon cancer is 100% by age 50
    D. Once a polyp is detected, total proctocolectomy is recommended
    E. There is no association with upper GI malignancy

11. Which of the following is true regarding colonic polyps?
    A. Tubulovillous adenomas have a lower malignancy risk than tubular adenomas
    B. Sessile serrated polyps should be resected
    C. The polyps in Peutz-Jeghers syndrome are hyperplastic
    D. Pseudopolyps are commonly found in FAP
    E. In an adenomatous polyp, the risk of malignancy is related to its location in the GI tract

12. A 75-year-old woman presents with mild diffuse abdominal pain and diarrhea that is positive on fecal immunochemical test. Her medical history is negative. Her WBC count is normal, as is her hematocrit. A CT scan shows mild thickening of the colonic wall at the splenic flexure with some associated pericolic fat stranding. Which of the following is the best next step in management?
    A. Diagnostic laparoscopy
    B. Exploratory laparotomy
    C. IV antibiotics and fluid hydration
    D. Colonoscopy
    E. Mesenteric angiography

13. A 65-year-old institutionalized patient presents with a 2-day history of abdominal distention, nausea, and obstipation. Physical examination is significant for marked distention with mild diffuse abdominal tenderness, no guarding, and no rebound. The WBC count is 10,000 cells/μL. Plain films reveal a massively dilated, inverted U-shaped (omega sign) loop of bowel. Management should consist of:
    A. Endoscopic detorsion
    B. Endoscopic detorsion followed by sigmoid colectomy during the same hospitalization
    C. Endoscopic detorsion followed by elective sigmoid colectomy in the case of a recurrence
    D. Exploratory laparotomy with sigmoid colectomy, on-table lavage, and primary anastomosis
    E. Exploratory laparotomy with sigmoid colectomy, proximal colostomy, and oversewn rectal stump

14. A 38-year-old woman presents with a 1-day history of nausea, vomiting, abdominal distention, and obstipation. The physical examination is significant for distention with a tympanic mass in the left upper quadrant and mild abdominal tenderness. She is hemodynamically stable with no leukocytosis or lactic acidosis. A plain abdominal radiograph reveals a markedly dilated, kidney-shaped loop of bowel with haustral markings that project from the right lower quadrant to the left upper quadrant. The diagnosis is confirmed with CT scan lacking evidence of bowel malperfusion. Which of the following is likely to be the best treatment option?
    A. Cecostomy tube placement
    B. Operative detorsion with cecopexy
    C. Right hemicolectomy with an ileostomy and mucus fistula
    D. Initial endoscopic detorsion with a subsequent right hemicolectomy
    E. Right colectomy with primary anastomosis

15. Which of the following is true regarding diverticular diseases of the lower GI tract?
    A. They occur most commonly in the descending colon
    B. The rectum can be affected
    C. Incidentally discovered cecal diverticula require surgical management
    D. Elective sigmoid resection should be preceded by a mechanical bowel preparation with oral and IV perioperative antibiotics
    E. They are associated with a long, redundant colon

16. A 50-year-old male is undergoing a screening colonoscopy under intravenous (IV) sedation. Near the end of the procedure, he briefly becomes unresponsive, requiring a sternal rub to arouse him. IV anesthetics are weaned off and the procedure is completed. In the recovery room, a chest x-ray is performed to rule out an aspiration event before discharge. There is no consolidation in the lungs, but free air is seen under the diaphragm. The patient has no complaints, the abdomen is soft, he would like to eat, and he has normal vital signs. Which of the following is the best next step?
    A. Exploratory laparotomy
    B. Diagnostic laparoscopy
    C. Serial abdominal exam for 6 hours
    D. Admit to hospital, IV antibiotics, and bowel rest
    E. Discharge home

17. Ten years after an abdominoperineal resection for locally advanced rectal cancer, a patient presents with a hernia adjacent to his stoma that causes him discomfort and interferes with the placement of his colostomy bag. It has been increasing in size over the last several months. Which of the following is true regarding this condition?
    A. Chronic obstructive pulmonary disease (COPD) is the strongest risk factor
    B. Treatment for this patient includes weight loss and a support device such as a hernia belt
    C. Stoma relocation is the superior treatment
    D. Prophylactic mesh placement at the initial operation decreases risk of this complication
    E. This complication is more common with loop ileostomy than end colostomy

18. A 47-year-old morbidly obese male underwent emergent sigmoidectomy with end colostomy creation yesterday morning for perforated diverticulitis. Evaluation of the colostomy on morning rounds reveals diffusely dusky mucosa. On examination with a test tube and light, the dusky area appears to be superficial to the fascia. Management consists of:
    A. Reexploration in the operating room (OR), resection of ischemic colon, and stoma relocation
    B. Reexploration in the OR, segmental colon resection, and placement of stoma at the same site
    C. Reexploration in the OR, on-table bowel prep, and primary colonic anastomosis
    D. Observation and reevaluate the colostomy in 12 to 24 hours
    E. IV antibiotics

19. A 75-year-old male with chronic constipation presents with severe abdominal pain and fever. CT scan shows free air and stranding in the colon. The colon and rectum appear to be dilated and filled with large masses of stool. Intraoperatively, a round perforation about 1 cm in diameter is found in the colon with thickened balls of stool protruding out. Which of the following is true regarding this patient?
    A. The perforation is most likely to occur at the splenic flexure
    B. It is associated with nonsteroidal antiinflammatory drug (NSAID) use
    C. It is best managed by primary closure and washout
    D. Anticholinergic agents could have prevented this condition
    E. The perforation is usually at the mesenteric border

20. A 71-year-old female with COPD is recovering from pneumonia in the intensive care unit (ICU). She is on a ventilator. Her abdomen is acutely distended, and she has not had a bowel movement in several days. Imaging demonstrates a cecum measuring 8 cm in diameter with gas pattern of distention extending to the rectum. There is no stool in the rectal vault. Her vital signs are stable. Her doctor would like to start neostigmine. Which of the following is true regarding the administration of neostigmine for this patient's condition?
    A. History of coronary artery disease is considered a contraindication
    B. History of second-degree heart block is considered a contraindication
    C. Neostigmine should not be given as a continuous infusion
    D. Neostigmine is effective in 20% of patients with this condition
    E. If a bolus of neostigmine is not successful, repeat boluses should be avoided

21. For the patient in question 20, neostigmine and endoscopic decompression fail to improve symptoms. She appears more distended and uncomfortable. Repeat x-ray shows cecum is now 10 cm in diameter. She is taken to the operating room. Intraoperatively, her colon appears edematous and dilated to 10 cm, but there are no signs of ischemic bowel identified. Which of the following is the most appropriate treatment option?
    A. Total abdominal colectomy with ileoanal anastomosis
    B. Proctocolectomy with ileal pouch–anal anastomosis
    C. Placement of cecostomy tube
    D. Transanal retrograde colonic insertion of a long multiperforated Faucher tube
    E. Subtotal colectomy with end ileostomy

22. A 32-year-old male diagnosed with ulcerative colitis 1 year ago presents to the emergency department with jaundiced skin. He is admitted and workup is consistent with primary sclerosing cholangitis. Which of the following is additionally recommended?
    A. Immediate screening colonoscopy
    B. Immediate colonoscopy with random biopsies
    C. Colonoscopy with random biopsies at 8 to 10 years after his UC diagnosis
    D. Screening colonoscopy at age 50
    E. Symptom-driven colonoscopy as needed

23. A 65-year-old woman presents with massive bleeding per rectum. Her initial blood pressure in the ED is 80/60 mmHg, with a heart rate of 120 beats per minute. After volume resuscitation, the blood pressure increases to 120/80 mmHg. A nasogastric aspirate is negative for blood. A bedside anoscopy is performed and hemorrhoidal bleeding is ruled out, and the patient remains hemodynamically stable. The next step in her management is:
    A. Colonoscopy
    B. Mesenteric arteriography
    C. Tagged red cell scan
    D. Upper endoscopy
    E. Exploratory laparotomy

24. A 35-year-old patient with a history of ulcerative colitis who has undergone restorative total proctocolectomy with an ileal pouch–anal anastomosis presents with a 3-day history of abdominal pain, increased bowel movements, hematochezia, and fever. Which of the following is true regarding this condition?
    A. Biopsy is typically not required
    B. This is an uncommon complication
    C. Use of probiotics is not helpful
    D. Urgent excision of the J-pouch is often necessary
    E. Ciprofloxacin is more effective treatment than metronidazole

25. Which of the following is true about familial adenomatous polyposis?
    A. Microsatellite instability is a major contributor to this disease
    B. It is not associated with extraintestinal manifestations
    C. Patients with the gene mutation should begin screening with flexible sigmoidoscopy at age 20
    D. Patients undergoing prophylactic proctocolectomy have a lower subsequent risk of developing periampullary carcinoma
    E. Upper endoscopy should be performed every 1 to 3 years

26. A 10-year-old boy with acute myelogenous leukemia presents with right lower quadrant abdominal pain and tenderness. He recently completed chemotherapy. His temperature is 102°F and WBC count is 900 cells/μL. A CT scan reveals inflammation and thickening of the right colon and stranding in the adjacent fat. Management consists of:
    A. IV antibiotics, bowel rest, and IV fluids
    B. Right hemicolectomy with primary ileotransverse colostomy
    C. Right hemicolectomy with ileostomy and mucous fistula
    D. Cecostomy
    E. Appendectomy

27. A 40-year-old man presents with a 5-day history of right lower quadrant abdominal pain, anorexia, and fever. On physical examination, he is focally tender in the right lower quadrant, and a mass is palpable. A CT scan shows a small (<1 cm) abscess surrounding an inflamed appendix. After fluid resuscitation and intravenous antibiotics, which of the following is the most appropriate management?
    A. CT-guided drainage followed by interval appendectomy
    B. Initial nonoperative management followed by interval appendectomy
    C. Laparoscopic appendectomy
    D. Open appendectomy
    E. Nonoperative management

28. A 55-year-old man is undergoing a screening colonoscopy. A benign-appearing 1-cm pedunculated polyp is removed from the sigmoid colon with a cold snare. Four hours later, severe left lower quadrant pain develops in the patient. A CT scan reveals free intraperitoneal air with minimal fat stranding around the sigmoid colon. The situation is best managed by:
    A. Diverting proximal colostomy
    B. Resection of sigmoid colon with an end colostomy and oversew of the rectum
    C. Resection of the sigmoid colon with primary anastomosis
    D. Primary closure of the perforation
    E. Broad-spectrum antibiotics and nasogastric decompression

29. Five days after appendectomy, liquid stool is noted to be coming out of the right lower quadrant wound. The patient is hemodynamically stable, afebrile, and tolerating an oral diet. Which of the following is true about this condition?
    A. The patient should have nothing by mouth and be placed on parenteral nutrition
    B. Octreotide should be started
    C. The patient should immediately undergo reexploration and a cecostomy
    D. The patient should immediately undergo reexploration and a right colectomy
    E. The condition resolves spontaneously in most instances

30. Which of the following is true regarding chemotherapy for colon carcinoma?
    A. The combination of 5-fluorouracil and leucovorin prolongs survival in stage IV colon cancer
    B. Radiation therapy is commonly used in combination with chemotherapy in the management of colon cancer
    C. Bevacizumab (Avastin) has not been shown to prolong survival in stage IV colon cancer
    D. 5-fluorouracil and leucovorin prolong survival in patients with stage III colon cancer
    E. Bevacizumab (Avastin) is a monoclonal antibody against epidermal growth factor receptor

31. A 40-year-old man undergoes an appendectomy for acute appendicitis. Final pathology reveals a 1.1-cm carcinoid at the base of the appendix. Lymph nodes are negative. Which of the following is true about this condition?
    A. No further treatment is necessary
    B. There is a significant chance that carcinoid syndrome will develop in the patient
    C. The patient should receive chemotherapy
    D. The patient should undergo reexploration and a right colectomy
    E. Most appendiceal carcinoids are 2.5 cm or larger when discovered

32. An important source of energy for colonocytes, particularly in the setting of diversion colitis, is:
    A. Ketone bodies
    B. Glucose
    C. Amino acids
    D. Propionate
    E. Glutamine

33. A 15-year-old boy presents to a colorectal clinic with a family history of familial polyposis. APC gene testing is performed, and the result is positive. Flexible sigmoidoscopy reveals eight polyps in the sigmoid. Colonoscopy reveals no other polyps. Polyps are consistent with adenomatous polyps without evidence of malignancy. Which of the following is the recommended management?

    A. Repeat sigmoidoscopy in 6 months
    B. Cyclooxygenase-2 inhibitors, repeat sigmoidoscopy in 6 months
    C. Total colectomy with ileorectal anastomosis
    D. Total proctocolectomy with continent ileostomy
    E. Restorative proctocolectomy with ileal pouch–anal anastomosis

34. The most common presentation for appendiceal adenocarcinoma is:

    A. Palpable abdominal mass
    B. Acute appendicitis
    C. Ascites
    D. Incidental finding during unrelated abdominal surgery
    E. Chronic anemia

35. The most common perianal lesion in Crohn's disease is:

    A. Fissures
    B. Skin tags
    C. Perianal abscess
    D. Perianal fistulas
    E. Hemorrhoids

36. A 10-year-old boy presents with symptoms and signs suggestive of acute appendicitis. An ultrasound shows enlarged hypoechoic mesenteric lymph nodes and an absence of a thickened or dilated blind-ending tubular structure. Which of the following is true about this condition?

    A. A diagnostic laparoscopy should be performed
    B. This condition usually causes more peritoneal irritation than appendicitis
    C. The WBC count tends to be higher than with appendicitis
    D. It occurs with equal frequency in adults and children
    E. It is usually associated with an antecedent upper respiratory tract infection

37. A 50-year-old woman presents with symptoms and signs of acute appendicitis. At surgery, there is a large amount of gelatinous ascites with peritoneal implants. This most likely represents:

    A. Benign ovarian tumor
    B. Appendiceal mucinous adenoma
    C. Tuberculous appendicitis
    D. *Salmonella enteritidis*
    E. *Yersinia enterocolitica*

38. A 75-year-old woman presents to clinic for follow-up after four episodes of uncomplicated diverticulitis in the past year, each of which required a 5-day hospitalization for IV antibiotics and bowel rest. The patient is a diabetic. Previous CT scans demonstrated inflammation in the sigmoid colon with fat stranding. Subsequent colonoscopy revealed diverticula throughout the majority of the transverse, descending, and sigmoid colon, but was negative for other pathology. Which of the following is the most correct surgical intervention?

    A. Total colectomy with ileoproctostomy
    B. Sigmoid colectomy with proximal margin at an area without any hypertrophy of the muscularis propria and distal margin where the taenia splay out
    C. Left colectomy with proximal margin where there is cessation of diverticula and distal margin where the taenia splay out
    D. Sigmoid colectomy with proximal margin at an area without any hypertrophy of the muscularis propria and distal margin at the rectosigmoid junction
    E. Left colectomy with proximal margin where there is cessation of diverticula and distal margin at the rectosigmoid junction

39. A hernia containing an appendix is known as:

    A. Petit hernia
    B. Amyand hernia
    C. Littre hernia
    D. Spigelian hernia
    E. Grynfeltt hernia

40. A 35-year-old man presents with a 1-day history of anorexia, right lower quadrant pain and tenderness, and low-grade fever. At surgery, the appendix appears normal. However, both the cecum and terminal ileum appear red and inflamed. Management would consist of:

    A. Right hemicolectomy
    B. Appendectomy
    C. Close wound without further intervention
    D. Biopsy of the cecal wall
    E. Biopsy of the terminal ileum

41. A 15-year-old boy presents with a 5-day history of right lower quadrant pain and a fever of 103°F. On examination, he has right lower and right upper quadrant tenderness. Total bilirubin is 3 mg/dL and alkaline phosphatase is 250 IU/L. CT with contrast demonstrates multiple densities in the right lobe of the liver, a phlegmon in the right lower quadrant, and stranding around the superior mesenteric vein with air bubbles within the vein. The clinical picture most likely represents:

   A. Amebic liver abscess
   B. Pylephlebitis
   C. Carcinoid syndrome
   D. Metastatic adenocarcinoma
   E. Inflammatory bowel disease (IBD)

42. The most common worldwide intestinal parasite causing appendicitis is:

   A. *Enterobius vermicularis*
   B. *Strongyloides stercoralis*
   C. *Ascaris lumbricoides*
   D. *Echinococcus granulosus*
   E. *Clonorchis sinensis*

43. Incidental appendectomy is BEST indicated in which of the following circumstances?

   A. During gastric bypass surgery in a 45-year-old man
   B. During hysterectomy in a 30-year-old woman
   C. During small bowel resection in a 30-year-old woman with Crohn's disease
   D. During laparoscopic cholecystectomy in a 25-year-old woman
   E. During a Whipple procedure in a 50-year-old man

Answers

1. C. This patient is presenting with a first episode of uncomplicated diverticulitis, which is generally limited to pericolonic inflammation and phlegmon. Mesalamine, rifaximin, and probiotics are not typically recommended to reduce risk of diverticulitis recurrence. However, patients with chronic smoldering disease may notice improvement in symptoms with these adjuncts. To rule out an associated malignancy, the American Society of Colon and Rectal Surgeons recommends that all patients with complicated diverticulitis should undergo colonoscopy at 6 to 8 weeks after resolution of symptoms if colonoscopy has not been performed in the past year. For uncomplicated diverticulitis, this recommendation should be individualized to the patient; however, most practitioners would recommend colonoscopy in those with high-risk findings on CT imaging (mesenteric lymphadenopathy) or those with clinical recovery that is atypical. The rate of colon cancer in the setting of diverticulitis ranges from 0.5% to 2.7% for uncomplicated disease, and as high as 11% for complicated diverticulitis. In the setting of a single episode of uncomplicated diverticulitis that has fully resolved, sigmoid colectomy is not recommended (B, D). This patient's symptoms appear to have resolved, so there is no indication for repeat imaging (E). In the case of persistent or recurrent symptoms, chronic smoldering diverticulitis should be considered in the differential diagnosis, as sigmoid resection is effective in resolution of pain in this setting.

References: Sharma PV, Eglinton T, Hider P, Frizelle F. Systematic review and meta-analysis of the role of routine colonic evaluation after radiologically confirmed acute diverticulitis. *Ann Surg.* 2014;259(2):263–272.

Tehranian S, Klinge M, Saul M, Morris M, Diergaarde B, Schoen RE. Prevalence of colorectal cancer and advanced adenoma in patients with acute diverticulitis: implications for follow-up colonoscopy. *Gastrointest Endosc.* 2020;91(3):634–640.

Hall J, Hardiman K, Lee S, et al. The American Society of Colon and Rectal Surgeons clinical practice guidelines for the treatment of left-sided colonic diverticulitis. *Dis Colon Rectum.* 2020;63(6):728–747.

2. A. This patient presents with a large bowel obstruction, most likely secondary to metastatic colon cancer given the imaging findings of bilateral lung nodules and liver masses. The first step in managing a large bowel obstruction is to rule out a closed-loop obstruction, which is surgical emergency. Patients with a competent ileocecal valve and an obstructing colonic mass should be considered to have a closed-loop obstruction and should undergo urgent surgical decompression (i.e., colostomy or ileostomy) or resection (C, D). Patients with evidence of small bowel dilation and no systemic signs of infection likely have an incompetent ileocecal valve and may be appropriate candidates for bridging therapy which can allow for proper staging and an elective oncologic resection. Colonic stenting has been increasingly utilized to manage left-sided large bowel tumors presenting with obstruction. As this patient does not have a tissue diagnosis, colonoscopy and stent placement will serve both diagnostic and therapeutic purposes. Uncovered stents are superior to covered stents in the management of large bowel obstruction as they are associated with fewer complications, lower rates of stent migration, and longer duration of patency (B). Chemotherapy should not be initiated without tissue diagnosis and impending obstruction (E).

Reference: Kaplan J, Strongin A, Adler DG, Siddiqui AA. Enteral stents for the management of malignant colorectal obstruction. *World J Gastroenterol.* 2014;20(37):13239–13245.

3. B. The colon is responsible for both water and electrolyte reabsorption. Water absorption averages 1 to 2 L per day but can be as much as 5 L. However, the small intestine (mostly jejunum) is where the majority of water absorption occurs (A). Sodium is absorbed actively via Na+,K+-ATPase with water following passively. Chloride is actively absorbed, not secreted, through a chloride–bicarbonate exchange (D). Bacteria fermentation in the colon produces short-chain fatty acids, which are a primary source of energy for colonocytes (E). Decreasing colonic pH (as occurs with lactulose) results in a decrease in ammonia reassertion (C).

4. D. For patients with peritoneal studding from appendiceal adenocarcinoma, cytoreductive surgery with hyperthermic intraperitoneal chemotherapy (HIPEC) has shown promise in patients without evidence of distant organ metastasis. In a large series in which complete cytoreduction was defined as tumor nodules less than 2.5 mm in diameter remaining after surgery, patients with complete cytoreduction and adenomucinosis pathology had a 5-year survival rate of 86%. Incomplete cytoreduction had a 5-year survival rate of only 20%. Systemic or intraperitoneal chemotherapy alone leads to lower survival rates (B, C, E). Offering no treatment to a patient with peritoneal studding secondary to appendiceal adenocarcinoma would not be appropriate (A). HIPEC is being used for colorectal, gastric, and ovarian cancer, as well as intraperitoneal mesothelioma.

References: Jaffe BM, Berger DH. Appendix. In: Brunicardi FC, Andersen DK, Billiar TR, et al., eds. *Schwartz's principles of surgery.* 8th ed. New York: McGraw-Hill; 2005:1119–1138.

Lally KP, Cox C, Andrassy RJ. Appendix. In: Townsend CM, Jr, Beauchamp RD, Evers BM, Mattox KL, eds. *Sabiston textbook of surgery: The biological basis of modern surgical practice.* 17th ed. Philadelphia: W.B. Saunders; 2004:1381–1400.

Sugarbaker PH, Chang D. Results of treatment of 385 patients with peritoneal surface spread of appendiceal malignancy. *Ann Surg Oncol.* 1999;6(8):727–731.

Sugarbaker PH, Jablonski KA. Prognostic features of 51 colorectal and 130 appendiceal cancer patients with peritoneal carcinomatosis treated by cytoreductive surgery and intraperitoneal chemotherapy. *Ann Surg.* 1995;221(2):124–132.

5. B. This patient is presenting with a first-time diagnosis of colon cancer. Preoperative CT scan of the abdomen and pelvis to evaluate tumor extension, lymphatic spread, and metastases is recommended for all colon cancer patients. Routine staging with CT scan of the chest is frequently performed but controversial, as metastatic pulmonary disease is uncommon. In a systematic review of 5873 patients that underwent preoperative staging chest CT, 9% had an indeterminate pulmonary nodule, of which only 10% were malignant. Carcinoembryonic antigen has low diagnostic yield for colon cancer, but is useful in assessing persistence of disease following resection. Transrectal endoscopic ultrasound (A) is useful in locoregional staging for rectal cancer but not colon cancer. PET/CT scans are not used routinely for staging of a newly diagnosed colon cancer (C–E) but be useful to assess rising CEA levels following initial surgical treatment.

References: National Comprehensive Cancer Network (NCCN). NCCN Guidelines for Patients. Version 2.2021: Colon Cancer. Updated January 21, 2021. Accessed March 7, 2022. https://www. nccn.org/patients/guidelines/content/PDF/colon-patient.pdf.

Nordholm-Carstensen A, Wille-Jørgensen PA, Jorgensen LN, Harling H. Indeterminate pulmonary nodules at colorectal cancer staging: a systematic review of predictive parameters for malignancy. *Ann Surg Oncol.* 2013;20(12):4022–4030.

6. E. The risk of the development of colon cancer in patients with UC increases with time. By 20 years, colon cancer will develop in approximately 10% of patients. Thus, surveillance colonoscopy is recommended. Colon cancer develops in UC in the absence of polyps. In addition, areas of dysplasia may not be readily apparent on standard colonoscopy. As such, once a patient has had UC for 8 years, colonoscopic surveillance is recommended annually thereafter. In addition to biopsies of areas of suspicion, random biopsies are recommended because flat dysplasia develops in these patients. The finding of even high-grade dysplasia is an indication for surgery. Repeat colonoscopy would be inappropriate (A). Some authors recommend surgery even for low-grade flat dysplasia because the risk of malignancy is also significantly increased; a recent metaanalysis demonstrated that these patients have a nine times increased risk of having colorectal cancer compared with patients who are dysplasia free. Dysplasia in a flat (nonpolypoid) lesion is concerning because it is more difficult to monitor with follow-up screening. The curative operation is a restorative proctocolectomy with an ileal pouch–anal anastomosis (B–D). In addition to dysplasia, the indications for colectomy in patients with UC include toxic megacolon, severe lower GI bleeding, and intractable disease that does not respond to medical management.

References: Ullman T, Croog V, Harpaz N, Sachar D, Itzkowitz S. Progression of flat low-grade dysplasia to advanced neoplasia in patients with ulcerative colitis. *Gastroenterology.* 2003;125(5):1311–1319.

Thomas T, Abrams KA, Robinson RJ, Mayberry JF. Meta-analysis: cancer risk of low-grade dysplasia in chronic ulcerative colitis. *Aliment Pharmacol Ther.* 2007;25(6):657–668.

7. B. Mucosal edema is the earliest finding on endoscopy. As the disease advances, friable mucosa and ulcerations develop (A). A "lead pipe" colon is a feature of longstanding UC seen on barium enema and is the result of a loss of haustral markings and shortening of the colon. Although crypt abscesses are almost always seen with UC, other inflammatory conditions of the colon can also present with crypt abscesses (E). Findings on gross appearance in Crohn's colitis that are not characteristic of UC include a thickened mesentery, thickened bowel wall, segmental disease, and "creeping fat" or "fat wrapping." On microscopic examination, Crohn's disease is transmural, whereas UC is limited to the mucosa and submucosa. Noncaseating granulomas are a hallmark feature of Crohn's disease, whereas crypt abscesses are characteristic of UC. Plasmacytosis (increase in plasma cells in lamina propria) can be found in both UC and Crohn's disease (C). Pseudopolyps are seen in both UC and Crohn's disease (D).

8. D. It is important to remember that appendiceal perforation is the most important variable in determining fetal mortality during pregnancy; thus, it is imperative to make the diagnosis early. Conversely, a general anesthetic increases the risk of premature labor. A recent large study was conducted comparing appendicitis in more than 3000 pregnant women with more than 94,000 nonpregnant women. The study found that the rate of negative appendectomy was higher in pregnant women compared with nonpregnant women (23% versus 18%). Rates of fetal loss and early delivery were considerably higher in women with complex appendicitis (6% and 11%, respectively) compared with negative (4% and 10%, respectively) and simple (2% and 4%, respectively) appendicitis. Complex appendicitis and a negative appendectomy remained risks for fetal loss on multivariate analysis. Interestingly, laparoscopy was associated with a higher rate of fetal loss compared with open appendectomy (odds ratio of 2.31) (B). Ultrasonography has been extremely useful in helping diagnose appendicitis. If findings are equivocal, magnetic resonance imaging (MRI) should be performed. One must strive to avoid unnecessary appendectomies that place the fetus at risk; however, delays in operative care for appendicitis likewise place the fetus at risk.

References: McGory ML, Zingmond DS, Tillou A, Hiatt JR, Ko CY, Cryer HM. Negative appendectomy in pregnant women is associated with a substantial risk of fetal loss. *J Am Coll Surg.* 2007;205(4):534–540.

Lim HK, Bae SH, Seo GS. Diagnosis of acute appendicitis in pregnant women: value of sonography. *AJR Am J Roentgenol.* 1992;159(3): 539–542.

9. D. Stage for stage, colonic malignancy in Lynch syndrome has the same prognosis as sporadic cancer. In a small number of sporadic colon cancers, microsatellite instability and inappropriate DNA methylation leads to impaired DNA mismatch repair, increasing the risk for developing colon cancer. Lynch syndrome (or HNPCC) arises because of errors in the mismatch repair genes that code for the DNA mismatch repair enzymes. It is an autosomal dominant syndrome with an increased risk of colorectal carcinoma and other malignancies, with a lifetime risk of approximately 80% for colon cancer, 20% for gastric cancer, and a high risk of endometrial and upper genitourinary tract cancer (A, B). The colon cancers are more commonly right sided (as opposed to left sided in sporadic cancer); as such, screening requires colonoscopy, which is recommended either at age 25 or 10 years less than the age at which colon cancer developed in other family members (whichever is earlier) (C). Patients with FAP should begin screening much earlier (age 10–12). Upper endoscopy screening is also recommended starting at age 50. The modified Amsterdam criteria for clinical diagnosis of HNPCC can be remembered by the 3-2-1-1 rule: 3 or more relatives with histologically verified cancers in the colon, endometrium small intestine, or pelvis; 2 or more successive generations affected; 1 or more relatives diagnosed before age 50 (E); and 1 should be a first-degree relative of the other two. Additionally, FAP must be ruled out to diagnose Lynch syndrome.

References: Stigliano V, Assisi D, Cosimelli M, et al. Survival of hereditary non-polyposis colorectal cancer patients compared with sporadic colorectal cancer patients. *J Exp Clin Cancer Res.* 2008; 27(1):39.

Watson P, Lin KM, Rodriguez-Bigas MA, et al. Colorectal carcinoma survival among hereditary nonpolyposis colorectal carcinoma family members. *Cancer.* 1998;83(2):259–266.

van der Post RS, Kiemeney LA, Ligtenberg MJL, et al. Risk of urothelial bladder cancer in Lynch syndrome is increased, in particular among MSH2 mutation carriers. *J Med Genet.* 2010;47(7):464–470.

10. B. Familial juvenile polyposis is an autosomal dominant (A) disorder (just like hereditary nonpolyposis colon cancer [HNPCC], FAP, and Peutz-Jeghers syndrome). It is a completely different entity from FAP. The polyps are hamartomas (also called juvenile polyps), not adenomas. Hamartomas are benign growths composed of histologically normal and mature cells found in abnormal locations and configurations. However, the hamartomas can degenerate into adenomas and malignancy, causing risk of colon cancer, but not to the same degree as with FAP. The lifetime risk is approximately 10% to 38% (versus 100% for FAP) (C). Because of this risk and because many polyps occur on the right side, colonoscopic (rather than flexible sigmoidoscopic) surveillance is recommended, beginning at approximately 10 to 12 years of age. Unlike FAP, in which the presence of polyps equates with a need for a restorative proctocolectomy, if a polyp is seen, it should be snared and sent to pathology (D). In most instances, it will be a hamartoma. If adenomatous changes are seen, then a colectomy should be performed, and if the rectum is spared, an ileorectal anastomosis can be done with close surveillance. Approximately 15% to 20% of Peutz-Jeghers syndrome patients develop stomach or duodenal cancers, so upper endoscopic surveillance is recommended by age 25 (E).

References: Dunlop MG, British Society for Gastroenterology, Association of Coloproctology for Great Britain and Ireland. Guidance on gastrointestinal surveillance for hereditary non-polyposis colorectal cancer, familial adenomatous polypolis, juvenile polyposis, and Peutz-Jeghers syndrome. *Gut.* 2002;51(Suppl 5):V21–V27.

Howe JR, Mitros FA, Summers RW. The risk of gastrointestinal carcinoma in familial juvenile polyposis. *Ann Surg Oncol.* 1998;5(8): 751–756.

11. B. Sessile serrated polyps often harbor dysplasia or carcinoma in situ and should be resected. Given their flat morphology, they are at risk of not being detected or undergoing incomplete removal and may contribute to interval cancer development. Patients with serrated polyposis syndrome (previously known as hyperplastic polyposis syndrome) can present with upward of 100 polyps in the colon, some of which are premalignant. Patients with this syndrome are considered to be at increased risk for colon cancer. Adenomatous polyps are considered neoplastic and are divided into three types: tubular (<5% risk of malignancy), tubulovillous (20% risk of malignancy), and villous (40% risk of malignancy) (A). Polyp size is also an important determinant, with polyps smaller than 1 cm having an extremely low risk of malignancy vs a nearly 50% risk of malignancy in polyps larger than 2 cm. The location of a polyp does not affect the risk of malignancy (E). Most colon cancers develop from adenomatous polyps. Peutz-Jeghers syndrome is characterized by hamartomatous polyps (C). They present with GI bleeding and intussusception. Although hamartomatous polyps are not considered premalignant, they can degenerate into adenomatous polyps, so there is a risk of malignancy. The polyps in Peutz-Jeghers syndrome occur primarily in the small intestine, but they can also occur in the colon and rectum. Patients have melanin spots on the buccal mucosa and lips. Because of the diffuse nature of polyps throughout the GI tract, surgery is only indicated if there is evidence of obstruction or bleeding or evidence that a polyp has undergone adenomatous change. Inflammatory polyps or pseudopolyps are islands of regenerating mucosa seen most often in IBD or after mucosal injury (D).

References: Correa P, Strong JP, Reif A, Johnson WD. The epidemiology of colorectal polyps: prevalence in New Orleans and international comparisons. *Cancer.* 1977;39(5):2258–2264.

Hyman NH, Anderson P, Blasyk H. Hyperplastic polyposis and the risk of colorectal cancer. *Dis Colon Rectum.* 2004;47(12):2101–2104.

12. C. Ischemic colitis occurs primarily in elderly patients at an average age of 70 years and may present with lower GI bleeding. Fecal immunochemical test has replaced the older fecal occult guaiac blood test because it has been shown to have superior adherence, usability, accuracy, sensitivity, and better detection of occult bleeding. Unlike acute small bowel ischemia, which develops in association with mesenteric arterial or venous occlusive disease, colonic ischemia is rarely the result of major vascular occlusion. Rather, it usually occurs as a result of a low-flow state such as severe dehydration. As such, mesenteric angiography is typically not helpful (E). It tends to develop in watershed areas of blood supply, such as the splenic flexure (most common), known as Griffith's point, where collaterals are present between the superior mesenteric artery and inferior mesenteric artery (specifically, the middle colic artery and the ascending branch of the left colic artery, respectively); Sudeck's critical point (rectosigmoid junction), where collaterals are present between the sigmoid artery and superior rectal artery; and the ileocecal area. In addition to advanced age, risk factors for ischemic colitis include underlying cardiovascular disease, diabetes, vasculitis, and hypotension. Most cases are mild and result in painless, bloody diarrhea. More severe cases can result in bacterial translocation with fever and leukocytosis or, rarely, full-thickness necrosis with peritonitis. The diagnosis is via a combination of the history and examination, plain films to rule out an acute abdomen and that sometimes will show signs of mucosal edema (thumb printing), and CT scan (nonspecific colonic wall edema and fat stranding). The surgeon needs to be aware that the differential diagnosis includes colon cancer and IBD. As such, colonoscopy should eventually be performed, although it is not necessary in the acute phase (D). The exception is ischemic colitis after aortic surgery, in which case the endoscopy assists in the diagnosis, and CT scan findings may be hard to interpret due to postsurgical changes. Most patients are treated medically with bowel rest and broad-spectrum antibiotics. Surgery is reserved for patients who deteriorate and/or have evidence of diffuse peritonitis or endoscopy in whom shows necrosis (A, B).

References: Balthazar EJ, Yen BC, Gordon RB. Ischemic colitis: CT evaluation of 54 cases. *Radiology.* 1999;211(2):381–388.

Schreuders EH, Grobbee EJ, Spaander MCW, Kuipers EJ. Advances in fecal tests for colorectal cancer screening. *Curr Treat Options Gastroenterol.* 2016;14(1):152–162.

13. B. This patient has a sigmoid volvulus. The common denominator in sigmoid volvulus is a large, redundant colon, which is frequently associated with chronic constipation. Individuals with chronic constipation (elderly or institutionalized), a high-fiber diet (leads to an elongated and redundant colon), or megacolon (Chagas disease) are predisposed. Patients present with symptoms and signs of an acute large bowel obstruction. The important issues are the following:

1. Establishing the correct diagnosis. This can generally be done by classic radiographic findings of a markedly dilated colon with a "bent inner tube" appearance or an omega sign.
2. Determining whether the patient already has an ischemic or dead bowel. This can be achieved via evidence of systemic toxicity (laboratory tests) and physical examination (peritonitis), and if these are present, the patient needs a laparotomy and sigmoid colectomy (D, E). Sometimes this is also seen at the time of endoscopy.
3. Understanding the value of endoscopic detorsion. This can be performed with either a rigid proctosigmoidoscope or a flexible endoscope.
4. Being aware that there is a high recurrence rate (as high as 40%). Thus, after detorsion, a recommendation should be made for a subsequent colectomy (A, C).
5. Distinguishing it from cecal volvulus, which cannot usually be endoscopically detorsed and requires surgery (right hemicolectomy).

Reference: Chung YF, Eu KW, Nyam DC, Leong AF, Ho YH, Seow-Choen F. Minimizing recurrence after sigmoid volvulus: Recurrence after sigmoid volvulus. *Br J Surg.* 1999;86(2):231–233.

14. E. Cecal or cecocolic volvulus is much less common than sigmoid volvulus. It occurs in younger patients. There are two types: axial ileocolic volvulus (90%) and cecal bascule (10%). In the former, the cecum rotates up and over to the left upper quadrant. Cecal bascule occurs when the cecum flips upward and anterior in a horizontal plane. It is thought to be due to a congenital anomaly leading to a lack of fixation of the cecum to the retroperitoneum, and as such, the terminal ileum, cecum, and ascending colon twist and can become ischemic. It can sometimes be hard to diagnose radiographically because the patient will often also demonstrate dilated loops of small bowel with air–fluid levels, giving the appearance of a small bowel obstruction. Unlike sigmoid volvulus, endoscopic decompression for cecal volvulus is very difficult (D). The treatment of choice is to perform a right colectomy with primary anastomosis; this is feasible despite no bowel preparation. There is a high recurrence rate after operative detorsion and cecopexy (B). If the right colon is already gangrenous (e.g., leukocytosis, acidosis, high fever, peritonitis), right hemicolectomy with ileostomy and mucus fistula is the treatment of choice (C). However, this patient's presentation makes this finding unlikely. Cecostomy tubes are inappropriate in a patient who is young and otherwise a good surgical candidate who would benefit from definitive treatment (A).

Reference: Habre J, Sautot-Vial N, Marcotte C, Benchimol D. Caecal volvulus. *Am J Surg.* 2008;196(5):e48–e49.

15. D. Sigmoid diverticular disease is thought to occur due to a low-fiber diet leading to constipation. A long, redundant colon, found in populations that have a high-fiber diet, increases the risk of developing volvulus (E). Sigmoid diverticula are considered false because they are composed of only mucosa and submucosa. They occur at points of weakness between the taeniae coli, where blood vessels penetrate the colonic wall. They occur most commonly in the sigmoid colon on the mesenteric side of the antimesenteric taenia (A). They occur due to increased intraluminal pressure, so they are considered pulsion diverticula. Because the taeniae splay out at the rectum, diverticula do not develop in the rectum (B). Asymptomatic diverticula (sigmoid or cecal) do not require surgical management (C). Patients deemed surgical candidates for sigmoid resection are best served with a mechanical bowel preparation with IV and oral perioperative antibiotics. This decreases the rate of surgical site infection by more than 50%.

Reference: Kim EK, Sheetz KH, Bonn J, et al. A statewide colectomy experience: the role of full bowel preparation in preventing surgical site infection. *Ann Surg.* 2014;259(2):310–314.

16. D. Pneumoperitoneum in a symptomatic patient almost always necessitates emergency surgery and is often due to visceral perforation (A, B). However, colonoscopy (less so with diagnostic versus therapeutic) can lead to benign pneumoperitoneum and is believed to be due to microperforation and/or the transmural passage of air secondary to insufflation. Patients with benign pneumoperitoneum, no abdominal pain, and no systemic signs of sepsis (fever, leukocytosis) can be treated with IV antibiotics and bowel rest. Due to the scarcity of benign pneumoperitoneum in the literature, these recommendations are based on several case reports and one prospective study. Serial abdominal exam should also be performed but in addition to admission, antibiotics and bowel rest (C). The patient should not be discharged home if there is concern for a perforated viscus (E).

Reference: Pearl JP, McNally MP, Elster EA, DeNobile JW. Benign pneumoperitoneum after colonoscopy: a prospective pilot study. *Mil Med.* 2006;171(7):648–649.

17. D. Parastomal hernias are a relatively common complication of stoma creation with an estimated occurrence rate as high as 50%, with end colostomy having the highest risk and loop ileostomy having the lowest risk (E). Other risk factors include older age, wound infection, obesity, malnutrition, immunosuppression, IBD, and COPD (A). While parastomal hernia can be asymptomatic, the estimated reoperation rate for patients with this condition is somewhere around 30%. A study published in the World Journal of Surgery in 2010 demonstrated a reduction of parastomal hernia rate from 55% to 7.8% with the placement of mesh during the index operation. Another study showed reduction of clinically significant parastomal hernia but no difference in CT detectable parastomal hernias with the use of mesh. Prophylactic mesh placement is being used more commonly as more studies suggest improved outcomes. Patients with asymptomatic parastomal hernia should be managed with a support device such as a hernia belt and weight loss. However, this patient is complaining of pain and difficulty applying his colostomy bag, which are both indications for repair or relocation of the stoma (B). Prosthetic mesh repair is considered the preferred surgical approach because relocating the stoma is associated with the same high risk of hernia formation as the initial stoma (C). A common repair is the Sugarbaker technique, in which mesh is placed around the ostomy as a flap valve.

References: Hiranyakas A, Ho YH. Laparoscopic parastomal hernia repair. *Dis Colon Rectum.* 2010;53(9):1334–1336.

Kann BR. Early stomal complications. *Clin Colon Rectal Surg.* 2008;21(1):23–30.

Tam KW, Wei PL, Kuo LJ, Wu CH. Systematic review of the use of a mesh to prevent parastomal hernia. *World J Surg.* 2010;34(11):2723–2729.

Vierimaa M, Klintrup K, Biancari F, et al. Prospective, randomized study on the use of a prosthetic mesh for prevention of parastomal hernia of permanent colostomy. *Dis Colon Rectum.* 2015;58(10):943–949.

18. D. Ischemia or necrosis of the stoma is a recognized complication of a colostomy creation. It is more likely to occur in situations in which the inferior mesenteric artery was ligated high, near the aorta, such that the stoma is relying on the marginal artery. It is important to evaluate the extent of ischemia before proceeding directly to the operating room. This is can be accomplished by placing a clear test tube into the ostomy and using a penlight to evaluate the mucosa down to the level of the fascia or via endoscopy. If the ischemia is evident down to the level of the fascia, the patient needs reexploration and revision; otherwise it may progress to full-thickness necrosis, perforation, and stool spillage into the peritoneum. The type of operation will depend on the extent of ischemia (A–C). In contrast, if the ischemia is superficial, it can be observed, and a mucocutaneous junction will form by secondary intention. This may lead to recession of the stoma or stricture but can be dealt with later when the patient recovers from surgery. In addition, it may be technically difficult, if not impossible, to gain additional length in a morbidly obese patient to refashion the stoma; thus, a return to the OR should be avoided if it can be done safely. There is no role for IV antibiotics (E).

Reference: Kim JT, Kumar RR. Reoperation for stoma-related complications. *Clin Colon Rectal Surg.* 2006;19(4):207–212.

19. B. This patient has a stercoral ulceration complicated by perforation. This is a rare condition occurring primarily in elderly patients suffering from chronic constipation. It is thought that a hard fecaloma leads to local ischemia, ulcer formation, and subsequent perforation. The antimesenteric border of the rectosigmoid colon is the most likely location owing to its unique characteristics including lower water content, poorer bloody supply, and higher pressure secondary to a narrowed intraluminal diameter (A–E). The diagnosis is suggested with the following four criteria: (1) a round antimesenteric colonic perforation >1 cm in diameter; (2) colon full of stool protruding through the perforation site; (3) evidence of multiple pressure ulcers and acute inflammation around the perforation; and (4) absence of external injury, diverticulitis, or obstruction due to neoplasms or adhesions. Patients most commonly present with diffuse abdominal pain and fever. The diagnosis is seldom made before surgery. Since inflammation and ulcer formation extend beyond the immediate bowel surrounding the perforation, a simple closure or limited colonic resection should be avoided (C). Thus, a formal colon resection with proximal colostomy (Hartmann procedure) is recommended. Stercoral ulcer perforation has a high mortality rate. Chronic constipation is a common problem affecting many people, but stercoral ulceration is rare; this suggests there may be additional predisposing factors contributing to this entity. Several reports have shown an association of NSAID use with the development of stercoral perforation. Additionally, anticholinergic agents will worsen chronic constipation and contribute to this complication (D).

References: Huang WS, Wang CS, Hsieh CC, Lin PY, Chin CC, Wang JY. Management of patients with stercoral perforation of the sigmoid colon: report of five cases. *World J Gastroenterol.* 2006;12(3):500–503.

Mauer CA, Renzulli P, Mazzucchelli L. Use of the accurate diagnostic criteria may increase incidence of stercoral perforation of the colon. *Dis Colon Rectum.* 2000;43(7):991–998.

Patel VG, Kalakuntla V, Fortson JK, Weaver WL, Joel MD, Hammami A. Stercoral perforation of the sigmoid colon: report of a rare case and its possible association with nonsteroidal antiinflammatory drugs. *Am Surg.* 2002;68(1):62–64.

Serpell JW, Nicholls RJ. Stercoral perforation of the colon. *Br J Surg.* 1990;77(12):1325–1329.

20. B. This patient has acute colonic pseudoobstruction or Ogilvie syndrome. It often occurs in critically ill patients without any signs of mechanical obstruction. The pathophysiology is not completely understood, is likely multifactorial, and is thought to occur secondary to paralysis of the bowel allowing for passive distention. Stable patients without any systemic signs of compromised bowel should initially undergo conservative management with bowel rest, nasogastric tube suction, decompressive rectal tube, and electrolyte repletion. Neostigmine is a reversible cholinesterase inhibitor that has been demonstrated in randomized controlled trials to have an improved response over placebo (reduction in cecum diameter of 5 cm compared to 2 cm). Up to 80% to 90% of patients have a favorable response to a single IV injection of 2 mg neostigmine (D). For those who do not respond, a second and third administration can be given. Alternatively, a continuous infusion of neostigmine at a rate of 0.4 to 0.8 mg/hour over 24 hours can be given and has been shown to have successful results (C). Contraindications to the use of neostigmine include acute urinary retention, acute coronary artery syndrome, asthma, bronchospasm, and second- or third-degree heart block (A). All patients being given neostigmine should be placed on cardiac monitoring, and a syringe prefilled with atropine should be placed at bedside and ready for immediate use. Endoscopic detorsion with or without placement of a decompression tube is a viable option in the absence of perforation, bowel ischemia, or peritonitis, particularly for those who do not respond to neostigmine and can aid in ruling out a mechanical obstruction.

References: Ponec RJ, Saunders MD, Kimmey MB. Neostigmine for the treatment of acute colonic pseudo-obstruction. *N Engl J Med.* 1999;341(3):137–141.

Van Der Spoel J, Oudemans-Van Straaten HM, Stoutenbeek CP. American Society for Gastrointestinal Endoscopy guideline on the role of endoscopy in the management of acute colonic pseudo-obstruction and colonic volvulus. *Gastrointest Endosc.* 2001;91(2):228–235.

Vogel JD, Feingold DL, Stewart DB, et al. Clinical practice guidelines for colon volvulus and acute colonic pseudo-obstruction. *Dis Colon Rectum.* 2016;59(7):589–600.

21. C. If conservative therapy fails in the management of Ogilvie syndrome or if there is any concern for compromised bowel, surgery should be considered. The three surgical options include tube colostomy, transanal insertion of a long multiperforated drainage tube, and total or subtotal colectomy with an ostomy. If during laparotomy there is no evidence of ischemic or perforated colon, then colectomy can be avoided (E). In this scenario, a right transverse or left lower quadrant sigmoid colostomy tube is often used with a success rate of 95%. This functions as a "blow-hole" colostomy at one or several points in the bowel and is more effective than a formal colostomy at providing pressure relief. A less effective option includes the transanal insertion of a large multiperforated tube (Faucher tube) guided to the proximal edge of dilated colon by the surgeon's hands (D). Next, the surgeon performs manual compressive maneuvers to milk the colonic content toward the tube. If there is any concern of compromised bowel, a total or subtotal colectomy should be performed. Primary anastomosis should be avoided because this has a high leak rate (A, B). This is a highly morbid procedure, with mortality estimated to be up to 40%.

References: Caves PK, Crockard HA. Pseudo-obstruction of the large bowel. *Br Med J.* 1970;2(5709):583–586.

Vanek VW, Al-Salti M. Acute pseudo-obstruction of the colon (Ogilvie's syndrome): An analysis of 400 cases. *Dis Colon Rectum.* 1986;29(3):203–210.

Vogel JD, Feingold DL, Stewart DB, et al. Clinical practice guidelines for colon volvulus and acute colonic pseudo-obstruction. *Dis Colon Rectum.* 2016;59(7):589–600.

22. B. PSC is a progressive and destructive disease of the entire biliary tree secondary to an inflammatory process. It is estimated that up to 80% of patients with PSC have IBD, with UC being most common. It has been demonstrated that PSC significantly increases the risk of colorectal cancer in these patients. UC patients should typically undergo screening colonoscopy with random biopsies starting 8 years from the time of their IBD diagnosis (C). However, patients diagnosed with PSC should receive a colonoscopy with random biopsies promptly at the time of PSC diagnosis and continue every 1 to 2 years thereafter. Patients without IBD or family history of colorectal cancer should begin screening at age 50 or after presenting with worrisome symptoms (D, E). Patients with family history of colorectal cancer should begin screening 10 years before the age of diagnosis of any first-degree relative with colorectal cancer.

References: Razumilava N, Gores GJ, Lindor KD. Cancer surveillance in patients with primary sclerosing cholangitis. *Hepatology.* 2011;54(5):1842–1852.

Zheng HH, Jiang XL. Increased risk of colorectal neoplasia in patients with primary sclerosing cholangitis and inflammatory bowel disease: a meta-analysis of 16 observational studies. *Eur J Gastroenterol Hepatol.* 2016;28(4):383–390.

23. A. The most common cause of lower GI bleeding, diverticulosis, accounts for more than one-half of cases. Rarely, massive lower GI bleeding can be the result of an upper GI source. Placing a nasogastric tube and aspirating for blood are important first steps after resuscitation. Likewise, hemorrhoids can rarely be the cause and can easily be ruled out with anoscopy while the patient is stabilized. The management algorithm depends on the patient's response to initial resuscitation. If the patient stabilizes, she should undergo colonoscopy as soon as a bowel preparation is completed (A). If the patient continues to bleed, the next step is to perform either mesenteric arteriography or a tagged red blood cell scan (nuclear scintigraphy) using technetium-99m (B, C). Arteriography can be both diagnostic and therapeutic (angioembolization). However, it is invasive and bleeding must be brisk (0.5–1 mL/min). It is also not as feasible to repeat the study in the case of a patient that stopped bleeding and rebleeds. Nuclear scanning detects bleeding at a much slower rate (only 0.1 mL/min), and since the radioactive agent remains labeled on the red blood cell for some time, repeat images can be obtained for up to 24 hours. If the patient cannot be stabilized and the source is not discovered, the patient should be taken to the operating room for an exploratory laparotomy with intraoperative endoscopy or colonoscopy (D–E). If the source cannot be localized, a total colectomy should be performed.

Reference: Farner R, Lichliter W, Kuhn J, Fisher T. Total colectomy versus limited colonic resection for acute lower gastrointestinal bleeding. *Am J Surg.* 1999;178(6):587–591.

24. E. Pouchitis is a nonspecific inflammation of the ileal reservoir that can occur after an ileoanal pouch creation or in a continent ileostomy reservoir. Pouchitis can be acute or can become chronic. Symptoms include increased diarrhea, hematochezia, abdominal pain, fever, and malaise. The diagnosis is established via a combination of the history, endoscopic findings, and histology from biopsy samples. Endoscopy with biopsy is important to rule out undiagnosed Crohn's disease (A). It is the most common long-term complication of this procedure, with an incidence as high as 30% to 55% (B). *Clostridium difficile*-associated pouchitis should be ruled out. The cause is unknown; it may be due to fecal stasis within the pouch, but emptying studies do not confirm this. A recent Cochrane study showed that ciprofloxacin is more effective than metronidazole for inducing remission of acute pouchitis. Most patients will respond rapidly to either oral preparations or enemas. Patients with chronic pouchitis may require ongoing suppressive antibiotic therapy. Salicylate and stool enemas have also been used with some success. Reintroduction of normal flora by probiotics has been shown to be useful in chronic cases (C). Rarely, the pouch requires excision, but this would not be done urgently (D).

References: Gionchetti P, Amadini C, Rizzello F, Venturi A, Poggioli G, Campieri M. Diagnosis and treatment of pouchitis. *Best Pract Res Clin Gastroenterol.* 2003;17(1):75–87.

Holubar SD, Cima RR, Sandborn WJ, Pardi DS. Treatment and prevention of pouchitis after ileal pouch-anal anastomosis for chronic ulcerative colitis. *Cochrane Database Syst Rev.* 2010;6:CD001176.

Madiba TE, Bartolo DC. Pouchitis following restorative proctocolectomy for ulcerative colitis: incidence and therapeutic outcome. *J R Coll Surg Edinb.* 2001;46(6):334–337.

Shen B, Achkar JP, Lashner BA, et al. A randomized clinical trial of ciprofloxacin and metronidazole to treat acute pouchitis. *Inflamm Bowel Dis.* 2001;7(4):301–305.

25. E. FAP is a rare autosomal dominant disease that accounts for approximately 1% of colon cancers. It is due to a mutation in the adenomatous polyposis coli (APC) tumor suppressor gene on chromosome 5q. Syndromes that are considered variants of FAP include attenuated FAP (delayed polyp growth), Turcot syndrome, and Gardner syndrome. If unrecognized or untreated, cancer can develop in all patients by age 35 to 40 years; in fact, polyps often begin at puberty. They eventually can develop thousands of polyps. As such, first–degree relatives of FAP patients who are APC positive should begin screening at age 10 to 12 years by flexible sigmoidoscopy (C). Relatives who are APC mutation negative

can wait until age 50 for screening because they are considered to have the same risk as the normal population. Adenomas can develop throughout the gastrointestinal (GI) tract in FAP patients, and in particular in the duodenum, and patients are at risk of the development of periampullary carcinoma. Therefore, upper endoscopy for surveillance every 1 to 3 years starting at age 25 to 30 years should be recommended. Prophylactic proctocolectomy does not decrease the risk of developing periampullary carcinoma, and it remains a common cause of morbidity in this patient population (D). Once the diagnosis of FAP has been made and polyps are developing, treatment is surgical. FAP may also be associated with extraintestinal manifestations such as congenital hypertrophy of the retinal pigment epithelium, desmoid tumors, epidermoid cysts, mandibular osteomas, and central nervous system tumors (B). In a small number of sporadic colon cancers, microsatellite instability leads to impaired DNA mismatch repair and thus an inability to ensure the fidelity of a copied DNA strand, increasing the risk for developing cancer (A).

26. A. In the neutropenic patient with leukemia who presents with acute abdominal pain, one must suspect neutropenic enterocolitis, which is commonly referred to as typhlitis. The typical patient presents with abdominal pain and tenderness, fever, and diarrhea in association with severe neutropenia (defined as an absolute neutrophil count <1000 cells/µL). A CT scan is helpful in ruling out perforation and in the case of typhlitis will show thickening of the cecal wall with pericolic stranding. Some reports have also shown the utility of ultrasonography in establishing the diagnosis via the demonstration of cecal thickening. The majority of patients respond to bowel rest and IV antibiotics. The mortality rate in children in contemporary series is 8% to 10%. Surgery should be reserved for patients with signs of perforation, although the need for surgical intervention is low (B–E).

References: Schlatter M, Snyder K, Freyer D. Successful nonoperative management of typhlitis in pediatric oncology patients. *J Pediatr Surg.* 2002;37(8):1151–1155.

Sloas MM, Flynn PM, Kaste SC, Patrick CC. Typhlitis in children with cancer: a 30-year experience. *Clin Infect Dis.* 1993;17(3):484–490.

27. E. Patients who present with a protracted history consistent with acute appendicitis and a palpable mass are likely to have a perforated and walled-off abscess. They are best managed by nonoperative therapy (IV antibiotics, bowel rest). Several large studies have shown a low recurrence rate in patients that undergo nonoperative management, so the paradigm in acute care surgery has now shifted such that interval appendectomy is not performed in most patients with a perforated appendicitis (B). Taking such a patient to the operating room for an open or laparoscopic appendectomy is acceptable (C, D). However, the intense inflammation and scarring will make the operation difficult and significantly increase the chances of having to perform an ileocecectomy (E). Additionally, routine CT-guided drainage of abscesses is not recommended particularly when the abscess is small (A).

Reference: Kaminski A, Liu ILA, Applebaum H, Lee SL, Haigh PI. Routine interval appendectomy is not justified after initial nonoperative treatment of acute appendicitis. *Arch Surg.* 2005;140(9):897–901.

28. D. In determining management of this case, one must consider the indications for the colonoscopy, the timing of the perforation, and the intraoperative findings. Because the polyp is pedunculated and benign appearing, one can presume that it has been completely removed and that further colon resection is not needed. The vast majority of colonic injuries, whether iatrogenic or from penetrating trauma, can be repaired primarily. Furthermore, this patient has presumably undergone a bowel prep, so the bacterial load is decreased. Resection with colostomy (A–C) would be reserved for patients with longstanding perforation and diffuse fecal contamination. Conservative management (E) would be inappropriate for a patient with an iatrogenic and symptomatic colonic perforation. The approach used for polypectomy should be considered by the surgeon and may impact surgical approach. If electrocautery was required during the initial polypectomy, unrecognized thermal injury may lead to failure of primary repair.

29. E. The patient has a cecal fistula. The most common causes are slippage of the suture or necrosis of the remaining appendiceal stump. Colocutaneous fistulas, being low-output fistulas, are not associated with losses of large amounts of fluid, electrolytes, or nutrients. Therefore, total parenteral nutrition is not necessary to maintain adequate nutrition (A). Spontaneous closure is the rule in the majority of patients. Cross-sectional imaging should be performed to rule out an intraabdominal abscess or fluid, as intraabdominal sepsis should be addressed. Surgery is not an appropriate initial management option (C, D). Patients can be fed a low-residue diet because absorption is mostly complete by the time the contents reach the cecum. Octreotide does not help in assisting closure of a cecal fistula (B). If the fistula fails to close, one must suspect the possibility of either a neoplasm in the cecum, IBD, tuberculosis, or distal obstruction.

Reference: Hale DA, Molloy M, Pearl RH, Schutt DC, Jaques DP. Appendectomy: a contemporary appraisal. *Ann Surg.* 1997;225(3):252–261.

30. D. Current guidelines indicate that stage I (node negative, invades submucosa) colon cancer does not need chemotherapy. The role of chemotherapy in stage II (node negative, invades subserosa or direct invasion of adjacent organ) colon cancer remains debatable. The combination of 5-fluorouracil and leucovorin prolongs survival in stage III colon cancer (positive lymph nodes, no distant metastasis) but not stage IV (A). Until recently, there was no effective chemotherapy for stage IV cancers. Two recent drugs have been approved for stage IV colon cancer. They have been shown to prolong life but not cure this advanced-stage cancer and are very costly (C). Cetuximab (Erbitux) is a monoclonal antibody that targets epidermal growth factor receptor. Bevacizumab (Avastin) is a monoclonal antibody against vascular endothelial growth factor A (E). Radiation therapy is not commonly used in the management of colon cancer but is used commonly in combination with chemotherapy for patients with rectal cancer (B).

31. D. Most carcinoids are found at the tip of the appendix. As such, they are not usually the cause of appendicitis but rather are incidental findings. Over 95% of carcinoid tumors of the appendix are less than 2 cm in size (E). Tumors less than 1 cm rarely extend outside of the appendix and are treated simply by appendectomy. A right colectomy is indicated for tumors larger than 1 cm with extension into the mesoappendix or the base and for those that are larger than 2 cm and located at the tip (A). In contrast, adenocarcinoma of any size and at any location in the appendix is treated with a right colectomy. Appendiceal carcinoids rarely cause carcinoid syndrome because widespread liver metastases are rare and there is no relation to tumor size and the development of carcinoid syndrome (B). There is no role for radiation or chemotherapy for appendiceal carcinoid (C). In one large series, the overall 5-year survival rate for localized lesions was 94%, 84.6% for regional invasion, and 33.7% for distant metastases. In approximately 15% of patients, noncarcinoid tumors at other sites were also evident.

References: Jaffe BM, Berger DH. Appendix. In: Brunicardi FC, Andersen DK, Billiar TR, et al., eds. *Schwartz's principles of surgery.* 8th ed. New York: McGraw-Hill; 2005:1119–1138.

Sandor A, Modlin IM. A retrospective analysis of 1570 appendiceal carcinoids. *Am J Gastroenterol.* 1998;93(3):422–428.

Stinner B, Kisker O, Zielke A, Rothmund M. Surgical management for carcinoid tumors of small bowel, appendix, colon, and rectum. *World J Surg.* 1996;20(2):183–188.

32. D. Diversion colitis can occur after fecal diversion. When the fecal stream is diverted, colonocytes are not exposed to intraluminal nutrients and the deficiency of these compounds can lead to mucosal atrophy and subsequent inflammatory colitis. Short-chain fatty acids (SCFAs) (acetate, butyrate, and propionate) are produced by bacterial fermentation of dietary carbohydrates such as lactulose. SCFAs are an important source of energy for the colonic mucosa, and their use is considered the first-line treatment (as rectal enema) for diversion colitis. The energy is used by colonocytes for processes such as active transport of sodium. Ketone bodies, glucose, or amino acids (glutamine) are not used as an energy source of colonocytes (A–C, E).

Reference: Harig JM, Soergel KH, Komorowski RA, Wood CM. Treatment of diversion colitis with short-chain-fatty acid irrigation. *N Engl J Med.* 1989;320(1):23–28.

33. E. In a patient who tests positive for the APC gene, screening via sigmoidoscopy is recommended starting at age 10 to 12 years. Once polyps are detected, the recommendation is to remove the entire colon and rectum (A). Cyclooxygenase-2 inhibitors were shown to slow the growth of polyps in patients with FAP in a randomized study, but recent studies indicated that these drugs increased the risk of death from cardiovascular events (B). The best option is a restorative proctocolectomy with an ileal pouch–anal anastomosis. Total abdominal colectomy with ileorectal anastomosis is another option, but it requires careful lifelong surveillance of the rectal mucosa for polyps (C). Total proctocolectomy with continent ileostomy may be another option. If possible, avoiding an ostomy should be considered in a young patient (D).

34. B. Primary adenocarcinoma of the appendix presents most commonly as acute appendicitis. For this reason, it is always important to check the final pathology of the appendiceal specimen. Patients are at increased risk of synchronous neoplasms, particularly in the colon; thus, examination of the large intestine should be done with full colonoscopy. Definitive treatment consists of a right colectomy regardless of the size of the tumor. If the final pathology reveals appendiceal cancer, the patient should be taken back for a right colectomy. In one series, the 5-year survival rate after curative resection was 61% and 31%. The remaining answer choices are not typically a common presentation of appendiceal adenocarcinoma (A, C–E).

References: Fujiwara T, Hizuta A, Iwagaki H, et al. Appendiceal mucocele with concomitant colonic cancer. Report of two cases. *Dis Colon Rectum.* 1996;39(2):232–236.

Ito H, Osteen RT, Bleday R, Zinner MJ, Ashley SW, Whang EE. Appendiceal adenocarcinoma: long-term outcomes after surgical therapy. *Dis Colon Rectum.* 2004;47(4):474–480.

35. B. The most common perianal lesion in Crohn's disease is a skin tag, followed by fissures (A). Fissures are tears in the anoderm, and most are superficial and in the posterior midline (poorer blood supply). A deep fissure or one in an unusual location (lateral) should raise concern for Crohn's disease. Crohn's disease does increase the risk of developing hemorrhoids as well as perianal abscesses and fistulas (C–E). Most patients with anal manifestations will have Crohn's disease elsewhere. Perianal involvement is extremely rare with UC.

36. E. The presentation and findings are consistent with acute mesenteric adenitis (pseudoappendicitis). It is associated with *Y. enterocolitica*, *Helicobacter jejuni*, *Campylobacter jejuni*, and *Salmonella* or *Shigella* species, and streptococcal infections of the pharynx. It occurs more commonly in children and is often preceded by an upper respiratory infection (D). It is a diagnosis of exclusion. Physical examination typically reveals more vague and diffuse tenderness, without significant guarding, as opposed to the localized tenderness seen in appendicitis (B). Leukocytosis is usually present in patients with acute mesenteric adenitis with WBC counts between 10 and 15 × 103 cells/μL, similar to those found in patients with appendicitis (C). CT may show generalized lymphadenopathy in the small bowel mesentery, but these findings are nonspecific. The diagnosis is often made intraoperatively. There is no need for nodal biopsy (A).

Reference: Abdel-Haq NM, Asmar BI, Abuhammour WM, Brown WJ. Yersinia enterocolitica infection in children. *Pediatr Infect Dis J.* 2000;19(10):954–958.

37. B. Pseudomyxoma peritonei is a confusing term because it has been applied to several different pathologies. It has been used in reference to any progressive process in which the peritoneal cavity becomes filled with a thick gelatinous substance. This gelatinous substance is thought to arise from mucus-secreting cells from a perforated, mucus-producing tumor, which can be either benign or malignant and can originate from the appendix, small bowel, or ovary. Even if these cells are benign, once it has spread throughout the peritoneum, the substance is difficult to eradicate, and with time, the patient's small bowel becomes mechanically obstructed. If the source is a malignant tumor, the 5-year survival rate is significantly reduced. The most common source of this condition is a benign mucinous cystadenoma of the appendix. The new terminology has been coined disseminated peritoneal adenomucinosis to define patients with mucinous peritoneal implants that arise from a benign adenoma of the appendix. This is the most common variety. A more aggressive form has

been called peritoneal mucinous carcinomatosis and features extensive proliferative epithelium, cytologic atypia, and a high mitotic rate. Treatment consists of aggressive removal of all peritoneal implants as well as an appendectomy. Intraperitoneal chemotherapy likewise shows promising results. The 5-year survival rate is approximately 50% but varies greatly by histology. Tuberculous peritonitis often presents as slowly progressive abdominal distention due to ascites, combined with fever, weight loss, and abdominal pain (C). Characteristic features at surgery are multiple whitish nodules scattered over the visceral and parietal peritoneum. Salmonella enteritidis typically presents with diarrhea, nausea, and vomiting with stool leukocytes (D). It can rarely lead to intestinal perforation, most commonly through an ulcerated Peyer patch. Yersinia infections can lead to mesenteric adenitis, colitis, and ileitis that can present in a similar fashion to acute appendicitis (E). Yersinia infections can also cause appendicitis. Meigs syndrome is seen in patients with a benign ovarian tumor (A) and presents with ascites and pleural effusion that resolve after resection of the tumor.

Reference: Wirtzfeld DA, Rodriguez-Bigas M, Weber T, Petrelli NJ. Disseminated peritoneal adenomucinosis: a critical review. *Ann Surg Oncol.* 1999;6(8):797–801.

38. B. Previously, it was recommended that all patients should undergo surgery after the second episode of uncomplicated diverticulitis. However, several large studies have refuted this, and it is now recommended that surgical intervention be offered on a case-by-basis basis, taking into account the number of episodes, age, comorbidities, severity of attacks, and impact on quality of life. In particular, a lower threshold for surgery is recommended for diabetic and immunocompromised (taking steroids) patients. In contrast, it is recommended that all cases of complicated diverticulitis be offered definitive surgical intervention after the acute condition has resolved. One of the principles of surgery for diverticulitis is that one only needs to resect inflamed, thickened colon, despite the presence of diffuse diverticula (A, C, E). Once the distal colon is removed, the intraluminal pressure will decrease and the majority of the proximal diverticula will resolve. Recurrence is primarily the result of an inadequate distal resection, which inadvertently may leave behind sigmoid diverticula. Because diverticula do not occur in the rectum, the distal resection margin should be taken at normal-appearing rectum (D). The rectum can be identified by the fact that the taenia splays out.

References: Bullard KM, Rothenberger DA. Colon, rectum, and anus. In: Brunicardi FC, Andersen DK, Billiar TR, et al., eds. *Schwartz's principles of surgery.* 8th ed. New York: McGraw-Hill; 2005:1055–1118.

Chapman J, Davies M, Wolff B, et al. Complicated diverticulitis: is it time to rethink the rules? *Ann Surg.* 2005;242(4):576–581.

Lipman JM, Reynolds HL. Laparoscopic management of diverticular disease. *Clin Colon Rectal Surg.* 2009;22(3):173–180.

Stocchi L. Current indications and role of surgery in the management of sigmoid diverticulitis. *World J Gastroenterol.* 2010;16(7):804–817.

39. B. An Amyand hernia is one containing the Appendix. The importance of an Amyand hernia is that it can be confused with a standard strangulated hernia. Management should consist of appendectomy without the use of mesh. It is named after Claudius Amyand, who performed the first appendectomy in London in 1746. The patient was an 11-year-old boy with a scrotal hernia that contained the appendix perforated by a pin. Petit hernia is a type of lumbar hernia located in the inferior lumbar triangle (A). It is bound by the iliac crest inferiorly, the external oblique muscle anteriorly, and the latissimus dorsi muscle posteriorly. Littre hernia is a hernia containing Meckel diverticulum (C). Spigelian hernia is a hernia through the linea semilunaris and between two layers of abdominal wall, making these difficult if not impossible to palpate (D). Grynfeltt hernia is another type of lumbar hernia found in the superior lumbar triangle, which is bound by the quadratus lumborum muscle on its floor, the internal oblique muscle anteriorly, and the 12th rib superiorly (E).

Reference: Logan MT, Nottingham JM. Amyand's hernia: a case report of an incarcerated and perforated appendix within an inguinal hernia and review of the literature. *Am Surg.* 2001;67(7):628–629.

40. C. Although only a minority of patients (10%) who present with terminal ileitis progress to Crohn's disease on long-term follow-up, the surgeon should always consider this diagnosis. The indications for resection would include free perforation, fistula, or stricture. The diagnosis can be confused with appendicitis. Provided the cecum is not inflamed, the appendix should be removed to avoid confusion in the future because recurrent abdominal pain may develop in the patient. However, in the presence of active inflammation of the cecum, appendectomy should not be performed because there is a higher risk of an enterocutaneous fistula formation (B). Similarly, biopsy should be avoided because this increases the risk for enterocutaneous fistula formation as well (D, E). Therefore, closure of the wound without further intervention is the correct management for this patient. This patient should subsequently receive a colonoscopy with random biopsies to look for evidence of inflammatory bowel disease.

41. B. Pylephlebitis is essentially an infectious inflammation of the portal venous system. These veins drain the gastrointestinal tract. It typically begins within the small veins draining an area of infection within the abdomen and is most often associated with diverticulitis and appendicitis. Extension of the thrombophlebitis into larger veins can lead to septic thrombophlebitis of the portal vein or its tributaries (superior mesenteric vein, splenic vein) as well as multiple small liver abscesses. Due to laminar flow patterns, the bacteria are more likely to lodge and form abscesses in the right lobe of the liver. Similarly, amebic liver abscesses also form in the right lobe but are usually singular (A). Patients with pylephlebitis are usually not jaundiced but have elevated liver enzymes (particularly alkaline phosphatase). Pylephlebitis was much more common in the preantibiotic era, but it has become very rare due to major advances in antibiotic and surgical treatment. Air bubbles or thrombi of the portal venous system are key findings of pylephlebitis on CT scan (D). The reported mortality rate is as high as 30% to 50%. Because of the rarity, established management protocols are lacking. The most prudent approach seems to be rapid administration of broad-spectrum antibiotics, removal of the infectious source (in this case by appendectomy), and anticoagulation (for the suspected thrombosed superior mesenteric vein). Neither carcinoid syndrome (C) nor IBD (E) are likely to present with elevated alkaline phosphatase and total bilirubin, and neither fits the clinical history of the patient.

References: Chang YS, Min SY, Joo SH, Lee SH. Septic thrombophlebitis of the porto-mesenteric veins as a complication of acute appendicitis. *World J Gastroenterol.* 2008;14(28):4580–4582.

Vanamo K, Kiekara O. Pylephlebitis after appendicitis in a child. *J Pediatr Surg.* 2001;36(10):1574–1576.

42. C. The association of parasites with appendicitis is somewhat controversial. The debate is whether the parasite is an incidental finding or the actual cause. Ascariasis is the most common parasite worldwide, with an estimated 1.4 billion persons infected. The majority of infections occur in the low- and middle-income countries (LMIC) of Asia and Latin America but are becoming more common in the United States owing to increased international travel and emigration from LMIC. *E. vermicularis* (pinworm) is the second most common parasite (A). Intestinal parasites can cause appendicitis by obstructing the lumen. Thus, it is always important to check the final pathology; therapy with a helminthicide is necessary postoperatively. Mebendazole, pyrantel pamoate, and albendazole are the drugs of choice. *S. stercoralis* (threadworm) can lead to pneumonitis, malabsorption, and bleeding ulcers (B). *E. granulosus* can lead to hydatid cyst disease (D). *C. sinensis* (Chinese liver fluke) can increase the risk of pigmented (brown) gallstones and cholangiocarcinoma (E).

43. C. When deciding whether to perform an incidental appendectomy during another procedure, one must factor in the lifelong risk of appendicitis versus the risks of appendectomy and the additional costs. Because the lifelong risk of appendicitis is only 8.6% in men and 6.7% in women, incidental appendectomy is rarely recommended. In a large study of patients undergoing cholecystectomy with and without incidental appendectomy, low-risk patients undergoing appendectomy showed a significant increase in nonfatal complications (odds ratio of 1.53). Particular circumstances in which incidental appendectomy (during the course of another operation) would be recommended are for children about to undergo chemotherapy (due to risk of subsequent typhlitis), in the disabled (i.e., para/quadriplegic) who cannot react normally to abdominal pain, Crohn's disease patients (because they have a significant risk of subsequent abdominal pain) whose cecum is free of macroscopic disease (to minimize risk of postoperative cecal fistula), and individuals who are about to travel to remote places where there is no access to medical/surgical care. The patients in the remaining answer choices (A, B, D, E) would not benefit from an incidental appendectomy.

Reference: Wen SW, Hernandez R, Naylor CD. Pitfalls in nonrandomized outcomes studies: the case of incidental appendectomy with open cholecystectomy. *JAMA.* 1995;274(21):1687–1691.

Alimentary Tract—Anorectal

11

MICHAEL A. MEDEROS, FORMOSA CHEN, AND BEVERLEY A. PETRIE

ABSITE 99th Percentile High-Yields

I. Anorectal Abscess: Cryptoglandular Abscess Infection of Glands in Crypts at Dentate Line
   A. Types: perianal (subcutaneous), intersphincteric, ischiorectal, supralevator
   B. Treatment considerations:
      1. Every anorectal abscess requires drainage; antibiotics not typically required unless overlying cellulitis or systemic signs of infection
      2. Approximately 30% of patients will develop a fistula-in-ano after incision and drainage
      3. "Outward" drainage when an abscess enters, or passes through, skeletal muscle (i.e., levator ani, external sphincter); best for subcutaneous (perianal) or ischiorectal abscesses (together account for 90%); all others (intersphincteric, supralevator) should be drained internally through the rectum/anal canal (e.g., incision of internal sphincter along length of abscess for intersphincteric abscess)
      4. "Horseshoe" abscess (bilateral abscesses arising from the deep postanal space); treatment includes external drainage of bilateral ischiorectal fossae and open posterior drainage or internal drainage of posterior abscess

II. Fistula-in-Ano: Chronic Form of Perianal Abscess in Which the Abscess Cavity Does Not Heal Completely; Instead, It Becomes an Inflammatory Tract With a Primary Opening (Internal Opening) in the Anal Crypt at the Dentate Line and a Secondary Opening (External Opening) in the Perianal Skin
   A. Types: submucosal/superficial, intersphincteric (20%–45%), transsphincteric (30%–60%), suprasphincteric (<20%), extrasphincteric (2%–5%)
   B. Treatment considerations:
      1. Ensure abscesses are drained and sepsis controlled prior to definitive measures
      2. Utilize techniques that will have the lowest risk of recurrence and sphincter dysfunction; evaluate all patients for baseline fecal incontinence prior to definitive therapy
      3. Rule out Crohn disease prior to definitive surgical management of complex fistulas; fistulas in Crohn respond to Crohn medical management (e.g., infliximab) and may worsen with surgery
      4. Surgical techniques: initial management either fistulotomy or seton placement
         a) Seton: initial management for undrained abscess related to fistula, and to mature a fistulous tract prior to definitive surgical intervention
         b) Fistulotomy: ideal for low or superficial simple fistulas involving less than one-third of the internal sphincter complex, and known internal/external openings
         c) Fistulectomy: associated with larger defects, higher risk of incontinence, and without higher healing rates compared to fistulotomy; usually not used
         d) Cutting seton: may be used for fistulas involving more than one-third of the internal sphincter in an attempt to superficialize the tract for fistulotomy
         e) Ligation of intersphincteric fistula tract (LIFT) procedure: ideal for transsphincteric fistulas with matured tracts

      f) Endorectal advancement flap: good option for high and complex anal fistulas; goal is to cover the internal opening with flap of mucosa, submucosa, and rectal wall

      g) Fibrin glue and plugs: relatively ineffective treatment; lowest risk of incontinence but associated with high rates of persistent or recurrent disease

III. Pilonidal Disease
   A. Acquired foreign body reaction to ruptured hair follicles in the intergluteal cleft; pilonidal disease does not involve the anal canal, differentiating it from fistula-in-ano
   B. Pilonidal disease without concurrent abscess can be treated with weight loss, shaving of intergluteal area, avoiding prolonged sitting, phenol application, and improving hygiene
   C. Acute pilonidal abscess requires incision and drainage (off midline)
   D. Definitive therapy should be performed after the inflammatory period has resolved; digital rectal exam should be performed to evaluate for retrorectal fullness
      1. Principles of definitive surgical management:
         a) Determine extent of pilonidal disease by identifying all "pits" and sinus tracts; a fistula probe and methylene blue are useful adjuncts
         b) Chronic sinus tracts may be unroofed and marsupialized with healing by secondary intention
         c) Extensive and complex pilonidal disease requires excision down to the sacrococcygeal fascia closure techniques include various advancement and rotational flaps; rhomboid flap reconstruction is associated with the lowest recurrence rate

IV. Anal Intraepithelial Neoplasia (AIN) and Squamous Cell Cancer (SCC)
   A. Human papillomavirus (HPV) high-risk strains: 16 and 18 (HPV 6 and 11 associated with condyloma acuminata)
   B. Low-grade squamous intraepithelial lesion (LSIL) = AIN-1
      1. Low-grade dysplasia, has the potential to progress to HSIL
      2. Surveillance in immunocompetent individuals; low risk for progression to HSIL
   C. High-grade squamous intraepithelial lesion (HSIL) = AIN-2 and AIN-3
      1. Premalignant lesion requiring intervention; 10% to 20% of lesions progress to SCC
      2. Managed with ablative or topical therapies (e.g., electrocautery, imiquimod, trichloracetic acid, 5-FU)
   D. Anal canal SCC (cannot be completely visualized with distraction of gluteal cheeks) management:
      1. Chemoradiation with modified Nigro protocol: 5-FU, mitomycin C, pelvic radiation (50–54 Gy) for all except T1N0 (2020 NCCN guidelines), which requires WLE
      2. Follow-up: physical exam (digital rectal exam, anoscopy, inguinal LN palpation) starting 8 to 12 weeks after cXRT
         a) If no evidence of disease on exam: follow with exams every 3 to 6 months for 5 years
         b) If persistent disease on exam: reexamine in 4 weeks, then every 3 months; if still persistent ≥6 months after cXRT, then biopsy, restage, and abdominoperineal resection (APR) (if not metastatic)
         c) If progressive disease on exam: biopsy, restage, and APR (if not metastatic)
      3. Metastatic: definitive chemo +/− radiation; immunotherapy (e.g., PDL1 inhibitors)
   E. Perianal SCC (previously anal margin): completely visualized on distraction of the gluteal cheeks and within 5 cm of the anal verge
      1. If Tis-T1, N0, well to moderately differentiated: may be amenable to wide local excision with 1-cm margins if negative margins can be achieved without affecting sphincter function
      2. Treat like anal canal SCC if tumor does not meet the above criteria

V. Rectal Prolapse
   A. Complete rectal prolapse (procidentia) is characterized by concentric mucosal folds/rings versus radial folds seen with incomplete (mucosal or hemorrhoidal) prolapse
   B. Requires colonoscopy to rule out other conditions prior to elective surgery to address prolapse
   C. Acute management of rectal prolapse is reduction; if can't reduce, use sugar to decrease edema and reattempt
   D. Surgery for definitive management
      1. Transabdominal approach for patients who are good surgical candidates (<10% recurrence)

a) Rectopexy (with or without mesh), add sigmoidectomy if redundant sigmoid colon or history of constipation

b) Perineal approach for patients with significant comorbid conditions or limited lifespan (up to 30% recurrence at 2 years)

    (1) Altemeier procedure: perineal rectosigmoidectomy (also indicated for incarcerated and/or strangulated complete prolapse)

    (2) Delorme procedure: mucosal stripping and muscle plication

VI. Rectal Adenocarcinoma

  A. Preop evaluation: surgeon exam, pelvic MRI or endorectal ultrasound, CT chest/abdomen/pelvis

    1. Pelvic MRI is the preferred imaging modality over endorectal ultrasound to determine depth of invasion and nodal involvement

  B. Neoadjuvant chemoradiation indications: tumors T3 or greater (stage 2), N+ (stage 3), and/or if decreasing tumor size may spare sphincter and avoid APR

  C. Adjuvant chemotherapy indications: stage 2 tumors with high-risk features (obstructive lesion, T4, poorly differentiated) and stage 3 rectal cancer (N+)

  D. Total mesorectal excision: excision of the rectum and all the pararectal lymph nodes within the mesorectum

    1. Lowers risk of local recurrence and should be performed in all low- and mid-rectal cancers

  E. Transanal local resection

    1. The major downside is that total mesorectal excision (removes local lymph nodes and decreases local recurrence) is not done with local excision; thus there is a higher local recurrence rate (7%–21% compared with 5%–10% for a transabdominal approach)

    2. Can be considered in patients at lowest risk for lymph node metastases; all of the following must be true to qualify: T1 tumor within 8 cm from the anal verge, ≤3 cm, mobile and nonfixed, <30% bowel circumference, no perineural or lymphovascular invasion, well-to-moderately differentiated, able to resect with >3 mm negative margins, no nodal involvement on imaging

    3. Intact <u>full-thickness</u> specimen with goal of 1.0 cm margins (although >3 mm margins are accepted)

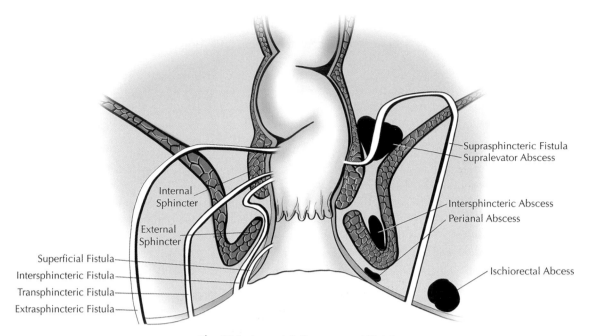

Fig. 11.1 Anorectal Abscesses and Fistulas.

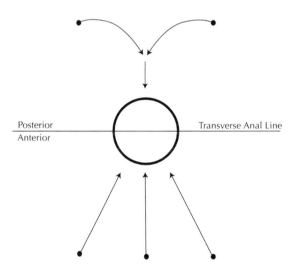

Goodsall rule relates the external opening of an anal fistula to the internal opening. If the external opening is posterior to the transverse anal line, then the fistula tract will follow a curved trajectory to its internal opening. If located anterior to the transverse anal line, a fisula will have a radial trajectory.

Fig. 11.2 Goodsall Rule.

Questions

1. A 32-year-old male presents with anal pain. He reports some staining of blood on tissue paper after bowel movements. On physical exam, his abdomen is soft and benign. He has no perirectal masses and is found to have a lateral perianal fissure. What is the most likely cause?
   A. Passage of a hard stool
   B. Receptive anal intercourse
   C. Crohn disease
   D. Ulcerative colitis
   E. Perirectal abscess

2. A 61-year-old male is referred by his primary care physician for persistent anemia. He reports a 20-pound unintentional weight loss and previous episodes of hematochezia. He undergoes colonoscopy in which a 5-cm fungating mass is found 10 cm from the anal verge. He is scheduled for surgery. Which of the following is the most important surgical factor for reducing the risk of local recurrence?
   A. Twelve or more lymph nodes harvested
   B. Total mesorectal excision
   C. Five-centimeter radial margin
   D. One-centimeter negative distal margin
   E. Proximal ligation of the inferior mesenteric vessels

3. A 45-year-old male is found to have a 2-cm lesion in the anal canal that is biopsied and found to be squamous cell carcinoma. There is no evidence of distant disease or adenopathy. What is the next best step in management?
   A. Abdominoperineal resection
   B. Wide local excision
   C. Chemotherapy and radiation
   D. Topical imiquimod
   E. Observation

4. A 30-year-old female with fistula-in-ano who was treated at an outside hospital 3 months ago now presents to you for further management. On exam, there is a seton with the external opening of the fistula lateral to the anus. On digital rectal exam, the internal opening is above the levator complex. What is the best treatment option?
   A. Endorectal mucosal advancement flap
   B. Fibrin glue
   C. Cutting seton
   D. Ligation of intersphincteric fistula tract
   E. Fistulotomy

5. A 68-year-old male presents to the emergency room with abdominal distension, obstipation, and weight loss. On CT scan, the patient is found to have colonic dilation, decompressed small bowel, and an obstructing mass in the rectum. On digital rectal exam, the mass is palpated at about 4 cm from the anal verge. What is the next best step in management?
   A. Rectal stent placement
   B. Loop colostomy creation
   C. Neoadjuvant chemoradiation
   D. Abdominoperineal resection
   E. Loop ileostomy creation

6. A 55-year-old male with cirrhosis complicated by esophageal varices presents with bright red blood per rectum. Nasogastric lavage reveals bilious fluid. Hematocrit is 25, and patient is given 2 units of blood. Colonoscopy demonstrates blood in the rectal vault and blue-tinted submucosal elevations in the distal rectum and anal canal. He is hemodynamically stable. What is the best treatment option next step?
   A. Medical management
   B. Transjugular intrahepatic portosystemic shunt (TIPS)
   C. Hemorrhoidectomy
   D. Injection sclerotherapy
   E. Balloon tamponade

7. Which of the following is true regarding hidradenitis suppurativa?
   A. It may mimic a complex anal fistula
   B. There is no role for topical clindamycin in perineal hidradenitis suppurativa
   C. Radical excision with skin grafting is typically necessary
   D. It may progress beyond the anal verge into the anal canal
   E. It is not associated with keloid formation

8. Twelve hours after hemorrhoidal banding, a 45-year-old man presents to the emergency department reporting rectal and abdominal pain and an inability to urinate. His temperature is 102°F and heart rate is 110 beats per minute. Management consists of:
   A. Placement of a Foley catheter
   B. Broad-spectrum IV antibiotics
   C. Broad-spectrum antibiotics and rectal examination with the patient under anesthesia
   D. Stool softeners and oral antibiotics
   E. In-and-out catheterization of bladder and stool softeners

9. A 50-year-old woman presents with rectal pain, incomplete rectal voiding, and bright red blood and mucus per rectum. Colonoscopy reveals a solitary rectal ulcer in the distal rectum on the anterior wall. A biopsy specimen of the ulcer shows chronic inflammation. Management consists of:
   A. Transanal excision of the ulcer
   B. Perineal rectosigmoidectomy
   C. Abdominal rectopexy
   D. High-fiber diet and defecation training
   E. Rectal fixation with prosthetic sling

10. The most common cause of a rectovaginal fistula is:
    A. Carcinoma of the rectum
    B. Crohn disease
    C. Obstetric injury
    D. Ulcerative colitis
    E. Radiation

11. Approximately 3 hours after a hemorrhoidectomy, a patient continues to have bleeding from the anus. The nurse has changed the pad multiple times and has attempted to pack the rectum with gauze. What is the next best step in management?
    A. Rubber banding the bleeding site
    B. Rectal packing with epinephrine gauze
    C. Suture ligation
    D. Ice packs
    E. Foley catheter balloon compression

12. A 60-year-old woman presents with severe perianal itching that is constant throughout the day. Examination reveals minimal erythema and excoriations in the perianal region. Which of the following is the best initial treatment?
    A. Exam under anesthesia
    B. Biopsy and/or culture
    C. Oral antibiotics
    D. Application of nonscented barrier cream
    E. Intravenous steroids

13. A 65-year-old woman presents to the emergency department with severe perianal pain for 12 hours that came on after straining during a bowel movement. Physical examination reveals an exquisitely tender perianal mass with bluish discoloration under the perianal skin. Management consists of:
    A. Stool softeners and sitz baths
    B. Rubber band ligation
    C. Stab incision and drainage with the patient under local anesthesia in the emergency department
    D. Elliptical excision of skin and drainage with the patient under local anesthesia in the emergency department
    E. Rectal examination with the patient under general anesthesia with incision and drainage

14. Which of the following is true regarding anogenital warts?
    A. Human papillomavirus (HPV) types 6 and 11 predispose to malignancy
    B. No association exists with squamous intraepithelial lesions
    C. Treatment depends on location and extent of disease
    D. Immunomodulator therapy is ineffective when used topically
    E. Vaccine against HPV does not prevent anogenital warts

15. Which of the following is true regarding chronic anal fissures?
    A. Topical diltiazem is first-line treatment
    B. Topical nitroglycerin and botulinum toxin injection have similar results as first-line therapies
    C. Topical nitrates are superior to topical diltiazem
    D. Anterior fissures are more common in men
    E. Lateral internal sphincterotomy is the-gold standard treatment

16. Hirschsprung disease presenting in an adult:
    A. Does not occur
    B. Is not associated with the RET mutation
    C. Is best diagnosed by a barium enema
    D. Requires a pull-through procedure for definitive management
    E. Can be treated with anorectal myomectomy

17. A 56-year-old male patient is found to have rectal adenocarcinoma just proximal to the dentate line. Which of the following is true about wide local excision (WLE) of such a lesion?
    A. WLE is an option provided the tumor is 4 cm or less
    B. Inguinal lymph node metastases do not occur with rectal cancers above the dentate line
    C. The presence of lymphatic invasion precludes WLE
    D. WLE is reasonable provided the invasion remains within the serosa
    E. WLE is not a recommended option

18. The recommended initial treatment of anal canal melanoma is:
    A. Abdominoperineal resection (APR)
    B. Wide local excision (WLE)
    C. WLE with regional lymph node dissection
    D. Radiation therapy
    E. Radiation therapy and chemotherapy

19. A 30-year-old male presents with redness, pain, and fluctuance in the intergluteal cleft, about 4 cm posterior to the anus. There is considerable hair adjacent to the lesion. Which of the following is the most appropriate management?
    A. Incision and drainage in the intergluteal cleft
    B. Incision and drainage lateral to the intergluteal cleft
    C. En bloc excision of the sinus tract with flap reconstruction
    D. Excision with primary closure
    E. Unroofing the tract and marsupializing

20. A 35-year-old man with leukemia and severe neutropenia presents with severe anal pain. Physical examination at the bedside demonstrates induration but no obvious fluctuance in the perianal region. Which of the following is the best management?
    A. Intravenous (IV) antibiotics only
    B. Bedside anoscopy and, if fluctuant mass detected, then bedside incision and drainage
    C. Bedside anoscopy and, if fluctuant mass detected, then operative incision and drainage
    D. Examination under anesthesia with wide debridement of perianal area
    E. Examination under anesthesia with biopsy of indurated areas and incision and drainage, even if no pus is detected

21. Which of the following is true regarding the blood supply to the rectum?
    A. The superior and middle rectal arteries arise from the inferior mesenteric artery
    B. The middle rectal veins drain into the internal iliac veins
    C. The inferior rectal veins drain into the inferior mesenteric vein
    D. The superior rectal veins drain into the inferior vena cava
    E. There is excellent collateralization between the superior and middle rectal arteries

22. An 80-year-old woman with multiple significant medical comorbidities presents with rectal prolapse. She has a history of chronic constipation. Colonoscopy findings are negative. Treatment would be best achieved via:
    A. Fixation of the rectum with prosthetic sling (Ripstein repair)
    B. Anterior resection with rectopexy
    C. Thiersch anal encirclement
    D. Resection of perineal hernia and closure of the cul-de-sac (Moschcowitz procedure)
    E. Perineal rectosigmoidectomy (Altemeier procedure)

23. Which of the following statements are true regarding perianal disease in association with Crohn disease?
    A. Anal fistulas tend to have a single tract
    B. Magnetic resonance imaging (MRI) is not particularly helpful
    C. The liberal use of multiple setons is helpful
    D. Infliximab is ineffective in healing these fistulas
    E. Aggressive use of fistulotomy provides the best chance of cure

24. A 23-year-old male who recently engaged in unprotected anoreceptive sexual intercourse presents with severe rectal pain with mucopurulent discharge. Which of the following etiologies is most likely?
    A. *Chlamydia trachomatis*
    B. *Neisseria gonorrhoeae*
    C. *Treponema pallidum*
    D. *Haemophilus ducreyi*
    E. *Shigella* species

25. Which of the following is true regarding fistula-in-ano?

A. Drainage of an anorectal abscess rarely results in a persistent fistula-in-ano

B. The internal opening is generally easily identifiable

C. Fistulas are categorized based on their relationship to the anal mucosa

D. Surgical treatment is determined by the internal and external opening of the fistula

E. Injecting hydrogen peroxide or methylene blue into the external opening is contraindicated

Answers

1. C. Typical anal fissures are predominantly located in the posterior midline (90%) and, less commonly, the anterior midline. The two leading theories for developing an anal fissure are relative ischemia of the posterior midline and high mechanical stress at the posterior location. Constipation, passage of large formed or hard stools, instrumentation, and receptive anal intercourse may cause tears in the anoderm in the posterior and anterior locations (A,B). Atypical fissures can form anywhere in the anal canal and are related to underlying conditions such as Crohn disease, tuberculosis, HIV, leukemia, and anal neoplasms. Ulcerative colitis generally does not affect the anus (D). Perirectal abscesses may be related to underlying fistula-in-ano but are not generally associated with anal fissures (E).

Reference: Lu KC, Herzig DO. Anal fissure. In: Steele SR, Hull TL, Saclarides TJ, Senagore AJ, Whitlow CB, eds. *The ASCRS textbook of colon and rectal surgery*. 3rd ed. Springer International Publishing; 2016:205–214.

2. B. Total mesorectal excision (TME) allows for a complete resection of the rectal tumor and draining of lymph nodes, achieving tumor-free circumferential and distal margins. In patients treated with TME, local recurrence rates were lower compared to those who underwent conventional surgery (9% versus 16%, respectively). Lymph node dissection is an important tenet of cancer surgery. A standard TME removes the pararectal nodes. Further, 12 nodes may not be harvested in resection for a mid- or low-rectal cancer, especially in patients who received neoadjuvant radiation (A). A lateral lymph node dissection of the common, external, and internal iliac nodes as well as the obturator nodes may have a small decrease in local recurrence when compared with standard TME in patients who did not receive neoadjuvant radiation, but the number of nodes harvested is not pertinent. A distal resection margin of 1 cm is recommended for low rectal cancers. The negative distal and radial margins can be achieved with a TME (C, D). Routine high (proximal) ligation of the inferior mesenteric vessels does seem to affect outcomes in the absence of obvious proximal inferior mesenteric nodal involvement (E).

Reference: Katz MHG. Proctectomy. In: American College of Surgeons, Katz MHG, eds. *Operative standards for cancer surgery: volume II: esophagus, melanoma, rectum, stomach, thyroid*. 1st ed. Lippincott Williams and Wilkins; 2018:134–145.

3. C. Anal squamous cell carcinoma (SCC) is categorized by its location: anal canal or perianal (previously anal margin).

Anal canal SCC includes lesions that are incompletely visualized with spreading of the gluteal cheeks, while perianal SCC includes lesions that are completely visualized with spreading of the gluteal cheeks to a radius of 5 cm from the anus. First-line treatment for locoregional anal canal SCC is chemoradiation with 50 to 54 Gy of radiation with 5-FU and mitomycin. Abdominoperineal resection is reserved for patients who have persistent or recurrent disease 6 months or greater after chemoradiation (A). Perianal SCC may be amenable to wide local excision for Tis-T1 lesions (select T2 lesions) if there is no significant involvement of the sphincter complex and 1 cm margins can be obtained (B). Lesions that do not meet those criteria, have evidence of nodal disease, or are poorly differentiated are treated like anal canal SCC with chemoradiation. Observation is an appropriate option for patients with a low-grade squamous intraepithelial lesion (AIN 1) since these lesions often regress and are less likely to progress to SCC. Conversely, high-grade squamous intraepithelial lesions (AIN 2/3) are considered premalignant and may be treated with ablative therapy or topical agents, such as imiquimod (D). SCC by definition is invasive cancer and should not be observed (E).

References: Samdani T, Nash GM. Anal cancer. In: Steele SR, Hull TL, Saclarides TJ, Senagore AJ, Whitlow CB, eds. *The ASCRS textbook of colon and rectal surgery*. 3rd ed. Springer International Publishing; 2016:357–371.

Ajani JA, Winter KA, Gunderson LL, et al. Fluorouracil, mitomycin, and radiotherapy vs fluorouracil, cisplatin, and radiotherapy for carcinoma of the anal canal: a randomized controlled trial. *JAMA*. 2008;299(16):1914–1921.

James RD, Glynne-Jones R, Meadows HM. Mitomycin or cisplatin chemoradiation with or without maintenance chemotherapy for treatment of squamous-cell carcinoma of the anus (ACT II): a randomised, phase 3, open-label, 2×2 factorial trial. *Lancet Oncol*. 2013;14(6).

4. A. Several treatments for fistula-in-ano have been described. Determining the type of fistula is important when deciding which treatment is best suited for the patient. "Low" fistulas include those that involve less than one-third of the internal sphincter complex. These fistulas are often amenable to fistulotomy with low risk of causing sphincter dysfunction (E). Fistulas that involve more than one-third of the internal sphincter complex are considered "high." Cutting setons are those that are periodically tightened, facilitating superficialization of the fistula tract for eventual fistulotomy/fistulectomy. However, this treatment is associated with a significant risk of anal incontinence for extrasphincteric fistulas (C). Fibrin glue acts as a sealant and has the lowest risk of anal incontinence of the options listed, but it is associated with a very low success rate and is not recommended (B). Endorectal mucosal advancement flaps are an option for complex fistulas (high transsphincteric, suprasphincteric, and extrasphincteric fistulas) with a success rate between 60% and 93%. The ligation of intersphincteric fistula tract (LIFT) procedure is another option for high transsphincteric fistulas, with a success rate of about 70%. However, this is not an option for an extrasphincteric fistula (D).

References: Santoro GA, Abbas MA. Complex anorectal fistulas. In: Steele SR, Hull TL, Saclarides TJ, Senagore AJ, Whitlow CB, eds. *The ASCRS textbook of colon and rectal surgery*. 3rd ed. Springer International Publishing; 2016:245–274.

Steele SR, Kumar R, Feingold D, Rafferty JL, Buie WD, The Standards Practice Task Force, the American Society of Colon and Rectal Surgeons. Practice parameters for the treatment of perianal abscess and fistula-in-ano. *Dis Colon Rectum*. 2011;54:1465–1474.

Williams JG, Farrands PA, Williams AB, et al. The treatment of anal fistula: ACPGBI position statement. *Colorectal Dis*. 2007;9 Suppl 4:18–50.

Jarrar A, Church J. Advancement flap repair: a good option for complex anorectal fistulas. *Dis Colon Rectum*. 2011;54:1537–1541.

5. B. Decompression is critical when addressing any obstructive lesions in any portion of the gastrointestinal tract. This patient with an obstructing rectal cancer will likely require neoadjuvant therapy; however, the obstruction must be addressed first (C). Rectal stents are for obstructive lesions in the mid to high rectum and serve as a bridge for surgery. However, stenting a low obstructing rectal cancer is associated with chronic pain, tenesmus, worse quality of life, and stent migration (A). In general, emergent resection of a locally advanced, obstructing rectal cancer without proper staging and omitting multimodality therapy should be avoided because this may potentially compromise oncologic outcomes (D). A proximal diverting ostomy is an ideal option for a low obstructing rectal cancer. A loop colostomy (e.g., transverse or sigmoid loop colostomy) will effectively relieve the obstruction (B). A loop ileostomy is a viable option if there is evidence of small bowel dilation, suggesting an incompetent ileocecal valve. However, a loop ileostomy would not relieve the obstruction in this case, where the ileocecal valve is competent, evidenced by the decompressed small bowel (E). A loop colostomy would provide effective venting whether there is small bowel dilation or not.

References: You YN, Hardiman KM, Bafford A, et al. The American Society of Colon and Rectal Surgeons clinical practice guidelines for the management of rectal cancer. *Dis Colon Rectum*. 2020;63(9):1191–1222.

Pisano M, Zorcolo L, Merli C, et al. 2017 WSES guidelines on colon and rectal cancer emergencies: obstruction and perforation. *World J Emerg Surg*. 2018;13(1):36.

6. D. The index of suspicion for rectal varices should be high in this patient with cirrhosis and portal hypertension. Rectal varices are the result of portosystemic shunting from the inferior mesenteric vein and superior rectal veins via the middle and inferior rectal veins due to underlying portal hypertension. Characteristics of rectal varices that help differentiate them from internal hemorrhoids are that they do not prolapse and they originate from the rectum. A submucosal varix often has a bluish-gray hue and may appear

serpentine. It is important to differentiate varices from hemorrhoids because certain interventions on a mistaken varix, like hemorrhoidectomy, could be catastrophic (C). Initial treatment for any acute gastrointestinal bleed includes prompt resuscitation and correction of coagulopathy. Nasogastric tube demonstrating nonbloody bilious fluid suggests that this patient does not have an upper GI bleed and so EGD would not be necessary (A). Patients with cirrhosis and stigmata of portal hypertension including rectal varices must first be medically optimized with sodium restriction and oral diuretics (furosemide, spironolactone). First-line endoscopic intervention includes injection sclerotherapy or endoscopic band ligation. However, large anorectal varices may not be amenable to banding. Pneumatic tamponade is a good measure to stop active bleeding and is used as a bridge to a definitive intervention (E). TIPS is a useful intervention to relieve the portal venous pressure and reduce variceal bleeding. However, it is associated with an increased risk of hepatic encephalopathy and should only be considered as a last resort (B). An alternative for persistent bleeding includes angioembolization. Surgery is rarely indicated.

Reference: Robertson M, Thompson AI, Hayes PC. The management of bleeding from anorectal varices. *Curr Hepatol Rep*. 2017;16(4):406–415.

7. A. Hidradenitis suppurativa is disease of the follicular epithelium, involving areas containing cutaneous apocrine sweat glands. It occurs in the armpits, groin, under the breasts, and between the buttocks. The typical appearance is of multiple open comedones with sinus tracts and small abscesses. Scarring can lead to keloid formation (E). It can mimic complex anal fistula disease but stops at the anal verge because there are no apocrine sweat glands in the anal canal (D). It can also mimic perianal Crohn disease. Initial treatment is with warm compresses and lifestyle changes such as weight loss, wearing loose-fitting clothes, cessation of smoking, and local hygiene. Topical antibiotics (e.g., clindamycin) and biologic therapy, such as adalimumab, have also been used with some success (B). If this fails, surgery may be needed to incise and drain acute abscesses and unroof fistulas with debridement of granulation tissue. Radical excision and skin grafting are almost never necessary (C).

Reference: Dunn KM, Rothenberger DA. Colon, rectum, and anus. In: Brunicardi F, Andersen DK, Billiar TR, Dunn DL, Hunter JG, Matthews JB, Pollock RE. eds. *Schwartz's principles of surgery*. 10th ed. McGraw Hill Education; 2015:1233.

8. C. Sepsis after the treatment of hemorrhoids has been described after banding, sclerotherapy, and stapled hemorrhoidectomy. Although very rare, it is life threatening. It is most common in immunocompromised patients. The patient usually presents within the first 12 hours after the procedure but can present in a delayed fashion. The most common symptoms are severe perineal pain, fevers, and urinary retention. Appropriate management of sepsis after hemorrhoidectomy includes hospital admission, fluid resuscitation, and IV antibiotics with coverage of gram-negative rods and anaerobes. Examination with the patient under anesthesia is recommended to rule out a necrotizing infection that may require debridement. Conservative management with medical management is not appropriate for a patient suspected of having sepsis (A,B,D,E).

References: Cirocco WC. Life threatening sepsis and mortality following stapled hemorrhoidopexy. *Surgery.* 2008;143(6):824–829.

McCloud JM, Jameson JS, Scott AND. Life-threatening sepsis following treatment for haemorrhoids: a systematic review. *Colorectal Dis.* 2006;8(9):748–755.

9. D. Solitary rectal ulcer syndrome is an uncommon disorder that can be confused with malignancy because the patient presents with rectal bleeding, pain, and evidence of straining during bowel movements. It is a benign process caused by an internal intussusception from chronic straining, leading to repetitive trauma to the mucosa. On proctoscopy, nodules or a mass may be found, in which case the term *colitis cystica profunda* is used. Biopsy should be performed to exclude malignancy. The diagnosis of an internal intussusception can be confirmed with anorectal manometry and defecography. Treatment is nonoperative and includes a high-fiber diet, defecation training to avoid straining, and laxatives or enemas. Either abdominal or perineal repair, as for a patient with rectal prolapse, is recommended for failure of medical management (B, C). Transanal excision of a rectal ulcer is considered in the management of rectal cancer after determining the extent of tumor invasion through the bowel wall and evaluating the adjacent lymph nodes (A). Rectal fixation with prosthetic sling can be considered in the case of rectal procidentia (E).

Reference: Felt-Bersma R, Cuesta M. Rectal prolapse, rectal intussusception, rectocele, and solitary rectal ulcer syndrome. *Gastroenterol Clin North Am.* 2001;30(1):199–222.

10. C. A rectovaginal fistula is most often due to an obstetric injury after a vaginal delivery in association with episiotomy, typically in primigravidas. Other causes include inflammatory bowel disease (Crohn disease more than ulcerative colitis) (B, D), carcinoma of the rectum (A), radiation therapy for pelvic malignancies (E), and, rarely, perianal abscesses and diverticulitis. It can also be iatrogenic during low anterior resections, particularly in women who have had a hysterectomy. Treatment for low fistulas is with an endorectal advancement flap, and for high fistulas (more likely due to neoplasm, Crohn disease, radiation), management is via a transabdominal approach with resection of the affected rectal segment.

11. C. Bleeding can occur immediately or, in the case of hemorrhoidal banding, after 7 to 10 days, when the necrotic stump sloughs off. Options for the management of bleeding include rectal packing with epinephrine gauze (B), ice packs (D), and balloon compression with a Foley catheter (E). The majority of bleeding is mild and resolves with simple measures. However, if bleeding is copious, the patient should be taken back to the operating/procedure room, where visualization is better, anesthesia is adequate, cautery can be used, and suture ligation can be performed.

References: Jongen J, Bock JU, Peleikis HG, Eberstein A, Pfister K. Complications and reoperations in stapled anopexy: learning by doing. *Int J Colorectal Dis.* 2006;21(2):166–171.

Ravo B, Amato A, Bianco V, et al. Complications after stapled hemorrhoidectomy: can they be prevented? *Tech Coloproctol.* 2002;6(2):83–88.

12. D. Pruritus ani is a common problem with a multitude of etiologies. The possible etiologies include perianal infection, surgically correctable causes (prolapsing hemorrhoids, fissure, neoplasm, fistula), antibiotic use, noninfectious dermatologic causes (seborrhea, psoriasis, contact dermatitis), and systemic diseases (jaundice, diabetes). However, the majority of pruritus ani is idiopathic and often related to local hygiene (both overzealous and inadequate hygiene). Treatment focuses on removal of irritant, maintaining good perianal hygiene, dietary adjustments, and avoiding scratching (A–C). Maintaining perianal hygiene is an important aspect of treatment. However, patients should be counseled that the perianal region should not be scrubbed vigorously and that use of scented products should be avoided as these can exacerbate the pruritus. Hypoallergenic and unscented moisturizing cream and barrier creams can be applied if dry skin is an issue (D). Biopsy and/or culture of the region may be necessary if the symptoms persist despite treatment (B). Hydrocortisone ointment can provide symptomatic relief but should not be used for prolonged periods due to risk of dermal atrophy that may lead to more pruritus (E).

Reference: Ansari P. Pruritus ani. *Clin Colon Rectal Surg.* 2016;29(1):38–42.

13. D. Hemorrhoids should be distinguished as being either internal or external. Internal ones arise above the dentate line and as such are insensate. They may cause painless bleeding during straining to defecate, may prolapse, or may even become strangulated. If they strangulate, they can cause pain due to intense spasm of the anal sphincter. External hemorrhoids originate below the dentate line, are covered with anoderm, and may cause discomfort such as itching, but generally only cause severe pain if they become thrombosed. Treatment of thrombosed external hemorrhoids, as in this case, consists of excision and drainage of the thrombosed hemorrhoid with the patient under local anesthesia. To prevent recurrence or inadequate drainage, it is important to excise an ellipse of skin and not simply perform a stab avulsion (C–E). Do not rubber band thrombosed external hemorrhoids because this is not well tolerated by patients secondary to severe pain (B). Nonoperative management is acceptable if the patient has had symptoms for more than 72 hours and the pain is already beginning to subside (A). Numerous studies have shown that local anesthesia is well tolerated.

Reference: Jongen J, Bach S, Stübinger SH, Bock JU. Excision of thrombosed external hemorrhoid under local anesthesia: a retrospective evaluation of 340 patients. *Dis Colon Rectum.* 2003;46(9):1226–1231.

14. C. Condyloma acuminata (anogenital warts) is caused by HPV. There are at least 66 types of HPV. Types 6 and 11 are found in benign anogenital warts, whereas types 16 and 18 behave more aggressively and are more frequently associated with dysplasia and malignant transformation (A). There is an association with squamous intraepithelial lesions and squamous cell carcinoma (B). Condylomas occur in the perianal region, the squamous epithelial of anal canal, and occasionally the mucosa of the distal rectum. The treatment depends on location and extent of disease. The options include caustic agents (podophyllin, trichloroacetic acid, nitric acid), cryotherapy, fulguration, surgical excisions, antineoplastic preparations (5-FU), laser therapy, interferon, immunomodulator therapy (imiquimod), cidofovir, and surgical excision (D). There are vaccines against HPV that potentially prevent anogenital warts (E).

Reference: Gordon PH. Condyloma acuminatum. In: Gordon PH, Nivatvongs S, eds. *Principles and practice of surgery for the colon, rectum, and anus.* 3rd ed. CRC Press; 2007:261–274.

15. E. Anal fissures are thought to develop as the result of the passage of hard stools, causing trauma to the anoderm distal to the dentate line and typically in the posterior location owing to its poorer blood supply. Anterior fissures are more common in women (D). Given their distal location, anal fissures cause exquisite pain with each defecation, often accompanied by blood on the toilet paper. In general, non-operative treatment starts by softening the stool with fiber, increased water intake, and sitz baths (i.e., topical agents are not always first-line treatment) (A). Numerous topical agents have been used with varying degrees of success, including 2% lidocaine jelly, nitroglycerin ointment (0.2%), topical diltiazem, and topical arginine (a nitric oxide donor). Topical nitrates do not have superior healing rates compared with diltiazem (C). In fact, nitrates are associated with side effects such as headaches in as many as 30% of patients, and thus topical diltiazem is used more frequently. Botulinum toxin injections have similar efficacy as nitroglycerin as first-line treatment (B). Surgery is generally reserved for those for whom medical management fails. Surgical management involves a lateral internal sphincterotomy. Though it can be performed on either side, the right side is more likely to avoid hemorrhoidal tissue. The internal sphincter should be divided and only the length of the fissure as this ensures the lowest rate of incontinence. Fissurectomy has inferior healing rates compared to lateral internal sphincterotomy based on two randomized trials.

Reference: Stewart DB Sr, Gaertner W, Glasgow S, Migaly J, Feingold D, Steele SR. Clinical practice guideline for the management of anal fissures. *Dis Colon Rectum.* 2017;60(1):7–14.

16. E. Hirschsprung disease rarely presents in adults (A). In this setting, the patient typically has a lifelong history of constipation and fecal impaction. A careful history will often reveal symptoms dating back to infancy. In most circumstances, Hirschsprung disease presenting in an adult consists of a short segment of aganglionosis. Although a barium enema can be diagnostic if an extremely dilated proximal colon, transitional zone, and contracted distal colon and rectum are seen, it may miss short-segment Hirschsprung disease if the rectal tube is introduced too far past the anal canal, bypassing the contracted segment (C). As such, the diagnosis is established by a rectal mucosal biopsy specimen demonstrating aganglionosis. As in children, Hirschsprung disease is associated with the *RET* mutation in a percentage of patients (B). Although pull-through procedures, such as the Soave or Duhamel operation, are performed in children and in those with long segments of aganglionosis, an anorectal myomectomy can be performed in adults with short-segment aganglionosis (D).

Reference: Wu J, Schoetz D, Coller J. Treatment of Hirschsprung's disease in the adult: report of five cases. *Dis Colon Rectum.* 1995;38(6):655–659.

17. C. The upper and middle rectum mostly drain into the inferior mesenteric nodes, whereas the lower rectum drains into both the inferior mesenteric nodes and internal iliac nodes. Rectal cancers just proximal to the dentate line can potentially spread to inguinal lymph nodes, so a careful inguinal examination for lymphadenopathy is an important part of the physical examination in these patients (B). WLE is an option in a limited number of cases for rectal adenocarcinoma (E). Indications for WLE in rectal adenocarcinoma include size <3 cm, T1 status (invades only submucosa) (D), less than 30% involvement of bowel wall, proximity within 8 cm of anal verge, mobile and nonfixed lesion, and well/moderately differentiated, no lymphovascular/perineural invasion or tumor budding on tissue biopsy, or nodal involvement on imaging. WLE needs a 1-cm radial and 2-mm deep margin. If WLE is contraindicated, abdominoperineal resection or low anterior resection is appropriate.

Reference: Whiteford MH. Local excision of rectal neoplasia. In: Steele SR, Hull TL, Saclarides TJ, Senagore AJ, Whitlow CB, eds. *The ASCRS textbook of colon and rectal surgery.* 3rd ed. Springer International Publishing; 2016:495–505.

18. B. Melanoma of the anal canal is extremely rare, and the overall prognosis is poor. Given its rarity, established management protocols are lacking. Radiation therapy and chemotherapy can be considered as adjuvant therapy depending on melanoma depth and staging (D, E). However, surgical resection is the initial treatment. A recent metaanalysis showed no stage-specific survival advantage of APR over WLE (A). As such, WLE is the recommended management. Lymph node dissection has not been shown to improve survival but may incur significant morbidities (C).

References: Droesch JT, Flum DR, Mann GN. Wide local excision or abdominoperineal resection as the initial treatment for anorectal melanoma? *Am J Surg.* 2005;189(4):446–449.

Singer M, Mutch MG. Anal melanoma. *Clin Colon Rectal Surg.* 2006;19(2):78–87.

19. B. Pilonidal disease is theorized to exist due to ruptured hair follicles in the intergluteal region. These ingrown hairs may become infected and present as an abscess in the sacrococcygeal region. However, this is one theory of the origin; the true etiology is still unknown. Pilonidal disease can either present acutely with an abscess or chronically (prior drainage). Acute disease is best treated with incision and drainage of the abscess lateral to the intergluteal cleft, as opposed to directly in the cleft because the latter creates constant friction in the wound and therefore heals poorly (A). The remaining answer choices are used for chronic disease (E). Although there is not a "gold standard" for chronic pilonidal cyst management, the preferred treatment option depends on whether the pilonidal cyst is simple or complex. Excision with primary closure off the midline for a simple, noninfected pilonidal cyst is the most appropriate treatment option (D). Complex pilonidal cysts may require an en bloc excision of the sinus tract with a flap reconstruction (C). A rhomboid flap is the favored approach.

Reference: Dunn KM, Rothenberger DA. Colon, rectum, and anus. In: Brunicardi F, Andersen DK, Billiar TR, Dunn DL, Hunter JG, Matthews JB, Pollock RE. eds. *Schwartz's principles of surgery.* 10th ed. McGraw Hill Education; 2015:1233.

20. A. Perianal pain may develop in neutropenic patients, yet the diagnosis of a perianal abscess may be difficult given the lack of inflammatory response to infection. In a severely neutropenic patient with no fluctuance, IV antibiotics alone is considered appropriate treatment. In patients who do not improve, or who subsequently develop fluctuance, an examination with the patient under anesthesia should be performed to rule out an abscess that requires drainage (B, C). Any areas of induration should be biopsied to exclude a leukemia infiltrate and cultured to aid in the selection of antimicrobial agents (E). Wide debridement of perianal area would not be indicated for a perianal abscess (D).

21. B. The superior rectal arteries arise from the inferior mesenteric artery, which provides blood to the upper rectum. The middle rectal artery arises from the internal iliac artery and the inferior rectal artery arises from the pudendal artery (branch of the internal iliac artery), which provide blood to the rest of the rectum and the anal canal (A). Rich collaterals exist between the rectal arteries such that they are relatively resistant to ischemia. Sudak's point marks the superior rectal and middle rectal junction. It is considered a watershed area and thus is unique in that it has a poor blood supply (E). The middle rectal arteries are the least consistent and are absent in as many as three-fourths of patients. The venous drainage follows the arterial supply (C). The superior rectal veins drain into the inferior mesenteric vein and then to the portal vein (D), whereas the middle and inferior rectal veins drain into branches of the internal iliac veins and into the inferior vena cava.

22. E. Procidentia (rectal prolapse) is much more common in women than men. It is most common in elderly women. In young men, it is more often associated with psychiatric disease. It involves all layers of the rectum and starts 6 to 7 cm from the anal verge. As a general rule, adults with rectal prolapse require surgery, whereas children can often be managed nonoperatively. Procedures are divided into abdominal and perineal procedures. In general, abdominal procedures are associated with a lower recurrence rate but a higher complication rate than perineal procedures. As such, abdominal procedures are used for younger, lower-risk patients, and perineal procedures are used for older, higher-risk patients (A, B). Recent studies have shown favorable results with the perineal rectosigmoidectomy in elderly high-risk patients. The perineal rectosigmoidectomy has a 15% recurrence rate and is a good option for older patients. Another well-accepted perineal operation is the Delorme procedure, which involves reefing the rectal mucosa. The Thiersch anal encirclement is no longer used (C). Moschcowitz procedure is more often performed for the management of vaginal prolapse (D).

Reference: Williams JG, Rothenberger DA, Madoff RD, Goldberg SM. Treatment of rectal prolapse in the elderly by perineal rectosigmoidectomy. *Dis Colon Rectum.* 1992;35(9):830–834.

23. C. Anal fistulas in association with Crohn disease tend to be complex and have multiple fistulous tracts (A). MRI is particularly helpful to detect the extent of the fistula tract and identify abscesses and to visualize the anal sphincter and pelvic floor muscle (B). These patients should also undergo sigmoidoscopy, colonoscopy, and small bowel follow-through

to determine the extent of disease. Antibiotics (metronidazole, ciprofloxacin) are used in treatment of fistulas to control symptoms and sepsis, but fistulas tend to recur when the antibiotics are discontinued. Immunomodulators (cyclosporine, tacrolimus, mercaptopurine, azathioprine, and infliximab) have been used as well with varying degrees of success. Of these, infliximab seems to be the most effective (D). The liberal use of setons is recommended. Aggressive use of fistulotomy should be avoided for low intersphincteric, suprasphincteric, or extrasphincteric fistulae because it is associated with delayed healing and an increased risk of incontinence (E).

References: Davis BR, Kasten KR. Anorectal abscess and fistula. In: Steele SR, Hull TL, Saclarides TJ, Senagore AJ, Whitlow CB, eds. *The ASCRS textbook of colon and rectal surgery.* 3rd ed. Springer International Publishing; 2016:215–244.

Gold SL, Cohen-Mekelburg S, Schneider Y, Steinlauf A. Perianal fistulas in patients with Crohn's disease, part 1: current medical management. *Gastroenterol Hepatol (NY).* 2018;14(8):470–481.

24. B. Proctitis typically presents with pain, tenesmus, rectal bleeding, diarrhea, and mucous discharge. It can be due to a bacterial infection, viral infection, trauma, radiation, or inflammatory bowel disease. Bacterial proctitis is often due to sexually transmitted disease and is associated with anal intercourse. *N. gonorrhoeae* is the most common bacterial cause, followed by *Chlamydia*, which tends to produce fewer symptoms (A). *T. pallidum, H. ducreyi,* and *Shigella* species are uncommon causes of proctitis (C–E). Bacterial proctitis can also be due to nonsexually transmitted diseases, primarily in association with inflammatory bowel disease. Treatment of bacterial proctitis is with antibiotics, whereas for proctitis in association with inflammatory bowel disease, the treatment includes steroids and 5-aminosalicylic acid enemas.

25. D. Drainage of an anorectal abscess provides a cure for the majority of patients, with 26% to 50% going on to develop a persistent fistula-in-ano (A). Most fistulas are cryptoglandular in origin. Other causes, though less common, include trauma, Crohn disease, malignancy, radiation, and infections (tuberculosis, actinomycosis, and chlamydia). The external opening of the fistula is usually obvious, whereas the internal one is often hard to identify (B). Fistulas are categorized based on their relationship to the anal sphincter complex (intersphincteric, transsphincteric, and suprasphincteric) (C). Surgical treatment is determined by the location of the internal and external openings and the course of the fistula tract (D) and may include simple fistulotomy, draining or cutting seton, fibrin glue injection, fibrin plug, ligation of intersphincteric fistula tract (LIFT) procedure, or anorectal advancement flap. Gently injecting hydrogen peroxide or methylene blue into the external opening may help identify the internal opening (E). The main goal of treatment is to treat and eliminate sepsis while at the same time maintaining continence.

Reference: Davis BR, Kasten KR. Anorectal abscess and fistula. In: Steele SR, Hull TL, Saclarides TJ, Senagore AJ, Whitlow CB, eds. *The ASCRS textbook of colon and rectal surgery.* 3rd ed. Springer International Publishing; 2016:215–244.

Breast 12

NAVEEN BALAN, JUNKO OZAO-CHOY,
AND CHRISTINE DAUPHINE

ABSITE 99th Percentile High-Yields

I. Breast Imaging
   A. Screening mammogram guidelines: q1-2 years with initiation at 45-50 years old
      1. 3D mammography or digital breast tomosynthesis for high-risk or dense breast patients
   B. Ultrasound (US) as part of diagnostic workup of breast symptom
      1. <30 years old: US can be used as solitary evaluation
      2. >30 years old: US and diagnostic mammogram must be used
   C. MRI
      1. *BRCA1/BRCA2* (and other hereditary breast syndromes): annual MRI from ages 25 to 29; those 30+ need annual MRI + mammogram (alternating q6 months)
      2. Gail risk with >20% lifetime cancer risk: annual MRI + mammogram (alternating q6 months)
      3. Useful in workup of axillary nodal metastasis with unknown breast primary

Category	Definition	Management	Example
BI-RADS 0	Need more information	Additional imaging	Abnormal screening mammogram
BI-RADS 1	Normal	Routine screening	Normal breast tissue
BI-RADS 2	Benign	Routine screening	Ovoid, smooth solid mass, stable findings
BI-RADS 3	Probably benign	Interval imaging (3–6 mo)	Benign-appearing clustered calcifications
BI-RADS 4	Suspicious	Biopsy	Indeterminate clustered calcifications
BI-RADS 5	Highly suggestive for cancer	Biopsy	Spiculated mass, branching calcifications
BI-RADS 6	Biopsy-proven cancer	Definitive Treatment	Mass with biopsy-proven malignancy

II. Benign Breast Disease
   A. Fibrocystic disease
      1. Pathologic diagnosis: microcysts, fibrosis, hyperplasia, apocrine metaplasia, and adenosis; commonly found on stereotactic breast biopsy of calcifications
   B. Mastitis/breast abscess
      1. Mastitis: oral antibiotics with gram-positive coverage; continue breastfeeding if lactating
      2. Abscess: smoking, nipple rings, nipple cleft are risk factors; aspiration is preferred, Incision and debridement (I&D) only if aspiration not possible/abscess is superficial, if multiple recurrences consider surgical excision
         a) IV antibiotics and hospitalization if severe; dicloxacillin for lactating patient
         b) Milk fistula (complication of I&D): fistula will resolve with cessation of breastfeeding
         c) Associated mass: biopsy to rule out malignancy; needed to confirm granulomatous mastitis (a chronic autoimmune inflammatory disorder); stain for AFB, fungi

C. Nipple discharge
  1. Physiologic: milky, green, gray, yellow, blue, bilateral, stimulation-induced
     a) Check TSH, prolactin if spontaneous bilateral milky discharge (if elevated, then MRI for prolactinoma)
  2. Pathologic: serous/bloody, unilateral, spontaneous; most common cause of unilateral bloody nipple discharge is intraductal papilloma (malignancy rate is 7%)
D. Mastalgia
  1. Clinical breast exam; diagnostic imaging only needed for focal breast pain; generalized mastalgia not associated with malignancy
  2. Reassure patient, use supportive bras, can also use danazol and tamoxifen if persistent
E. Abnormal imaging with discordant benign pathology
  1. Pathologic finding discordant from BIRADS 5 imaging, then surgical excision required

III. Breast Cancer
  A. Lumpectomy: for nonrecurrent ductal carcinoma in situ (DCIS) or invasive cancer (followed by radiation in most) with small/isolated lesions amenable to breast conservation and without pathogenic mutation for hereditary breast cancer
  B. Mastectomy: for DCIS or invasive cancer with locally advanced/multiple lesions, recurrence/pathogenic mutation for hereditary cancer, or contraindication to radiation (prior radiation treatment, connective tissue disorder, homozygous ATM gene mutation)
  C. Sentinel lymph node biopsy: perform with mastectomy/lumpectomy
     1. Blue dye: contraindicated in pregnancy; Lymphazurin—rare anaphylaxis; methylene blue—can cause tissue/skin necrosis
     2. Sulfur colloid (technetium Tc 99m): radiotracer used in lymphoscintigraphy
     3. Resect all radio "hot" (>10% of hottest node), blue, and/or palpable LNs; no minimum required
     4. False-negative rate decreases with more lymph nodes harvested postneoadjuvant chemo
     5. Higher nodal identification with both dye and radiotracer injection in subareolar space
  D. Axillary lymph node dissection:
     1. Indicated if any SLNs positive postneoadjuvant, >2 positive SLNs in lumpectomy, any positive nodes in mastectomy, inflammatory breast cancer, if unable to find nodes on SLNB for invasive cancer
     2. Increased risk of lymphedema, chronic pain, thoracodorsal (latissimus dorsi—unable to adduct arm), and long thoracic nerve injury (serratus anterior—winged scapula)
  E. Neoadjuvant chemotherapy: given for locally advanced breast cancer in order to attempt breast conservation therapy (lumpectomy), inflammatory breast cancer, node-positive disease, and strongly considered in triple-negative or *HER2+* cancer
  F. Early breast cancer (T1-T2, N0, M0): lumpectomy + SLNB + radiation versus mastectomy + SLNB; +/− chemotherapy/endocrine therapy based on receptor status/gene signature profile
  G. Locally advanced breast cancer (T3-T4, N1/N2): neoadjuvant chemotherapy, then surgery followed by radiation therapy; endocrine therapy based on receptor status (gene signature not indicated); additional adjuvant chemotherapy if *HER2+* and/or residual disease

IV. Special Considerations

Lesion	History	Imaging/histology	Management
Simple cyst	Painful, enlarges with menses	Oval or round, well-circumscribed, anechoic on US	Aspiration if symptomatic; if bloody, send for cytology
Complex cyst	Painful, palpable mass	Thickened wall, septations, solid features, intracystic mass, bloody	Core needle biopsy of the solid components or wall
Fat necrosis	Prior trauma	Lucent centered calcifications	Core needle biopsy usually not needed unless diagnosis is uncertain
Fibroadenoma	Mobile, enlarging mass, usually young patients	Well circumscribed, smooth, develops central popcorn calcifications as mass involutes with age	Surgical excision if growing or symptomatic; no routine excision <2 cm
Phyllodes tumor	Rapidly growing mass	Leaf-like projections with epithelial and stromal components (benign and malignancy types)	Wide local excision with 1 cm margins; if malignant, no axillary evaluation needed because nodal spread is rare
Intraductal papilloma	Unilateral bloody nipple discharge	Branching fibrovascular core, overlying epithelial and myoepithelium; most common cause of unilateral bloody discharge	Surgical excision to rule out concomitant malignancy (peripheral papillomas have higher risk of malignancy)
Paget disease	Eczematoid changes to nipple	Large cells with pale cytoplasm and prominent nucleoli	Full-thickness skin biopsy of involved nipple then central lumpectomy vs mastectomy, if invasive cancer or DCIS is also found, then treat as such
Radial scar (complex sclerosing lesion)	Detected abnormality on screening	Spiculated with central lucency, fibroelastic core with surrounding radiating ducts/lobules	Excisional biopsy to rule out malignancy
Atypical ductal/lobular hyperplasia/LCIS		Atypical hyperproliferation of ductal or lobular epithelium	Excisional biopsy, no margins needed; consider 5 y of antiestrogen therapy after excision to lower risk of subsequent cancer
DCIS		Branching, pleomorphic, or widespread calcifications on mammogram, subtypes (comedo, cribriform, papillary, pseudopapillary)	- Mastectomy vs lumpectomy - SNLB if: mastectomy, lumpectomy in UOQ, or central lumpectomy with removal of nipple - 2-mm margins needed during excision
Invasive cancer	Abnormal screening; Palpable mass	Spiculated mass, pleomorphic or widespread calcifications, invasion of cancer cells	- Mastectomy vs lumpectomy with radiation - SLNB vs ALND - No ink on tumor for margin

A. Inflammatory breast cancer (can be misdiagnosed as mastitis)
1. Clinical: erythema, peau d'orange changes, usually breast inflammation that has failed medical management and has rapidly progressed over the course of weeks
2. Negative skin biopsy does not rule out the diagnosis; still need to perform core needle biopsy of underlying mass or lymph node; pan-CT required to evaluate for distant metastases (20%–35% of patients)
3. Pathology: skin biopsy shows dermal lymphovascular tumor emboli and obstruction of dermal lymphatics (cause of edema and peau d'orange)
4. Treatment: neoadjuvant chemotherapy, modified radical mastectomy without immediate reconstruction, adjuvant radiation (no role for SLNB even if clinical response).
B. Male breast cancer
1. Consider genetic testing for all men with breast cancer, otherwise treat as with women; no need for prophylactic bilateral mastectomy in males with BRCA (different than women)
2. Tamoxifen is superior to anastrozole for hormone therapy

C. Breast cancer during pregnancy
   1. First trimester: if no abortion, mastectomy + SLNB versus ALND, chemotherapy safe in 2nd trimester or later, but radiation/endocrine/trastuzumab therapy must be postpartum
   2. Second to early 3rd trimester neoadjuvant chemotherapy (if indicated), then mastectomy versus lumpectomy + SLNB versus ALND + radiation/endocrine/trastuzumab postpartum
D. Invasive breast cancer in patients >70 years of age
   1. For luminal A (strongly ER/PR-positive, *HER2*-negative) cancers, may omit radiation postlumpectomy if negative margins and negative SLNB; may omit SLNB if poor operative candidate
E. ACOSOG Z0011
   1. SLNB for T1/T2, clinically node-negative cancer in patients who proceed directly to breast conservation therapy (lumpectomy) without prior chemotherapy
      a) If more than two nodes return positive → need completion ALND
      b) must then get chemotherapy and radiation for equivalent survival

V. Medications
   A. Endocrine therapy
      1. Selective estrogen receptor modulator (SERM): block effect of estrogen on tissue
         a) Tamoxifen: increased venous thromboembolism risk, increased risk of endometrial adenocarcinoma, pre- or postmenopausal
         b) Raloxifene: prevent osteoporosis, lower rate of uterine cancer, postmenopausal
      2. Aromatase inhibitor (AI): blocks conversion of androgens to estrogens in peripheral tissues in postmenopausal women; decreases bone density (serial DEXA scans for osteoporosis)
      3. Anastrozole outperforms tamoxifen for postmenopausal patients, can cause myalgias; switch to letrozole or exemestane if not tolerated (other AIs)
   B. Chemotherapy
      1. Anthracyclines (doxorubicin [Adriamycin]): irreversible cardiotoxicity
      2. Taxols (paclitaxel): numbness, tingling, burning of hands/feet
   C. *HER2* receptor inhibitor (trastuzumab): reversible cardiotoxicity; cannot be used in pregnancy

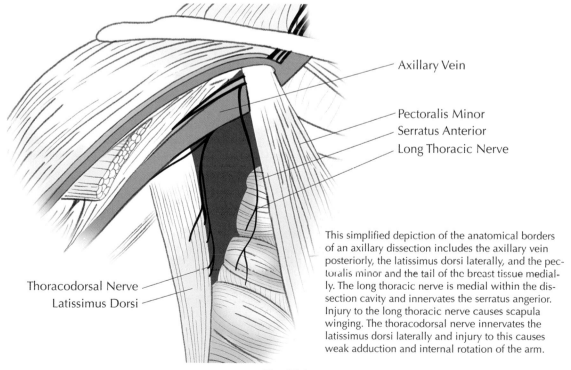

This simplified depiction of the anatomical borders of an axillary dissection includes the axillary vein posteriorly, the latissimus dorsi laterally, and the pectoralis minor and the tail of the breast tissue medially. The long thoracic nerve is medial within the dissection cavity and innervates the serratus anterior. Injury to the long thoracic nerve causes scapula winging. The thoracodorsal nerve innervates the latissimus dorsi laterally and injury to this causes weak adduction and internal rotation of the arm.

Axillary Vein

Pectoralis Minor
Serratus Anterior
Long Thoracic Nerve

Thoracodorsal Nerve
Latissimus Dorsi

Fig. 12.1

Questions

1. A 56-year-old woman with cT1N0 invasive ductal carcinoma (IDC) of the left breast (ER+/PR+/HER2-) undergoes lumpectomy with sentinel node biopsy. Pathology demonstrates a 1 mm caudal margin and confirms no lymph node involvement. A 21-gene assay recurrence score is 8 (low). Which of the following describes the next best management?
   A. Reexcision of the caudal margin, radiation therapy, endocrine therapy
   B. Radiation therapy and endocrine therapy
   C. Chemotherapy, radiation therapy, endocrine therapy
   D. Radiation therapy alone
   E. Endocrine therapy alone

2. A 50-year-old woman undergoes further mammographic workup of an abnormality detected on screening. Subsequent diagnostic mammographic views are coded BI-RADS 5, and a core needle biopsy is performed, showing usual ductal hyperplasia, apocrine metaplasia, and adenosis. Which of the following statements is TRUE regarding the next step in management?
   A. Excision of the mammographic abnormality should be performed
   B. Excision of the mammographic abnormality should be performed, followed by chemoprophylaxis with tamoxifen
   C. Excision is not necessary, but chemoprophylaxis with tamoxifen is recommended
   D. Neither excision nor chemoprophylaxis is recommended
   E. Breast MRI should be performed to determine need for further excision and/or chemoprophylaxis

3. Which of the following is true regarding Poland syndrome?
   A. It typically presents as a bilateral condition
   B. Women are more commonly affected than men
   C. It can be associated with excess hair in the chest/axillary region
   D. It is due to an x-linked autosomal recessive genetic disorder
   E. It typically presents with abnormal digits on the ipsilateral upper extremity

4. A 45-year-old woman with ER-negative, PR-negative, HER2-negative right invasive ductal breast cancer that is 3 cm in size and positive axillary lymph nodes also has fullness in the right supraclavicular area. Ultrasound-guided fine-needle aspiration of a supraclavicular node reveals metastatic breast cancer. Which of the following is describes the best management of this patient?
   A. Chemotherapy followed by modified radical mastectomy and chest wall radiation extended to supraclavicular fossa
   B. Chemotherapy, followed by modified radical mastectomy with excision of supraclavicular node and standard chest wall radiation
   C. Modified radical mastectomy with excision of supraclavicular node, followed by chemotherapy and standard chest wall radiation
   D. Modified radical mastectomy with excision of supraclavicular node, followed by chemotherapy and chest wall radiation extended to supraclavicular fossa
   E. Palliative chemotherapy only, no role for surgical resection

5. A 78-year-old woman with mild dementia, chronic obstructive pulmonary disease (COPD), diabetes, end-stage renal disease, and a prior lower extremity amputation for peripheral vascular disease has an episode of severe chest pain 1 day after undergoing core biopsy of a 1.5-cm left breast mass. EKG shows an acute MI. Angiogram demonstrates a critical stenosis of the left anterior descending artery, and a drug-eluting stent is placed. She is subsequently placed on antiplatelet therapy. Her biopsy results later reveal invasive ductal carcinoma that is low grade, 90% estrogen receptor (ER) and progesterone receptor (PR) positive, and HER2 negative. Her axilla is clinically negative. What is the BEST therapeutic approach to this patient?
   A. Plan lumpectomy and sentinel node biopsy for 12 weeks post stent placement
   B. Plan mastectomy and sentinel node biopsy for 12 weeks post stent placement
   C. Refer for neoadjuvant chemotherapy, with plan for subsequent lumpectomy and sentinel node
   D. Refer for palliative chemotherapy as she is not a surgical candidate
   E. Initiate neoadjuvant endocrine therapy, with plan for subsequent lumpectomy

6. A 50-year-old female presents to your clinic complaining of generalized, nonfocal cyclical breast pain in her left breast. Her clinical breast examination is normal, and she has a negative screening mammogram within the past 6 months. You advise her that:
   A. Breast pain is frequently associated with breast cancer
   B. Oral contraceptives are not associated with breast pain
   C. Pharmacologic agents are not recommended in the treatment of breast pain
   D. The fit of her bra is an important consideration as a cause of breast pain
   E. Breast pain is not very responsive to treatment

7. Which of the following is TRUE of sentinel lymph node (SLN) biopsy?
   A. Identification of SLNs by either the blue dye or radioactive colloid is successful in the vast majority of cases
   B. SLN biopsy should not be performed in women with breast cancer and confirmed-nodal disease who are undergoing neoadjuvant therapy
   C. There is no role in DCIS
   D. Utilization of the technetium radiocolloid is contraindicated in pregnancy
   E. The false-negative rate is extremely low

8. Which of the following is TRUE regarding radiotherapy for the treatment of breast cancer after breast conservation?
   A. Radiotherapy should be performed even if no lymph nodes are positive for cancer
   B. Radiotherapy is recommended as treatment for a positive margin after lumpectomy
   C. Whole breast radiotherapy is most effective when given concurrently with chemotherapy
   D. Radiotherapy is less efficacious with small tumors compared to larger ones
   E. Higher energy radiation exerts more damage to the skin

9. Which of the following is TRUE regarding chemotherapy for the treatment of breast cancer?
   A. Neoadjuvant chemotherapy has been shown to have better outcomes for ER-positive, HER2-negative breast cancer compared with adjuvant chemotherapy
   B. In patients with ER-negative, PR-negative, HER2-negative (triple-negative) breast cancer, complete response to neoadjuvant chemotherapy is achieved in the vast majority of patients
   C. 21 gene assay recurrence score may be used to guide chemotherapy treatment in node-negative early-stage ER+ breast cancer
   D. Chemotherapy is most effective in infiltrating ductal cancers that have low Ki67
   E. Chemotherapy is indicated if the breast cancer is proven to be invasive

10. Which of the following is TRUE regarding positive lymph nodes in breast cancer?
    A. Involvement of internal mammary lymph nodes is considered stage IV disease
    B. In the setting of breast conservation, completion axillary lymph node dissection should be performed if the sentinel lymph node biopsy is positive
    C. In a patient with a core biopsy-proven positive lymph node and no primary lesion detected, axillary lymph node dissection and serial 6-month mammograms are recommended
    D. In the setting of mastectomy with a positive sentinel lymph node, radiotherapy to the axilla can be considered instead of performing axillary lymph node dissection
    E. Following neoadjuvant chemotherapy for a 6-cm primary breast cancer with associated 3-cm nodes, if all lesions have disappeared on ultrasound imaging axillary dissection is no longer necessary

11. A 52-year-old woman with a body mass index (BMI) of 25 is recommended to undergo a mastectomy for a 9-cm segmental distribution of calcifications that were shown to be DCIS on core needle biopsy. The calcifications are about 1 cm from the nipple. Physical exam and ultrasound of the axilla are negative. The patient has a small breast contour and desires reconstruction of her breast. In addition to sentinel node biopsy, which of the following would be the BEST management?
    A. Nipple-sparing mastectomy with immediate tissue expander placement
    B. Nipple-sparing mastectomy with delayed reconstruction
    C. Skin-sparing mastectomy with immediate tissue expander placement
    D. Skin-sparing mastectomy with delayed reconstruction
    E. Total mastectomy with delayed reconstruction after adjuvant therapy

12. After a modified radical mastectomy, a 45-year-old woman reports new-onset weakness in the ipsilateral arm when pulling down on a cord to adjust the blinds in her home. On examination, she has difficulty when attempting to internally rotate and adduct her arm. What is the best explanation for her deficits?
    A. Transection of the intercostobrachial nerve
    B. Application of surgical clips across the long thoracic nerve
    C. Transection of the thoracodorsal nerve
    D. Cautery injury to the supraclavicular nerve
    E. Retractor injury to the medial pectoral nerve

13. A 35-year-old woman presents with burning pain and redness along the anterolateral right breast. On exam, a firm tender cord could be palpated just below the skin from the shoulder tracking down toward the lateral breast. Which of the following is TRUE regarding the initial management of this disease?
    A. Mammogram and ultrasound should be performed
    B. Systemic anticoagulation should be initiated
    C. Antibiotics covering gram-positive bacterial strains should be administered
    D. A short course of oral corticosteroid therapy should be prescribed
    E. An incisional biopsy of the skin should be performed

14. Which of the following statements is true regarding the lymphatic anatomy of the breast?
    A. Axillary lymph nodes are organized into three levels with respect to the pectoralis major muscle
    B. In a standard axillary dissection for breast cancer, only level I and II nodes are removed
    C. Approximately 30% of the lymphatic drainage from the breast goes to the contralateral lymph nodes
    D. Rotter nodes are technically level I nodes
    E. Batson plexus is a network of lymphatics that drain the subareolar portion of the breast

15. Which of the following is true regarding gynecomastia?
    A. It is considered a risk factor for male breast cancer
    B. Alcohol is not a risk factor
    C. It is uncommon after age 50
    D. It is due to accumulation of subareolar fat.
    E. It is associated with use of proton-pump-inhibitors (PPI)

16. Which of the following is least likely to contribute to the development of breast infection (mastitis/abscess)?
    A. Nipple ring insertion
    B. Granulomatous mastitis
    C. Smoking
    D. Hidradenitis
    E. Alcohol intake (>2 drinks/day)

17. A 44-year-old woman presents with a palpable tender mobile mass in the upper outer quadrant of her left breast. The overlying skin is normal and there is no adenopathy on exam. Ultrasound examination reveals a 2.5-cm cystic lesion. An ultrasound-guided cyst aspiration is performed. Which of the following is true?
    A. The fluid should be sent for cytologic examination only if it is blood tinged
    B. Straw-colored fluid should prompt a core needle biopsy
    C. The presence of septations is associated with a low recurrence rate of the cyst after aspiration
    D. Thickness of the cyst wall does not correlate with cancer risk
    E. Viscous gel-like fluid is a poor prognostic sign

18. Nipple discharge is most suspicious of breast cancer in which of the following women?
    A. A 35-year-old woman with bilateral brown discharge that is only visible with squeezing of the nipple
    B. A 45-year-old woman with unilateral serous discharge that is spontaneous
    C. A 30-year-old woman who is lactating and notices unilateral bloody nipple discharge that is spontaneous
    D. A 50-year-old woman with greenish-colored discharge bilaterally that is sometimes spontaneous
    E. A 40-year-old woman with bilateral milky discharge that occurs spontaneously onto her bra

19. Which of the following statements is TRUE regarding tamoxifen therapy?
    A. It has been shown to reduce the risk of developing breast cancer by 90% in patients that are considered high risk
    B. Its primary serious side effect is loss of bone mineral density
    C. In ER-positive invasive breast cancer, optimal duration of therapy for patients under 50 is 10 years
    D. It is more effective when administered concurrently with chemotherapy
    E. Treatment with tamoxifen is safe in the second and third trimesters of pregnancy

20. Which of the following is most characteristic of a malignant lesion as seen on ultrasound imaging?
    A. Taller-than-wide measurements
    B. Hypoechoic mass
    C. Anechoic mass
    D. Homogenous internal structure
    E. Bilateral edge shadowing

21. A 45-year-old premenopausal woman undergoes stereotactic core needle biopsy of calcifications seen on screening mammogram. The biopsy reveals atypical ductal hyperplasia (ADH). Which of the following is TRUE about the management of this patient?
    A. Tamoxifen should be prescribed
    B. The lesion should be completely excised with a negative margin
    C. No further excision is required if the calcifications were completely removed
    D. Prophylactic bilateral mastectomy should strongly be considered
    E. Sentinel lymph node biopsy should be performed along with excision of the lesion

22. A 50-year-old woman has undergone stereotactic needle biopsy of a 4 cm area of abnormal calcifications, showing high-grade ductal carcinoma in situ (DCIS). Which of the following choices is the most appropriate treatment for this patient?
    A. Lumpectomy alone
    B. Modified radical mastectomy
    C. Lumpectomy and sentinel lymph node biopsy
    D. Lumpectomy and sentinel lymph node biopsy, followed by whole breast radiotherapy
    E. Lumpectomy and sentinel lymph node biopsy with intraoperative radiotherapy

23. BRCA1 and BRCA2 are:
    A. Protooncogenes
    B. Cyclin-dependent kinase
    C. Tumor suppressor genes
    D. Mismatch repair genes
    E. Tyrosine kinases

24. Which of the following is TRUE of invasive lobular carcinoma of the breast?
    A. It is more commonly associated with pleomorphic lobular carcinoma in-situ (LCIS) as opposed to nonpleomorphic LCIS
    B. Lobular cancers are typically hormone receptor-negative
    C. Breast conservation therapy is contraindicated
    D. Invasive lobular cancers typically appear on mammogram and ultrasound as a discrete mass
    E. Lobular cancers comprise 40% of all invasive breast cancers

25. A 28-year-old lactating woman presents with a 2-day history of right breast pain and redness that is progressively worsening. On examination, a 4-cm area of skin adjacent to the nipple-areolar complex is erythematous and tender, with some focal edema and no detectable fluctuance. Focused ultrasound confirms the absence of a fluid collection. The appropriate initial management would consist of:
    A. Image-guided core needle biopsy
    B. Cessation of breast-feeding and/or pumping
    C. Incision and drainage
    D. Oral antibiotics
    E. Mammography

26. A 40-year-old woman presents with a 10-cm right breast mass. She notes that it has been rapidly growing, and the weight of the mass causes her right breast to rest lower than her left. Pathology from a core needle biopsy revealed a fibroepithelial lesion with notable leaflike projections of the stroma. Which of the following statements is true of this lesion?
    A. Stromal hypercellularity is the pathologic feature that typically distinguishes this lesion from fibroadenoma
    B. It commonly demonstrates an aggressive growth pattern similar to breast cancer, infiltrating surrounding tissues as it enlarges
    C. Sentinel lymph node biopsy has become standard in malignant cases
    D. The addition of radiotherapy is recommended in most patients to prevent recurrence after lumpectomy
    E. Surgical margins of at least 2 cm are recommended

27. A 55-year-old woman was found on routine mammography to have a new, 1.7 cm, stellate lesion with a translucent area in the central portion. Which of the following best describes appropriate management of this lesion?
    A. Observation only
    B. Repeat mammography in 6 months
    C. MRI of the breast
    D. Image-guided core needle biopsy followed by wire-localized excision
    E. Image-guided core needle biopsy, followed by wire-localized wide excision with a negative margin

28. Which of the following is TRUE regarding intraductal papilloma?
    A. The presence of bloody discharge is concerning for atypia or malignant regions within the papilloma
    B. Peripherally located papillomas (distant from the nipple) are associated with an increase in subsequent breast cancer risk
    C. The most common presenting symptom is a nontender, smooth, mobile nodule beneath the nipple-areolar complex
    D. When associated with bloody discharge, excision with a small margin is recommended
    E. Breast MRI is indicated prior to excision to rule out malignancy

29. A 50-year-old woman presents to her primary doctor with a palpable mass in the upper outer quadrant of her right breast. It has been present and unchanged for 3 months, and she has no personal or family history of breast or ovarian cancer. On examination, there is a 1.5-cm firm, nontender mass with no associated skin or nipple abnormalities and no lymphadenopathy. Mammography is performed and there is no evidence of mass, asymmetry, or calcification. It is reported as normal. What is the next appropriate step?
    A. Observation, with repeat physical exam in 3 months
    B. Order a repeat mammogram in 3 to 6 months
    C. Order MRI of the breast
    D. Order focused breast ultrasound
    E. Excision of the mass

30. MRI of the breast is best indicated in which of the following scenarios?
    A. 45-year-old woman with a 1-cm area of microcalcifications that is excised and pathology demonstrates atypical ductal hyperplasia
    B. 45-year-old, average-risk woman with focal breast pain and normal mammogram and ultrasound
    C. 45-year-old woman with infiltrating carcinoma found in an axillary node with a negative mammogram and ultrasound
    D. 45-year-old woman with microcalcifications that are excised and pathology demonstrates DCIS with comedo necrosis
    E. 45-year-old woman with a 1-cm area of microcalcifications that is excised and pathology demonstrates lobular carcinoma in situ

31. A 45-year-old woman presents with a 10 mm area of suspicious microcalcifications on mammogram. Stereotactic core needle biopsy reveals only LCIS. Wire localized excisional biopsy successfully removes all calcifications but there is classic LCIS at the margins. Which of the following is the most appropriate NEXT step in management?
    A. Bilateral prophylactic mastectomies, with or without reconstruction
    B. Reexcision to clear margins
    C. No further therapy
    D. Sentinel lymph node biopsy to stage the ipsilateral axilla
    E. Lifelong tamoxifen

32. A 48-year-old female is being evaluated for a new left breast mass that was found on mammogram. She reports having two alcoholic drinks per day, is an active smoker with a five-pack-per-year smoking history, and has a mother who was diagnosed with breast cancer at age 65. Her past medical history is significant for atypical ductal hyperplasia that was excised 6 years previously. Which of the following factors is associated with the highest risk of breast cancer in this patient?
    A. Age
    B. Mother with a history of breast cancer
    C. Daily alcohol intake
    D. Smoking
    E. History of atypical ductal hyperplasia

33. Which histologic type of DCIS is most likely to progress to invasive ductal cancer?
    A. Comedo
    B. Micropapillary
    C. Papillary
    D. Cribriform
    E. Solid

34. A 45-year-old woman undergoes breast-conservation therapy for DCIS. The final pathology shows no evidence of invasion and a 0.2 mm cranial margin. The NEXT appropriate step is:
    A. No further surgery; should initiate radiation therapy
    B. No further surgery; should initiate tamoxifen
    C. Reexcision of the close margin only
    D. Reexcision of the close margin and perform sentinel node biopsy
    E. Mastectomy

35. A woman with a history of glioblastoma, left lower limb osteosarcoma as a teenager and breast cancer at the age of 40 is likely to have which of the following:
    A. Cowden syndrome
    B. Li-Fraumeni syndrome
    C. Peutz-Jeghers syndrome
    D. Ataxia-telangiectasia
    E. *BRCA2* mutation

36. A 21-year-old woman with a strong family history of breast cancer has just learned she is a carrier of a *BRCA1* germline mutation. Which of the following is TRUE regarding this mutation?
    A. Breast cancers associated with *BRCA1* mutations are typically hormone receptor negative
    B. *BRCA1* mutations are considered "gain of function" mutations
    C. *BRCA* mutations account for nearly half of all breast cancers
    D. Her lifetime risk of developing breast cancer can be reduced by half if she takes tamoxifen
    E. Male relatives of the patient have a 100-fold risk of developing breast cancer if they are carriers of the mutation

37. A 56-year-old woman is diagnosed with a 1.5 cm breast cancer, which is estrogen and progesterone receptor negative with no overexpression of *HER2/neu*. Her axillary exam is normal. Aside from axillary evaluation by sentinel lymph node biopsy, what is the most appropriate recommendation for breast cancer therapy?
    A. Lumpectomy alone
    B. Lumpectomy plus hormonal therapy
    C. Lumpectomy plus radiotherapy
    D. Lumpectomy plus chemotherapy
    E. Lumpectomy plus radiotherapy and chemotherapy

38. Which of the following patients with a 1.5-cm invasive ductal breast cancer would be the most appropriate for breast-conserving therapy?
    A. 33-year-old woman who is 10 weeks pregnant at diagnosis
    B. 58-year-old woman who has a history of lumpectomy in the same breast for previous T1N0 breast cancer
    C. 55-year-old woman with ipsilateral palpable lymph nodes that appear abnormal on ultrasound
    D. 52-year-old woman with scleroderma
    E. 50-year-old woman with synchronous, multicentric ipsilateral invasive lobular cancer

39. Which of the following is the most important predictor of 10-year disease-specific survival for breast cancer?

A. Primary tumor size
B. Histologic grade
C. Total number of positive lymph nodes
D. Estrogen-receptor status
E. Age at time of diagnosis

40. A 55-year-old woman presents with 1 month of breast erythema and swelling. On physical examination and mammogram, there is no evidence of a breast mass. However, there is diffuse skin thickening and edema associated with a 3-cm lymph node in the axilla. A trial of broad-spectrum antibiotics has been ineffective. A core needle biopsy reveals infiltrating carcinoma that is 10% estrogen-receptor positive and *HER2/ neu* negative. Which of the following statements is TRUE regarding her management?

A. Tamoxifen should be initiated immediately
B. Modified radical mastectomy should be performed as soon as possible to increase chances of survival
C. Radiation therapy should be performed concurrently with chemotherapy to improve response rates
D. Chemotherapy alone should be initiated immediately
E. Antibiotics should be continued because of the infectious signs

41. Batson plexus provides a potential metastatic route of breast cancer to:

A. Supraclavicular nodes
B. Bone
C. Liver
D. Adrenal glands
E. Lung

42. A 65-year-old female underwent left modified radical mastectomy followed by chemotherapy and radiation therapy for a stage II breast cancer when she was 40 years old. She has had long-standing swelling of her ipsilateral arm and recently developed raised purple nodules along the anterior upper arm. Which of the following is TRUE regarding treatment of this lesion?

A. Treatment of this condition is largely conservative
B. Bevacizumab (angiogenesis inhibitor) plus paclitaxel has emerged as the treatment of choice
C. Concurrent Adriamycin-based chemotherapy and radiation are considered the optimal treatment strategy
D. Surgical resection is the optimal primary treatment modality
E. Laser and radiofrequency ablation treatments, followed by low-dose radiation therapy

43. A 58-year-old postmenopausal woman with a history of right breast cancer presents with a new 1.2-cm nodule within the scar of her lumpectomy incision. Her prior therapy included a negative sentinel node biopsy, radiotherapy, and chemotherapy, and she is currently taking tamoxifen. Core needle biopsy reveals recurrent infiltrating ductal carcinoma that is hormone receptor-positive and *HER2* negative. Which of the following is TRUE regarding her condition?

A. Sentinel node biopsy cannot be performed again
B. Lumpectomy (excision of skin with margin) is recommended if patient desires breast conservation
C. Tamoxifen should be continued for an additional 5 years
D. She should undergo bilateral mastectomy
E. Mastectomy is recommended

44. A 65-year-old woman presents with a longstanding history of a scaly eczematoid rash involving her right nipple and extending onto the areola. The rash has not resolved despite daily applications of steroid cream. Other than the skin changes on the nipple, the physical examination of the breast is unremarkable. A mammogram is negative. Which of the following is TRUE regarding this condition?

A. A new steroid cream should be administered
B. A punch biopsy of the skin is recommended
C. If nipple discharge is present, cytologic examination of the discharge is frequently diagnostic
D. This lesion is precancerous
E. Mastectomy is rarely required to treat this condition

45. Which of the following is TRUE of breast lymphoma?

    A. Primary breast lymphoma is predominantly a T-cell lymphoma

    B. Secondary breast lymphomas are much more common than primary breast lymphoma

    C. Primary breast lymphoma does not respond well to the chemotherapy that is standardly used for nonbreast lymphoma

    D. Breast lymphoma has a predilection for central nervous system recurrence

    E. Treatment of breast lymphoma tends to require mastectomy with node dissection in most cases

46. The primary serious adverse reaction to trastuzumab that requires monitoring is which of the following?

    A. Hepatic toxicity

    B. Renal toxicity

    C. Cardiac toxicity

    D. Pulmonary toxicity

    E. Bone marrow toxicity (aplastic anemia)

Answers

1. B. Genomic profiling has emerged as an important adjunct in determining which early breast cancer patients benefit from adjuvant chemotherapy. There are multiple assays available and are generally utilized in ER-positive, *HER2*-negative, node-negative invasive breast cancers to provide "low" versus "high" systemic recurrence risk scores. For high scores, chemotherapy has demonstrated a survival benefit over endocrine therapy alone; whereas for low scores, endocrine therapy alone has similar survival to endocrine plus chemotherapy. This patient has a low recurrence score, eliminating benefit from chemotherapy (C). Additionally, following breast conservation therapy with lumpectomy and SLNB, radiation is recommended to reduce local recurrence risk (E). While excision of DCIS is recommended to have a 2 mm margin, resection of invasive cancer only requires no ink on tumor (A). Adjuvant endocrine therapy reduces the risk of cancer recurrence for hormone receptor-positive cancers (D).

    Reference: NCCN National Comprehensive Cancer Network Clinical Practice Guidelines in Oncology; Breast Cancer – BINV-2 and BINV-6 pages of Version 2.2021. http://www.nccn.org

2. A. Radiologic-pathologic discordance is an important concept in determining further management of breast lesions after a percutaneous breast biopsy. Core needle biopsies inherently have a degree of sampling error when performed, and can underestimate the lesion since only a small part is sampled. If the pathologic result is not concordant (i.e., consistent) with the radiologic finding, then surgical excision is mandated to evaluate the entire tissue. Specifically, if mammographic findings are highly suspicious for malignancy and are coded as BI-RADS 5, but core biopsy results are benign, then excisional biopsy should be performed as this indicates a discordance between the imaging and pathology. (C, D) Ductal hyperplasia, apocrine metaplasia, and adenosis are elements of fibrocystic change, a benign breast disease that does not mandate chemoprophylaxis with tamoxifen (which is recommended for atypical lesions that increase

future breast cancer risk) (B, C). Breast MRI has no role in discordance of BI-RADS 5 imaging and benign core biopsy findings (E).

3. E. Poland syndrome is a sporadic congenital disorder that classically affects the unilateral breast (A), chest wall, and upper extremity. It is present in at least 1 in 100,000 individuals, occurs more commonly on the right than left (2:1 to 3:1), and affects men more often than women (3:1) (B). Underdevelopment or absence of the pectoralis, serratus, and latissimus dorsi muscles, symbrachydactyly (fused, missing, and/or shortened digits), shortened forearm, dextrocardia, rib abnormalities, absent axillary hair (C), athelia, diminished subcutaneous fat localized over the ipsilateral chest wall, and renal agenesis or hypoplasia (rare) have all been described as characteristics of Poland syndrome. The cause is thought to be due to interruption in the vascular supply to the affected chest wall and upper extremity in utero (not a genetic disorder) resulting in hypoplasia of the chest wall muscles (D).

4. A. Involved supraclavicular nodes denote an N3c nodal stage, which is a stage III breast cancer. Breast cancer would be stage IV if more distant nodes (contralateral, periaortic, hilar) are involved or cancer has metastasized to bone, brain, lung, visceral organ, etc., for which palliative chemotherapy would be indicated (E). Regarding treatment of supraclavicular nodes, chemotherapy and radiation to the supraclavicular fossa without surgical resection of the supraclavicular node is the recommended approach (B, C). Resection of the supraclavicular node may be recommended if not fully treated by chemotherapy and radiation but it would not be the planned definitive therapy (C, D).

5. E. In elderly patients and in patients with multiple comorbidities that, in and of themselves, limit a patient's survival, the standard treatment algorithms may be altered to reduce potential adverse effects of treatment that have lower margins of benefit in patients with limited life spans. Given her recent myocardial infarction, immediate surgical risk is extremely high (A, B). Therefore, a 3- to 6-month course of aromatase inhibitor therapy followed by reimaging to assess response is the best course of action. This patient has a luminal A type breast cancer (strongly ER/PR-positive, *HER2*-negative, and low grade) that would likely demonstrate a low genomic profile signature signaling no benefit for chemotherapy (C, D) Furthermore, cardiac toxicities related to chemotherapy (doxorubicin) would likely be higher risk for this patient with cardiac morbidities.

6. D. Breast pain is a common breast complaint among women and is a common reason for referral to specialty breast clinics although primary care physicians are able to work up and treat breast pain (E). Breast pain is typically not associated with breast cancer although focal breast noncyclic breast pain in patients without recent breast imaging may warrant at least a screening mammogram or focused breast ultrasound (A). Oral contraceptives, hormone therapy, psychiatric agents (serotonin and norepinephrine reuptake inhibitor, and antipsychotics) as well as cardiovascular agents (spironolactone, digoxin) are known to cause mastalgia in some patients (B). If breast pain is nonfocal and cyclical, conservative treatments such as smoking cessation, diet modification and decrease in caffeine intake, evaluating the fit of the patient's bra are important first considerations (D). For continued and severe breast pain, pharmacologic agents such as vitamin E, evening primrose oil, NSAIDs, tamoxifen, and danazol are other options for treatment (C). The majority of patients with breast pain will find relief in this treatment algorithm.

Reference: Cornell LF, Sandhu NP, Pruthi S, Mussallem DM. Current management and treatment options for breast pain. *Mayo Clin Proc.* 2020;95(3):574–580.

7. A. Sentinel lymph node biopsy is typically indicated as an axillary staging procedure for patients with clinically node-negative breast cancer. The success rate for identifying the sentinel nodes when using both a blue dye and radioactive colloid is 95% or higher (A), and the false-negative rate (inaccurately determining the axilla to be negative for metastatic cancer) is around 10% (E). The clinical recurrence rate in the axilla after negative sentinel lymph node biopsy is 0.3%. By definition, DCIS is noninvasive and therefore cannot be associated with positive nodes in the axilla. However, when DCIS is found on core biopsy, the remaining lesion may contain invasive cancer (i.e., upstage), so sentinel node biopsy is recommended in cases where the upstage rate is highest (high-grade DCIS, comedonecrosis, association with a mass lesion, >2 cm) or if breast lymphatics will be removed/disrupted at the primary surgery (mastectomy or lumpectomy in upper outer quadrant of the breast) precluding performance of sentinel node biopsy at a second procedure if invasive cancer is unexpectedly found (C). In women with invasive breast cancer and biopsy-proven nodal disease, SLNB is still considered after neoadjuvant therapy if the nodal bed is radiologically and clinically negative as a subset of patients will have downstaged nodal disease following neoadjuvant therapy (B). Radioactive technetium is low dose, and has been observed as safe for use in pregnancy (D). It is actually the blue dyes that require caution in pregnancy.

Reference: Boughey JC, Suman VJ, Mittendorf EA, et al. Sentinel lymph node surgery after neoadjuvant chemotherapy in patients with node-positive breast cancer: the ACOSOG Z1071 (Alliance) clinical trial. *JAMA.* 2013;310(14):1455–1461.

8. A. Radiotherapy works by directly damaging DNA within cells, not by inducing ischemia. It exerts most of its effect during the M phase of the cell cycle by inducing formation of free oxygen radicals. As such, radiation therapy is more efficacious with smaller tumors that have a higher oxygen potential (D). Higher energy radiation has a skin-preserving effect as the maximal ionizing potential is not reached until the radiation beam reaches deeper structures (E). Additionally, it has been shown to be most effective when used sequentially after chemotherapy instead of concurrently (C). Nearly all patients undergoing lumpectomy for invasive and noninvasive breast cancer are candidates for radiotherapy. NSABP B17 established that radiotherapy significantly reduces local recurrence when administered after lumpectomy (A). Postmastectomy radiotherapy is generally indicated for locally advanced disease (T4, 4-cm tumor size or greater, and 4 or more lymph nodes positive). In general, positive margins should be excised and radiotherapy not relied upon to clear margins (B). ACOSOG Z0011 trial demonstrated that patients with early invasive breast cancer (T1 and T2) undergoing breast-conserving therapy do not need completion axillary dissection if the sentinel lymph node biopsy is positive as there is no difference in mortality.

Reference: Giuliano AE, McCall LM, Beitsch PD, et al. ACOSOG Z0011: a randomized trial of axillary node dissection in women with clinical T1-2 N0 M0 breast cancer who have a positive sentinel node. *J Clin Oncol.* 2010;28(18_suppl):CRA506-CRA506. doi:10.1200/jco.2010.28.18_suppl.cra506.

9. C. Chemotherapy plays an important role in treating occult distant metastatic disease in invasive cancer. However, not all invasive cancers benefit from chemotherapy (E). Those that are low-grade, small, lymph-node negative, and have low S-phase fractions (<5%) or Ki67 (<20%) (markers of proliferation) have minimal to no benefit over endocrine therapy alone (D). Gene expression profile assays, such as the 21 gene assay, that test which genes are being expressed in cancer tissue have been able to categorize patients into groups that will likely benefit from chemotherapy versus those that will not (C). Chemotherapy timed preoperatively versus postoperatively has the same survival outcome for all cancer subtypes (A). However, newer research may be demonstrating benefits for triple-negative and *HER2*-positive cancers. In triple-negative breast cancer, a complete pathologic response (no more tumors seen at surgery) after neoadjuvant chemotherapy is approximately 40% (B).

10. D. In general terms, having grossly positive axillary lymph nodes is an indication for axillary dissection. However, the ACOSOG Z0011 trial established equivalent survival with axillary dissection and no axillary dissection in patients with early-stage breast cancer undergoing lumpectomy and radiation therapy who have three or fewer positive nodes (B). The AMAROS trial further established that women with early breast cancer and no clinically palpable nodes could undergo radiotherapy in place of axillary dissection if lymph nodes were determined to be positive (D).

However, for patients with locally advanced disease and palpable lymph nodes, axillary dissection remains an important component of treatment to prevent local recurrence (E). In a patient with an isolated positive node, magnetic resonance imaging (MRI) looking for a primary is indicated, if no primary is found, most would recommend mastectomy (C). Involvement of internal mammary lymph nodes represents advanced local disease (cN2b or cN3) not metastatic disease (A).

Reference: Giuliano AE, McCall LM, Beitsch PD, et al. ACOSOG Z0011: a randomized trial of axillary node dissection in women with clinical T1-2 N0 M0 breast cancer who have a positive sentinel node. *J Clin Oncol.* 2010;28(18_suppl):CRA506-CRA506. doi:10.1200/jco.2010.28.18_suppl.cra506.

11. C. Nipple-sparing mastectomy is contraindicated in patients with extensive intraductal cancer, associated nipple discharge, Paget disease, or cancer within a 2-cm distance of the nipple (A, B). Whereas total mastectomy would be an oncologically sound operation, this patient desires reconstruction and has no contraindications to immediate placement of expanders and sparing the skin (D, E).

12. C. Modified radical mastectomy includes, by definition, a resection of level I and II axillary nodes along with the entire breast parenchyma under skin flaps. Several important nerves reside in the axilla, injury to which can lead to significant motor and sensory deficits. Avoidance of intraoperative use of neuromuscular blockade during anesthesia and careful identification of the long thoracic and thoracodorsal nerves are key to avoiding inadvertent injury. The intercostobrachial nerve is the lateral cutaneous branch of the second intercostal nerve. Resection does not lead to any motor loss, but it can cause loss of sensation over the medial aspect of the upper arm (A). The long thoracic nerve courses along the lateral chest wall in the midaxillary line on the serratus anterior muscle to innervate it. The serratus anterior muscle abducts and laterally rotates the scapula and holds it against the chest wall. Injury to the long thoracic nerve results in a winged scapula (B). The thoracodorsal nerve courses lateral to the long thoracic nerve on the latissimus dorsi muscle, following the course of the subscapular artery. It innervates the latissimus dorsi muscle. The latissimus dorsi muscle adducts, extends, and medially rotates the upper arm. Injury to this nerve generally does not cause a major disability, but it can lead to difficulty in arm adduction and medial rotation. Furthermore, preservation of this nerve and vessels is important if a subsequent latissimus dorsi flap is being considered. The medial pectoral nerve runs lateral to or through the pectoral minor muscle, actually lateral to the lateral pectoral nerve, with both innervating the pectoralis minor and major muscles. Injury to the medial pectoral nerve may lead to atrophy of the clavicular portion of the pectoralis muscles, resulting in atrophy of the pectoralis muscle (E). The anterior branches of the supraclavicular nerve are sensory nerves that supply a limited area of skin over the upper aspect of the breast, and therefore injury would not result in a motor deficit (D).

13. A. Mondor disease is a thrombophlebitis involving one or more of the superficial anterior chest wall veins (lateral thoracic vein, thoracoepigastric vein, or the superficial epigastric vein). Similar to superficial thrombophlebitis that presents elsewhere, it usually causes an acute onset of pain and tenderness. It is a result of an inflammatory-thrombotic process and not an infectious or autoimmune disease (C, D). Risk factors include recent trauma or surgery to the local area, heavy lifting, tight clothing, and underlying malignancy. Mondor disease typically presents over the lateral aspect of the breast and eventually turns into a palpable cord or hard mass. The veins most commonly involved include the lateral thoracic vein, the thoracoepigastric vein, and, less frequently, the superficial epigastric vein. The disorder is benign, self-limited, and not itself malignant or a risk factor for breast cancer. Mammography and ultrasound are typically performed to exclude underlying malignancy. Otherwise, the diagnosis is largely clinical and biopsy is not necessary (E). Treatment consists of nonsteroidal antiinflammatory drugs and warm compresses. Antibiotics, systemic anticoagulation, and corticosteroids are not warranted (B).

Reference: Mayor M, Burón I, de Mora JC, et al. Mondor's disease. *Int J Dermatol.* 2000;39(12):922–925.

14. B. Axillary lymph nodes are classically organized into six anatomic groups based on their anatomic location (lateral, pectoral, scapular, central, subclavicular, and interpectoral). However, a more clinically useful classification is into levels based on their location relative to the pectoralis minor muscle, with level I being located lateral (most inferior) to the muscle border, level II being located behind the pectoralis minor, and level III nodes medial (A). Rotter nodes are interpectoral (between the pectoralis major and minor muscles) and are technically level II nodes (D). In a standard axillary dissection, level I and II nodes are removed. There are approximately 20 to 30 lymph nodes in the average axilla, and the lymphatic drainage is fairly predictable, following a hierarchical pattern to the first echelon of nodes, followed by secondary and then tertiary echelons. This pattern is the basis of the principle for sentinel lymph node biopsy. Most of the lymphatic drainage of the breast is to the axilla, with drainage to the contralateral breast being rare (C). For this reason, it is not standard to remove (or even check for) sentinel nodes in the ipsilateral supraclavicular and internal mammary or contralateral lymph node stations. The network of lymphatics that drains the subareolar region is called Sappey, and it is important because this is the principle behind subareolar injection of blue dye and radiocolloid for sentinel lymph node mapping. Batson plexus is instead a network of venous drainage that is thought to be a route for metastasis to the spine (E).

15. E. Gynecomastia is an asymptomatic condition resulting from the abnormal benign proliferation of glandular breast tissue concentrically behind the nipple areolar complex in men. It is not considered a risk factor for breast cancer (A). After examination, it is not uncommon to find that most patients, in fact, have pseudogynecomastia, which is an accumulation of subareolar fat without a proliferation in glandular tissue (D). There are three stages where gynecomastia is more common - infancy, puberty, and after age 50. The stimulation of breast growth is attributed to an imbalance of the effects of estrogen versus testosterone. Older patients are more vulnerable to this imbalance and thus up to 70% of patients older than 50 have senescent gynecomastia (C). Spironolactone increases the metabolism and clearance of testosterone; marijuana alters the hypothalamic-pituitary-gonadal axis; uremia related to ESRD causes prolonged half-life of luteinizing hormone (LH), which leads to decreased secretion of LH and decreased testosterone levels; and cimetidine increases plasma prolactin levels, all of which are well-described causes of gynecomastia. It is also associated with PPI. Alcohol is a risk factor for both gynecomastia and breast cancer (B). Mammography is excellent in differentiating true gynecomastia from malignant disease with a sensitivity and specificity exceeding 90%. However, the positive predictive value for cancer is low, as would be expected with such a low incidence of malignancy in this patient population. If the patient is bothered by the appearance of gynecomastia, antiestrogens such as tamoxifen are frequently used with success. Rarely, patients will require surgical removal.

References: Johnson RE, Murad MH. Gynecomastia: pathophysiology, evaluation, and management. *Mayo Clin Proc.* 2009;84(11):1010–1015.

16. E. Nonlactational breast infections predominantly occur when there is an obstruction or pseudo obstruction of the lactiferous duct. The most common organism remains *Staphylococcus aureus*. Trauma to the nipple, which includes the placement of nipple rings, causes scarring and obstruction (A). Granulomatous mastitis is an inflammatory lesion of the breast, which may be autoimmune in nature, but is often recurrent and associated with superinfections of the inflammatory mass (B). Smoking causes a change in the epithelium of the breast duct (keratinizing squamous metaplasia) that leads to keratin plugs that obstruct the ducts (C). Hidradenitis is a skin infection that is caused by obstruction of the apocrine sweat glands, which often occurs in the periareolar, axillary, and inframammary regions of the breast (D). Alcohol does not have a known direct association with breast abscess.

17. A. Breast cysts are overwhelmingly a benign entity, occurring most frequently in women between the ages of 35 and 50. The typical presentation is that of a painful smooth, mobile firm mass that often fluctuates in size according to the timing of a woman's menstrual cycle. The exact etiology is largely unknown, but it is clear that hormones play a role in the course of disease. Breast cysts largely disappear after menopause, so the presence of a cyst in a postmenopausal woman should raise concern. The vast majority of breast cysts are termed "simple cysts" and do not require any action at all. The presence of a simple cyst does not elevate an individual's risk of subsequent breast cancer. Aspiration is primarily recommended if a woman is symptomatic, or if the cyst was inadvertently discovered on mammographic imaging, and the sonographer cannot definitively determine a sonographic lesion to be cystic or concordant with the mammographic abnormality. Though most fluid aspirated from breast cysts is straw-colored and watery, a viscous gel-like aspirate is common and not worrisome unless it contains blood (B, E). There is no need to send cyst aspirate for cytologic evaluation unless it is bloody. In the case of bloody aspirate, core needle biopsy should also be performed on the cyst wall. If suspicious features such as intracystic septations, thickened walls, and intracystic mass are present, these cysts are called "complicated cysts," and core needle biopsy is recommended (D). Recurrence of a simple breast cyst (or perhaps an enlargement of a different nearby cyst) is common after aspiration, and no feature predicts high or low risk of cyst recurrence (C). However, if a cyst recurs within 2 weeks of the aspiration procedure, this should spark suspicion and consideration for biopsy.

18. B. Nipple discharge is considered "pathologic" if it is serous or bloody in color, unilateral, emanating from a single duct only, copious in amount, or spontaneous. When a woman experiences pathologic discharge after the age of 50, it is particularly more worrisome. Brown, green, white (milky), yellow, and blue discharge is more commonly "physiologic" and can usually be expressed from multiple ducts and/or bilaterally on examination. Bloody and serous types should raise concern for malignancy. Breast-feeding women can commonly have blood-tinged milk in the first weeks of pregnancy. This condition requires only observation, as it is most often self-limited. In the case of pathologic discharge, mammography and breast ultrasound should be performed in an attempt to identify an occult malignancy causing the discharge. If negative, ductal excision is recommended as both diagnostic and therapeutic. Malignant lesions are found in fewer than 10% of cases. From this list of patients, choice B is the most suspicious for breast cancer (A, C–E).

19. C. Tamoxifen is a selective estrogen-receptor modulator (SERM) that acts competitively at the estrogen receptor to halt cell division. Indications for its use are to reduce cancer risk in high-risk patients and as a cancer therapy in men and women with estrogen receptor-positive noninvasive and invasive breast cancer (D). It is also considered beneficial in women who suffer from cyclical mastalgia who have severe symptoms that have failed other measures. In the NSABP-P01 trial, high-risk patients (5-year Gail risk >1.67% or lobular carcinoma in situ [LCIS]) experienced a 50% risk reduction in subsequent noninvasive and invasive breast cancers. A 90% risk reduction is associated with prophylactic mastectomy, not tamoxifen (A). The decision to give tamoxifen must always weigh the possible benefit against the potential side effects. Tamoxifen is associated with the development of endometrial adenocarcinoma and with an increased risk of venous thromboembolism and cataract formation (B). It should be administered for 10-years following surgical resection in premenopausal women with breast cancer (C). If a woman is pregnant, tamoxifen therapy should be halted to avoid fetal exposure (can cause craniofacial malformations and ambiguous genitalia) and reinitiated after pregnancy and lactation (E).

20. A. On ultrasound, lesions that are anechoic are fluid filled (i.e., cysts), and lesions that are hypoechoic are solid (C). Benign and malignant masses can appear hypoechoic, but having a homogeneous internal structure is a benign characteristic (B, D). Bilateral edge shadowing is also a typically benign finding on ultrasound as echoes are deflected off a smooth-bordered rounded mass and appear as dark shadows below each edge of a lesion (E). Taller-than-wide measurements denote a lesion that is infiltrative of the natural elements of the breast, which run parallel to the chest wall. Lesions that are benign are typically wider-than-tall and grow along the natural elements of the breast.

21. A. Atypical ductal hyperplasia, along with atypical lobular hyperplasia and flat epithelial hyperplasia, is classified as a "proliferative lesion with atypia." As such, it is associated with up to five times higher relative risk of breast cancer than normal breast tissue. The risk is higher with multifocal lesions. Stromal fibrosis and apocrine metaplasia do not have an increased risk for breast cancer and thus do not need any additional workup (D). Though ADH is a benign diagnosis, it is morphologically similar to low-grade ductal carcinoma-in-situ and must be less than 2 mm in size to be termed ADH. Surgical excision is recommended if ADH is diagnosed on core biopsy because of reported rates of upstaging (finding cancer) of 20% to 30% (C). It is not important to have a negative margin, but excision of the initial abnormal area must be contained in the surgical specimen for pathologic evaluation (B). Incorrect targeting (i.e., not seeing the clip on specimen radiograph) should spark consideration for retargeting and reexcision. Tamoxifen is a standard recommendation after excisional biopsy confirms the absence of cancer. Patients enrolled in the NSABP P-01 trial were randomized to tamoxifen versus placebo, and those who took tamoxifen had a 50% reduction in subsequent invasive and noninvasive carcinoma of the breast. Axillary staging is not indicated given that ADH is benign, and bilateral prophylactic mastectomy should not be recommended for this relatively low-risk lesion (E).

22. D. From the NSABP B-17 trial, lumpectomy plus radiotherapy was established as superior to lumpectomy alone, given the significant reduction of ipsilateral breast tumor recurrence rates with the addition of radiotherapy (A, C). Sentinel lymph node biopsy is not absolutely indicated for DCIS when performing lumpectomy. However, it is often performed in cases of high-grade DCIS, and in those with suspicion for microinvasion, mass present on imaging, and/or negative hormone receptors, to reduce the need for second surgeries if occult invasive disease is found within the specimen. Additionally, in most cases of lumpectomy (and all cases of mastectomy), the lymphatic drainage has been removed along with the tumor, and thus sampling the sentinel node would be impossible. Planned axillary dissection (as part of a modified radical mastectomy) would not be indicated for in situ disease (B). Intraoperative radiotherapy is now considered appropriate according to ASTRO guidelines for partial breast irradiation for "low-risk" DCIS that is 2.5 cm or smaller, low or intermediate grade, and with margins greater than 3 (yes, three) mm. However, this scenario describes a larger lesion that is high-grade and is therefore not appropriate for IORT (E)

23. C. *BRCA1* and *BRCA2* are examples of tumor suppressor genes, which normally regulate and inhibit growth of abnormal cells. A mutation in both copies of a tumor suppressor gene such as the *BRCA* gene (usually one inherited and one acquired) leads to loss of this protective function and unregulated growth of abnormal cells goes unchecked. On the other hand, protooncogenes (such as ras) typically code for proteins that stimulate cell growth, and mutations in these genes lead to upregulated cell division and therefore cancer (A). Mismatch repair genes code for proteins that recognize DNA errors and repair them, making them a type of tumor suppressor gene. Mutations in mismatch repair genes

can then lead to cancer formation. A common example is the *MSH2* and *MLH1* associated with Lynch syndrome (D). Tyrosine kinases and cyclin-dependent kinases are groups of enzymes that are important for cell regulation and play key roles in development of many cancers (B, E).

24. A. Invasive lobular cancers comprise only 15% of all invasive breast cancers and arise from the terminal lobular components of the lactiferous ducts (E). These cancers are typically hormone receptor positive and tend to occur in postmenopausal women (B). Histologically, lobular cancers grow in a linear pattern infiltrating between tissue planes rather than distorting them. This growth pattern explains why lobular cancer can be very indiscrete on mammogram and ultrasound (poorly defined borders) (D). Although it can be difficult to determine the extent of the lesion and mastectomy is often recommended for lobular cancers, breast conservation is an acceptable option and is associated with low rates of recurrence (C). Pleomorphic LCIS is an aggressive form of LCIS and has higher chance of having underlying lobular carcinoma. Nonpleomorphic LCIS has a higher chance of harboring ductal carcinoma.

25. D. Mastitis commonly complicates lactation and is characterized by erythema, warmth, and tenderness of the breast. It can often be associated with fever and malaise. The majority of patients present without an associated abscess. The etiology is thought to be due to bacteria ascending in the ductal tree of the breast through the nipple, coupled with relative milk stasis from intermittent clogging of ducts and long intervals between feedings. The initial treatment includes the administration of antibiotics covering *S. aureus* (dicloxacillin), hot compresses with breast massage, and continuation of breastfeeding or pumping to evacuate static milk (B). Hand evacuation may be necessary if the breast is too tender to allow feeding or pumping. Incision and drainage or percutaneous aspiration are usually not warranted in the absence of a clear area of fluctuance or a fluid collection seen on ultrasound (C). Mammography is typically not helpful in the workup of mastitis, often resulting in false-positive findings (mass, skin thickening). However, if symptoms and signs of redness and skin thickening persist, mammography and core needle biopsy with or without skin biopsy should be performed to rule out inflammatory breast carcinoma (A, E).

26. A. The described lesion is a phyllodes tumor, also historically referred to as cystosarcoma phyllodes. These tumors are rare, accounting for fewer than 1% of breast neoplasms, and consist of both an epithelial component and a cellular, spindle cell stromal component that forms a characteristic leaflike structure (hence the term *phyllodes*). They are predominantly benign, but borderline malignant and malignant variants occur in up to 40% of cases. Phyllodes tumors typically occur in women during the fifth decade of life and commonly present as a fast-growing, firm, mobile mass in the breast. At large sizes, the contours of the tumor are often visible beneath a thin stretched layer of skin, and the size and weight of the tumor cause the breast to take on the shape of a "teardrop." On imaging, phyllodes tumors appear similar to fibroadenomas, with distinct well-circumscribed margins and macrolobulations (B). Core needle biopsy is the standard for obtaining a tissue diagnosis, particularly in a woman over 40 years of age. However, benign phyllodes tumors can still be difficult to distinguish from fibroadenoma with core sampling alone, most often being reported as a "fibroepithelial lesion," which require excision in order to make the diagnosis. Distinguishing features of benign phyllodes from fibroadenoma are largely based on stromal hypercellularity and morphology. Recent studies suggest that the best way to distinguish the two lesions is by the proportion of individual long spindle nuclei (>30% is reliable for phyllodes tumors) amid dispersed stromal cells. Excision with a clear margin of breast tissue is the treatment of choice for the vast majority of phyllodes tumors, even malignant ones as long as a margin greater than 1 cm is achievable (E). For larger, borderline and malignant lesions, mastectomy may be required, but this is not common. Borderline malignant and malignant forms of the disease are associated with high local recurrence rates and metastasis via a hematogenous route, most commonly to the lungs. Therefore, sentinel node biopsy and axillary dissection are not indicated, given that phyllodes tumors very rarely metastasize to lymph nodes (C). Radiotherapy is not generally used after lumpectomy (as it is in breast cancer) since phyllodes are most often benign and, even in malignant variants, radiotherapy has questionable benefit (D). Chemotherapy has not been proven effective with these tumors and is typically not recommended.

References: Chen WH, Cheng SP, Tzen CY, et al. Surgical treatment of phyllodes tumors of the breast: retrospective review of 172 cases. *J Surg Oncol*. 2005;91(3):185–194.

Krishnamurthy S, Ashfaq R, Shin HJ, Sneige N. Distinction of phyllodes tumor from fibroadenoma: a reappraisal of an old problem. *Cancer*. 2000;90(6):342–349.

27. D. Radial scars (RSs) (<1 cm) and complex sclerosing lesions (CSLs) (>1 cm) are, in and of themselves, benign and are classified as proliferative lesions without atypia (papillomatosis and sclerosing adenosis are two other examples). As such, they are associated with a mildly increased risk of subsequent breast cancer (1.5–2 times normal). These lesions can mimic carcinomas of the breast on mammography given their stellate appearance. However, presence of a translucent central area of fat within the lesion is the classical finding on imaging. Although these lesions have a specific appearance on mammography, core needle biopsy is necessary to exclude malignancy (A–C). Histologically, RS and CSL are characterized by a fibroelastic core from which ducts and lobules radiate. Though biopsy rarely reveals atypia, carcinoma-in-situ or invasive cancer, upstaging is not uncommon after excision. Therefore, when core biopsy demonstrates RS or CSL, excisional biopsy of the entire lesion is generally recommended (E). It is notable that newer studies have suggested that excisional biopsy may not be necessary in cases where vacuum-assisted needle cores provide large volume biopsy specimens, atypical epithelial hyperplasia is absent, and when mammographic findings are consistent with histologic findings. Regardless, it is important for the radiologist and pathologist to alert the surgeon to the presence of an RS due to its increased risk of associated and subsequent malignancy.

References: Alleva DQ, Smetherman DH, Farr GH Jr, Cederbom GJ. Radial scar of the breast: radiologic-pathologic correlation in 22 cases. *Radiographics*. 1999;19 Spec No(suppl_1):S27–S35; discussion S36–S37.

Cawson JN, Malara F, Kavanagh A, Hill P, Balasubramanium G, Henderson M. Fourteen-gauge needle core biopsy of mammographically evident radial scars: is excision necessary?: is excision necessary? *Cancer*. 2003;97(2):345–351.

Fasih T, Jain M, Shrimankar J, Staunton M, Hubbard J, Griffith CDM. All radial scars/complex sclerosing lesions seen on breast screening mammograms should be excised. *Eur J Surg Oncol*. 2005;31(10):1125–1128.

Jacobs TW, Byrne C, Colditz G, Connolly JL, Schnitt SJ. Radial scars in benign breast-biopsy specimens and the risk of breast cancer. *N Engl J Med*. 1999;340(6):430–436.

28. B. Intraductal papilloma is a benign intraepithelial tumor of the breast ductal tissues. When it occurs as a single centrally located lesion, it is classified as a nonproliferative lesion of the breast and confers no subsequent increased risk of breast cancer (adenosis, fibrosis, and squamous/apocrine metaplasia are other examples). A papilloma can grow as large as a few centimeters in diameter and most commonly presents with spontaneous, unilateral bloody or serosanguinous nipple discharge (C). It is the most common cause of bloody discharge, which does not increase the likelihood of associated malignancy (A). When excised, no margin is required (D). Intraductal papillomas may be localized to the periphery, sparing the main duct; these are often multiple and are associated with a small increase in subsequent breast cancer risk. Although invasive and noninvasive carcinomas must be ruled out with diagnostic mammogram and focused ultrasound examination (even with a negative mammography), malignancy accounts for fewer than 10% of cases of bloody nipple discharge (E).

29. D. It is important to note that mammography alone is insufficient to determine whether to perform further diagnostic workup of a palpable breast mass. Reportedly up to 10% of palpable malignancies can be missed if reliant only on the results of a mammogram as a result of varying breast density because some breast cancers can be mammogram occult. Therefore, choosing to observe, reevaluate or repeat the mammogram in 3 months would delay the diagnosis of a possible malignancy (A, B). Ordering additional breast imaging is the standard approach when there is a palpable finding and the initial mammogram is negative. Focused breast ultrasound is the recommended study to further assess the palpable area. There is no role for MRI at this point given the information provided (C). If the lesion is confirmed on ultrasound and is solid, core needle biopsy is then indicated. All breast imaging reports follow a standardized reporting system and use a well-established lexicon of descriptive terms. The Breast Imaging Reporting and Data System (BI-RADS) category classification for mammograms uses a 0- to 6-point scale as follows: 0, assessment incomplete and additional imaging required; 1, negative; 2, benign finding; 3, probably benign finding; 4, suspicious abnormality; 5, highly suspicious of malignancy; 6, known biopsy-proven malignancy. Recommendations by category for nonpalpable findings are as follows: 0, should obtain additional studies (such as ultrasonography); 1 and 2, continue routine screening; 3, short-term follow-up mammogram in 6 months; 4, perform needle biopsy; 5, biopsy and treatment; 6, continue with treatment plan.

References: Eberl MM, Fox CH, Edge SB, Carter CA, Mahoney MC. BI-RADS classification for management of abnormal mammograms. *J Am Board Fam Med*. 2006;19(2):161–164.

Kerlikowske K, Smith-Bindman R, Ljung BM, Grady D. Evaluation of abnormal mammography results and palpable breast abnormalities. *Ann Intern Med.* 2003;139(4):274–284.

30. C. MRI has very few absolute indications for diagnostic workup of breast lesions. Perhaps the most established is evaluating for a primary breast cancer in a patient with known nodal metastasis and no obvious lesion within the breast. Having ADH or LCIS in a group of calcifications would require wire-localized excisional biopsy, and MRI has no role (A, E). A focus of DCIS requires wide excision, followed by adjuvant treatments (D). In dense breasts, there could be a potential role for MRI to assess extent of disease, but having "C" as an option would obviate "D" as a choice. MRI does not have a role in the evaluation of breast pain (B).

31. C. LCIS is a lobular neoplasia that is noninvasive and originates from the terminal lobular region of the lactiferous ducts. LCIS found on core-needle biopsy requires lumpectomy or wide-excision to rule out concurrent invasive cancer. Unlike ductal carcinoma in situ, it is often not associated with calcifications and is instead most often an incidental finding on biopsy. There are two subtypes, classic and pleomorphic. LCIS is not considered to be a premalignant lesion (i.e., does not itself progress to cancer), and therefore wide excision with negative margins is not necessary for classic LCIS (C) and neither is radiotherapy. However, negative margins are required for pleomorphic LCIS as this form is considered to be much more aggressive (B). It is a noninvasive lesion and does not require nodal evaluation (D). It is, however, a marker for the subsequent development of cancer, most often invasive, in either the ipsilateral or contralateral breasts. This risk is reportedly 7 to 10 times the average woman's risk, but not high enough to warrant bilateral prophylactic mastectomy (A). Management of LCIS after excision entails close surveillance. Tamoxifen or raloxifene will be offered for 5 years (but not lifelong), but many patients decline given side effects (E).

References: Frykberg ER. Lobular carcinoma in situ of the breast. *Breast J.* 1999;5(5):296–303.

Sonnenfeld MR, Frenna TH, Weidner N, Meyer JE. Lobular carcinoma in situ: mammographic-pathologic correlation of results of needle-directed biopsy. *Radiology.* 1991;181(2):363–367.

32. E. The most common risk factors for breast cancer are female sex, age, family history of breast cancer (specifically a primary relative), genetic mutations (*BRCA* genes, *PALB2, p53*), personal history of breast cancer, receiving therapeutic dose of radiation to chest wall before age 30, prior breast biopsy showing ductal or lobular atypia or lobular carcinoma-in-situ, obesity, first pregnancy after age 30, menses beginning before age 12 or ending after age 55, daily alcohol intake of two drinks or more, smoking, physical inactivity, and having dense breast tissue on mammography. The highest risk is associated with gene mutation carriers, where lifetime risk can be upwards of 80%. In the scenario presented above, the patient's age does not particularly put her at risk, since most breast cancers occur after the age of 60. A woman in her 40s has a breast cancer risk of 1 in 69 compared to 1 in 29 for a woman in her 60s (A). Having a primary relative with breast cancer (without associated gene mutation) elevates a woman's personal risk by a factor of 2 (B). Daily alcohol intake of 3 drinks or more increases a woman's risk by 1.5 times (C). The effect of smoking on breast cancer risk

remains controversial. It is generally understood, but not definitively proven, that smoking is a significant risk factor and, as such, smoking cessation is usually recommended to reduce risk (D). Having a history of ductal or lobular atypia is associated with 3.5 to 5 times increased risk, and a history of lobular carcinoma-in-situ (LCIS) carries a 7 to 10 times increased risk. Most of the remaining risk factors are related to increased exposure to estrogen and include an increased number of menstrual cycles such as young age at menarche, old age at menopause, and nulliparity.

33. A. DCIS is further classified histologically into micropapillary, papillary, cribriform, solid, and comedo subtypes. The former three being considered less aggressive than the latter two. The comedo subtype is considered the most aggressive, and because cells turn over more quickly, they can quickly outgrow their blood supply and the center of the duct may become plugged with dead cellular debris, often referred to as comedo necrosis (B–E). Comedo DCIS tends to also have a higher cytologic grade and is more likely to produce microcalcifications that deposit around necrotic tissue.

Reference: Nakhlis F, Morrow M. Ductal carcinoma in situ. *Surg Clin North Am.* 2003;83(4):821–839.

34. C. Consensus guidelines in 2016 recommend a 2-mm margin as adequate for DCIS treated with whole-breast radiation. This is in contrast to invasive ductal carcinoma where "no ink on tumor" is considered satisfactory for an oncologic resection. Radiotherapy alone or tamoxifen alone would be inadequate to treat the above patient (A, B). Sentinel node would only be indicated if the lumpectomy demonstrated invasive cancer or if the patient had opted for a mastectomy for the index operation (D). Mastectomy for positive margins is reserved for cases where multiple margins are positive or when margins remain positive after multiple reexcisions (E).

Reference: Morrow M, Van Zee KJ, Solin LJ, et al. Society of Surgical Oncology–American Society for Radiation Oncology–American Society of Clinical Oncology consensus guideline on margins for breast-conserving surgery with whole-breast irradiation in ductal carcinoma in situ. *Pract Radiat Oncol.* 2016;6(5):287–295.

35. B. All of the choices provided are inherited disorders that carry an increased lifetime risk of developing breast cancer. Cowden syndrome is caused by a mutation in *PTEN* and is characterized by multiple hamartomatous lesions as well as cancer of the breast, endometrium, kidney, and thyroid (A). Li-Fraumeni syndrome is caused by mutations in *p53* and is associated with breast cancer, sarcomas, glioblastoma, and adrenocortical cancers. Peutz-Jeghers syndrome is caused by mutations in *STK11* gene and classically is associated with the presence of hyperpigmented mucocutaneous spots, bowel hamartomas, and cancers of the gastrointestinal tract, pancreas, liver, breast, endometrium, and ovary (C). Ataxia-telangiectasia is caused by mutation of the *ATM* gene and, along with neurologic and vasculocutaneous findings for which this disorder is named, it carries an increased risk of breast cancer, lymphoma, and leukemia (D). *BRCA2* mutations are associated with breast, ovarian, fallopian tube, pancreas, prostate, and skin (melanoma) cancers (E).

References: Bland KL, Beenken SW, Copeland EM. Breast. In: Brunicardi FC, Andersen DK, Billiar TR, et al., eds. *Schwartz's principles of surgery.* 8th ed. New York: McGraw-Hill; 2005:453–500.

Iglehart S, Kaelin C. Breast. In: Townsend CM, Jr, Beauchamp RD, Evers BM, Mattox KL, eds. *Sabiston textbook of surgery: the biological basis of modern surgical practice.* 17th ed. Philadelphia: W.B. Saunders; 2004:867–928.

36. A. Hereditary breast cancers (caused by mutations in *BRCA, PTEN, ATM, STK11, PALB2,* and *p53* genes) collectively account for only 10% of all breast cancers (C), with *BRCA* mutations accounting for 25% of all hereditary breast cancers. The mutations result in "loss of function" of the tumor suppression that *BRCA* genes normally provide (B). *BRCA1* mutations confer a 55% to 65% lifetime risk for breast cancer and a 35% to 45% lifetime risk for ovarian cancer. *BRCA2* mutations confer a lifetime risk of 40% to 55% for breast cancer and a 15% to 25% lifetime risk for ovarian cancer (D). Breast cancers in women with *BRCA1* mutations tend to be hormone receptor-negative and are often triple-negative. Therefore, the use of tamoxifen as chemoprevention is not generally recommended to reduce risk (D). Prophylactic bilateral mastectomy is the risk-reducing strategy most recommended, resulting in 90% overall risk reduction. Male breast cancer risk is typically elevated to 100-fold risk in individuals who have *BRCA2* mutations, not *BRCA1* (E).

Reference: Fossland VS, Stroop JB, Schwartz RC, Kurtzman SH. Genetic issues in patients with breast cancer. *Surg Oncol Clin N Am.* 2009;18(1):53–71.

37. E. This question addresses the appropriate adjuvant therapy for early-stage triple-negative breast cancer. First, all patients for whom lumpectomy is performed for invasive cancer should undergo radiotherapy to reduce local recurrence and achieve a similar survival outcome to mastectomy. Second, hormonal therapy is not indicated in patients who are hormone receptor negative. Chemotherapy is indicated for all triple-negative breast cancer because of the more aggressive nature of the disease and lack of other systemic therapy options. Taken together, this patient requires the last option of radiotherapy and chemotherapy, without hormonal therapy (A–D). For triple-negative cancers that are 2 cm or greater or node-positive, consideration should be given to neoadjuvant chemotherapy.

38. C. Breast conservation, by way of lumpectomy, can be adequately performed to treat T1 and smaller T2 breast cancers as long as adjuvant radiotherapy is administered to reduce the risk of local recurrence. Contraindications to receiving radiotherapy therefore drive the contraindications of having a lumpectomy. Radiotherapy cannot be safely administered in pregnancy, so women who are diagnosed in their first 2 semesters are often recommended mastectomy (A). Women in their third trimester can often undergo operative therapy and wait until after childbirth to initiate radiotherapy. Women with locally recurrent breast cancer, where radiation therapy was previously completed, are also typically advised to undergo mastectomy because a second round of radiotherapy to the same breast would exceed maximal recommended doses (B). Active connective tissue disorders, such as scleroderma, may lead to increases in radiotherapy-related complications and therefore are considered relative to absolute contraindications to radiation (D). *Multicentric* cancers (being located in separate quadrants of the breast) can also preclude lumpectomy, particularly if

there is insufficient breast tissue to allow for two separate wide excisions (E). It is important to note that *multifocal* cancers refer to multiple foci of breast cancer in the same quadrant and are amenable to breast-conserving therapy. The best choice is the woman with ipsilateral involved nodes because axillary dissection is performed separately and does not limit the ability to perform breast conservation.

Reference: Morrow M, Strom EA, Bassett LW, et al. Standard for breast conservation therapy in the management of invasive breast carcinoma. *CA Cancer J Clin.* 2002;52(5):277–300.

39. C. Large tumor size, poor histologic grade, and estrogen-receptor status can certainly denote a poorer prognosis but the strongest predictor is the presence of regional metastatic disease (A, B, D). Younger patients also tend to have more aggressive, higher grade, receptor-negative breast cancers, but nodal status is still more predictive (E). In more recent years, gene expression profiles have surpassed nodal status in early-stage breast cancer in the ability to predict cancer recurrence (i.e., need for systemic therapy).

40. D. Inflammatory breast cancer comprises only 1% of all breast cancers and is characterized by erythema and skin edema (called peau d'orange) that result from malignant obstruction of subdermal lymphatics. It is often mistaken initially with mastitis, and failure to respond to conventional antibiotic therapy is an indication to obtain tissue for analysis. Absence of a palpable mass is common; therefore, biopsy should be performed of the abnormal skin and abnormal lymph nodes to confirm the diagnosis. The best prognosis results from early treatment with systemic chemotherapy (i.e., neoadjuvant chemotherapy) followed by either surgery or radiotherapy depending on resectability (A, C). The surgical therapy of choice is modified radical mastectomy because there is no role for sentinel node biopsy in inflammatory cancer or in patients with clinically positive nodes (B). Concurrent chemotherapy and radiotherapy have been shown to be inferior to sequential therapy. There is no role to continue antibiotics because the erythema is due to inflammatory cancer, not ongoing infection (E). The 5-year survival rate is still only 30% to 50%.

Reference: Cristofanilli M, Buzdar AU, Hortobágyi GN. Update on the management of inflammatory breast cancer. *Oncologist.* 2003;8(2):141–148.

41. B. Batson plexus is a venous network that runs in the paravertebral space and drains abdominopelvic and thoracic regions. The veins are valveless and therefore have been implicated in the metastatic spread of prostate, breast, and colon malignancies to bone, particularly the pelvis, vertebral bodies, and skull. The Batson venous plexus also explains why patients may have bone metastases without first having pulmonary metastases because tumor cells enter the plexus and deposit in the vertebrae without first passing through the lungs (A, C–E).

Reference: Mundy GR. Mechanisms of bone metastasis. *Cancer.* 1997;80(S8):1546–1556.

42. D. Purple nodular lesions occurring on an arm with long-standing lymphedema present is angiosarcoma, or lymphangiosarcoma, otherwise referred to as Stewart-Treves syndrome. Classically, the patient has undergone axillary dissection and radiotherapy for cancer treatment and develops lymphedema. The local immune response is impaired, allowing for development of this aggressive malignancy within the breast or ipsilateral arm. The diagnosis is established via open biopsy because fine-needle aspiration alone may not be sufficient. Characteristic features include pleomorphic nuclei, frequent mitosis, necrosis, and stacking up of the endothelial cells lining neoplastic vessels (particularly with high-grade lesions). The tumor is highly aggressive with a propensity for early metastasis to the lungs. Treatment consists of early wide surgical debridement, which may require amputation of the limb. Prognosis is poor with most patients surviving less than 2 years.

References: Heitmann C, Ingianni G. Stewart-Treves syndrome: lymphangiosarcoma following mastectomy. *Ann Plast Surg.* 2000;44(1):72–75.

Sher T, Hennessy BT, Valero V, et al. Primary angiosarcomas of the breast. *Cancer.* 2007;110(1):173–178.

Vorburger SA, Xing Y, Hunt KK, et al. Angiosarcoma of the breast: angiosarcoma of the breast. *Cancer.* 2005;104(12):2682–2688.

43. E. In breast cancer local recurrence, the receipt of prior radiotherapy precludes the option of breast conservation the second time around (B). Therefore, mastectomy is routinely indicated in local recurrence after lumpectomy and whole breast radiation. Repeat sentinel node biopsy has been shown to have adequate identification and false-negative rates, so axillary dissection can usually be avoided in this group if the lymph nodes remain clinically negative (A). Breast cancer recurrence is a different issue than having two separate primary breast cancers in one's lifetime. Typically, occurrence of cancer within a prior surgical incision is indicative of local recurrence, which is more common in BRCA-positive patients. However, bilateral mastectomy is not indicated but may be considered if BRCA positive (D). Lastly, the local recurrence occurred while the patient was taking tamoxifen, so the patient should preferably be switched to a different agent. Given her postmenopausal status, aromatase inhibitor would be a better option (C).

44. B. Paget disease of the breast is a rare cancer of the nipple involving intraepithelial invasion of Paget cells (large, pale vacuolated cells) at the nipple surface causing an eczematoid appearance that is often confused for a contact dermatitis (A). Failure to respond to topical treatments should raise concern for Paget disease, and full-thickness skin punch biopsy (not shave) is the biopsy method of choice. Nipple

discharge is rarely present, and cytologic evaluation of ductal fluid has no role in the diagnostic evaluation since the Paget cells are within the epithelial layer (C). Paget disease is a cancerous lesion and is often simultaneously associated with extensive ductal carcinoma in situ or invasive ductal cancer extending deep to the visible lesion (D). Paget disease is most commonly treated with mastectomy given the extent of the underlying cancer (E).

Reference: Kollmorgen DR, Varanasi JS, Edge SB, Carson WE III. Paget's disease of the breast: a 33-year experience. *J Am Coll Surg.* 1998;187(2):171–177.

45. D. Breast lymphoma is a rare disease. The majority of cases are B-cell lymphomas, and the most common type is diffuse large B-cell lymphoma (40%–70%) (A). Breast lymphomas are equally divided into primary and secondary (B). Treatment depends on whether the lesion is localized or diffuse as well as on the grade of lymphoma. With localized and low-grade lymphomas, primary excision may be all that is necessary, while standard combination therapy with CHOP (cyclophosphamide, doxorubicin, vincristine, prednisone) along with radiation therapy is recommended for intermediate- or high-grade lymphoma (C, E). Several studies have noted an unusual predilection for distant dissemination for breast lymphoma to the central nervous system.

References: Brogi E, Harris NL. Lymphomas of the breast: pathology and clinical behavior. *Semin Oncol.* 1999;26(3):357–364.

Wong WW, Schild SE, Halyard MY, Schomberg PJ. Primary non-Hodgkin lymphoma of the breast: the Mayo Clinic Experience. *J Surg Oncol.* 2002;80(1):19–25.

46. C. Herceptin (trastuzumab) is a humanized IgG1 kappa monoclonal antibody that selectively binds with high affinity to the epidermal growth factor receptor 2 (*HER2*) protein. Overexpression of *HER2*/neu (found in approximately 15%–20% of breast cancers) is associated with a worse prognosis and an increased risk of recurrence but provides a specific target for the treatment of breast cancer. Trastuzumab is associated with cardiac failure manifesting as a decreased left ventricular ejection fraction (LVEF). Thus, serial assessments of the LVEF need to be performed while administering trastuzumab, particularly if given in conjunction with other agents that are cardiotoxic (such as anthracyclines) (A, B, D, E).

Reference: Seidman A, Hudis C, Pierri MK, et al. Cardiac dysfunction in the trastuzumab clinical trials experience. *J Clin Oncol.* 2002;20(5):1215–1221.

Endocrine Surgery

13

MICHAEL A. MEDEROS AND JAMES WU

ABSITE 99th Percentile High-Yields

I. Thyroid
  A. Workup of new thyroid nodule
    1. Initial workup:
       a) TSH (hot nodules rarely cancerous)
       b) Neck ultrasound (risk of malignancy estimated by TIRADS or ATA scoring systems)
    2. Indications for thyroid fine-needle aspirate (FNA) based on size + estimated risk on ultrasound
       a) Do not biopsy lesions less than 1 cm
    3. FNAB categorized by Bethesda category
       a) Bethesda III & IV are indeterminate thyroid nodules; options include repeat FNA, observation, diagnostic lobectomy, or genomic classifier testing (Afirma, Thyroseq)
       b) Genomic classifier testing: high NPV, mediocre PPV
  B. Papillary and follicular carcinoma considerations
    1. Extent of surgery based on size (<1 cm: lobectomy, 1–4 cm: lobe vs total, >4 cm: total)
       a) Total thyroidectomy indicated if there are nodal metastases, gross extrathyroidal extension
    2. Postoperative radioactive iodine only needed for high-risk disease after total thyroidectomy (nodal metastases, extrathyroidal extension)
    3. Follicular thyroid carcinoma spreads hematogenously (most common in bone and lung)
  C. Medullary thyroid carcinoma considerations
    1. Workup includes: calcitonin, CEA, RET mutation testing
    2. Rule out pheochromocytoma prior to surgery, check calcium for hyperparathyroidism (MEN 2A/MEN 2B)
    3. Extent of surgery should include prophylactic bilateral central neck dissection
    4. Does not take up radioactive iodine, so radiation therapy and chemotherapy are ineffective
  D. Graves disease
    1. Treatment options: antithyroid medication, radioactive iodine, total thyroidectomy
    2. Surgery favored: in association with thyroid nodules, or ophthalmic disease (radioactive iodine will worsen eye disease)
    3. Lugol solution or potassium iodide given one week before surgery will decrease thyroid vascularity
    4. Patients can experience postthyroidectomy thyrotoxicosis, treat with beta-blockade preoperatively

II. Parathyroid
  A. Hyperparathyroidism
    1. Indications for parathyroidectomy for primary hyperparathyroidism
       a) Symptomatic disease: osteoporosis or fragility fracture, or kidney stones
       b) Asymptomatic disease: age <50, serum Ca >1 mg/dL above normal range, vertebral compression fractures, osteoporosis, silent nephrolithiasis, nephrocalcinosis, urine Ca >400 μg/24 hours AND high stone risk profile, CrCl less than 60 ml/min
    2. Should rule out familial hypocalciuric hypercalcemia (FHH) with 24-hour urine calcium (high urine Ca rules this out)

3. A chloride/phosphate ratio of more than 33 and evidence of significant hypercalciuria bolster the diagnosis
4. MEN 1 and MEN 2A should have a 3.5 gland parathyroidectomy with bilateral thymectomy due to greater incidence of supernumerary and ectopic glands, or total parathyroidectomy with autotransplantation into forearm

B. Hypercalcemic crisis
1. First-line treatment is IV normal saline fluid resuscitation followed by bisphosphonates
2. Calcium of 14–15 mg/dL (in association with high PTH and palpable neck mass) is highly concerning for parathyroid carcinoma (rare)

C. Intraoperative considerations
1. Miami criterion for successful parathyroidectomy: >50% drop in PTH at 10 minutes post excision (check again 20 minutes post excision if criterion not met)
2. Location of ectopic superior glands: tracheoesophageal groove & retroesophageal > intrathyroidal, carotid sheath, in cervical thymus
3. Ectopic inferior glands (more variable): thymus > tracheoesophageal groove, intrathyroidal
    a) Perform cervical thymectomy if unable to locate inferior gland
4. If unable to locate parathyroid, complete operation and perform postoperative localization studies
5. Correcting hyperparathyroidism doesn't improve osteoporosis t-score but it decreases the rate at which it drops

III. Adrenal

A. Incidentaloma
1. Majority are benign, nonfunctioning (<10 Hounsfield units)
2. Perform biochemical workup to rule out functional tumor
    a) Cushing: low-dose dexamethasone suppression test, late-night salivary cortisol, or serum DHEA-S
    b) Aldosteronoma: plasma aldosterone concentration, plasma renin activity (renin-aldosterone ratio >20), BMP to check potassium
    c) Pheochromocytoma: 24-hour urine metanephrines
3. If nonfunctional, rule out malignancy
    a) Higher malignancy risk: size >4 cm, >30 Hounsfield units, heterogeneity, >50% washout
    b) Role of FNA for adrenal mass is very limited
        (1) If (+) cancer history, consider biopsy to rule out adrenal metastasis
        (2) Primary adrenal cortical carcinoma cannot be diagnosed with FNA
        (3) FNA of unsuspected pheochromocytoma can trigger catecholamine surge
    c) Consider adrenalectomy for lesions >4 to 5 cm (except myelolipoma) or lesions with suspicious radiographic features regardless of size

B. Cushing disease versus primary hypercortisolism
1. Twenty-four-hour urine cortisol, ACTH level, high-dose dexamethasone suppression test
2. Patients with subclinical hypercortisolism may have normal 24-hour cortisol levels; if there is high suspicion, proceed with low-dose dexamethasone suppression testing

C. Pheochromocytoma
1. Associated syndromes: von Hippel-Lindau, MEN 2, neurofibromatosis 1 (von Recklinghausen disease)
2. Alpha-blockade prior to initiating beta-blockers

D. Hyperaldosteronism (Conn syndrome)
1. Hypertension, hypokalemia, alkalosis
2. Aldosterone to renin ratio ≥30 (90% sensitive), plasma aldosterone concentration >10
3. Unilateral adenoma > bilateral adrenal hyperplasia; adenomas are usually small

E. Adrenal cortical carcinoma considerations
1. High attenuation (>20 Hounsfield units), >4 cm, heterogenous appearance on CT
2. Often are functional: hypercortisolism, hyperaldosteronism, hyperandrogenism
3. Open adrenalectomy; laparoscopic adrenalectomy is currently contraindicated (higher rate of local recurrence, poorer disease-free survival)
4. Mitotane for positive margins, vascular or capsular invasion, rupture/spillage, unresectable/recurrent/metastatic disease (most commonly liver & lung)
5. Associated syndrome: Li-Fraumeni (p53)

F. Adrenal metastases
1. Lung, kidney, melanoma, breast most common; often bilateral
2. Bilateral adrenalectomy may benefit select patients
    a) Evaluate for and correct adrenal insufficiency prior to bilateral adrenalectomy to prevent perioperative adrenal crisis; 30% of patients have entire gland replaced with tumor

IV. Thyroiditis

Thyroiditis	Hyper-/hypothyroid	Cause & associations	Treatment
Hashimoto (chronic or lymphocytic) thyroiditis	Hypothyroid May have thyrotoxicosis with transient hyperthyroidism due to gland destruction	• Autoimmune, (HLA) -DR3, -DR5, & -B8 • Antithyroid peroxidase (anti-TPO) antibodies (90%); antithyroglobulin antibodies (20%–50%) • Female > male, 30–60 years old, painless goiter • Risk of primary thyroid lymphoma	• Levothyroxine • Thyroidectomy reserved for large goiters with compressive symptoms
Postpartum thyroiditis	Hyperthyroid with decreased uptake on RAI scan due to follicular cell destruction → euthyroid period → transient hypothyroidism → euthyroid (recovery)	• Autoimmune, may have higher antithyroid titers • Painless	• No treatment unless symptoms are severe • Hyperthyroid—beta-blockers (propranolol if breastfeeding) • Hypothyroid—levothyroxine
Acute (suppurative) thyroiditis	Euthyroid	• Bacterial (*Staphylococcus aureus* and *Streptococcus pyogenes*) > fungal > parasitic • Painful	• Ultrasound-guided fine-needle aspiration with Gram stain and culture to determine etiology, antibiotics
Subacute granulomatous (de Quervain) thyroiditis	Hyperthyroid with decreased uptake on RAI scan due to gland destruction → euthyroid period → transient hypothyroidism → euthyroid (recovery)	• Preceded by viral URI • Female > male, painful goiter, fatigue, weight loss	• Supportive care, NSAIDs, steroids
Riedel (fibrous) thyroiditis	Hypothyroid	• Firm, nontender, extensive fibrosis that may compress adjacent structures • May have elevated serum IgG4	• Glucocorticoids, tamoxifen, levothyroxine • Surgery reserved for severe compressive symptoms

V. Bethesda Classification

Category	Cytopathology	Malignancy rate	Management
I	Nondiagnostic/inadequate	0%–20%	Repeat FNA with ultrasound guidance
II	Benign	0%–3%	Clinical and sonographic follow-up
III	Atypia of undetermined significance/follicular lesion of undetermined significance (FLUS)	5%–15%	Repeat FNA, molecular testing, or lobectomy
IV	Follicular neoplasm/suspicious for follicular neoplasm, e.g., Hürthle cell (oncocytic) type	15%–30%	Molecular testing and lobectomy
V	Suspicious for malignancy	60%–75%	Near-total thyroidectomy or lobectomy
VI	Malignant	97%–99%	Near-total thyroidectomy or lobectomy

IV. Hyperparathyroidism

Type	Cause	Serum Ca/Phos	Urine Ca	Treatment
Primary	Parathyroid adenoma (85%) or hyperplasia Lithium-induced parathyroid hyperplasia	↑/↓	↑ (calcium creatinine clearance ratio >0.02 suggestive)	Adenoma—parathyroidectomy of affected gland Hyperplasia—3.5-gland excision or 4-gland excision with autotransplantation
Secondary	Chronic renal failure, hyperphosphatemia Vitamin D deficiency	↓/↑	-	Phosphate binders & dietary modification, calcium supplementation, vitamin D, cinacalcet 3.5-gland parathyroidectomy for calciphylaxis, bone pain, intractable pruritus, persistent anemia, or pathologic fractures
Tertiary	Persistent hyperfunctioning parathyroid glands after kidney transplantation	↑/↓	↑	3.5-gland parathyroidectomy
Parathyroid carcinoma		↑↑/↓	↑	Parathyroidectomy with en bloc ipsilateral thyroidectomy + isthmusectomy & ipsilateral central neck dissection (lateral neck dissection only if evidence of gross LN involvement). Repeat neck exploration for recurrent disease.

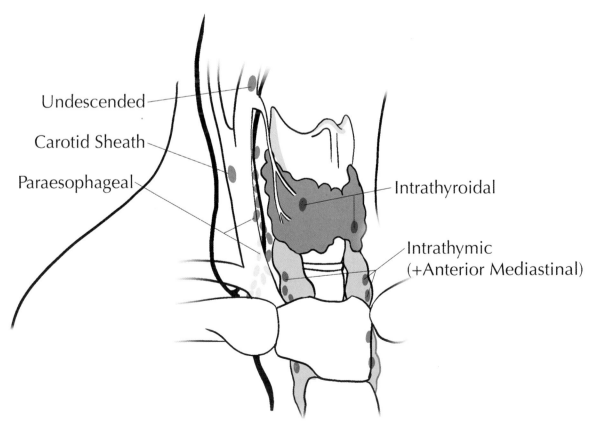

Fig 13.1 Location of Lost Parathyroid Glands.

Questions

1. A 55-year-old male has recalcitrant hypertension despite taking three antihypertensive medications. He is subsequently found to have an aldosterone to renin ratio greater than 30. A CT reveals a 1-cm left adrenal lesion and a 2-cm right adrenal lesion. What is the next best step in management?
   A. Right adrenalectomy
   B. Left adrenalectomy
   C. Bilateral adrenalectomy
   D. Selective venous sampling
   E. ^{11}C-metomidate scan

2. A 52-year-old obese male who underwent CT scan 2 months ago following a car collision was incidentally found to have a 3-cm left adrenal mass. Which of the following is the next appropriate step?
   A. Laparoscopic left adrenalectomy
   B. Surveillance CT performed at 6 months and then annually for 1 to 2 years
   C. No further testing necessary
   D. PET CT
   E. Overnight low-dose (1 mg) dexamethasone suppression test

3. A 40-year-old female presents with incidentally discovered mild elevation in serum calcium. She is otherwise healthy. A PTH level is elevated as well. Both ultrasound and sestamibi scan of the neck are negative. Which of the following is true about this condition?
   A. It may represent tertiary hyperparathyroidism
   B. A 24-hour urine calcium is indicated
   C. She should proceed to neck exploration
   D. It should be treated with cinacalcet
   E. Selective venous sampling is indicated

4. A 40-year-old female presents with incidentally discovered hypercalcemia to 11.7 mg/dL. She is otherwise healthy. A PTH level is elevated as well. Both ultrasound and sestamibi scan of the neck are negative. Urine calcium is elevated. What is the most appropriate next step?
   A. Proceed to neck exploration
   B. Treatment with cinacalcet
   C. Selective venous sampling
   D. MRI of the neck
   E. Observation

5. Following total thyroidectomy for follicular cancer, a 65-year-old female presents to the emergency department 4 days later complaining of circumoral numbness and tingling of her fingers. Phosphate level is normal. Which of the following is true about this condition?
   A. It likely represents hungry bone syndrome (HBS)
   B. It may lead to a shortened QT on ECG
   C. The risk can be reduced by routine postoperative calcium and vitamin D supplementation
   D. Most patients are symptomatic
   E. It is more common with thyroidectomy for benign lesions

6. A 45-year-old man with episodic severe hypertension is found to have an elevated plasma metanephrine level and a serum calcium level of 11.5 mg/dL. Which of the following would be indicated in the workup?
   A. CT scan of the sella turcica
   B. Calcitonin level
   C. Serum gastrin level
   D. Serum prolactin level
   E. A 24-hour urine cortisol

7. Which of the following laboratory findings is characteristically associated with primary hyperparathyroidism?
   A. Elevated serum phosphate
   B. Increased serum chloride
   C. Decreased urinary calcium
   D. Metabolic alkalosis
   E. Elevated calcium with a decreased PTH

8. A 60-year-old woman presents with fatigue, weakness and confusion. She has history of kidney stones and pathologic fractures. On physical she has a palpable neck mass. Her serum calcium level is 14.8 mg/dL. The most likely diagnosis is:
   A. Parathyroid adenoma
   B. Parathyroid hyperplasia
   C. Parathyroid cancer
   D. Breast cancer with bone metastasis
   E. Secondary hyperparathyroidism

9. During neck exploration for primary hyperparathyroidism, only three parathyroid glands are identified, all of which appear normal in size. Which of the following would be appropriate?
   A. Perform a transcervical thymectomy
   B. Remove all three glands and reimplant one in the forearm
   C. Remove two and a half glands and then close
   D. Perform median sternotomy to look for ectopic parathyroid
   E. Obtain biopsy samples of all three parathyroid glands and then close

10. After total thyroidectomy and postoperative iodine ablation for a 5-cm follicular thyroid cancer, the best test to monitor for recurrent disease is:
    A. Serum thyroid-stimulating hormone (TSH)
    B. Serum calcitonin
    C. Serum thyroglobulin
    D. ^{131}I scan
    E. Cross-sectional CT or MRI

11. Which of the following is true regarding adrenal cortical carcinoma?
    A. Associated evidence of hormonal excess is common
    B. The diagnosis is generally made by CT-guided needle biopsy
    C. Staging is based on tumor histology
    D. Because of malignant potential, adrenal masses larger than 3 cm should be excised
    E. Laparoscopic adrenalectomy is the preferred approach for surgical resection

12. Malignancy within a thyroglossal duct cyst is typically:
    A. Follicular thyroid
    B. Papillary thyroid
    C. Squamous cell
    D. Anaplastic thyroid
    E. Hürthle cells

13. After a total thyroidectomy, the right vocal cord is noted to be fixed in a paramedian position. This most likely represents:
    A. Injury to the recurrent laryngeal nerve (RLN)
    B. Injury to the internal branch of the superior laryngeal nerve
    C. Injury to the external branch of the superior laryngeal nerve
    D. Trauma from endotracheal intubation
    E. Compression from hematoma

14. The most common pituitary neoplasm associated with MEN 1 secretes:
    A. ACTH
    B. Prolactin
    C. Growth hormone
    D. Thyroid-stimulating hormone
    E. Follicle-stimulating hormone

15. Which of the following features of Graves disease does not improve with antithyroid therapy?
    A. Tremor
    B. Anxiety
    C. Graves dermopathy
    D. Gastrointestinal disturbance
    E. Exophthalmos

16. A 56-year-old male presents with refractory hypertension despite being started on hydrochlorothiazide and lisinopril by his primary care physician. His blood pressure is 182/92 mmHg. Laboratory studies are remarkable for an aldosterone-renin ratio of 25 and hypokalemia. Which of the following is the next best step?
    A. Triamterene
    B. Amiloride
    C. Spironolactone
    D. Phenoxybenzamine
    E. Eplerenone

17. A 40-year-old female presents with a 4 cm thyroid nodule that is biopsy-proven papillary thyroid carcinoma. The patient is taken to surgery, and final pathologic evaluation reveals a 4-cm papillary thyroid carcinoma with microscopic invasion of the perithyroidal tissue, but no vascular invasion. A 1-cm lymph node in the lateral neck is positive. Which of the following answer choices correctly pairs *this* patient's American Thyroid Association (ATA) risk stratification with her pathologic findings?
    A. Low risk; no vascular invasion
    B. Intermediate risk; tumor 4 cm
    C. Intermediate risk; positive lymph node <3 cm
    D. High risk; tumor 4 cm
    E. High risk; microscopic invasion of perithyroidal tissue

18. A 46-year-old female with a 3-cm palpable right-sided thyroid nodule has a fine-needle aspirate (FNA) performed, which is reported as nondiagnostic. What is the best next step?
    A. Repeat FNA
    B. Core needle biopsy
    C. Right thyroid lobectomy
    D. Total thyroidectomy
    E. Ultrasound in 6 months

19. A 51-year-old male with a 2-cm palpable right-sided thyroid nodule has an FNA performed, which is reported as follicular lesion of undetermined significance (FLUS). Which of the following is true about this condition?
    A. Repeat FNA is not recommended
    B. Molecular testing does not influence management
    C. Right thyroid lobectomy is an acceptable option
    D. Total thyroidectomy is the next best step
    E. Ultrasound follow-up in 6 months is the best option

20. The thyroid gland is derived from which embryologic structure?
    A. First pharyngeal arch
    B. Third pharyngeal pouch
    C. Third pharyngeal arch
    D. Fourth pharyngeal pouch
    E. Fourth pharyngeal arch

21. Which of the following cancers most commonly metastasizes to the thyroid?
    A. Parathyroid gland
    B. Kidney
    C. Lung
    D. Breast
    E. Esophagus cancer

22. Two patients are diagnosed with pheochromocytoma. In one patient, the mass is located in the adrenal gland and in the other, the mass is localized to the organ of Zuckerkandl. Which enzyme accounts for the difference in the serum levels of epinephrine in the two patients?
    A. Tyrosine hydroxylase
    B. Dopamine-beta-hydroxylase
    C. Phenylethanolamine N-methyltransferase (PNMT)
    D. Dihydroxyphenylalanine (DOPA)-decarboxylase
    E. Catechol-O-methyltransferase (COMT)

23. A 45-year-old woman with rheumatoid arthritis on chronic steroids has not been able to get a refill on her medications including atenolol, methotrexate, and prednisone. She arrives at the emergency department with a fever, hypotension, nausea, and dizziness. The next best step is:
    A. Intravenous (IV) antibiotics
    B. IV hydrocortisone
    C. IV fluids
    D. Administer oral methotrexate
    E. Complete blood count, basic metabolic panel, and cortisol level

24. A 45-year-old male presents with a 2-day history of nausea, vomiting, and marked abdominal distention. He has no prior surgical history. Before this, he's had watery diarrhea for about a month. On exam, he has diffuse tenderness without rebound or guarding. Computed tomography (CT) scan demonstrates markedly dilated loops of small bowel with an abrupt transition in the mid jejunum with distal collapse. In addition, there are two, 2-cm solid masses in the right lobe of the liver. At surgery, at the point of obstruction, there is a small mass in the mid ileum with surrounding fibrosis, causing tethering and kinking of the small bowel mesentery. The two lesions in the right lobe of the liver are not palpable. A segmental small bowel resection is performed. Additionally, which of the following is recommended?
    A. Cholecystectomy
    B. Ultrasound-guided liver biopsy
    C. Liver resection
    D. Appendectomy
    E. No additional procedure

25. Which of the following is true regarding Hürthle cell carcinoma?
    A. It is considered a subtype of follicular carcinoma
    B. Lymph node metastasis is exceedingly rare
    C. Diagnosis of malignancy is usually made by FNA
    D. Residual disease is effectively treated with iodine 131 (^{131}I)
    E. Histologically they demonstrate Orphan Annie cells

26. A patient presents with fatigue and bone pain. Serum calcium level is 11.1 mg/dL and parathyroid hormone (PTH) is elevated. Which is the least acceptable method of localization?
    A. Operative exploration
    B. CT scan
    C. Technetium-99m sestamibi imaging
    D. Magnetic resonance imaging (MRI)
    E. Ultrasound scan

27. Which of the following is true regarding follicular thyroid cancer?
    A. It is the most common thyroid malignancy
    B. It most commonly spreads via a hematogenous route
    C. Prophylactic nodal dissection is recommended
    D. It is best managed by hemithyroidectomy
    E. Multicentricity is common

28. A 45-year-old woman presents with symptomatic primary hyperparathyroidism. During surgery, it is noted that all four glands are markedly enlarged. Which of the following is the best recommendation?
    A. Removal of three and a half glands for parathyroid hyperplasia, leaving half of a gland in place
    B. Removal of all four glands
    C. Terminate the surgery and treat with medical management
    D. Biopsy all four glands
    E. Remove one gland, and biopsy the other three

29. Which of the following is true regarding laparoscopic adrenalectomy?
    A. It is the procedure of choice for small functional adenomas
    B. It is contraindicated for pheochromocytoma
    C. It is contraindicated for bilateral pheochromocytoma
    D. It is contraindicated for pheochromocytomas larger than 5 cm
    E. It is a well-established option for malignant tumors

30. A 65-year-old woman with a history of Hashimoto thyroiditis presents with fever, dysphagia, and a painless thyroid mass that has enlarged over a short period of time. This most likely represents:
    A. Lymphoma
    B. Follicular cancer
    C. Anaplastic thyroid cancer
    D. Acute suppurative thyroiditis
    E. Medullary thyroid cancer (MTC)

31. Which of the following is LEAST likely associated with hyperparathyroidism?
    A. Cholelithiasis
    B. Pancreatitis
    C. Osteoclastomas
    D. Diarrhea
    E. Peptic ulcer disease

32. Which of the following is true regarding the parathyroid glands, and/or the location of ectopic superior/inferior glands?
    A. The inferior glands arise from the fourth branchial pouch and the superior ones from the third pouch
    B. The superior glands are more likely to be found in an ectopic position
    C. The superior glands are more likely to be found in the thymus
    D. Three glands are more common than five glands
    E. Ectopic superior glands are more likely to be found in the retro- or paraesophageal space

33. Which of the following is not an indication for parathyroidectomy in a patient with asymptomatic primary hyperparathyroidism?
    A. Serum calcium of 11.6 mg/dL
    B. Creatinine clearance less than 60 mL/min
    C. Age younger than 50 years
    D. Bone density at the hip of 1.5 standard deviations below matched controls
    E. High risk of forming kidney stones

34. A 45-year-old-woman presents with truncal obesity and hypertension. A 24-hour urine-free cortisol level is markedly elevated and a low-dose dexamethasone suppression test fails to suppress the elevated plasma cortisol levels. Plasma adrenocorticotropic hormone (ACTH) levels are also markedly elevated. A high-dose dexamethasone suppression test also fails to suppress the urinary-free cortisol level. Which of the following would most likely demonstrate the cause of her symptoms?
    A. CT scan of the sella turcica
    B. Petrosal sinus sampling for ACTH
    C. Chest CT
    D. MRI of the sella turcica
    E. CT scan of the abdomen

35. Calcified clumps of cells on histology are consistent with:
    A. Papillary cancer
    B. Hürthle cell cancer
    C. Follicular cancer
    D. Medullary thyroid cancer
    E. Anaplastic cancer

36. Which of the following is true regarding pheochromocytoma?
    A. Risk of malignancy is higher in patients with familial tumors
    B. Malignancy is determined histologically by the number of mitoses
    C. Familial tumors are more likely to be unilateral
    D. Metaiodobenzylguanidine scanning is useful for localizing extra adrenal pheochromocytomas
    E. Urine metanephrine has the highest sensitivity

37. The most common type of thyroid cancer in children is:
    A. Papillary
    B. Follicular
    C. Medullary
    D. Hürthle cell
    E. Anaplastic

38. Which of the following is true regarding secondary hyperparathyroidism?
    A. Serum calcium levels are markedly increased
    B. It is usually associated with a parathyroid adenoma
    C. PTH levels are typically normal
    D. Can be caused by severe vitamin D deficiency
    E. Most patients will eventually require parathyroidectomy

39. Which of the following is true regarding tertiary hyperparathyroidism?
    A. It is usually due to an underlying parathyroid carcinoma
    B. It is most commonly seen after successful kidney transplantation
    C. The serum calcium level is usually normal or low
    D. Distinguishing between secondary and tertiary hyperparathyroidism is essential because the management differs
    E. It only occurs in patients with chronic renal insufficiency

40. The most common extra adrenal site of pheochromocytoma is the:
    A. Rectum
    B. Bladder
    C. Neck
    D. Organ of Zuckerkandl
    E. Sacrum

41. Which of the following is true regarding neuroblastoma?
    A. It is the third most common abdominal malignancy in children
    B. Prognosis is better for older children than those diagnosed before 1 year of age
    C. It is associated with aniridia and hemihypertrophy
    D. In the mediastinum, they are most often located anteriorly
    E. Amplification of the *N-myc* oncogene has an unfavorable prognosis

42. During thyroidectomy, the superior thyroid arteries were ligated a centimeter away from the thyroid capsule as opposed to immediately adjacent to it. This technical error would most likely result in which of the following complications?
    A. Loss of voice projection
    B. Loss of airway
    C. Hoarseness
    D. Aspiration
    E. Ineffective cough

43. A 45-year-old woman with a history of a goiter presents to the emergency department with a high fever, heart rate of 130 beats per minute, tremors, sweating, and exophthalmos. Which of the following can exacerbate symptoms?
    A. Aspirin
    B. Propylthiouracil
    C. Beta-blocker
    D. Methimazole
    E. Steroids

44. Which of the following is true regarding substernal goiter?
    A. Surgical resection should be reserved for patients with tracheal deviation
    B. Most are primary mediastinal goiters with a blood supply arising from intrathoracic vessels
    C. Most can be resected by a cervical incision
    D. Most are highly responsive to prolonged thyroid suppression
    E. Because of the risk of tracheomalacia, most patients should have a prophylactic tracheostomy at the time of resection

45. The most common cause of primary adrenal insufficiency in the United States is:
    A. Autoimmune
    B. Tuberculosis
    C. Metastatic disease
    D. Adrenal hemorrhage
    E. Exogenous steroid use

46. The most common cause of Cushing syndrome aside from exogenous corticosteroid administration is:
    A. Adrenal cortical carcinoma
    B. Adrenal adenoma
    C. Corticotropin (ACTH)-producing pituitary adenoma
    D. Ectopic ACTH syndrome
    E. Ectopic corticotropin-releasing hormone syndrome

47. Which of the following is true regarding the renin-angiotensin system?
    A. The juxtaglomerular cells are located within the renal efferent arteriole
    B. The juxtaglomerular cells secrete aldosterone in response to decreased blood pressure
    C. The juxtaglomerular cells detect changes in chloride concentration in the renal tubule
    D. Renin catalyzes the conversion of angiotensinogen to angiotensin I
    E. Angiotensin I directly stimulates the production of aldosterone

48. Which of the following is true regarding the anatomy/blood supply to the adrenal glands?
    A. Venous drainage has more anatomic variability than arterial blood supply
    B. Catheter-based venous hormonal sampling is easier to perform on the right adrenal vein
    C. On the right, the adrenal vein drains into the right renal vein
    D. Right adrenalectomy is more likely to lead to life-threatening hemorrhage than left adrenalectomy
    E. The majority of the arterial blood supply arises from the celiac trunk

49. A 70-year-old man is found to have an incidental mass in his right adrenal gland on CT scan. He has no history of malignancy and has a normal blood pressure. The findings of the remainder of the history and physical examination are negative. Plasma free metanephrines are negative. The serum potassium level is normal. Urinary free cortisol is normal, and a 1-mg overnight dexamethasone suppression test shows a low cortisol level (1.5 µg/dL) the following morning. The mass is 4.5 cm on CT scan, has smooth borders, and has a low attenuation value. Which of the following is true regarding this condition?
    A. The patient should undergo a CT-guided needle biopsy
    B. The patient should undergo a laparoscopic adrenalectomy
    C. The patient should undergo an open adrenalectomy
    D. A repeat CT scan should be performed in 6 months
    E. The mass is most likely malignant

50. Which of the following is true regarding the histology of the adrenal gland?
    A. The zona glomerulosa is the inner layer of the adrenal cortex
    B. Cells in the zona fasciculata produce cortisol
    C. Cells in the zona reticularis produce aldosterone
    D. Medullary cells are chromaffin negative
    E. The zona reticularis is the middle layer of the adrenal cortex

51. A 38-year-old female with stage 2 chronic kidney disease is diagnosed with primary hyperparathyroidism. Preoperative localization studies indicate a single enlarged left inferior parathyroid gland. She undergoes minimally invasive single gland parathyroidectomy under local anesthesia. An enlarged gland is identified and removed. Intraoperative PTH levels are sent 10 minutes later, and a 40% drop in PTH from baseline is noted. Which of the following is true?
    A. One should proceed to four-gland exploration
    B. Repeat PTH level should be obtained at 20 minutes
    C. It is acceptable to close the wound
    D. The vein from where the PTH was sampled does not affect PTH decline
    E. The PTH decline is affected by the patient's kidney disease

52. The hallmark of multiple endocrine neoplasia type 2 (MEN 2) is:
    A. Unilateral pheochromocytoma
    B. Bilateral pheochromocytoma
    C. Medullary carcinoma of the thyroid
    D. Menin mutation
    E. Four-gland parathyroid hyperplasia

53. The most common cause of congenital adrenal hyperplasia is:
    A. 11β-Hydroxylase deficiency
    B. 3-Hydroxydehydrogenase deficiency
    C. 21-Hydroxylase deficiency
    D. 17-Hydroxylase deficiency
    E. Congenital adrenal lipoid hyperplasia

54. A 45-year-old man with a history of primary hyperparathyroidism presents for an enlarged thyroid nodule. Further workup reveals an elevated calcitonin level. Which of the following is true regarding the most likely condition?
    A. Bilateral prophylactic central node dissection is indicated in addition to total thyroidectomy
    B. Radiotherapy is an effective treatment modality
    C. Plasma or urine metanephrines do not need to be checked prior to intervention
    D. The likelihood of nodal metastases is low
    E. Chemotherapy is effective for residual disease

55. The most accurate test for hyperthyroidism is:
    A. Free thyroxine (T_4)
    B. Total T_4
    C. Total triiodothyronine (T_3)
    D. Thyroid-stimulating hormone (TSH)
    E. Thyroid scan

56. Which of the following is true regarding the blood supply to the thyroid/parathyroid glands?

A. The parathyroid glands are usually supplied by the superior thyroid arteries

B. The inferior thyroid artery is the first branch of the external carotid artery

C. The RLNs are at risk of injury during ligation of the superior thyroid arteries

D. The external branch of the superior laryngeal nerve is at risk of injury when the inferior laryngeal arteries are ligated

E. The thyroid ima artery usually arises from the aorta

57. Which of the following is true regarding the laryngeal nerves?

A. The external branch of the superior laryngeal nerve provides sensation to the larynx

B. Bilateral injury to the superior laryngeal nerves often results in acute airway obstruction

C. The right RLN separates from the vagus after crossing the subclavian artery

D. The recurrent laryngeal nerve is both motor and sensory to the larynx

E. The RLNs provide motor function to the cricothyroid

58. A nonrecurrent laryngeal nerve:

A. Does not exist

B. Is more common on the left

C. Can occur in conjunction with a recurrent nerve on the right

D. Loops around the aorta on the right side

E. Is less prone to injury during surgery than a recurrent nerve

59. Which of the following is a direct effect of parathyroid hormone?

A. Stimulates hydroxylation of cholecalciferol in the kidney

B. Stimulates reabsorption of phosphate by the kidney

C. Stimulates reabsorption of bicarbonate by the kidney

D. Stimulates absorption of calcium by the small intestine

E. Stimulates hydroxylation of 25-hydroxyvitamin D in the kidney

60. Lateral aberrant thyroid in most instances represents:

A. Metastatic papillary carcinoma

B. Metastatic follicular carcinoma

C. Metastatic Hürthle cell carcinoma

D. A congenital lesion related to thyroid descent

E. An extension of a thyroglossal duct cyst

61. A 45-year-old woman presents with a 1.5-cm right thyroid nodule. FNA findings are consistent with papillary carcinoma. Her history is significant for radiation therapy for lymphoma as a child. Optimal management of this patient would consist of:

A. Right hemithyroidectomy

B. Right hemithyroidectomy plus central lymph node dissection

C. Total thyroidectomy

D. Total thyroidectomy plus right modified radical neck dissection

E. Total thyroidectomy with postoperative [131]I

Answers

1. D. Primary hyperaldosteronism is secondary to the release of excess aldosterone from one or both adrenal glands. The diagnosis is made biochemically, ideally after discontinuation of antihypertensives, with an aldosterone to renin ration of 20 to 30. Once a biochemical diagnosis is made, a thin-cut adrenal CT should be the initial method of localization. In the case of a unilateral adrenal lesion, some surgeons advocate proceeding with adrenalectomy if the lesion is >1 cm and the contralateral adrenal gland is normal on CT. Alternatively, some surgeons recommend routine adrenal venous sampling in most patients, especially those older than 40 years old as they are more likely to have nonfunctioning adrenal adenomas. In the setting of bilateral adenomas on CT, adrenal venous sampling should be performed (A, B). It would be inappropriate to perform bilateral adrenalectomy without further attempts at localizing the source (C). Functional nuclear medicine studies can also aid with lateralization but is typically performed if venous sampling is unsuccessful (E). Further, if this patient's hyperaldosteronism is due to hyperplasia, it would be treated medically.

Reference: Yeh MW, Livhits MJ, Duh Q. The adrenal glands. In: Townsend CM Jr, Beauchamp RD, Evers BM, Mattox KL. *Sabiston textbook of surgery: the biological basis of modern surgical practice.* 20th ed. Elsevier; 2016:963–995.

2. E. Incidentalomas are discovered in 1% to 4% of imaging studies that are evaluating an unrelated issue. The majority of incidentalomas are nonfunctioning adenomas (60%). The remaining tumors in a patient that do not have a history of malignancy include pheochromocytoma, cortisol-producing adenoma, aldosteronoma, adrenocortical carcinoma, and myelolipoma. There should be a high level of suspicion for adrenal metastasis in a patient with a history of malignancy and/or bilateral lesions. All adrenal incidentalomas should undergo biochemical testing to evaluate for subclinical Cushing syndrome, pheochromocytoma, and aldosteronoma (E). A functional incidentaloma is an indication for adrenalectomy. For patients with negative biochemical testing and size <3 cm can effectively be monitored with surveillance cross sectional imaging to evaluate for growth (B). Annual biochemical testing is often performed as well for up to 5 years. Indications for adrenalectomy for nonfunctioning incidentalomas include size >5 cm. For patients with 3 to 5 cm nonfunctioning incidentalomas, adrenalectomy can be considered for patients with few surgical risk factors and those with concerning radiographic features (irregular borders, central necrosis, high vascularity, and internal calcifications) (A). PET CT is not part of the initial workup (D). No further testing would be incorrect (C).

Reference: Yeh MW, Livhits MJ, Duh Q. The adrenal glands. In: Townsend CM Jr, Beauchamp RD, Evers BM, Mattox KL. *Sabiston textbook of surgery: the biological basis of modern surgical practice.* 20th ed. Elsevier; 2016:963–995.

3. B. Surgery is indicated in asymptomatic patients under the age of 50 that are suspected to have primary hyperparathyroidism. Familial hypocalciuric hypercalcemia (FHH) causes mild increase in serum calcium and can initially be misdiagnosed as primary hyperparathyroidism. It is a benign condition due to mutations in *CASR*, which encodes a calcium receptor. The lack of calcium signal increases the PTH level, which increases renal calcium reabsorption. Thus, part of the workup of primary hyperparathyroidism is to obtain a 24-hour urine calcium. Hypercalciuria with a high PTH level and high serum calcium level confirms primary hyperparathyroidism. A low urine calcium level suggests FHH. Once FHH is ruled out, four-gland neck exploration can be performed without the need for further imaging (C). Tertiary hyperparathyroidism typically occurs in patients with renal failure, most of whom have undergone kidney transplantation (A). Cinacalcet is indicated for patients with secondary hyperparathyroidism (D). Selective venous sampling is an invasive procedure that is indicated in patients with recurrent hyperparathyroidism, when other forms of imaging fail to identify the abnormal gland (E).

4. A. Noninvasive localization studies should always be employed before taking a patient to surgery for primary hyperparathyroidism. Indications for parathyroidectomy in the asymptomatic patient include serum calcium >1 mg/dL above normal, age <50, evidence of end-organ dysfunction (decreased creatinine clearance or low bone density). In this young patient, with hypercalcemia greater than 1 mg/dL above normal, surgery should be offered (E). However, it is not uncommon for patients to have negative noninvasive localization studies. In a patient who has not had previous neck exploration, he/she can be taken to surgery for parathyroid exploration. Ultimately, patients with negative imaging remain candidates for parathyroidectomy given the high rate of false-negative imaging. Patients with negative noninvasive localization studies who have had a previous

neck exploration for primary hyperthyroidism and have persistent or recurrent hyperparathyroidism pose a more difficult scenario. These patients may benefit from invasive localization via venous sampling prior to remedial neck exploration (C). MRI is rarely indicated as primary imaging for localization. It is reserved patients who are not candidates for other imaging (e.g., pregnant patients). It may be useful in the setting of a surgical reexploration of the neck. However, this patient has not had a previous exploration and already has negative imaging with modalities that carry greater sensitivity and specificity than MRI (D). Cinacalcet is indicated for patients with secondary hyperparathyroidism due to chronic kidney disease (B).

Reference: Wilhelm SM, Wang TS, Ruan DT, et al. The American Association of Endocrine Surgeons guidelines for definitive management of primary hyperparathyroidism. *JAMA Surg.* 2016;151(10):959–968.

5. C. Transient hypocalcemia following thyroidectomy is a known complication and can occur in 2% to 53% of patients undergoing total thyroidectomy. The etiology is likely multifactorial and includes reversible ischemia to the parathyroid glands, hypothermia to the glands, and endothelin-1 release (known to suppress PTH production). Additionally, iatrogenic removal of one or several parathyroid glands is possible during thyroidectomy and can contribute to postoperative hypocalcemia. Patients with hypocalcemia can present with neuromuscular excitability, tetany (Chvostek sign), circumoral paresthesia, seizures, QT prolongation on ECG, and cardiac arrest (B). However, most patients with transient hypocalcemia following thyroid surgery are asymptomatic (D). Independent predictors of hypocalcemia following thyroidectomy include low postoperative PTH level, female gender, and patients with a malignant neoplasm (E). Several studies have demonstrated that the routine use of postoperative administration of calcium and vitamin D can reduce the incidence and/or severity of hypocalcemia. HBS is extremely rare. It has also been proposed as a possible contributing factor but occurs more frequently after parathyroid surgery. However, similar to PTH, thyroid hormone can also provide a stimulus to break down bone, and once this stimulus is removed, the bones attempt to deplete their calcium by removing it from serum, which can lead to HBS. This typically presents with hypophosphatemia and hypomagnesemia and is usually seen in patients with severe preoperative bone disease (A).

References: Alhefdhi A, Mazeh H, Chen H. Role of postoperative vitamin D and/or calcium routine supplementation in preventing hypocalcemia after thyroidectomy: a systematic review and meta-analysis. *Oncologist.* 2013;18(5):533–542.

Grodski S, Serpell J. Evidence for the role of perioperative PTH measurement after total thyroidectomy as a predictor of hypocalcemia. *World J Surg.* 2008;32(7):1367–1373.

6. B. The elevated plasma metanephrine indicates a high suspicion for pheochromocytoma. Further workup for this should include a CT or MRI scan of the abdomen to detect an adrenal mass. The elevated calcium suggests hyperparathyroidism. The patient should have a PTH level measured and, if it is elevated, should undergo a sestamibi scan. Given these findings, the patient most likely has MEN type 2, which is characterized by pheochromocytoma, hyperparathyroidism, and MTC. Screening for MTC involves measuring the serum calcitonin level. MEN type 1 is characterized by hyperparathyroidism, pituitary tumor, and pancreatic tumors. CT of the sella turcica may be used to look for a pituitary tumor such as prolactinoma (A). An elevated prolactin level will also support a diagnosis of prolactinoma (D). Elevated gastrin level is associated with gastrinoma (C). A 24-hour urine cortisol level can be used in the workup for Cushing syndrome (E).

7. B. PTH inhibits phosphate reabsorption at the proximal convoluted tubule, thereby lowering phosphate levels (A). It also inhibits the Na^+/H^+ antiporter. This leads to an inhibition of bicarbonate excretion in the urine, resulting in a mild metabolic acidosis and corresponding hyperchloremia (D). This subsequently results in an elevated chloride-to-phosphate ratio (>33). PTH levels are increased (E). Hypercalcemia typically results in hypercalciuria, with the exception being in patients with familial hypocalciuric hypercalcemia (C).

8. C. Parathyroid carcinoma is extremely rare and accounts for less than 1% of cases of primary hyperparathyroidism. It should be suspected in the setting of severe symptoms of hypercalcemia, in association with very high serum calcium (usually 14.6–15.0 mg/dL) and PTH, history of kidney stones and pathologic fractures, and a palpable neck mass (A, B). Benign causes of hyperparathyroidism very rarely result in a palpable neck mass and are less likely to cause a hypercalcemic crisis. Determination of malignancy is difficult because, similar to other endocrine malignancies, there are not any classic histologic features that reliably distinguish parathyroid malignancy from benign disease. Thus, one must look for evidence of local invasion at the time of surgery as well as enlarged lymph nodes. Treatment is surgical and involves en bloc resection of the parathyroid tumor with the ipsilateral thyroid gland, as well as a modified radical lymph node dissection if nodal metastasis is present. Recently, cinacalcet was approved by the US Food and Drug Administration and is effective in controlling the hypercalcemia associated with parathyroid carcinoma. Breast cancer with bone metastasis may be associated with a paraneoplastic syndrome in which a high level of PTH-related protein is found. This is unlikely to present with a palpable neck mass (D). Secondary hyperparathyroidism is associated with a low level of serum calcium (E).

Reference: Shane E. Parathyroid carcinoma. *J Clin Endocrinol Metab*. 2001;86(2):485–493.

Sharretts JM, Kebebew E, Simonds WF. Parathyroid cancer. *Semin Oncol*. 2010;37(6):580–590.

9. A. On occasion, despite careful neck exploration, only three parathyroid glands will be encountered. A careful search for the ectopic gland should be conducted (B, C). The inferior glands are more likely to be ectopic than the superior ones. Most inferior glands are to be found within 2 cm of the inferior thyroid pole. If not found, the next step is to perform a cervical thymectomy and send the tissue for frozen section. If still glands are not found, the carotid sheath should be opened. Intraoperative ultrasonography should then be used to determine whether there is an intrathyroidal parathyroid gland. If ultrasonography is not available, ipsilateral thyroid lobectomy should be considered. Another useful modality in

this setting is intraoperative gamma probe detection. Likewise, intraoperative PTH assays can assist in determining whether the pathologic gland has been removed. Ectopic parathyroid glands are only rarely found in the mediastinum, so a median sternotomy is not recommended unless all other options are explored (D). Biopsy may result in ischemia of the parathyroid glands (E).

10. C. Serum thyroglobulin levels are the most useful modality to monitor patients for recurrence of differentiated thyroid cancer (papillary and follicular) after total thyroidectomy and radioactive iodine ablation. Thyroglobulin is a glycoprotein that is the primary component of colloid matrix within the thyroid follicle. Thyroglobulin levels in patients who have undergone total thyroidectomy should be 3 ng/mL or less when the patient is receiving thyroid hormone replacement therapy and less than 5 ng/mL when thyroid hormone supplementation is withheld. Serum thyroglobulin levels seem to be most predictive of recurrence when patients are hypothyroid as documented by a high TSH level (A). An increase above these levels is highly suggestive of metastatic disease. The recommendation after thyroidectomy is to check thyroglobulin levels initially at 6-month intervals after surgery. If the thyroglobulin levels are elevated, an ^{131}I scan is recommended (D). Recurrence of MTC is determined by calcitonin levels (B). Routine cross-sectional surveillance imaging via CT or MRI is not currently recommended. Periodic ultrasound in addition to thyroglobulin is recommended by the NCCN for select patients with a high risk for recurrence (E).

References: Baudin E, Do Cao C, Cailleux AF, et al. Positive predictive value of serum thyroglobulin levels, measured during the first year of follow-up after thyroid hormone withdrawal, in thyroid cancer patients. *J Clin Endocrinol Metab*. 2003;88(3):1107–1111.

Duren M, Siperstein AE, Shen W, et al. Value of stimulated serum thyroglobulin levels for detecting persistent or recurrent differentiated thyroid cancer in high- and low-risk patients. *Surgery*. 1999;126(1):13–19.

Lal G, Clark OH. Thyroid, parathyroid and adrenal. In: Brunicardi FC, Andersen DK, Billiar TR, et al., eds. *Schwartz's principles of surgery*. 8th ed. New York: McGraw-Hill; 2005:1395–1470.

11. A. Adrenocortical carcinomas are rare. They should be suspected in the presence of large tumors (>5–6 cm) or if the CT scan shows evidence of necrosis, hemorrhage, or local invasion. Approximately 60% of patients with adrenocortical carcinoma present with hormonal excess, including Cushing syndrome and virilization. There are no distinctive histologic or cytologic features that distinguish adrenocortical carcinoma from an adenoma (C). Thus, one must rely on evidence of local invasion, lymph node metastasis, or distant metastasis. CT-guided needle biopsy is not recommended (B). The best chance for cure is surgical resection. Open adrenalectomy is the standard of care for surgical resection for adrenal cortical carcinoma as the laparoscopic approach is associated with higher local recurrence rates and poorer disease-free survival (E). Adrenal masses that are hormonally active should be excised. In the absence of hormonal activity and in the absence of CT scan features suggestive of malignancy, resection is recommended for asymptomatic masses if they are larger than 5 to 6 cm (D).

Reference: Ng L, Libertino JM. Adrenocortical carcinoma: diagnosis, evaluation and treatment. *J Urol*. Published online 2003:5–11.

12. B. The frequency of thyroid carcinoma among patients with a surgically removed thyroglossal duct cyst in one large series was 0.7%. The majority is papillary cancer that is found incidentally after a Sistrunk procedure (performed for the cyst) (A, C–E). If discovered incidentally, the patient should subsequently undergo a total thyroidectomy because additional cancer is usually found within the thyroid gland as well.

Reference: Heshmati HM, Fatourechi V, van Heerden JA, Hay ID, Goellner JR. Thyroglossal duct carcinoma: report of 12 cases. *Mayo Clin Proc.* 1997;72(4):315–319.

13. A. The RLN innervates the intrinsic muscles of the larynx, except the cricothyroid muscles, which are innervated by the external branch of the superior laryngeal nerve (C). The internal branch of the superior laryngeal nerve provides sensory input for the pharynx (B). Injury to one RLN leads to paralysis of the ipsilateral vocal cord. The cord becomes fixed in either the paramedian position or the abducted position. If the cord becomes fixed in the paramedian position, the patient will have a weak voice, whereas if it becomes fixed in the abducted position, the patient will have a hoarse voice and an ineffective cough. If both RLNs are injured, an airway obstruction may develop acutely in the patient. Trauma from endotracheal intubation or compression from hematoma does not typically cause vocal cord paralysis (D, E).

14. B. Pituitary tumors are the third most common tumors in MEN 1. The majority are prolactinomas (A, C–E). They may cause bitemporal hemianopsia due to local compression of the optic chiasm resulting in loss of peripheral vision or may lead to amenorrhea and galactorrhea in women or hypogonadism in men. Women are more likely to present early in the course of the disease as they are more likely to have hormonal symptoms. Men typically present later with mass-effect of the tumor (visual changes, headaches, etc.).

15. E. Graves disease is the most common cause of hyperthyroidism in the United States and is due to antibodies targeting thyrotropin receptors, which increase production of thyroid hormone. Patients present with anxiety, rapid or irregular heart rate, heat intolerance, weight loss, thinning hair, decreased libido, diarrhea, thick and shiny skin (Graves dermopathy), and exophthalmos. The preferred therapy is radioactive iodine ablation, but medical therapy with propylthiouracil (PTU) or methimazole is also available. Exophthalmos develops in about 10% of patients and is the only symptom that is resistant to antithyroid therapy and even worsens after radioactive iodine ablation (A–D). Some studies suggest that the use of prednisone before antithyroid therapy can help improve exophthalmos.

References: Bartalena L, Marcocci C, Bogazzi F, et al. Relation between therapy for hyperthyroidism and the course of Graves' ophthalmopathy. *N Engl J Med.* 1998;338(2):73–78.

Shiber S, Stiebel-Kalish H, Shimon I, Grossman A, Robenshtok E. Glucocorticoid regimens for prevention of Graves' ophthalmopathy progression following radioiodine treatment: systematic review and meta-analysis. *Thyroid.* 2014;24(10):1515–1523.

Stein JD, Childers D, Gupta S. Risk factors for developing thyroid-associated ophthalmopathy among individuals with Graves' disease. *JAMA.* 2015;133(3):290–296.

16. C. Primary hyperaldosteronism should be suspected in patients with hypertension and hypokalemia. Primary hyperaldosteronism results from autonomous aldosterone secretion, which, in turn, leads to suppression of renin secretion. The diagnosis is made by demonstrating a combination of inappropriate potassium excretion in the urine (kaliuresis), low plasma renin, and a high aldosterone-to-renin ratio (>20). While it was previously believed that an adrenal adenoma (Conn syndrome) was the most common cause of primary hyperaldosteronism, we now know that nearly 60% of cases are due to idiopathic bilateral adrenal hyperplasia (IBAH). It is important to clearly establish the etiology because the management is different. An adrenal adenoma should be removed with a unilateral adrenalectomy but IBAH is managed with medical therapy alone using a mineralocorticoid replacement such as spironolactone or eplerenone. Amiloride and triamterene are also potassium-sparing diuretics but are less optimal (A, B). A double-blind randomized controlled study demonstrated the superiority of spironolactone in controlling hypertension compared with eplerenone (E). Bilateral adrenalectomy is considered in cases of severe refractory hypertension. However, this has a high risk of complications and will subject the patient to lifelong dependence of mineralocorticoids (fludrocortisone) and steroids. Phenoxybenzamine is an alpha-1 receptor antagonist used in the preoperative management of pheochromocytoma (D).

References: Kaplan NM. The current epidemic of primary aldosteronism: causes and consequences. *J Hypertens.* 2004;22(5):863–869.

Stowasser M. Update in primary aldosteronism. *J Clin Endocrinol Metab.* 2009;94(10):3623–3630.

Parthasarathy HK, Ménard J, White WB, et al. A double-blind, randomized study comparing the antihypertensive effect of eplerenone and spironolactone in patients with hypertension and evidence of primary aldosteronism. *J Hypertens.* 2011;29(5):980–990.

17. C. The AJCC/TNM staging system does not adequately predict the risk of recurrence in differentiated thyroid cancer. Thus, the ATA developed a 3-tiered clinic-pathologic risk stratification for recurrence in 2009 with modifications in 2015. For papillary thyroid carcinoma, low-risk patients include those having intrathyroidal tumors without extrathyroidal extension, vascular invasion, metastases, aggressive histology, and clinical N0 or ≤5 N1 micrometastases (<0.2 cm in largest dimension). Intermediate-risk patients include those with microscopic invasion into the perithyroidal tissue, aggressive histology, ascular invasion, and clinical N1 or >5 pathologic N1 nodes with all involved nodes <3 cm in largest dimension. High-risk patients are those with macroscopic invasion of perithyroidal tissue, incomplete tumor resection, distant metastases, and pathologic N1 disease with any node >3 cm in largest dimension. This patient has intermediate disease based on 2 factors: microinvasion into perithyroidal tissue and a metastatic lymph node <3 cm (C). Macroinvasion or incomplete resection is high-risk, not microinvasion (E). Tumor size is not a component of the ATA risk stratification system (B, D). The absence of vascular invasion is a low-risk feature, but this patient had other factors that make her intermediate risk (A).

Reference: Haugen BR, Alexander EK, Bible KC, et al. 2015 American Thyroid Association management guidelines for adult patients with thyroid nodules and differentiated thyroid cancer: the American Thyroid Association Guidelines Task Force on Thyroid Nodules and Differentiated Thyroid Cancer. *Thyroid.* 2016;26(1):1–133.

18. A. The most important test in the evaluation of a solitary thyroid nodule is FNA. This can be performed with ultrasound guidance if the lesion is difficult to palpate. Before the routine use of FNA, there was a high rate of benign thyroid surgical resections. With current practice, the percentage of thyroid nodules resected that are found to be malignant is over 50%. The Bethesda system for reporting thyroid cytopathology classifies nodules into six groups: (1) nondiagnostic or unsatisfactory, (2) benign, (3) atypia of undetermined significance or follicular lesion of undetermined significance, (4) follicular neoplasm or suspicious for a follicular neoplasm, (5) suspicious for malignancy, and (6) malignant. Patients with a nondiagnostic or unsatisfactory FNA should have a repeat FNA performed (B–E).

References: Cibas ES, Ali SZ, NCI Thyroid FNA State of the Science Conference. The Bethesda System for Reporting Thyroid Cytopathology. *Am J Clin Pathol*. 2009;132(5):658–665.

Yassa L, Cibas ES, Benson CB, et al. Long-term assessment of a multidisciplinary approach to thyroid nodule diagnostic evaluation. *Cancer*. 2007;111(6):508–516.

19. C. FNA results are classified into six different groups based on the Bethesda criteria. The management of FNA that is reported as FLUS is somewhat controversial. The current recommendation is to perform a repeat FNA (A). The risk of malignancy of FLUS has historically been around 5% to 15%. However, more recent series have found a malignancy rate closer to 30%. These authors recommend proceeding to thyroid lobectomy. Thus, the decision as to whether to repeat the FNA or proceed to thyroid lobectomy depends on patient risk factors for malignancy; the institutional rate of malignancy with FLUS; ultrasound features of the lesion; and more recently, molecular testing (not always available and expensive) (B, E). Follicular neoplasms will require a surgical lobectomy, and FNA demonstrating malignancy or suspicion for a malignant process will require a total thyroidectomy (D). Core needle biopsy has been proposed as an additional adjunctive tool, particularly in cases of nondiagnostic FNA but there have not been any conclusive studies to demonstrate its usefulness, nor is it considered the current standard of care. It may be considered for patients that are hesitant to proceed with surgical resection.

References: Cibas ES, Ali SZ, NCI Thyroid FNA State of the Science Conference. The Bethesda System for Reporting Thyroid Cytopathology. *Am J Clin Pathol*. 2009;132(5):658–665.

Yoon JH, Kim EK, Kwak JY, Moon HJ. Effectiveness and limitations of core needle biopsy in the diagnosis of thyroid nodules: review of current literature. *J Pathol Transl Med*. 2015;49(3):230–235.

20. A. The thyroid gland is one of the earliest endocrine glands to develop. It arises from the first and second pharyngeal arches. The superior parathyroid gland develops from the fourth pharyngeal pouch while the inferior parathyroid gland develops from the third pharyngeal pouch (B, D). An easy way to remember this is that the "**P**arathyroid derives from the **P**ouch." The third pharyngeal arch helps in the development of the stylopharyngeus muscle while the fourth pharyngeal arch allows for the development of the cricothyroid muscle (C, E).

21. B. The most common primary tumor to metastasize to the thyroid is renal cell carcinoma. Other primary cancers that metastasize to the thyroid gland, in descending order, include lung, breast, and esophageal cancer (C–E). Parathyroid gland carcinoma does not metastasize to the thyroid gland (A).

References: Nakhjavani MK, Gharib H, Goellner JR, van Heerden JA. Metastasis to the thyroid gland. A report of 43 cases. *Cancer*. 1997;79(3):574–578.

Stevens TM, Richards AT, Bewtra C, Sharma P. Tumors metastatic to thyroid neoplasms: a case report and review of the literature. *Patholog Res Int*. 2011;2011:238693.

22. D. The synthesis of catecholamines is a complex process and is governed by various enzymes. Tyrosine hydroxylase is considered the rate-limiting step and converts L-tyrosine to L-dopa, which is then converted to dopamine by dopa-decarboxylase (A). Dopamine is converted to norepinephrine by dopamine-beta-hydroxylase and norepinephrine is converted to epinephrine by PNMT (B, C). COMT metabolizes both norepinephrine and epinephrine (E). With the exception of PNMT, all the other enzymes have the name of the precursor as part of their nomenclature, which allows for an easy way to remember the key steps. PNMT is rarely present outside of the adrenal medulla, which accounts for why extra-adrenal pheochromocytomas do not synthesize a high level of norepinephrine. The brain stem, retina, and cardiac tissue may also contain PNMT.

Reference: Ziegler MG, Bao X, Kennedy BP, Joyner A, Enns R. Location, development, control, and function of extraadrenal phenylethanolamine N-methyltransferase. *Ann N Y Acad Sci*. 2002;971(1):76–82.

23. C. Fever, hypotension, nausea, and dizziness in a patient taking chronic steroids that suddenly stopped taking all medications should raise concern for acute adrenal insufficiency. When the diagnosis is suspected, treatment should begin immediately before confirmatory tests become available (E). Initial treatment consists of IV normal saline volume resuscitation. This is then followed by either administration of 4 mg of dexamethasone or 100 mg of hydrocortisone (B). Dexamethasone is preferred because it will not interfere with cosyntropin stimulation testing, which should be done the next morning to confirm the diagnosis. IV antibiotics are not used in acute adrenal insufficiency (A). Cessation of methotrexate does not present with the aforementioned symptoms (D).

24. A. This patient has metastatic midgut neuroendocrine tumor (NET). The finding of fibrosis and tethering of the mesentery is highly suggestive of a carcinoid tumor. The accompanying diarrhea, combined with likely liver metastasis, is highly suggestive of carcinoid syndrome. Compared to the foregut, midgut, and hindgut, NETs have a greater 5-year survival rate. Chemotherapy has not been shown to have a significant role in increasing disease-free survival. Symptom control is achieved with somatostatin analogs such as octreotide. Some of the few accepted lifelong indications for the use of octreotide, endorsed by the American Association of Oncology, include patients with peptide/amine-induced syndromes with clinical symptoms and for patients with progression of metastatic disease even without a syndrome. This patient will require postoperative octreotide, given his history of watery diarrhea. Octreotide promotes biliary sludging and leads to a high rate of symptomatic cholelithiasis and as such, cholecystectomy is recommended at the time of surgery (E). This indication becomes stronger in patients that are planned to undergo hepatic artery embolization secondary to metastasis to the liver. Liver biopsy or resection is not appropriate during an emergency surgery (particularly when the lesion is not readily palpable) and his disease is likely amenable to less morbid procedures such as radiofrequency ablation and/or hepatic artery embolization (B, C). There is no indication to perform an appendectomy in the above patient (D).

Reference: Öberg K, Kvols L, Caplin M, et al. Consensus report on the use of somatostatin analogs for the management of neuroendocrine tumors of the gastroenteropancreatic system. *Ann Oncol.* 2004;15(6):966–973.

25. A. Hürthle cell carcinoma accounts for less than 10% of thyroid malignancies and is considered a subtype of follicular cancer. Like follicular cancer, the presence of malignancy is established by the demonstration of vascular or capsular invasion. FNA and frozen section do not reliably establish malignancy (C). The tumors contain sheets of eosinophilic cells packed with mitochondria, which are derived from oncocytic or oxyphilic cells of the thyroid gland. Hürthle cell carcinomas differ from follicular cell carcinomas in that they are often multifocal and bilateral, are more likely to metastasize to local nodes and distant sites, and are associated with a higher mortality rate (B). Residual disease is not effectively treated with radioactive iodine because Hürthle cell carcinomas do not take up radioactive iodine (D). Orphan Annie cells are a hallmark of papillary carcinoma (E). Unlike differentiated thyroid cancer, nodal metastases predict a worse outcome in widely invasive Hürthle cell carcinoma, as does extrathyroidal extension.

Reference: Stojadinovic A, Ghossein RA, Hoos A, et al. Hürthle cell carcinoma: a critical histopathologic appraisal. *J Clin Oncol.* 2001;19(10):2616–2625.

26. D. Technetium-99m sestamibi imaging is the most widely used and accurate modality, with sensitivity greater than 80% for detection of parathyroid adenomas. High-resolution ultrasonography in particular is complementary. The other imaging techniques are thought to be more useful when sestamibi scanning fails to identify the parathyroid pathology, for the workup of recurrent hyperparathyroidism, or when surgical exploration fails to identify the parathyroid lesion (A, C). Ultrasonography has an overall lower sensitivity, although it may be most useful in identifying intrathyroidal parathyroids (E). Some institutions utilize 4-D parathyroid protocol CT, which has demonstrated higher sensitivities than sestamibi and neck ultrasound (B). The combination of 4-D CT and ultrasound has demonstrated a sensitivity of 94% and specificity of 96% for localizing hyperfunctioning parathyroid glands. MRI generally not used in localization studies unless other methods are contraindicated (e.g., pregnancy).

Reference: Quinn CE, Udelsman R. The parathyroid glands. In: Townsend CM Jr, Beauchamp RD, Evers BM, Mattox KL, eds. *Sabiston textbook of surgery: the biological basis of modern surgical practice.* 20th ed. Elsevier; 2016:122–136.

27. B. Follicular cancer is the second most common thyroid cancer, and it spreads primarily via a hematogenous route with the lung as its primary site of metastasis (A). Multicentricity is uncommon (E). Unlike papillary carcinoma, accurate diagnosis using FNA is not possible because cytologic features cannot distinguish a benign follicular lesion from a follicular carcinoma. To establish malignancy, demonstration of capsular or vascular invasion on histology is necessary. Thus, if FNA demonstrates a follicular neoplasm, the patient should undergo a thyroid lobectomy to determine malignancy. Once histologic confirmation of malignancy is made, total thyroidectomy is recommended with or without postoperative ¹³¹I. Total thyroidectomy also permits the detection of subsequent metastasis using nuclear scanning (D). Postoperative radioactive iodine following total thyroidectomy is indicated for all tumors larger than 4 cm, gross extrathyroidal extension of the tumor regardless of size, lymph node metastases, and for high-risk features including tall-cell or columnar-cell variant (D). An added advantage of postoperative radiation is that it allows for continued monitoring for recurrence with thyroglobulin. Prophylactic nodal dissection is not required (C).

28. A. Surgical management of a solitary parathyroid adenoma consists of resection of the single enlarged gland. After resection of the candidate parathyroid thyroid gland for adenoma, intraoperative parathyroid hormone (PTH) is routinely measured to ensure an appropriate drop post resection. On rare occasions, double adenomas are present. For four-gland hyperplasia, resection of 3.5 glands is recommended. Alternatively, resection of all four glands with reimplantation of half of one gland into the brachioradialis muscle in the forearm can be performed. Removing all four glands without reimplantation increases the risk for hypoparathyroidism (B). Medical management is not appropriate for primary hyperparathyroidism (C). On occasion, distinguishing between adenoma and hyperplasia may be difficult if two glands are enlarged and the other two appear normal or slightly enlarged. In this circumstance, removal of the two enlarged glands and biopsy of an additional gland may be performed to rule out four-gland hyperplasia. However, in the presence of one enlarged gland, there is no role for biopsy of the other three glands because this may result in ischemia of the remaining parathyroid glands (D, E). Another frequent dilemma occurs when only three glands are found, and all appear normal. If an studies unless other methods are contraindicated inferior one is missing, it may be found in the thymus, angle of the mandible, at the skull base, superior to the superior parathyroid glands, or, rarely, within the thyroid gland. If the ectopic gland is not found, transcervical thymectomy is recommended. If the superior gland is missing, it may be found within the thyroid gland, in the paraesophageal or retroesophageal grooves, or caudal to the inferior glands. Although ectopic glands are found in the mediastinum on rare occasion, median sternotomy is not recommended at initial exploration.

Reference: Quinn CE, Udelsman R. The parathyroid glands. In: Townsend CM Jr, Beauchamp RD, Evers BM, Mattox KL, eds. *Sabiston textbook of surgery: the biological basis of modern surgical practice.* 20th ed. Elsevier; 2016:45–55.

29. A. Laparoscopic adrenalectomy has become the procedure of choice for small- and medium-sized functional and benign adrenal tumors. Pheochromocytoma is not a contraindication to the laparoscopic approach and may be used successfully for unilateral or bilateral tumors (B, C). Tumor size alone is not a contraindication to the laparoscopic approach. For a large tumor that is clearly malignant based on CT scan evidence of local invasion or lymph node metastasis, the laparoscopic approach is contraindicated (E). Open adrenalectomy is preferred for pheochromocytomas larger than 6 cm. (D).

References: Assalia A, Gagner M. Laparoscopic adrenalectomy. Br J Surg. 2004;91(10):1259–1274.

Brunt LM, Moley JF. In: Townsend CM, Jr, Beauchamp RD, Evers BM, Mattox KL, eds. *Sabiston textbook of surgery: the biological basis of modern surgical practice.* 17th ed. Philadelphia: W.B. Saunders; 2004:1023–1070.

Laimore TC, Moley JF. The multiple endocrine neoplasia syndromes. In: Townsend CM, Jr, Beauchamp RD, Evers BM, Mattox KL, eds. *Sabiston textbook of surgery: the biological basis of modern surgical practice.* 17th ed. Philadelphia: W.B. Saunders; 2004:1071–1090.

Lal G, Clark OH. Thyroid, parathyroid and adrenal. In: Brunicardi FC, Andersen DK, Billiar TR, et al., eds. *Schwartz's principles of surgery.* 8th ed. New York: McGraw-Hill; 2005:1395–1470.

30. A. Hashimoto thyroiditis is an autoimmune disorder that leads to destruction of thyroid follicles by both cell- and antibody-mediated immune processes, including activation of helper lymphocytes and antibody formation against thyroglobulin and thyroid peroxidase. It is the leading cause of hypothyroidism and most commonly affects young females. It results in a lymphocytic infiltration. Treatment of Hashimoto thyroiditis is with thyroid hormone replacement. Hashimoto thyroiditis is associated with primary thyroid lymphoma. The chronic antigenic stimulation coupled with a chronic proliferation of lymphoid tissue in the thyroid is thought to lead to the development of lymphocytic transformation. In a patient with Hashimoto thyroiditis, lymphoma should be suspected in the setting of a rapidly enlarging thyroid mass (B–E). Patients additionally may report fever, cervical lymphadenopathy, dysphagia, and hoarseness. FNA may suggest the diagnosis, but flow cytometry (with core needle biopsy) is required to confirm the diagnosis. The treatment recommendation is chemotherapy using CHOP (cyclophosphamide, doxorubicin, vincristine, and prednisone) and radiation therapy in most cases of thyroid lymphoma. Hashimoto thyroiditis also does increase the risk of thyroid cancer.

Reference: Ansell SM, Grant CS, Habermann TM. Primary thyroid lymphoma. *Semin Oncol.* 1999;26(3):316–323.

31. D. Hyperparathyroidism is classically associated with "stones (calcium phosphate or oxalate kidney stones), moans (not feeling well), groans (vague abdominal pain, peptic ulcer disease, pancreatitis, gallstones, and constipation), bones (bone pain, osteoporosis, osteitis fibrosa cystica, brown [osteoclastic] tumors), and psychiatric overtones (depression, fatigue)." Pancreatitis tends to occur in patients with a very high serum calcium level (>12.5 mg/dL). The increased incidence of cholelithiasis is due to increased biliary calcium, leading to formation of calcium bilirubinate stones. Diarrhea is not typically associated with hyperparathyroidism but constipation is (A–C, E).

32. E. In one large autopsy study, 84% of patients had four parathyroid glands, 13% had more than four glands, and only 3% had three glands (D). The superior parathyroid glands are derived from the fourth branchial pouch, which also gives rise to the thyroid gland. The third branchial pouch gives rise to the inferior parathyroid glands and the thymus (A). Ectopic inferior glands are more likely to be found within the thymus than the superior glands, whereas the superior glands are more likely to be found in the retro- or paraesophageal position (B, C). Given the longer descent of the inferior glands, they are overall much more likely to be in an ectopic position.

33. D. Patients with symptomatic hyperparathyroidism should undergo surgery. Symptoms are defined as having evidence of kidney stones; neuromuscular, neuropsychological, or bone symptoms; hypercalcemic crisis; or a history of pancreatitis or peptic ulcer (E). Conversely, controversy exists as to whether every patient who is asymptomatic should undergo parathyroidectomy. Natural history studies of patients with asymptomatic hyperparathyroidism indicate that one-fourth to one-third of patients without symptoms will progress to the development of symptoms over 15 years. Current guidelines for surgery in asymptomatic patients include at initial evaluation: age less than 50, serum calcium level more than 1 mg/dL above the upper limit of reference value, reduced creatinine clearance (<60 mL/min), evidence of renal stones or nephrocalcinosis, evidence of bone mass reduction more than 2.5 standard deviations below matched controls, fragility fractures, and unwillingness or inability to undergo continued follow-up (A–C, E).

Reference: Quinn CE, Udelsman R. The parathyroid glands. In: Townsend CM Jr, Beauchamp RD, Evers BM, Mattox KL, eds. *Sabiston textbook of surgery: the biological basis of modern surgical practice.* 20th ed. Elsevier; 2016:78–92.

34. C. Measurement of elevated 24-hour urinary cortisol levels is a very sensitive (95%–100%) and specific (98%) modality for diagnosing Cushing syndrome, and as such it should be the first test used to establish the diagnosis of Cushing syndrome. If the level is elevated, a low-dose dexamethasone suppression test should be performed. Suppression rules out Cushing syndrome. Failure to suppress cortisol levels establishes the diagnosis of Cushing syndrome. ACTH levels should then be measured. Low ACTH levels indicate a primary adrenal source of cortisol, and thus the next step would be to obtain an abdominal CT scan (E). A high ACTH level suggests either a pituitary or ectopic source of ACTH production. A high-dose dexamethasone suppression test should then be performed because a pituitary source of ACTH will result in some ACTH and cortisol suppression. If cortisol production is suppressed, pituitary MRI should be performed (D). CT scan is less sensitive in demonstrating a pituitary mass (A). Failure to suppress cortisol production with high-dose dexamethasone suggests an ectopic ACTH tumor. The most common causes of ectopic ACTH production are bronchial tumors and small cell lung cancer. Thus, the study of choice would be a chest CT scan. Petrosal sinus sampling of ACTH is an invasive procedure to determine which side of the pituitary gland an ACTH-producing tumor is located (B).

35. A. Psammoma bodies are calcified deposits representing clumps of sloughed cells. It is considered diagnostic of papillary carcinoma (B–E). Another histologic characteristic of papillary carcinoma is Orphan Annie nuclei.

36. D. Pheochromocytomas occur either sporadically, as part of multiple endocrine neoplasia (MEN) type 2A and MEN type 2B, in association with von Hippel-Lindau disease, and with von Recklinghausen disease. The diagnosis of a benign or a malignant pheochromocytoma cannot be accurately determined by the histologic appearance but rather is based on evidence of local invasion or the presence or absence of metastasis (B). The risk of malignancy is lower in patients with familial tumors than in patients with sporadic tumors, although familial tumors are more likely to be bilateral (A, C). The diagnosis of pheochromocytoma is established by demonstrating an increased level of catecholamines and their metabolites in the plasma and urine. Plasma metanephrine levels have the highest sensitivity for pheochromocytoma (99% sensitivity) and are used by most as the initial screening test (E).

37. A. Papillary cancer is the most common thyroid malignancy in adults and children (B–E). The rate of malignancy in thyroid nodules is higher in children. In adults, approximately 5% of thyroid nodules are malignant, whereas in children, the rate is approximately 25%. Prognosis in children overall is excellent.

References: Gauger PG, Doherty GM. The parathyroid gland. In: Townsend CM, Jr, Beauchamp RD, Evers BM, Mattox KL, eds. *Sabiston textbook of surgery: the biological basis of modern surgical practice.* 17th ed. Philadelphia: W.B. Saunders; 2004:985–1000.

Hanks JB. The thyroid. In: Townsend CM, Jr, Beauchamp RD, Evers BM, Mattox KL, eds. *Sabiston textbook of surgery: the biological basis of modern surgical practice.* 17th ed. Philadelphia: W.B. Saunders; 2004:947–984.

Lal G, Clark OH. Thyroid, parathyroid and adrenal. In: Brunicardi FC, Andersen DK, Billiar TR, et al., eds. *Schwartz's principles of surgery.* 8th ed. New York: McGraw-Hill; 2005:1395–1470.

38. D. Secondary hyperparathyroidism is seen in the majority of cases in association with chronic renal failure (B). Rarely, it occurs secondary to intestinal malabsorption of calcium and vitamin D in the absence of kidney failure (D). The underlying etiology is a chronic overstimulation of the parathyroid glands. Renal failure leads to a decreased level of calcitriol (vitamin D_3), an elevation in phosphate, and a drop in serum calcium levels (A). This leads to increased PTH secretion. PTH levels are typically very high, ranging from 500 to 1500 pg/mL (normal is ≤65 pg/mL) (C). As renal failure progresses, there is a decrease in vitamin D and calcium receptors, leading to parathyroid gland resistance to calcitriol and calcium. This vicious cycle worsens as renal failure worsens. Patients with secondary hyperparathyroidism are generally hypocalcemic or normocalcemic. The typical parathyroid gland pathology is four-gland hyperplasia. Medical management has historically consisted of a low-phosphate diet, phosphate binders, and oral supplementation with calcium and vitamin D. More recently, cinacalcet has been approved by the US Food and Drug Administration for the treatment of secondary hyperparathyroidism due to chronic renal failure. Cinacalcet is a calcimimetic agent. It increases the sensitivity of the calcium-sensing receptor to activation by extracellular calcium and thus directly lowers PTH levels. The majority of patients with secondary hyperparathyroidism can be managed medically. The recent introduction of cinacalcet will likely lead to an even further reduction in the need for surgical management. In general, surgery is indicated for failed medical management (E). Indications include intractable bone pain, severe pruritus, calciphylaxis, and progressive renal osteodystrophy. Surgical treatment consists of

removal of all four glands with autoimplantation of parathyroid tissue in the forearm muscle or removal of three and a half glands.

References: Block GA, Martin KJ, de Francisco ALM, et al. Cinacalcet for secondary hyperparathyroidism in patients receiving hemodialysis. *N Engl J Med.* 2004;350(15):1516–1525.

Lindberg JS, Culleton B, Wong G, et al. Cinacalcet HCl, an oral calcimimetic agent for the treatment of secondary hyperparathyroidism in hemodialysis and peritoneal dialysis: a randomized, double-blind, multicenter study. *J Am Soc Nephrol.* 2005;16(3):800–807.

Shoback DM, Bilezikian JP, Turner SA, McCary LC, Guo MD, Peacock M. The calcimimetic cinacalcet normalizes serum calcium in subjects with primary hyperparathyroidism. *J Clin Endocrinol Metab.* 2003;88(12):5644–5649.

Slatopolsky E, Brown A, Dusso A. Pathogenesis of secondary hyperparathyroidism. *Kidney Int Suppl.* 1999;73:S14–S19.

39. B. Tertiary hyperparathyroidism most commonly occurs in the setting of a patient who has had long-standing secondary hyperparathyroidism in whom subsequently autonomously functioning parathyroid glands develop that continue secreting PTH despite high serum calcium levels (C). The most common clinical scenario in which it develops is the patient who has undergone renal transplantation (A, E). Distinguishing between secondary and tertiary hyperparathyroidism is not critical because the initial management is medical, and surgery is indicated for failure of medical management (D). Surgical treatment consists of removal of 3½ glands rather than all 4 glands with autoimplantation of parathyroid tissue in the forearm muscle in cases in which all four glands are enlarged.

Reference: Kebebew E, Duh QY, Clark OH. Tertiary hyperparathyroidism: histologic patterns of disease and results of parathyroidectomy: histologic patterns of disease and results of parathyroidectomy. *Arch Surg.* 2004;139(9):974–977.

40. D. The "rule of tens" regarding pheochromocytoma (10% bilateral, 10% extra adrenal, 10% familial, 10% multifocal, 10% malignant) was taught for generations. It was ultimately disproved in the year 2000 after a series of reports described novel germline mutations causing pheochromocytoma. We now recognize that 20% to 40 % of pheochromocytomas arise as a result of an underlying familial syndrome and that clear genotype-phenotype correlations exist. The organ of Zuckerkandl is a para-aortic structure located at the take-off of the inferior mesenteric artery or at the aortic bifurcation. It consists of a small mass of chromaffin cells that are derived from the neural crest. In the fetal circulation, it is important in the regulation of blood pressure via the secretion of catecholamines but then regresses. Pheochromocytoma may rarely be found in the bladder and can present with symptoms during voiding (B). The remaining choices are very rare locations for pheochromocytoma (A, C, E).

Reference: Disick GIS, Palese MA. Extra-adrenal pheochromocytoma: diagnosis and management. *Curr Urol Rep.* 2007;8(1):83–88.

41. E. Neuroblastoma is the most common abdominal malignancy in children and the third most common overall and is of neural crest origin (A). It most often presents as an abdominal mass, and most patients have advanced disease at presentation. For stage I disease, surgical resection is the best treatment. The overall survival rate is less than 30% (C). The tumor may cross the midline, and a majority of patients show signs of metastatic disease at presentation. Because these tumors are derived from the sympathetic nervous system, catecholamines and their metabolites will be produced at increased levels. Prognosis is based on age at presentation (older or younger than 1 year of age), tumor biology, and tumor histology. Children less than 1 year of age have more advanced disease (B). Amplification of the *N-myc* oncogene has an unfavorable prognosis. High-risk groups have only a 20% long-term survival rate. In infants, spontaneous regression has been well described. In the mediastinum, they most often present in the posterior mediastinum (the most common location for neurogenic mediastinal tumors) (D). Neuroblastoma is associated with many different syndromes, including dancing eyes–dancing feet syndrome (cerebellar ataxia, nystagmus, and involuntary movements), catecholamine release, periorbital metastasis leading to proptosis and periorbital ecchymosis, skin metastasis that gives the appearance of a blueberry muffin, and severe diarrhea (due to release of vasoactive intestinal polypeptide). Aniridia and hemihypertrophy, however, are associated with Wilms tumor.

Reference: Meitar D, Crawford SE, Rademaker AW, Cohn SL. Tumor angiogenesis correlates with metastatic disease, N-myc amplification, and poor outcome in human neuroblastoma. *J Clin Oncol.* 1996;14(2):405–414.

42. A. The external branch of the superior laryngeal nerve lies on the inferior pharyngeal constrictor muscle and descends alongside the superior thyroid artery before innervating the cricothyroid muscle. Injury to the external superior laryngeal nerve results in an inability to tense the ipsilateral vocal cord and difficulty hitting high notes, projecting the voice, and voice fatigue during a prolonged speech. Injury to the internal branch of the superior laryngeal nerve results in loss of sensory input from the pharynx and subsequent ineffective cough and/or aspiration (D, E). Injury to the recurrent laryngeal nerve can cause vocal cord collapse and hoarseness (C). Bilateral recurrent laryngeal nerve can result in loss of airway (B).

References: Gauger PG, Doherty GM. The parathyroid gland. In: Townsend CM, Jr, Beauchamp RD, Evers BM, Mattox KL, eds. *Sabiston textbook of surgery: the biological basis of modern surgical practice.* 17th ed. Philadelphia: W.B. Saunders; 2004:985–1000.

Hanks JB. The thyroid. In: Townsend CM, Jr, Beauchamp RD, Evers BM, Mattox KL, eds. *Sabiston textbook of surgery: the biological basis of modern surgical practice.* 17th ed. Philadelphia: W.B. Saunders; 2004:947–984.

Lal G, Clark OH. Thyroid, parathyroid and adrenal. In: Brunicardi FC, Andersen DK, Billiar TR, et al., eds. *Schwartz's principles of surgery.* 8th ed. New York: McGraw-Hill; 2005:1395–1470.

43. A. In the follicular cell, inorganic iodide is trapped and transported across the basement membrane. Iodide is oxidized to iodine. It is then coupled with tyrosine moieties. This leads to the formation of monoiodotyrosine or diiodotyrosine, catalyzed by thyroid peroxidase. Two diiodotyrosine molecules couple to form T_4, and one monoiodotyrosine and one diiodotyrosine combine to form T_3, both of which are bound to thyroglobulin. In the periphery, approximately 70% to 75% of T_3 and T_4 is bound to thyroid-binding globulins (not to be confused with thyroglobulin), and most of the remainder is bound to thyroid-binding prealbumin and albumin, leaving only a small amount of unbound or active thyroid hormone. T_4 is relatively inactive but is present in

larger amounts. T_4 is converted to the more active form of T_3 in the liver, kidneys, pituitary, and other tissues. Thus, treatment of thyroid storm involves inhibiting several steps: (1) addressing the ABCs by determining whether an airway is needed, administering 100% oxygen, and starting aggressive fluid hydration; (2) decreasing new hormone synthesis; (3) inhibiting the release of thyroid hormone; and (4) blocking the peripheral effects of thyroid hormone. Propylthiouracil and methimazole both inhibit oxidation of iodide to iodine and inhibit the thyroid peroxidase–mediated coupling of iodotyrosines (D). Propylthiouracil also inhibits the conversion of T_4 to T_3 (B). Beta-blockers such as propranolol are useful in controlling the adrenergic response to thyroid storm (C). Propranolol also inhibits peripheral conversion of T_4 to T_3. Steroids also inhibit the conversion of T_4 to T_3 in the periphery (E). Aspirin is contraindicated in thyroid storm because it is thought to decrease protein binding of thyroid hormones. Thus, it may increase the levels of unbound T_3 and T_4.

Reference: Nayak B, Burman K. Thyrotoxicosis and thyroid storm. *Endocrinol Metab Clin North Am.* 2006;35(4):663–686.

44. C. Substernal goiter is divided into primary and secondary forms. Primary forms, defined as ones that originate in the mediastinum with blood supply from intrathoracic vessels, are very rare (B). Most substernal goiters are extensions from cervical goiters. Most surgeons recommend resection for the mere presence of a substernal goiter because most are symptomatic, and those that are not can cause progressive compression of the trachea (A). In addition, they may harbor an unsuspected malignancy. The majority can be successfully removed with a cervical collar incision. Sternotomy is very rarely needed nor is tracheostomy because most can be intubated, even in the face of tracheal compression, with a pediatric endotracheal tube (E). They are not typically responsive to prolonged thyroid suppression (D).

References: Gauger PG, Doherty GM. The parathyroid gland. In: Townsend CM, Jr, Beauchamp RD, Evers BM, Mattox KL, eds. *Sabiston textbook of surgery: the biological basis of modern surgical practice.* 17th ed. Philadelphia: W.B. Saunders; 2004:985–1000.

Hanks JB. The thyroid. In: Townsend CM, Jr, Beauchamp RD, Evers BM, Mattox KL, eds. *Sabiston textbook of surgery: the biological basis of modern surgical practice.* 17th ed. Philadelphia: W.B. Saunders; 2004:947–984.

Hedayati N, McHenry CR. The clinical presentation and operative management of nodular and diffuse substernal thyroid disease. *Am Surg.* 2002;68(3):245–251; discussion 251–252.

Lal G, Clark OH. Thyroid, parathyroid and adrenal. In: Brunicardi FC, Andersen DK, Billiar TR, et al., eds. *Schwartz's principles of surgery.* 8th ed. New York: McGraw-Hill; 2005:1395–1470.

45. A. Adrenal insufficiency has primary and secondary causes. The most common cause of primary adrenal insufficiency in the United States is autoimmune adrenal atrophy. The most common cause worldwide is tuberculosis (B). Other less common causes include infections (fungal cytomegalovirus, human immunodeficiency virus), adrenal hemorrhage, metastases, and infiltrative disorders (amyloidosis) (C, D). The most common cause of secondary adrenal insufficiency is exogenous glucocorticoid therapy, followed by bilateral adrenal resection and pituitary tumors (E). Symptoms and signs of acute adrenal insufficiency include fever, nausea and vomiting, abdominal pain, hypotension, hyponatremia, and hyperkalemia. As such, it can readily be confused with septic shock. The most specific test for adrenal insufficiency is the ACTH stimulation test. Cortisol levels are measured at 1, 30, and 60 minutes. Blood and urine cortisol levels normally rise with ACTH; failure to rise is indicative of adrenal insufficiency.

Reference: Arlt W, Allolio B. Adrenal insufficiency. *Lancet.* 2003;361(9372):1881–1893.

46. C. Progressive truncal obesity is the most common symptom of Cushing syndrome, but it is not specific. Relatively specific findings include proximal muscle weakness, wide purple striae, spontaneous ecchymoses, and hypokalemic metabolic alkalosis. Hirsutism and acne are also associated with Cushing syndrome but are not specific. Cushing syndrome is most often due to exogenous corticosteroid administration. The most common pathology associated with Cushing syndrome is an ACTH-producing pituitary adenoma, which is referred to as *Cushing disease.* Causes of Cushing syndrome are divided into ACTH dependent (ACTH-producing pituitary adenoma, ectopic ACTH syndrome, and ectopic corticotropin-releasing hormone syndrome) and ACTH independent (adrenal carcinoma, adrenal adenoma, and adrenal hyperplasia) (A, B, D, E).

47. D. The juxtaglomerular cells are modified smooth muscle cells located in the afferent arteriole of each glomerulus (A). They synthesize the precursor prorenin, which is cleaved into the active proteolytic enzyme renin. Renal hypoperfusion, decreased plasma sodium, and increased sympathetic activity are the major stimuli for renin secretion (B, C). Renin initiates a sequence of steps that begins with cleavage of angiotensinogen (a protein produced in the liver) to form angiotensin I. Angiotensin I is then converted to angiotensin II by angiotensin-converting enzyme, found primarily in the lung. Angiotensin II causes systemic vasoconstriction and stimulates aldosterone synthesis and release by the adrenal gland, leading to sodium and water retention and expansion of the plasma volume (E). In the glomerulus, it leads to vasoconstriction of the efferent arteriole. This leads to increased glomerular pressure in an attempt to maintain the glomerular filtration rate despite systemic hypoperfusion.

48. D. The arterial blood supply to the adrenal glands is highly variable, whereas the venous drainage is more constant (A). The adrenal glands are supplied by three primary sources: the inferior phrenic artery, adrenal branches directly off the aorta, and branches from the renal artery (E). Additional branches may arise from the intercostal and gonadal arteries. A single left adrenal vein empties into the left renal vein and is a relatively longer vein than the single right adrenal vein, which is very short and enters the posterior aspect of the inferior vena cava (C). Adrenalectomy (open and laparoscopic) is more challenging on the right side because of (1) the need to retract the liver (for a laparoscopic approach), (2) the need to mobilize the duodenum, and (3) the short, posteriorly located adrenal vein that drains into the inferior vena cava, posing a risk of inferior vena cava hemorrhage. Likewise, venous sampling of the right adrenal vein is more challenging (B).

Reference: Corcione F, Esposito C, Cuccurullo D, et al. Vena cava injury. A serious complication during laparoscopic right adrenalectomy. *Surg Endosc.* 2001;15(2):218.

49. D. Incidentally discovered adrenal masses are quite common and are termed *adrenal incidentalomas.* Most are nonfunctioning cortical adenomas. The differential diagnosis includes a functional tumor (pheochromocytoma, aldosteronoma, cortisol producing), metastatic cancer (from lung, breast, melanoma), and adrenocortical carcinoma. A careful history and physical examination should be performed to detect evidence of hormonal excess (hypertension, virilization, Cushing disease). If the patient has hypertension and a low potassium level, plasma aldosterone, and renin levels should be obtained. If there is no evidence of hormonal excess, the following studies should still be obtained to rule out a functional tumor: plasma free metanephrines to rule out pheochromocytoma and a 1-mg overnight dexamethasone suppression test to rule out a cortisol-producing tumor (in normal patients, this will markedly suppress endogenous cortisol production to a level <1.8 µg/dL). Characteristics on the CT scan should also be determined. A mass with smooth borders, that is, homogeneous, and low attenuation (using Hounsfield units) is very likely benign, whereas an irregular mass with evidence of local invasion, that is, inhomogeneous, and a high attenuation score is of much more concern for malignancy (E). Fine-needle aspiration biopsy is not helpful in distinguishing a benign adrenal adenoma from a malignant adrenocortical carcinoma because it is even difficult to distinguish the two on histologic examination. Fine-needle aspiration biopsy would only be useful in the patient with a history of malignancy to rule out an adrenal metastasis (A). Surgery is generally recommended for functional adrenal adenomas, pheochromocytomas, masses that have CT scan features suggestive of malignancy, and masses larger than 5 cm. Once surgery is indicated, laparoscopic adrenalectomy has replaced open adrenalectomy for most indications. Open adrenalectomy is still preferred for very large tumors (>6 cm) and, in particular, when malignancy is suspected (B, C). For nonfunctional adrenal adenomas that do not fit the above criteria, repeat CT scan in 6 months may be performed.

Reference: Grumbach MM, Biller BMK, Braunstein GD, et al. Management of the clinically inapparent adrenal mass ("incidentaloma"). *Ann Intern Med.* 2003;138(5):424–429.

50. B. The adrenal gland is divided into the outer cortex and the inner medulla. The cortex is further subdivided into three layers ("GFR": glomerulosa, fasciculata, reticularis). The zona glomerulosa is the outermost layer and is responsible for aldosterone production (A). The middle layer, the zona fasciculata, produces glucocorticoids. The zona reticularis is the inner layer of the adrenal cortex (E). Adrenal androgens are produced by the deepest cortical layer, the zona reticularis (C). Cells of the adrenal medulla produce epinephrine (80%) and norepinephrine (20%). Medullary cells are chromaffin positive (D).

51. B. In patients with primary hyperparathyroidism secondary to a single adenoma, removal of the enlarged gland is considered the preferred treatment and biochemical cure is typically confirmed intraoperatively. The Miami criteria outlines targeted PTH values after gland resection, and the criterion to conclude surgery is a greater than 50% drop in PTH level after gland removal. Serum PTH has a half-life estimated to be 3 minutes. PTH sampling should first be performed at 10 minutes after gland removal and can be repeated after 20 minutes if the PTH level does not decrease by more than 50%. Previously, it was thought that older age, high body mass index, and poor renal function can lead to an insufficient decline in PTH level during surgical resection, but a recent *JAMA Surgery* study demonstrated that these factors did not have a significant impact on PTH half-life, and as such the Miami Criteria can be used in these patients as well (E). It would be inappropriate to proceed to a four-gland exploration or to close the wound without confirming biochemical cure (A, C). If the baseline PTH level is sampled from the internal jugular vein ipsilateral to a single adenoma, then the PTH level can take longer to drop; therefore, longer wait times may be appropriate in this setting (D).

References: Calò PG, Pisano G, Loi G, et al. Intraoperative parathyroid hormone assay during focused parathyroidectomy: the importance of 20 minutes measurement. *BMC Surg.* 2013;13(1):36.

Leiker AJ, Yen TWF, Eastwood DC, et al. Factors that influence parathyroid hormone half-life: determining if new intraoperative criteria are needed. *JAMA Surg.* 2013;148(7):602–606.

52. C. The hallmark of MEN 2 is MTC. Eventually, nearly 100% of patients with MEN 2 develop MTC, whereas only approximately 40% develop pheochromocytoma and one-third have parathyroid hyperplasia (A, B, E). MTC is characteristically multifocal and bilateral and presents at a young age. MTC is associated with C-cell hyperplasia. It is caused by mutations in the RET protooncogene (not menin) that are present in all thyroid C cells and thus lead to multifocal MTC (D).

53. C. Congenital adrenal hyperplasia results from inherited enzyme deficiencies that can lead to ambiguous genitalia, postnatal virilization, and problems with salt metabolism. The most common enzyme defect is 21-hydroxylase deficiency (>90% of cases). In the complete form, the deficiency leads to a decrease in both cortisol and aldosterone. This leads to ambiguous genitalia in females (due to androgen excess), salt wasting with hypernatremia, and hypokalemia. The remaining answer choices can also cause congenital adrenal hyperplasia but are less commonly found (A, B, D, E).

54. A. A patient with a history of primary hyperparathyroidism, newly enlarging thyroid nodule, and elevated calcitonin level likely has multiple endocrine neoplasm-2A. These patients are at risk for developing medullary thyroid carcinoma (MTC). The characteristics of MTC that affect surgical approach include the following: (1) MTC is more aggressive than other thyroid cancers with higher recurrence and mortality rates. (2) MTC does not take up radioactive iodine, and radiation therapy and chemotherapy are ineffective (B, E). (3) MTC is multicentric in 90% of MEN 2 patients. (4) In patients with palpable disease, more than 70% have nodal metastases (D). (5) The ability to measure postoperative stimulated calcitonin levels has allowed assessment of the adequacy of surgical extraction. The two main factors affecting survival are stage and age at diagnosis (D). A key factor in survival is early detection via calcitonin screening in at-risk patients. In one large study, biochemical cure predicted a survival rate of 97.7% at 10 years. Management of MTC includes total thyroidectomy with routine central node dissection (A). It should be noted that MEN 2A is rare, and in fact, most MTCs

are sporadic. Sporadic cases are less likely to be multicentric than those associated with MEN 2. Microscopically, a characteristic feature of MTC is the finding of abundant collagen and amyloid. Prior to addressing the MTC in a patient with suspected MEN 2, pheochromocytoma must be excluded/managed prior to prevent hypertensive crisis (C).

References: Kebebew E, Ituarte PH, Siperstein AE, Duh QY, Clark OH. Medullary thyroid carcinoma: clinical characteristics, treatment, prognostic factors, and a comparison of staging systems. *Cancer.* 2000;88(5):1139–1148.

Modigliani E, Cohen R, Campos JM, et al. Prognostic factors for survival and for biochemical cure in medullary thyroid carcinoma: results in 899 patients. The GETC Study Group. Groupe d'étude des tumeurs à calcitonine. *Clin Endocrinol (Oxf).* 1998;48(3):265–273.

55. D. TSH is the most accurate test in hyperthyroidism, with significant suppression in hyperthyroid states. In most states of hyperthyroidism, free T_4, total T_4, and total T_3 are elevated (A–C). Thyroid scan is not used in the initial workup for hyperthyroidism (E).

56. E. The thyroid gland is supplied by paired superior thyroid arteries from the external carotid arteries and the inferior thyroid arteries from the thyrocervical trunk. The superior thyroid artery is the first branch of the external carotid artery (B). During thyroidectomy, care must be taken when ligating the superior thyroid arteries to avoid injury to the external branch of the superior laryngeal nerve (D). To avoid injury, ligating the artery and vein separately and close to the thyroid gland is recommended. In approximately 3% of individuals, a thyroidea ima artery also provides blood to the thyroid gland and arises either from the aorta or the innominate artery. When ligating the inferior thyroid arteries, care must be taken to avoid injury to the RLNs (C). The inferior thyroid arteries usually supply the parathyroid glands (A). Ligation of the main trunk of the inferior thyroid arteries during total thyroidectomy can lead to parathyroid gland ischemia. There are three main pairs of veins draining the thyroid gland: the superior, middle, and inferior thyroid veins. The middle veins are the least constant. The superior and middle veins drain into the internal jugular veins, whereas the inferior veins drain into the brachiocephalic veins.

57. C. The superior laryngeal nerve and RLN arise from the vagus nerve. The superior laryngeal nerve divides into two branches and is both motor and sensory to the larynx (D). The internal branch is sensory to the supraglottic larynx, and, although rare, injury during thyroid surgery would lead to aspiration (A). The external branch innervates the cricothyroid muscle. Injury to the external superior laryngeal nerve causes an inability to tense the ipsilateral vocal cord. This does not cause hoarseness, but rather results in voice fatigue, and in singers creates difficulty in hitting high notes. It has been referred to as the nerve of Amelita Galli-Curci or "high note" nerve after the opera singer who underwent thyroid goiter surgery in the 1930s and lost her ability to sing afterward. The left RLN loops around the aorta at the ligamentum arteriosum. The right RLN loops around the right subclavian artery. The RLN innervates the intrinsic muscles of the larynx with the exception of the cricothyroid muscle, which is innervated by the external laryngeal nerve (E).

Injury to one RLN leads to paralysis of the ipsilateral vocal cord, which becomes fixed in the paramedian or abducted position. Bilateral RLN injury may lead to airway obstruction and complete loss of the voice (B).

58. C. A nonrecurrent laryngeal nerve is rare and occurs much more commonly on the right (A, B). It branches off the vagus nerve in the neck and heads directly to the larynx, as opposed to arising from the vagus after passing the subclavian artery (D). The anomalous location, as opposed to its normal position in the tracheoesophageal groove, makes it more prone to injury (E). On the right, a patient can have both a nonrecurrent nerve and a recurrent nerve. Nonrecurrent left laryngeal nerves have been reported but are extremely rare. The recurrent laryngeal nerve is most vulnerable to injury during the last 2 to 3 cm of its course but also can be damaged if the surgeon is not alert to the possibility of nerve branches and nonrecurrent nerves, particularly on the right side.

59. E. PTH increases the bone resorption by stimulating osteoclasts and inhibiting osteoblasts, leading to the release of calcium and phosphate into the circulation. At the kidney, PTH limits calcium excretion at the distal convoluted tubule via an active transport mechanism and inhibits phosphate and bicarbonate reabsorption, the latter leading to a mild metabolic acidosis (B, C). PTH also enhances hydroxylation of 25-hydroxyvitamin D to 1,25-hydroxyvitamin D in the kidney, which in turn directly increases intestinal calcium absorption (not a direct effect of PTH) (D). Cholecalciferol is hydroxylated to 25-hydroxyvitamin D in the liver. This is not regulated by PTH (A).

60. A. Lateral aberrant thyroid is a term used to denote what appears to be ectopic thyroid tissue found within the neck. In most instances, it actually represents metastatic thyroid cancer within a lymph node, most often of the papillary type. It is not typically associated with the remaining answer choices (B–E).

Reference: Jong D, Demeter S, Jarosz J. Primary papillary thyroid carcinoma presenting as cervical lymphadenopathy: the operative approach to the "lateral aberrant thyroid. *Am Surg*. 1993;59:172–176.

61. C. The accepted management of low-risk papillary thyroid cancer is either right hemithyroidectomy or total thyroidectomy with or without postoperative [131]I. In patients with papillary carcinoma with a history of radiation exposure, there is a higher rate of multicentricity. As such, total thyroidectomy is the recommended procedure (A, B). Postoperative radioactive iodine following total thyroidectomy is indicated for tumors larger than 4 cm, gross extrathyroidal extension of the tumor regardless of size, lymph node metastases, and for high-risk features including tall-cell or columnar-cell variant (E). An added advantage of postoperative radiation is that it allows for the continued monitoring for recurrence with thyroglobulin. Prophylactic *central* neck node dissection is gaining popularity as well. Modified radical neck dissection would not be indicated unless there were obvious lateral neck nodes (D).

References: Guerrero MA, Clark OH. Controversies in the management of papillary thyroid cancer revisited. *ISRN Oncol*. 2011;2011:303128.

Hay ID, Thompson GB, Grant CS, et al. Papillary thyroid carcinoma managed at the Mayo Clinic during six decades (1940–1999): temporal trends in initial therapy and long-term outcome in 2444 consecutively treated patients. *World J Surg*. 2002;26(8):879–885.

Skin and Soft Tissue 14

ERIC O. YEATES, AREG GRIGORIAN, AND CHRISTIAN DE VIRGILIO

ABSITE 99th Percentile High-Yields

I. Most Common Skin Cancers
   A. Basal cell carcinoma: most common skin cancer and overall cancer
      1. Majority found on head and neck, more commonly on upper lip
      2. Typically appears as a shiny, pearly skin nodule with rolled borders
      3. Treatment
         1. Excision with 4 to 5 mm margins for low risk, and 1 to 2 cm for high risk
         2. Low risk is trunk and extremity lesions <2 cm and head and neck lesions <1 cm; high risk is not meeting low risk criteria, immunocompromised, perineural invasion, morpheaform sclerosing, or micronodular
         3. Mohs micrographic surgery can be used for cosmetically sensitive areas (i.e., face)
   B. Squamous cell carcinoma (SCC): 2nd most common skin cancer (most common in transplant patients)
      1. Found on sunexposed skin, more likely on bottom lip
      2. UV and immunosuppression are risk factors
      3. Appears as ulcer or red/brown skin plaque
      4. Similar diagnoses: Bowen disease is SCC in situ, Marjolin ulcer is aggressive SCC originating from burns, scars, or chronic wounds
      5. Higher risk of metastases than BCC
      6. Treatment same as BCC
   C. Melanoma: third most common skin cancer, majority of skin cancer deaths
      1. UV exposure and congenital nevi are most common risk factors
      2. Uncommon locations: intraocular, anal
      3. Four main subtypes (all melanomas arise from melanocytes in epidermis)
         1. Superficial spreading: most common, moderately aggressive
         2. Nodular melanoma: second most common, very aggressive, vertical growth, often metastasized at diagnosis
         3. Lentigo maligna: least aggressive
         4. Acral lentiginous: very aggressive, more common in people of color, found on palms, soles of feet, and subungual
      4. Treatment
         a) For stages 1 to 2, no preoperative workup needed after history and exam
         b) For melanoma in situ of face: treat with MOHS and 5 mm margins
         c) Wide local excision: margins based on thickness (0.5 cm for in situ, 1 cm for ≤1 mm, 1 to 2 cm for 1 to 2 mm, 2 cm for ≥2 mm)
         d) Sentinel lymph node biopsy (SLNB) if ≥ 1 mm thick or ≥ 0.75 mm with ulceration
         e) Multicenter Selective Lymphadenopathy Trial (MSLT-1): SLNB led to decreased recurrence of melanoma compared to WLE alone
         f) MSLT-2: completion lymph node dissection had less disease in regional nodes at 3 years but did not improve melanoma-specific survival in patients with sentinel lymph node metastases

g) Targeted therapies: dabrafenib or vemurafenib for unresectable or metastatic melanoma in patients with BRAF mutations (increases risk of skin SCC); ipilimumab is a monoclonal antibody to CTLA-4 used in metastatic melanoma; both classes improve survival in stage-4 disease

II. Soft-Tissue Sarcomas: Over 50 Different Subtypes
   A. Most common subtypes (most common presentation is asymptomatic mass)
      1. Adults: Malignant fibrous histiocytoma (#1), liposarcoma, leiomyosarcoma
      2. Children: Rhabdomyosarcoma (#1), osteosarcoma, Ewing sarcoma
      3. Most sarcomas spread hematogenous
      4. Select sarcomas spread via lymphatics: Synovial, Clear cell, Angiosarcoma, Rhabdomyosarcoma, Epithelioid (SCARE)
      5. Diagnosis
         a) MRI (use T2 and gadolinium) and x-ray in extremity, CT for retroperitoneum
         b) Core needle biopsy (CNB) is first-line modality to work-up
         c) If CNB indeterminate: incisional (if >3 cm) or excisional biopsy (if <3 cm); excisional biopsy should include an elliptical incision along longitudinal axis of extremity
      6. 5-year survival of all stages is 65%
      7. Prognosis and staging based on mitotic index, necrosis, and tumor grade
      8. Staging should include CXR to rule out lung metastases (most common site for metastasis)
      9. Treatment
         a) Resection with 2 to 3 cm margins if possible; resection alone (w/o radiation) is OK for low-grade sarcomas, <5 cm with clear 1 to 2 cm margins
         b) Consider neoadjuvant chemo-XRT if it could allow limb salvage
         c) Consider adjuvant radiation for high grade, positive margins, large

III. Other Commonly Tested Skin and Soft Tissue Tumors

Tumor	Description	Treatment
Merkel cell carcinoma	Neuroendocrine origin, red or blue nodule, most infected by Merkel cell polyomavirus, UV exposure and immunocompromised states also risk factors, highly aggressive	WLE with 1–2 cm margins with SLNB, adjuvant radiation
Dermatofibrosarcoma protuberans	Firm, flesh-colored, red plaque often mistaken for keloid or hypertrophic scar; histologically identified by finger-like projections of spindle cells	WLE with 2–3 cm margins, can consider Mohs for face, radiation if negative margins not possible
Kaposi sarcoma	Vascular sarcoma caused by HHV8, occurs in immunocompromised hosts (i.e., AIDS)	Not curable, HAART for control
Desmoid tumors	Arise from fibroblasts, similar to very low-grade fibrosarcoma, most common in women in 30s, can occur after surgery or trauma, locally aggressive; associated with familial adenomatous polyposis (FAP) and Gardner syndrome; in sporadic forms, it has a female predominance in the postpartum period	Surgery or active surveillance (now controversial with surveillance preferred for non–favorable locations), neoadjuvant or adjuvant chemotherapy can be considered

Questions

1. Which of the following is true regarding necrotizing soft-tissue infections (NSTI)?
   A. Type I necrotizing fasciitis is polymicrobial
   B. Mortality rates are higher in pediatric cases
   C. The Laboratory Risk Indicator for Necrotizing Fasciitis (LRINEC) score is highly sensitive for NSTI
   D. Clostridium species is the most common pathogen identified
   E. Crepitus and bullae are early skin findings

2. A 43-year-old male presents with a 2 cm lesion on her upper lip, just above the vermillion border. A biopsy reveals a common skin cancer. Which of the following is true regarding her diagnosis?
   A. This is most likely a squamous cell carcinoma given the location
   B. Wide local excision with 5-mm margins should be performed
   C. XRT should be performed given the size and location of the lesion
   D. An ultrasound of the neck should be performed to rule out lymph node metastases
   E. This patient would be a good candidate for Mohs micrographic surgery

3. A 42-year-old female presents with a painless growing mass in her left inner thigh. An MRI reveals a 6 × 5 cm mass that is concerning for a soft-tissue sarcoma. A core-needle biopsy is indeterminate. Which of the following is the next best step in management?
   A. Excisional biopsy
   B. Resection with 2 cm margins
   C. Incisional biopsy through longitudinal incision
   D. Incisional biopsy at the tumor edge
   E. Repeat imaging in 6 months

4. Which of the following is least likely to be associated with lymphedema?
   A. Recurrent episodes of cellulitis
   B. "Buffalo hump" appearance of the dorsum of the foot
   C. Hyperpigmentation of the skin
   D. Peau d'orange appearance of the skin
   E. Thickening and squaring of toes

5. Which of the following is true regarding sarcoma?
   A. Kaposi sarcoma is a common cause of death in patients with AIDS
   B. Embryonal subtype is a rare childhood rhabdomyosarcoma
   C. Embryonal subtype has the worst prognosis in childhood rhabdomyosarcoma
   D. Osteosarcoma arises from stromal cells
   E. Osteosarcoma is one of the rarest malignant bone tumors

6. A 19-year-old male presents with severe pain in the second digit of the right hand. He has a fever of 103°F. He has recently been biting his nails. On exam, he is tender lateral to the nail fold of the digit, and it appears swollen and red. Which of the following is the best management?
   A. Warm compresses and oral antibiotic coverage for skin flora
   B. Incision and drainage at the mid-digital pulp
   C. Incision at lateral nail fold
   D. Incision at lateral nail fold plus oral antibiotic coverage for skin flora
   E. Incision at lateral nail fold plus oral antibiotic coverage for skin flora and anaerobic bacteria

7. A 45-year-old male with human papillomavirus (HPV) presents to clinic to discuss his care after being diagnosed with Bowen disease of the anus. Which of the following is true regarding his condition?
   A. This is considered an invasive cancer
   B. Wide local excision should be performed
   C. It can be managed initially with imiquimod
   D. HPV 6 and 11 are the most common subtypes leading up to this condition
   E. Negative margins prevent local recurrence

8. A 65-year-old female presents with a 5-cm rubber-like mass located on the right side of her back that has recently been causing pain. It has been slowly growing for the past year. On imaging, she has an unencapsulated mass with a lenticular shape. It has alternating streaks of fibrous and fatty tissue and is located between the subscapular region at the inferior pole of the scapula and the serratus anterior muscle over the thoracic rib cage. Which of the following is true regarding this condition?
   A. This is a malignant condition
   B. It is a benign tumor composed of adipose tissue
   C. Biopsy is necessary even when radiologic findings are typical
   D. Simple excision should be performed
   E. Wide local excision should be performed

9. A 21-year-old male presents to the emergency department (ED) with pain in his upper buttock. On exam, he has a tender mass at the intergluteal region overlying the natal cleft with a sinus tract draining purulent fluid. A single strand of hair is seen protruding from the tract. He reports that he has been treated for this condition several times. Which of the following is most correct?
   A. Control of hair growth at the intergluteal cleft is unlikely to prevent recurrence
   B. Incision and drainage should be performed in the ED
   C. Surgical excision of the sinus tract and marsupialization of the wound should be performed in the OR
   D. The pathogenesis likely involves apocrine glands
   E. CT scan of the pelvis should be performed

10. The most common cause of primary lymphedema is:
   A. Congenital lymphedema
   B. Lymphedema praecox
   C. Lymphedema tarda
   D. Filariasis
   E. Malignancy

11. A 29-year-old male presents with left wrist pain. He has a mass at the volar wrist that has been growing in size for the past 4 months and recently started causing him pain. The mass is compressible, freely moving but tethered in place, and transilluminates. Which of the following is true regarding this condition?
   A. It affects the volar wrist more commonly than it does the dorsal wrist
   B. It is unlikely to resolve without intervention
   C. Ligation of the tethering pedicle is required to achieve the lowest recurrence rate
   D. Simple aspiration is the preferred treatment option
   E. The pain is likely secondary to compression of the terminal branches of the posterior interosseous nerve

12. A 76-year-old female with a history of chronic lymphocytic leukemia (CLL) presents with a painless blue, firm nodule on the right shoulder. It first appeared several weeks prior and was pink in color. It now has overlying ulceration and measures 2 cm in diameter. Immunohistochemistry analysis of a skin sample demonstrates polyomavirus genome. Which of the following is the best next step in management?
   A. Expectant management
   B. Wide local excision with 1-cm margin and adjuvant radiation
   C. Wide local excision with 1-cm margin, sentinel lymph node biopsy (SLNB), and adjuvant radiation
   D. Wide local excision with 2-cm margin and adjuvant chemoradiation
   E. Neoadjuvant chemoradiation followed by wide local excision with 2-cm margin

13. Which of the following is true regarding dermatofibrosarcoma protuberans (DFSP)?
   A. Gross clinical margins are helpful in guiding width of excision
   B. The tumor is not radiosensitive
   C. If it occurs on the neck, wide local excision is the surgical treatment of choice
   D. Local recurrence rate is lower with Mohs micrographic surgery compared with wide local excision
   E. Sentinel lymph node biopsy should be performed

14. Which of the following is true regarding SLNB in melanoma?

    A. A 0.5-mm deep melanoma with ulceration does not require SLNB

    B. SLNB is unnecessary for melanoma that has more than a 4-mm thickness

    C. There is a survival benefit for completion lymphadenectomy following a positive SLNB

    D. Blue dye used for lymph node mapping should be injected outside of the planned wide local excision

    E. All nodes whose radioactivity count is greater than or equal to 10% of that of the hottest node should be removed

Answers

1. A. There are two types of necrotizing fasciitis (NF). Type I NF is the most common type and is polymicrobial with both aerobic and anaerobic organisms. It most commonly affects the elderly, diabetics, and the immunocompromised. Type II NF is monomicrobial, with the most common pathogens being group A strep, followed by *Staphylococcu aureus*. *Clostridium* is now considered a rare pathogen in NSTI (D). Type II NF typically occurs in younger, healthier patients that may have a history of IV drug use, trauma, or recent surgery. Though many NSTIs start with a breach in the skin/mucosa which facilitates organism entry into soft tissues, this is not always the case. A nonpenetrating injury can cause a strain or hematoma leading to an inflammatory response with influx of leukocytes. In a susceptible host with transient bacteremia, organisms can be introduced at the injury site. NSTIs can be difficult to diagnose due to their wide range of presentations and symptoms. Early findings are nonspecific but may include pain out of proportion to exam, ecchymosis, and erythema. Crepitus, bullae, and necrosis are late skin findings (E). NSTI is a clinical diagnosis that is aided by laboratory values and imaging. The Laboratory Risk Indicator for Necrotizing Fasciitis (LRINEC) score, which includes WBC, sodium, glucose, hemoglobin, CRP, and creatinine, is widely; used but not a perfect test. In a recent metaanalysis, an LRINEC score ≥6 had sensitivity of 68% and specificity of 85% (C). CT scan has been shown to be relatively sensitive and specific and notably superior to plain radiography. In suspected cases of NSTI, early surgical intervention with debridement of all necrotic tissue is the single most important treatment to reduce mortality. An early second look operation is also recommended. The mortality for NSTI has been unchanged for the last 100 years (25%–30%) but it is consistently lower in pediatric patients compared to adults (B).

    References: Fernando SM, Tran A, Cheng W, et al. Necrotizing soft tissue infection: diagnostic accuracy of physical examination, imaging, and LRINEC score: a systematic review and meta-analysis. *Ann Surg.* 2019;269(1):58–65.

    Stevens DL, Bryant AE. Necrotizing soft-tissue infections. *N Engl J Med.* 2017;377(23):2253–2265.

2. E. Given the lesion is located on the upper lip, just above the vermillion border, this is most likely a basal cell carcinoma (BCC), the most common malignancy in the United States. Squamous cell carcinoma is more commonly on the lower lip (A) and involve the vermillion. Although lip cancers in general have a male preponderance, upper lip cancers are similar for both sexes or even more common in women. Though wide local excision is the correct management for many BCC, this lesion is in a cosmetically sensitive area and maximal tissue preservation should be attempted (B, C). Mohs micrographic surgery utilizes multiple frozen sections of tissue to achieve complete resection with improved cosmetic results. BCC rarely metastasizes and imaging of regional lymph node basins is not routinely performed (D).

    Reference: Murray C, Sivajohanathan D, Hanna TP, et al. Patient indications for Mohs micrographic surgery: a systematic review. *J Cutan Med Surg.* 2019;23(1):75–90.

3. C. Diagnosis of a soft-tissue sarcoma in an extremity should start with an MRI to rule out vascular involvement prior to a biopsy. Core needle biopsy is highly accurate and is the preferred method for tissue diagnosis. If core needle biopsy is indeterminate and there is still a high suspicion for a sarcoma, an excisional biopsy (if less <3 cm) or incisional biopsy (if >3 cm) should be performed (A, B, E). A longitudinal elliptical incision along the long axis of the extremity should be used so that it can later be included during the formal resection (D). This is true for either incisional or excisional biopsies.

    Reference: Okada K. Points to notice during the diagnosis of soft tissue tumors according to the "Clinical Practice Guideline on the Diagnosis and Treatment of Soft Tissue Tumors." *J Orthop Sci.* 2016;21(6):705–712.

4. C. Distinguishing between chronic venous stasis and lymphedema on physical examination can be difficult, particularly early in their course. Lymphoscintigraphy is the diagnostic test of choice for lymphedema. Both patient groups will report heaviness and fatigue in the limb, which tends to worsen at the end of a day of prolonged standing. Venous stasis tends to be more pitting and lymphedema nonpitting. Venous stasis tends to spare the foot and toes, whereas lymphedema involves them. The swollen dorsum of the foot has a buffalo hump appearance, and toes look squared off (B, E). Recurrent cellulitis is a common complication of lymphedema (A). In advanced lymphedema, the skin develops a peau d'orange appearance (similar to inflammatory disease of the breast), lichenification, and hyperkeratosis (D).

Hyperpigmentation of the skin, due to hemosiderin deposition, is seen in venous insufficiency and not usually with lymphedema.

5. D. Kaposi sarcoma is considered the most common malignancy in AIDS but is rarely a cause of death (A). It is a vascular and cutaneous sarcoma most commonly occurring in the oral and pharyngeal mucosa and often presents with hemoptysis and dysphagia. Rhabdomyosarcoma is the most common soft-tissue sarcoma in childhood with the embryonal subtype being the most common and with a good prognosis (B). Alveolar subtype has the worst prognosis (C). Osteosarcoma is derived from mesenchymal stromal cells and is considered the most common malignant bone tumor in adults (E).

Reference: Ottaviani G, Jaffe N. The epidemiology of osteosarcoma. In: Jaffe N, Bruland O, Bielack S., eds. *Pediatric and adolescent osteosarcoma. Cancer treatment and research.* Vol. 152. Springer; 2009:3–13.

6. E. This patient has acute paronychia, which is an inflammation involving the proximal or lateral fingernail folds. It presents with sudden onset of pain at the nail fold with erythema and swelling. Acute paronychia is a clinical diagnosis but must be differentiated from a felon, which can have lasting consequences if not managed early. A felon is an abscess of the digital pulp and does not involve the nail bed. The appropriate management for a felon is an incision and drainage of the digital pulp at the midline to avoid injuring digital nerves (two sensory nerves medially and two sensory nerves laterally) (B). In contrast, most cases of acute paronychia are treated with warm compresses (A). In more severe cases (e.g., fever of 103°F), incision and drainage should be performed by placing a surgical blade under the cuticle margin and extending it laterally along the side of the affected nail fold. Oral antibiotics should be given for 5 days after drainage and should include coverage for skin flora, particularly with the use of an antistaphylococcal agent (C). However, in a patient with a history of nail-biting or in a patient with hand trauma and oral contact (e.g., punching the face), antibiotics should also cover oral flora including anaerobic bacteria (D).

References: Brook I. Paronychia: a mixed infection. Microbiology and management. *J Hand Surg Br.* 1993;18(3):358–359.

Clark DC. Common acute hand infections. *Am Fam Physician.* 2003;68(11):2167–2176.

7. C. Bowen disease is squamous cell carcinoma in situ (not invasive) of the perianal margin and is most commonly caused by HPV-16 and 18 (A, D). High-grade lesions are more likely to be symptomatic and present as a scaly, erythematous, pigmented plaque that may have a moist surface. Ulceration is suggestive of malignant transformation. Patients with known HPV infection should undergo screening for anal intraepithelial neoplasia (AIN). Some regard high-grade AIN as Bowen disease. Screening is often done in the operating room (OR) using Lugol solution, which is selectively taken up by normal perianal tissue but not by AIN because it lacks glycogen, giving it a characteristic tanned appearance and allowing for tissue biopsy. Previously, it was standard for all patients with high-grade AIN or Bowen disease to undergo wide local excision (B). However, this has come under scrutiny as several reports have reported a high rate of recurrence (up to 40%) even with negative margins and particularly in

patients with HPV (E). This is likely due to the fact that the remaining perianal skin continues to harbor HPV leading to continued transformation of normal cells. Initial treatment of Bowen disease includes imiquimod or topical 5-FU. Surgical excision can be considered for patients with severe symptomatic disease such as refractory pruritus. Patients should receive frequent biopsies to look for invasive cancer.

References: Brown SR, Skinner P, Tidy J, Smith JH, Sharp F, Hosie KB. Outcome after surgical resection for high-grade anal intraepithelial neoplasia (Bowens disease): surgical resection of high-grade anal intraepithelial neoplasia. *Br J Surg.* 1999;86(8):1063–1066.

Gordon PH, Nivatvongs S. *Principles and practice of surgery for the colon, rectum, and anus.* 3rd ed. CRC Press; 2007.

8. D. Elastofibroma dorsi is a benign, slow-growing process that is often mistaken for a soft-tissue sarcoma. Some consider it to be a reactive process; therefore, it is sometimes termed a pseudotumor. There has never been a report of malignant transformation (A). They are almost exclusively found in the subscapular or infrascapular region between the scapula and rib cage. Elastofibroma dorsi occurs more commonly in women older than 55. They are frequently right sided, often unilateral, and typically asymptomatic. The pathogenesis is thought to be due to repetitive microtrauma, but this has not been proven conclusively. Biopsy is unnecessary when radiologic findings are typical (C). MRI is the preferred imaging modality and will demonstrate a mass with streaks of fibrous and fatty tissue located beneath the scapula. Patients with asymptomatic lesions do not require intervention. Symptomatic patients should undergo simple excision (not wide local excision) (E). Local recurrence does not occur. A lipoma is a benign tumor composed of adipose tissue (B).

References: Vastamäki M. Elastofibroma scapulae. *Clin Orthop Relat Res.* 2001;392(392):404–408.

Daigeler A, Vogt PM, Busch K, et al. Elastofibroma dorsi-differential diagnosis in chest wall tumours. *World J Surg Oncol.* 2007;5(1):15.

Muratori F, Esposito M, Rosa F, et al. Elastofibroma dorsi: 8 case reports and a literature review. *J Orthop Traumatol.* 2008;9(1):33–37.

9. B. This patient has a pilonidal cyst with recurrent intergluteal abscess formation. Pilonidal cysts occur most commonly at the upper border of the intergluteal cleft and most commonly in young males. The pathophysiology is unclear but likely has to do with clogged hair follicles (D). Occasionally, hair may be seen protruding from the sinus tract. Inflamed apocrine glands are thought to be the culprit in patients with hidradenitis suppurativa. The diagnosis is made clinically and not with imaging or laboratory studies (E). Patients with an acute infection will present with a tender abscess draining purulent fluid at the pilonidal cyst site. This should be managed as all other cutaneous abscesses are treated, with incision and drainage (C). This will most likely recur, so the patient should have a referral to see a colorectal surgeon to discuss definitive repair after the acute condition has resolved. Although there is not a "gold standard" for chronic pilonidal cyst management, the preferred treatment option depends on if the pilonidal cyst is simple or complex. Excision with primary closure off the midline for a simple, noninfected pilonidal cyst is the most appropriate treatment option. Complex pilonidal cysts will require an en bloc excision of the sinus tract with a flap reconstruction. A rhomboid flap is the favored approach. Interestingly, there have been several studies demonstrating that control of intergluteal hair growth, either with clippers or laser treatment, will lead to decreased recurrence of disease (A).

References: Humphries AE, Duncan JE. Evaluation and management of pilonidal disease. *Surg Clin North Am.* 2010;90(1):113–124.

Khan MAA, Javed AA, Govindan KS, et al. Control of hair growth using long-pulsed alexandrite laser is an efficient and cost effective therapy for patients suffering from recurrent pilonidal disease. *Lasers Med Sci.* 2016;31(5):857–862.

Khanna A, Rombeau JL. Pilonidal disease. *Clin Colon Rectal Surg.* 2011;24(1):46–53.

10. B. Lymphedema is divided into primary (with no cause) and secondary (there is a known cause). Primary lymphedema is subdivided into three types: congenital, praecox, and tarda. Congenital lymphedema is present at birth (A). A familial version of congenital lymphedema is called Milroy disease. Lymphedema praecox develops during childhood or teenage years and accounts for 80% to 90% of cases of primary lymphedema and is 10 times more common in women (praecox is primary). It starts usually in the foot or lower leg. Lymphedema tarda is defined as starting after age 35 (C). Secondary lymphedema is more common than primary lymphedema. Worldwide infestation by Wuchereria bancrofti (filariasis) is the most common cause, whereas in the United States, the most common cause is post–axillary node dissection typically done for underlying breast cancer (D, E).

11. C. This patient has a ganglion cyst, which is also colloquially known as a "Bible cyst" because they were historically managed by slamming a book (the Bible) on the cyst allowing for decompression. The etiology has not been elucidated but is likely multifactorial. The leading theory is a simple herniation of the joint capsule. It consists of connective tissue from the synovial membrane of the joint or tendon sheath and most commonly affects the dorsal wrist (A). Most patients are asymptomatic but pain, discomfort, and paresthesia can occur. Compression of the terminal branches of the posterior interosseous nerve may be responsible for pain in the case of dorsal ganglion cysts while compression of the branches of the median or ulnar nerve contributes to the paresthesia experienced by patients with volar ganglion cysts (E). About 50% of cases resolve spontaneously within several months to 2 years (B). Intervention is indicated for patients that have pain or that are bothered by the cosmetic appearance. Simple aspiration or surgical excision alone has a high recurrence rate (up to 50%). To achieve a recurrence rate less than 10%, surgical excision with ligation of the pedicle is required and is now considered the gold standard in the treatment of a ganglion cyst.

References: Meena S, Gupta A. Dorsal wrist ganglion: current review of literature. *J Clin Orthop Trauma.* 2014;5(2):59–64.

Rizzo M, Berger RA, Steinmann SP, Bishop AT. Arthroscopic resection in the management of dorsal wrist ganglions: results with a minimum 2-year follow-up period. *J Hand Surg Am.* 2004;29(1):59–62.

12. C. Merkel cell carcinoma (MCC) is a rare but aggressive skin cancer of neuroendocrine origin arising from specialized touch receptor cells in the epidermis of the skin. It occurs in elderly, light-skinned patients and those with a history of sun exposure or immunosuppression, particularly CLL. The clinical features can be remembered by the mnemonic "AEIOU": Asymptomatic, Expanding rapidly, Immunosuppression, Older than 50 years old, and UV-exposed area. It often first appears as a pink nodule and progresses to a violaceous blue color with or without ulceration. About 80% of patients with MCC have Merkel cell polyomavirus genome found in tissue samples. It is unclear how this leads to the progression of MCC as Merkel cell polyomavirus is ubiquitous and found on most human skin. Wide local excision with 1- to 2-cm negative margins is the mainstay of treatment (A). Because there is a high propensity of lymph node spread, patients (with the exception of head and neck MCC) without palpable lymphadenopathy should have SLNB performed at the time of surgery (B). Additionally, all patients should receive adjuvant radiation to control local recurrence (10% recurrence rate with radiation and 50% without) (E). Chemotherapy is likely going to play an important role in the future, but as of yet, there are no conclusive studies to recommend this as a standard treatment modality for all patients with MCC (D).

References: Medina-Franco H, Urist MM, Fiveash J, Heslin MJ, Bland KI, Beenken SW. Multimodality treatment of Merkel cell carcinoma: case series and literature review of 1024 cases. *Ann Surg Oncol.* 2001;8(3):204–208.

Heath M, Jaimes N, Lemos B, et al. Clinical characteristics of Merkel cell carcinoma at diagnosis in 195 patients: the AEIOU features. *J Am Acad Dermatol.* 2008;58(3):375–381.

Santos-Juanes J, Fernández-Vega I, Fuentes N, et al. Merkel cell carcinoma and Merkel cell polyomavirus: a systematic review and meta-analysis. *Br J Dermatol.* 2015;173(1):42–49.

13. D. DFSP is considered the second most common cutaneous soft-tissue sarcoma following Kaposi sarcoma. It is a locally aggressive cancer with low metastatic potential. The majority of patients have a unique chromosomal translocation (t:17;22), leading to overexpression of PDGFB, a tyrosine kinase. It can occur at any age but most commonly presents in the fourth decade of life. DFSP first appears as a firm nodule that slowly enlarges and most commonly affects the trunk. Core needle biopsy is used for tissue diagnosis. The mainstay of treatment is wide local excision. Since it has an infiltrating growth pattern, extension beyond the clinical margins is common; thus good clinical margins are not helpful (A). This may help explain the high rate of local recurrence following surgery. DFSP occurring in the head and neck is better served with Mohs microscopic surgery to achieve superior cosmesis (C). Like most sarcomas, DFSP is radiosensitive and radiation therapy has been demonstrated to decrease local recurrence (B). However both systemic and local metastases are rare and thus, sentinel lymph node biopsy is not necessary (E). A recent metaanalysis demonstrated a lower recurrence rate with Mohs microscopic surgery compared with wide local excision (1.1% versus 6.3%). The prognosis of DFSP is excellent, with a 10-year survival close to 100%.

References: Gloster HM Jr. Dermatofibrosarcoma protuberans. *J Am Acad Dermatol.* 1996;35(3):355–374.

Foroozan M, Sei JF, Amini M, Beauchet A, Saiag P. Efficacy of Mohs micrographic surgery for the treatment of dermatofibrosarcoma protuberans: systematic review: Systematic review. *Arch Dermatol.* 2012;148(9):1055–1063.

Kreicher KL, Kurlander DE, Gittleman HR, Barnholtz-Sloan JS, Bordeaux JS. Incidence and survival of primary dermatofibrosarcoma protuberans in the United States. *Dermatol Surg.* 2016;42 Suppl 1:S24–31.

14. E. Lymph node metastases are not uncommon in melanoma. SLNB can provide accurate staging in melanoma and is recommended for all melanoma larger than 1 mm deep or for those with overlying ulceration regardless of depth (A, B). Most surgeons perform SLNB using a radioactive tracer, blue dye, or both. There has not been any conclusive data to show that any one particular agent is better than the other. Ironically, the radioactive tracer is considered to be safe in pregnancy but the blue dye is not. The radioactive tracer can be mapped with a Geiger counter, and the lymph node that takes up the largest amount of tracer (hot node) is assumed to be the sentinel lymph node. All nodes whose radioactivity count is greater than or equal to 10% of that of the hottest node should be removed because it is possible to have more than one sentinel lymph node. The most common blue dye used is isosulfan blue. Since the dye can stay around the skin for several months, it is recommended that the dye be injected within the boundary of the planned wide local excision, so it is also removed with the specimen (D). Rarely, isosulfan blue dye has been associated with a severe anaphylactic reaction. Additionally, all grossly suspicious lymph nodes should be removed as well. Although the role of SLNB has been firmly established in current practice, completion lymphadenectomy is a point of debate in the surgical community. Recently, the Multicenter Selective Lymphadenectomy Trial (MSLT-2)

trial showed that there was no melanoma-specific survival benefit in patients with positive SLNB who underwent completion lymphadenectomy compared with those that were observed, though there was improved regional control at 3 years (C). Palpable lymph nodes will require a therapeutic lymph node dissection. However, this should first be confirmed with a fine needle aspiration (FNA) biopsy.

References: Bilimoria KY, Balch CM, Bentrem DJ, et al. Complete lymph node dissection for sentinel node-positive melanoma: assessment of practice patterns in the United States. *Ann Surg Oncol.* 2008;15(6):1566–1576.

Coit DG, Andtbacka R, Anker CJ, et al. Melanoma, version 2.2013: featured updates to the NCCN guidelines. *J Natl Compr Canc Netw.* 2013;11(4):395–407.

Morton DL, Thompson JF, Cochran AJ, et al. Final trial report of sentinel-node biopsy versus nodal observation in melanoma. *N Engl J Med.* 2014;370(7):599–609.

Raut CP, Hunt KK, Akins JS, et al. Incidence of anaphylactoid reactions to isosulfan blue dye during breast carcinoma lymphatic mapping in patients treated with preoperative prophylaxis: results of a surgical prospective clinical practice protocol. *Cancer.* 2005;104(4):692–699.

Surgical Critical Care 15

ERIC O. YEATES AND DENNIS KIM

ABSITE 99 Percentile High-Yields

I. Acute Respiratory Distress Syndrome
   A. 2012 Berlin definition: replaces criteria from American-European Consensus Conference (AECC)
      1. Onset within 7 days of insult
      2. Bilateral opacities on chest x-ray or chest CT
      3. PaO_2/FiO_2 (PF) <300 with minimum PEEP 5 (Mild 200–300, Moderate 100–200, Severe <100)
      4. Must not be fully explained by cardiac failure or fluid overload (physician's best estimation); no need for invasive pulmonary artery catheter but can use echocardiogram
   B. Management considerations
      1. Tidal volume
         a) 6 ml/kg of ideal body weight
         b) Plateau pressure <30 cm of water
         c) Allow permissive hypercapnia
      2. Minimal PEEP and FiO_2 to match an acceptable arterial oxygenation (55–80 mmHg)
      3. Prone positioning
         a) Improves oxygenation and reduces ventilator-associated lung injury
         b) Improves mortality in moderate to severe ARDS
         c) Absolute contraindication: unstable spine fracture
         d) Relative contraindications: elevated ICP, severe facial trauma, hemodynamic instability, pregnancy, single anterior chest tube with air leak, unstable femur or pelvis
      4. Paralysis
         a) Consider in patients with PF <150
         b) Cisatracurium for 48 hours reduces mortality and barotrauma and increases the number of ventilator-free days
      5. Inhaled nitric oxide (iNO): improves oxygenation, but does not reduce mortality, may increase the risk of renal impairment
      6. Conservative fluid management: along with use of furosemide can decrease duration of mechanical ventilation, no improvement in mortality
      7. Continuous high-volume hemofiltration: may improve oxygenation, reduce duration of mechanical ventilation, and improve survival
      8. Early glucocorticoids: may decrease duration of mechanical ventilation and reduce mortality, but still controversial

II. Central Line Considerations
   A. Infection and DVT rates by location
      1. Femoral vein > internal jugular vein > subclavian vein
      2. Subclavian highest pneumothorax and failure rate
      3. If coagulopathic, use compressible site, avoid subclavian and IJ if possible

4. Avoid subclavian for patients that may need hemodialysis access in the future (central venous stenosis)
5. Air embolism
6. Prevention: trendelenburg during placement to increase CVP and decrease pressure gradient, avoid placing during inspiration, avoid short subcutaneous path to decrease risk during removal
    B. Management: Durant maneuver -> left lateral decubitus and Trendelenburg, encourages air bubble to move from right ventricular outflow tract to right atrium, can attempt aspiration

III. Commonly Used Sedation and Analgesic Medication in the ICU

Medication	Mechanism	Pharmacokinetics	Side effects	Miscellaneous
Lorazepam (Ativan)	GABA agonist	Metabolized by liver, no active metabolites	Delirium, renal dysfunction (propylene glycol)	Safer than other benzodiazepines in liver disease
Midazolam (Versed)	GABA agonist	Metabolized by liver, active metabolites (renal excretion)	Delirium	Fastest onset of benzodiazepines
Diazepam (Valium)	GABA agonist	Metabolized by liver, active metabolites (renal excretion)	Delirium	Longest acting of benzodiazepines
Propofol (Diprivan)	GABA agonist	Metabolized by liver, redistributes in fat	Hypotension, propofol infusion syndrome (PRIS)	PRIS: acute bradycardia with metabolic acidosis, rhabdomyolysis, hyperlipidemia, fatty liver
Dexmedetomidine (Precedex)	α2 agonist	Metabolized by liver	Hypotension, bradycardia, hypertension	No respiratory depression, has analgesic effects, less delirium
Fentanyl (Sublimaze)	μ agonist	Highly fat soluble, metabolized by liver	Respiratory depression, constipation	Accumulates with prolonged infusion, most potent
Morphine (Roxanol)	μ agonist	Metabolized by liver, active metabolites (renal excretion)	Respiratory depression, constipation	Least potent, morphine-6-glucuronide more potent than morphine
Hydromorphone (Dilaudid)	μ agonist	Metabolized by liver	Respiratory depression, constipation	Can use if patient develops tachyphylaxis to fentanyl
Ketamine	NDMA antagonist	Metabolized by liver	Hallucinations, cystitis, liver toxicity	When used for anesthesia, stimulates circulatory system, protective airway reflexes preserved

IV. Commonly Used Vasopressors in ICU

Medication	α	β1	β2	DA	V	Uses
Epinephrine						Cardiogenic shock, septic shock, anaphylaxis
Low dose	+	++	++			
High dose	++	+	+			
Norepinephrine	++	+				Septic shock (1st line), most other types of shock
Vasopressin					+	Septic shock (2nd line), pulmonary hypertension
Phenylephrine	+					Neurogenic shock
Dobutamine		+				Cardiogenic shock

Medication	α	$\beta1$	$\beta2$	DA	V	Uses
Dopamine						Neonatal hypotension, formerly for AKI
Low dose		+		++		
Medium dose	+	++		++		
High dose	++	+		+		
Isoproterenol		+	+			Bradycardia, formerly to treat asthma

V. Types of Shock and Related Physiologic Parameters

Physiologic state	CI	CVP/PCWP	SVR	Exam findings
Normal	2.4–4.0 L/min	0–5/6–12 mmHg	800–1200 dyn*sec/cm^5	
Hypovolemic shock (hemorrhagic, hypovolemic)	↓	↓	↑	Cool extremities, dry mucous membranes, tachycardia
Cardiogenic shock (MI, arrhythmia, heart failure)	↓	↑	↑	Cool extremities, lung crackles
Obstructive shock (PE, tension pneumothorax, tamponade	↓	↑	↑	Cool extremities, decreased breath sounds, tracheal deviation, distended neck veins
Septic shock	↑	↓	↓	Warm extremities, febrile
Neurogenic shock	↓	↓	↓	Warm extremities, bradycardia, spinal trauma

Questions

1. A 75-year-old male undergoes an emergent exploratory laparotomy and bowel resection for a small bowel obstruction. Two days later, he remains in the ICU intubated for hypoxic respiratory failure. On rounds, his nurse reports that he is Confusion Assessment Method (CAM)—ICU positive. Which of the following is true regarding his diagnosis?
   A. This condition will likely not affect his mortality
   B. Benzodiazepines and dexmedetomidine have a similar risk of contributing to this condition
   C. Quetiapine may improve his condition
   D. CAM-ICU may be used on patients with any Richmond Agitation Sedation Scale (RASS) score
   E. Haloperidol is contraindicated for this condition

2. Which of the following is true regarding the intraaortic balloon pump (IABP)?
   A. A sudden drop in urine output in a patient with an IABP should prompt an immediate chest x-ray
   B. The balloon inflates during early systole and deflates during diastole
   C. Coronary blood flow is unchanged
   D. IABP can be removed regardless of the platelet count
   E. Heparinization is required at all times with an IABP in place due to thrombotic risk

3. A 55-year-old male sustains severe multisystem injuries, including multiple rib fracture and a traumatic brain injury with subdural hematoma, after a motor vehicle collision. He remains intubated for multiple days and develops ventilator-associated pneumonia, acute renal failure, and septic shock and requires placement of a nontunneled hemodialysis catheter at bedside. His INR is 2.4. Which of the following is true regarding central line placement in this patient?
   A. The use of prophylactic antibiotics reduces catheter-associated infection
   B. Placement in the subclavian vein placement is ideal in this patient
   C. Placement of a central line in the internal jugular vein is contraindicated in a patient with intracranial hemorrhage
   D. Placement in the subclavian vein has the highest risk of pneumothorax
   E. Placement in the femoral vein has a lower risk of central line-associated bloodstream infection (CLABSI) compared to subclavian vein placement

4. A 68-year-old (70-kg) male nursing home resident is admitted for an altered mental status. His vital signs demonstrate orthostatic hypotension. Laboratory studies reveal a serum sodium level of 168 mEq/L, a serum potassium level of 4.0 mEq/L, a serum chloride level of 118 mEq/L, an HCO_3 level of 28 mEq/L, a blood urea nitrogen (BUN) of 30 mg/dL, and a serum creatinine level of 1.6 mg/dL. His free water deficit is:
   A. 3 L and all of it should be replaced over the next 12 hours
   B. 4 L and all of it should be replaced over the next 24 hours
   C. 5 L and 2.5 L should be replaced over the next 24 hours
   D. 7 L and 3.5 L should be replaced over the next 24 hours
   E. 10 L and 5 L should be replaced over the next 24 hours

5. Which of the following electrocardiographic changes is least likely to occur with hypokalemia?
   A. ST segment depression
   B. T-wave inversion
   C. Second- or third-degree atrioventricular block
   D. Premature ventricular complexes
   E. U waves

6. A 42-year-old woman with metastatic breast cancer is lethargic and has mental status changes. Her serum calcium is 14.5 mg/dL, serum alkaline phosphatase is 2000 IU/L, BUN is 42 mg/dL, and serum creatinine is 1.1 mg/dL. Initial treatment of the hypercalcemia should be:
   A. Mithramycin
   B. Bisphosphonates
   C. Loop diuretics
   D. Thiazide diuretics
   E. Normal saline infusion

7. A 75-year-old man becomes hypotensive (systolic blood pressure of 70 mmHg) after repair of an inguinal hernia. Urine output is low, and he is unresponsive to fluid administration. A pulmonary artery catheter is inserted. Cardiac output is 3 L/min; systemic vascular resistance (SVR) is 2140 dynes/sec × cm²; SvO$_2$ is 55%; pulmonary capillary wedge pressure (PCWP) is 24 mmHg. Which of the following is most likely to elevate the systolic blood pressure?
   A. 500 mL of Ringer's lactate to improve preload
   B. Lasix (furosemide) 20 mg intravenously to improve urine output
   C. Nitroprusside at 0.5 µg/kg/L/min to decrease the SVR
   D. Dobutamine at 5 to 10 µg/min for inotropic support
   E. Neo-Synephrine (phenylephrine) at 1 µg/L per min to increase blood pressure

8. Nosocomial pneumonia among intensive care unit patients:
   A. Has the same mortality rate as does community-acquired pneumonia (CAP)
   B. Is the most common nosocomial infection
   C. Can be avoided by early tracheostomy
   D. Is directly related to the duration of intubation
   E. Can be prevented by early institution of prophylactic IV antibiotics

9. Blood samples for the determination of mixed venous oxygen saturation (SvO$_2$) are ideally obtained from:
   A. Right atrium
   B. Pulmonary artery
   C. Pulmonary vein
   D. Two peripheral veins mixed together
   E. Central venous pressure line

10. Which of the following variables has the least influence on oxygen delivery?
    A. Hemoglobin
    B. Cardiac contractility
    C. Heart rate
    D. Carbon monoxide concentration
    E. Partial pressure of dissolved oxygen in the blood

11. Pulmonary artery occlusion pressure (PAOP) reflects which of the following physiologic variables?
    A. Cardiac output
    B. Pulmonary arterial pressure
    C. Left atrial pressure
    D. Pulmonary compliance
    E. Systemic vascular resistance (SVR)

12. Argatroban:
    A. Activates antithrombin
    B. Is cleared by the kidneys
    C. Is reversed with fresh-frozen plasma
    D. Can be monitored by the activated partial thromboplastin time
    E. Has a 3-hour half-life

13. A 54-year-old man who weighs 100 lbs comes to the ED after vomiting for 3 days and losing 10 lb. His serum electrolytes are as follows: sodium 136 mEq/L, potassium 3.1 mEq/L, chloride 88 mEq/L, and carbon dioxide 37 mEq/L. Which one of the following would be most helpful in determining the cause of his acid-base disorder?
    A. Urine sodium
    B. Urine creatinine
    C. Urine chloride
    D. Urine pH
    E. Urine potassium

14. Which of the following is true regarding medications commonly used for sedation in the intensive care unit?
    A. Propofol is associated with tachycardia
    B. Midazolam can lead to propylene glycol toxicity when given as a continuous infusion
    C. Dexmedetomidine has a similar method of action to clonidine
    D. Lorazepam has active metabolites leading to a longer duration of action
    E. Ketamine inhibits protective airway reflexes

15. A 70-year-old male with chronic obstructive pulmonary disease (COPD) presents to the emergency department (ED) after a stab wound to the left anterior thoracoabdominal region. His vitals are stable. The patient develops progressively worsening shortness of breath and noninvasive positive pressure ventilation (NPPV) with bilevel positive airway pressure (BiPAP) is started for a presumed COPD exacerbation. The patient's blood pressure then abruptly drops to 70/40 mmHg. Which of the following statements is true?
    A. This complication could have been prevented with a higher expiratory pressure on BiPAP
    B. The cardiopulmonary compromise is likely secondary to obstructive shock
    C. Immediate endotracheal intubation is mandatory
    D. BiPAP is contraindicated with COPD
    E. A nasogastric tube should have been placed before initiation of BiPAP

16. A 24-year-old obese male with a traumatic brain injury is 6 hours post procedure from a percutaneous dilatational tracheostomy tube placement. The nurse calls to state that the tracheostomy tube was accidentally dislodged. Which of the following is recommended?
    A. Immediately reinsert the tube
    B. Immediately reinsert the tube using ultrasound guidance
    C. Bag patient and urgently transport to the operating room for open reinsertion
    D. Perform bedside cricothyroidotomy
    E. Endotracheal intubation

17. A 50-year-old female was admitted to the intensive care unit (ICU) 36 hours ago with worsening hypoxic respiratory failure secondary to pulmonary contusion following a motor vehicle collision. The most recent chest radiograph shows new bilateral pulmonary infiltrates. Current arterial blood gas shows a PaO_2 of 70 mmHg. Current ventilator settings include a FiO_2 of 60% and a positive end-expiratory pressure (PEEP) of 8 cm H_2O. She has no history of heart disease. Which of the following is true regarding this condition?
    A. An objective surrogate for pulmonary artery capillary wedge pressure (PAWP) is necessary to make a diagnosis of ARDS
    B. Prone ventilation should be initiated
    C. Inhaled nitric oxide will confer a mortality benefit
    D. High-frequency oscillatory ventilation (HFOV) is associated with improved survival
    E. Neuromuscular blockade is associated with an increase in ventilator days

18. A 52-year-old male is preadmitted for a coronary artery bypass graft for three-vessel disease. While attempting to obtain a pulmonary artery capillary wedge pressure with the balloon inflated, the patient begins to cough and has a small amount of hemoptysis. However, this resolves quickly, and the patient shows no other signs of distress. Which of the following is the next best step in management?
    A. Deflate the balloon, withdraw the catheter into the right ventricle and refloat into the pulmonary artery
    B. Deflate the balloon and remove the pulmonary artery catheter entirely
    C. Leave the balloon inflated and prepare the patient for a catheter-based angiography
    D. Take immediately to the operating room for emergent thoracotomy
    E. Hyperinflate the balloon and advance the catheter as much as possible

19. A 68-year-old male has new onset of an irregular, narrow complex tachycardia with a ventricular rate of 125 beats per minute. A single dose of metoprolol is administered with minimal affect. The patient subsequently becomes diaphoretic and the blood pressure drops to 72/35 mmHg. What is the next best step in management?
    A. Unsynchronized cardioversion
    B. Synchronized cardioversion
    C. Defibrillation
    D. Amiodarone push followed by a continuous drip
    E. Intravenous (IV) push of adenosine

20. Which of the following is true regarding septic shock?
    A. It is characterized by poor perfusion of end organs
    B. Maintaining hemoglobin level greater than 10 g/dL is recommended
    C. In early septic shock, whole body oxygen consumption is decreased
    D. Positive fluid balance is associated with increased mortality
    E. The liver can serve as a continued source of inflammatory products

21. A 27-year-old male (75 kg) with severe peritonitis due to perforated appendicitis develops hypotension requiring pressors following laparotomy. He has low systemic vascular resistance and high cardiac output. Over the past 12 hours his urine output dropped to less than 10 cc/hour despite receiving adequate IV fluids. His creatinine increased from a baseline of 0.9 mg/dL on admission to 2.2 mg/dL. He is not acidotic nor hyperkalemic and does not appear to be volume overloaded. Which of the following is true for this patient?
    A. Hemodialysis (HD) should be initiated
    B. HD is better than CRRT at removing inflammatory mediators
    C. Early initiation of continuous renal replacement therapy (CRRT) will improve survival
    D. CRRT will require vascular access that differs from that of HD
    E. The timing of initiating CRRT does not change the length of hospital stay

22. A 21-year-old man who was the driver in a head-on collision has a pulse of 140 beats per minute, respiratory rate of 36 breaths per minute, and systolic blood pressure of 70 mmHg. His trachea is deviated to the left, with palpable subcutaneous emphysema and absent breath sounds over the right hemithorax. The next best step in the management of this patient is:
    A. Resuscitative thoracotomy
    B. Ultrasonography or chest radiograph to confirm diagnosis
    C. Intubation and ventilation
    D. Tube thoracostomy
    E. Needle thoracostomy

23. In hemorrhagic shock, which of the following is the most accurate sign of adequate fluid resuscitation?
    A. An increase in blood pressure
    B. An increase in urine output
    C. An increase in arterial oxygenation
    D. A decrease in thirst
    E. A decrease in tachycardia

24. A 50-year-old woman who is septic from ascending cholangitis is transferred to the surgical ICU. She undergoes cholecystectomy and common bile duct exploration after a failed endoscopic sphincterotomy. Because of hypotension and marginal urine output, a Swan-Ganz catheter is placed. Which of the following readings is least consistent with the patient's clinical course?
    A. Central venous pressure 5 cm H_2O
    B. SVR 300 dynes $\times$ sec $\times$ cm^2
    C. Cardiac index 2.0 L/min/cm^2
    D. Pulmonary capillary wedge pressure 10 cm H_2O
    E. SvO$_2$ 86%

25. Prolonged QT intervals are seen in association with:
    A. Hypomagnesemia
    B. Hypercalcemia
    C. Hyperphosphatemia
    D. Hyperkalemia
    E. Hypokalemia

26. Acute symptoms of hypermagnesemia are treated by:
    A. Fluid hydration with normal saline
    B. IV insulin
    C. Calcium chloride
    D. Dextrose
    E. Dialysis

27. A morbidly obese 48-year-old male is admitted to the ICU following an open cholecystectomy via a midline incision. The patient's PaO$_2$ is 50 mmHg on a FiO$_2$ of 60% and PEEP of 5 cm H_2O. After increasing PEEP to 10 cm H_2O, which of the following parameters is likely to increase?
    A. Arterial partial pressure of carbon dioxide (PaCO$_2$)
    B. Cardiac output
    C. Functional residual capacity (FRC)
    D. Left ventricular end-systolic volume
    E. Pulmonary edema

28. Which of the following is most commonly associated with transfusion-transmitted bacterial infection?
    A. *Staphylococcus aureus*
    B. *Staphylococcus epidermidis*
    C. β-Hemolytic streptococcus
    D. *Bacillus fragilis*
    E. Gram-negative organisms

29. Intraabdominal hypertension is defined as intraabdominal pressures that exceed:
    A. 12 cm H_2O
    B. 16 cm H_2O
    C. 20 cm H_2O
    D. 25 cm H_2O
    E. 30 cm H_2O

30. After an elective low anterior resection for rectal cancer, palpitations develop in a 59-year-old man with a history of congestive heart failure and an ejection fraction of 20% in the ICU. On the electrocardiogram, he is noted to be in a ventricular tachycardia (VT) at a rate of 150 beats per minute. On evaluation, he has altered mental status and his blood pressure is 95/65 mmHg. The best initial treatment for this arrhythmia would be:
    A. Epinephrine 1 mg IV push
    B. Amiodarone 150 mg IV over 10 minutes
    C. Immediate defibrillation with 360 J
    D. Synchronized cardioversion with 150 J
    E. Diltiazem 15 mg IV over 2 minutes

31. In patients with acute kidney injury, the most immediate threat to the patient is:
    A. Acidosis
    B. Hyperkalemia
    C. Platelet dysfunction
    D. Fluid overload
    E. Malnutrition

32. Which of the following is true regarding hepatorenal syndrome?
    A. Type II is rapidly progressive with a poor prognosis
    B. It is associated with intense renal vasodilation
    C. It is associated with splanchnic vasoconstriction
    D. The urine sodium is typically less than 10 mEq/L
    E. Type I is relatively stable

33. A 19-year-old man presents to the ED after a motor vehicle collision. The patient is alert and oriented but is unable to move his arms and legs. Results of a focused assessment with sonography for trauma (FAST) scan and chest and pelvic radiographs are all negative. On physical examination, the patient has a blood pressure of 80/60 mmHg and a heart rate of 70 beats per minute. His feet are warm and pink, and he is noted to have priapism. Which of the following is the next best step in management?
    A. Phenylephrine
    B. Intravenous fluid administration
    C. Dobutamine
    D. Epinephrine
    E. Norepinephrine

Answers

1. **C.** The CAM-ICU is one of the most commonly used tools for assessing for delirium in the ICU and can be used on intubated and nonintubated patients. The CAM-ICU algorithm first requires the patient to be sufficiently awake (RASS ≥ –3) (D). Next, it tests for inattention and disorganized thinking. Delirium is common in the ICU and has been shown to be an independent predictor of mortality (A). Prevention strategies include avoiding certain medications and early mobilization during interruptions in sedation. For example, patients receiving dexmedetomidine over benzodiazepines had a lower incidence of delirium (B). There is no medication that has conclusively been demonstrated to decrease the risk of the development of delirium in ICU patients. However, antipsychotics including haloperidol and quetiapine can be used to treat the symptoms of hyperactive delirium (E).

    References: Ely EW, Shintani A, Truman B, et al. Delirium as a predictor of mortality in mechanically ventilated patients in the intensive care unit. *JAMA.* 2004;291(14):1753–1762.

    Reade MC, Finfer S. Sedation and delirium in the intensive care unit. *N Engl J Med.* 2014;370(5):444–454.

2. **A.** The IABP is a circulatory assist device indicated for use in cardiogenic shock. Preoperatively, IABP is indicated for low cardiac output (CO) states including unstable angina refractory to medical therapy. Intraoperatively, it can be used to permit weaning from cardiopulmonary bypass when inotropic agents alone are not sufficient. Postoperatively, IABP is used primarily for low CO states refractory to medical management. IABPs are most commonly inserted into the femoral artery and the radiopaque tip of the balloon is positioned just below the aortic knob and just distal to left subclavian artery. IABPs work by inflating in diastole and deflating in early systole (B). This indirectly assists the heart by decreasing afterload and augmenting diastolic aortic pressure and increasing coronary blood flow (C). Contraindications include moderate/severe aortic regurgitation and aortic dissection. There are a number of known complications with IABPs, including hemolysis due to mechanical damage to red blood cells. Additionally, IABP migration or malpositioning can occur and cover the renal vessels, decreasing urine output. Though heparinization is recommended when possible to prevent thrombotic complications, the risk of bleeding should be weighed, especially in patients who recently underwent major cardiac surgery (E). Before removal of IABP, the platelet count, PT, and PTT should be normal (D).

    References: Krishna M, Zacharowski K. Principles of intra-aortic balloon pump counterpulsation. *Contin Educ Anaesth Crit Care Pain.* 2009;9(1):24–28.

    Pucher PH, Cummings IG, Shipolini AR, et al. Is heparin needed for patients with an intra-aortic balloon pump? *Interact Cardiovasc Thorac Surg.* 2012;15(1):136–139.

3. **D.** The choice of central line placement site is important in complex ICU patients that may have various contraindications. In a randomized control trial comparing complications between central line placement sites, subclavian placement had a lower risk of bloodstream infection and thrombosis compared to the internal jugular vein and femoral vein but had a higher rate of pneumothorax (E). In contrast, a Cochrane analysis found no difference in the risk of CLABSI between femoral, subclavian, and internal jugular vein site insertions (E). Subclavian placement should also be avoided in patients that may need hemodialysis access in the future and those with coagulopathy, as it is difficult to control bleeding with direct pressure in this area (B). Intracranial hemorrhage and/or elevated intracranial pressures are not a contraindication to catheterization of the internal jugular veins (C). There is also no high-level evidence supporting prophylactic antibiotics prevents catheter-associated infection (A).

Reference: Marik PE, Flemmer M, Harrison W. The risk of catheter-related bloodstream infection with femoral venous catheters as compared to subclavian and internal jugular venous catheters: a systematic review of the literature and meta-analysis. *Crit Care Med.* 2012;40(8):2479–2485.

4. D. Free water deficit = (serum sodium − 140)/(140) × total body water. Total body water is 50% of lean body mass in men and 40% in women. The free water deficit calculates to be 7 L, half of which should be replaced over the next 24 hours. The correction must be made slowly to avoid neurologic complications such as cerebral edema.

5. C. Electrocardiographic changes associated with hypokalemia include U waves, T-wave flattening, ST-segment changes, and arrhythmias (A, B, D, E). Atrioventricular block is more common with hypercalcemia and hyperkalemia. Hypokalemia is a common electrolyte abnormality in surgical patients, occurring because of inadequate supplementation with total parenteral nutrition and excessive IV fluids.

6. E. The treatment of hypercalcemia of malignancy should begin first with inducing calciuresis. This is accomplished by saline volume expansion. Once volume has been expanded, the next step is to administer loop diuretics because this similarly induces calciuresis (loops lose calcium) (C). Thiazide diuretics will have the opposite effect (D). Mithramycin acts directly on bones, lowering calcium levels, but the effect takes more than 24 hours (A). In contrast, bisphosphonate drugs are indicated in addition to IV hydration and loop diuretics in patients with cancer. This class includes zoledronic acid (superior) and pamidronate, which inhibits osteoclast activity, resulting in lower calcium levels in patients with bony metastasis. However, these agents may take 48 to 72 hours before reaching full therapeutic effect (B). Additionally, calcitonin lowers serum calcium levels within hours by inhibiting bone resorption that is occurring from metastatic disease; calcitonin is indicated in hypercalcemic crises. Corticosteroids are most useful in hypercalcemia related to sarcoidosis and multiple myeloma. They may be useful in patients with bony metastasis, but they take as long as 1 week to work.

Reference: Major P, Lortholary A, Hon J, et al. Zoledronic acid is superior to pamidronate in the treatment of hypercalcemia of malignancy: a pooled analysis of two randomized, controlled clinical trials. *J Clin Oncol.* 2001;19(2):558–567.

7. D. The patient is in cardiogenic shock as evidenced by low cardiac output, elevated SVR, and elevated PCWP. He has already shown to not have a persistent response to fluids so an additional bolus is unlikely to be helpful (A). Inotropic support in the form of dobutamine is indicated to improve cardiac contractility and cardiac output, while decreasing afterload. Alternative inotropes (vasoactive agents) include epinephrine and a phosphodiesterase inhibitor, such as milrinone. Given the patient's elevated PCWP, it is unlikely that further fluid resuscitation to increase preload is necessary. Furosemide (Lasix) is not a good option because his low urine output reflects poor forward flow versus volume overload (B). Nitroprusside is a vasodilator and could potentially improve cardiac output, but blood pressure is unlikely to improve without ionotropic agents (C). It should not be used as the next step in treating this patient. Phenylephrine

(Neo-Synephrine) is an α1-agonist that will increase SVR (afterload) and can increase blood pressure. However, the patient is already maximally vasoconstricted as you would expect in cardiogenic shock and as evidenced by the high SVR. Phenylephrine would be a poor choice in a patient with cardiogenic shock (E).

8. D. Nosocomial pneumonia is the second most common nosocomial infection (the most common is urinary tract infection) and the most common nosocomial infection among ventilated patients (B). The risk of ventilator-associated pneumonia increases 5% per day and is as high as 70% at 30 days. The 30-day mortality rate from nosocomial pneumonia can be as high as 40%, which is significantly higher than CAP (A). Nosocomial pneumonias are frequently polymicrobial, and gram-negative rods are the predominant organisms. The criteria for diagnosis include fever; cough; development of purulent sputum in conjunction with radiologic evidence of an infiltrate; suggestive Gram stain findings; and positive sputum, tracheal aspirate, pleural fluid, or blood cultures. Prophylactic use of IV antibiotic has not been shown to reduce rates of nosocomial infection or to improve survival (E). However, there are some data to suggest that oral decontaminant regimens (gentamicin/colistin/vancomycin 2% in Orabase gel every 6 hours) can reduce the rate of ventilator-associated pneumonia. However, this is not yet the standard of care. Although early tracheostomy can reduce the number of days on the ventilator, it does not lead to reduced rates of pneumonia (C).

Reference: Bergmans DC, Bonten MJ, Gaillard CA, et al. Prevention of ventilator-associated pneumonia by oral decontamination: a prospective, randomized, double-blind, placebo-controlled study. *Am J Respir Crit Care Med.* 2001;164(3):382–388.

9. B. SvO2 is an indirect measurement of oxygen delivery. It is measured from a blood sample obtained from the pulmonary artery. A true SvO2 includes blood from the vena cava and the coronary sinus (A, C–E). SvO2 is a marker for adequacy of resuscitation and reversal of hypoxemia. However, mixed venous gas is most commonly sampled from the superior vena cava using a central venous catheter.

10. E. Oxygen delivery (DO_2) is determined solely by the cardiac output and the oxygen content of blood (CaO_2), so anything that affects these two variables is going to have a direct effect on the DO_2. Because cardiac output is determined by the stroke volume and heart rate, a change in cardiac contractility will directly influence DO_2 (B, C). The oxygen content of blood can be defined by the equation $CaO_2 = (Hg \times 1.34 \times SaO_2) + (PaO_2 \times 0.003)$, where Hg is the concentration of hemoglobin, SaO_2 is the percent saturation of hemoglobin, 1.34 is the oxygen-carrying capacity of 1 g of hemoglobin, PaO_2 is the partial pressure of oxygen dissolved in the blood, and 0.003 is the measure of O_2 (in mL) dissolved in 1 dL of blood per mmHg of pressure. So hemoglobin and carbon monoxide (which decreases the percent saturation of hemoglobin by oxygen) will both affect oxygen delivery as well (A, D). The PaO_2 only contributes 1% to 2% of the total oxygen content (E). However, it is important to keep in mind that the SaO_2 is partly reliant on the PaO_2 as can be demonstrated by the oxyhemoglobin dissociation curve.

11. C. PAOP or pulmonary artery wedge pressure (PAWP) provides an indirect estimate of both left atrial and left ventricular diastolic pressure (A–B, D–E). These pressures can be measured using a Swan-Ganz or pulmonary artery catheter, which is a flexible balloon-tipped catheter that is inserted into the pulmonary artery and inflated, thereby occluding pulmonary artery pressures and reflecting left heart pressures. In diastole, there are no valves between the open mitral valve and closed pulmonic valves. In this unobstructed pathway between the left ventricle and the closed pulmonic valves, as well as the relatively low compliance of the pulmonary artery circulation, there exists a column of blood from the catheter tip in the pulmonary artery through the pulmonary capillary bed, pulmonary vein, left atrium, and left ventricle. The measured pressure approximates the pressure in the LV during end-diastole and is used as a measure of LV preload. With the balloon wedged and the ventricles in systole, PAWP now measures pressures reflected by the LA provided there are no significant mitral valve abnormalities. Swan-Ganz catheters provide both direct and indirect measurements of cardiac performance and these measurements are contingent upon when during the cycle the measurements are taken as well as whether or not the catheter is wedged.

12. D. Argatroban and lepirudin are both direct thrombin inhibitors and used for heparin-induced thrombocytopenia (HIT) and thrombosis (A–C, E). Both can be monitored by the activated partial thromboplastin time and both have relatively short half-lives (60–90 minutes for lepirudin and 40–50 minutes for argatroban). Neither can be reversed and neither requires the presence of antithrombin to be effective. Argatroban is cleared by hepatic metabolism, whereas lepirudin is cleared by the kidneys. In addition to being used for HIT, argatroban is approved in patients with or at risk of HIT who are undergoing percutaneous coronary intervention. Argatroban has a short half-life (40–50 minutes) and reaches a steady state with IV infusion at 1 to 3 hours. Because it is cleared by hepatic metabolism, it is the drug of choice for patients with HIT and renal insufficiency.

13. C. With a bicarbonate level of 37, this patient has a metabolic alkalosis. The cause of metabolic alkalosis can be determined by whether it is chloride responsive or resistant (A–B, D–E). Chloride-responsive cases (urine chloride <15 mEq/L) are much more common in surgical patients and result from vomiting (gastrointestinal loss of hydrogen ions), diuretics (genitourinary loss of chloride), and volume depletion (aldosterone-stimulated hydrogen ion loss in urine). Conversely, chloride-resistant types (urine chloride >25 mEq/L) result from mineralocorticoid excess or potassium depletion.

14. C. Benzodiazepines (particularly lorazepam and midazolam) are commonly used medications for long-term sedation in the intensive care unit (ICU). While they are equally efficacious when administered in doses of equivalent potency, they differ in onset of action and duration. Midazolam is highly lipophilic and has a quick onset of action when compared with lorazepam. Duration of action is much more multifactorial. Initially, it is also determined heavily by lipophilicity because of rapid redistribution from the central nervous system to the peripheral tissues. However, as tissue levels build up with continuous infusion, the duration of effect lengthens. Midazolam, in particular, also has active metabolites, which further prolong its duration; this effect is worsened by hepatic or renal failure. In contrast, lorazepam has no active metabolites, but mobilization to and from the peripheral tissues is much slower (D). With prolonged usage at high doses, lorazepam can lead to propylene glycol toxicity because it is included in the diluent. However, this is not used in the formulation of midazolam (B). For the above reasons, benzodiazepines are poor choices for prolonged sedation in the ICU. Propofol, which is believed to work on the GABA receptor, is a highly lipophilic anesthetic with a very quick onset and short duration. It quickly distributes to tissues and is rapidly metabolized by the liver, leading to a short duration of action. However, it has significant cardiovascular effects including hypotension and bradycardia (A). Ketamine is a potent sedative that blocks glutamate NMDA receptors within sensory nerve endings. It creates a dissociative anesthetic effect where patients remain conscious without inhibition of respiratory drive or protective airway reflexes (E). Unlike propofol, ketamine is considered to have analgesic properties. However, because of significant psychoactive effects, its use is limited. Dexmedetomidine and clonidine are both selective alpha-2 receptor antagonists, though the former has a much higher affinity for alpha-2 receptors than clonidine. Dexmedetomidine is a sedative with anxiolytic and analgesic properties without significant respiratory depression. Patients transition easily from undisturbed sedation to being aroused with stimuli.

References: Mihic S, Harris R. Hypnotics and sedatives. In: Brunton LL, Chabner BA, Knollmann BC, eds. *Goodman & Gilman's: the pharmacological basis of therapeutics.* 12th ed. McGraw-Hill; 2015:101–119.

Sokol S, Patel BK, Lat I, Kress JP. Pain control, sedation, and use of muscle relaxants. In: Hall JB, Schmidt GA, Kress JP, eds. *Principles of critical care.* 4th ed. McGraw-Hill; 2014:76–84.

15. B. Traumatic pneumothorax should be suspected in all patients with a penetrating thoracoabdominal injury. The addition of NPPV increases intrathoracic pressure and may convert a pneumothorax into a tension pneumothorax, which can subsequently decrease venous return and result in obstructive shock (as demonstrated in the above case). Similarly, endotracheal intubation also increases intrathoracic pressure and can result in shock (C). In a stable patient without classic exam findings for pneumothorax (decreased breath sounds, tympanic chest), a chest x-ray can be performed to look for the collapsed lung. This can be followed by insertion of a tube thoracostomy (chest tube). NPPV can be delivered using continuous positive airway pressure (CPAP) or BiPAP, with the former providing continuous positive pressure support on a single setting and the latter providing different amounts of pressure support during the expiratory and inspiratory phases. The theoretical benefit of BiPAP is that it allows for a lower amount of pressure support during the expiratory phase, which can help patients blow off carbon dioxide. In patients with COPD, this is particularly useful because they are at increased risk for hypercapnia (D). NPPV is a useful adjunct for respiratory failure if used in select patients without contraindications. It is currently recommended for first-line treatment of acute respiratory failure from COPD and congestive heart failure (CHF) with pulmonary edema (A). There are some data to suggest a trial of NPPV should be attempted first in select patients with acute hypoxic respiratory failure as this may prevent intubation. However, failure to improve within the first 1 to 2 hours of treatment should prompt conversion to intubation. Contraindications to NPPV include: cardiac or respiratory arrest, inability to cooperate and protect the airway or clear secretions, severely impaired consciousness, nonrespiratory organ failure, facial trauma or deformity, high risk of aspiration, recent upper gastrointestinal (GI) anastomosis, anticipated prolonged duration of mechanical ventilation, bullous lung disease such as emphysema (can result in pneumothorax), or hypotension (intrathoracic pressure can decrease venous return and thus cardiac output). Placement of a nasogastric tube can potentially complicate NPPV by impairing its ability to form an effective seal and increasing the risk of pressure ulcer formation, and it has not been definitively shown to decrease risk of aspiration (E).

References: Garpestad E, Brennan J, Hill NS. Noninvasive ventilation for critical care. *Chest*. 2007;132(2):711–720.

Keenan SP, Sinuff T, Burns KEA, et al. Clinical practice guidelines for the use of noninvasive positive-pressure ventilation and noninvasive continuous positive airway pressure in the acute care setting. *CMAJ*. 2011;183(3):E195–214.

Siddiqui FM, Felton T, Stevens A, Slater R. An unusual contraindication to the use of non-invasive ventilation in A&E. *Emerg Med J*. 2010;27(8):615.

16. E. The percutaneous method of tracheostomy placement has become widely used in critically ill patients because there is no need to transport the patient; the complications seem to be equivalent or lower to open tracheostomy, and the cost of the procedure is reduced. Initially, there was concern about the safety of this relatively novel method, especially in obese patients. However, a single-center study with over 3000 patients demonstrated that percutaneous tracheostomy placement had a lower complication rate. The study also indicated no higher complication rates for obese patients, especially with the advent of longer tracheostomy tubes. Early tracheostomy dislodgment is a relatively rare but potentially fatal complication associated with tracheostomy tube placement. Before the development of a mature tract, it is possible to inadvertently place the tracheostomy into the subcutaneous tissue, which would manifest with subcutaneous emphysema and oxygen desaturation. While replacement during this time period is possible in experienced hands, immediate endotracheal intubation is the recommended management (A–C, D). Although ultrasonography or a tracheostomy obturator does facilitate easier placement, it is still possible to place the tracheostomy tube in false tissue tracts (B).

Reference: Dennis BM, Eckert MJ, Gunter OL, Morris JA Jr, May AK. Safety of bedside percutaneous tracheostomy in the critically ill: evaluation of more than 3,000 procedures. *J Am Coll Surg*. 2013;216(4):858–865.

17. B. Acute respiratory distress syndrome (ARDS) was redefined in 2012 under the Berlin Definition into a three-tiered grading system consisting of mild ($PaO_2/FiO_2 = 200–300$ mmHg), moderate ($PaO_2/FiO_2 = 100–200$ mmHg), and severe ($PaO_2/FiO_2 < 100$ mmHg). The purpose of the consensus meeting was to correlate a new naming system with predicted mortality and to remove some outdated requirements (inclusion of the PAWP in the definition). In place of

the PAWP, clinical suspicion and a known inciting factor of ARDS in the last 7 days are sufficient for inclusion in the definition (A). Based on these criteria, this patient would fall into moderate ARDS ($PaO_2/FiO_2 = 117$ mmHg). A lung-protective strategy of ventilation using <6 mL/kg of tidal volume and higher levels of PEEP continues to be the mainstay of treatment. In addition, prone ventilation for more than 12 hours per day has also shown a mortality benefit when instituted early in moderate to severe ARDS but not in mild ARDS. While inhaled nitric oxide will improve a patient's oxygenation, there have been no studies to date that have definitively proven that it confers a mortality benefit (C). Also, there are some data to indicate that its use could potentially increase the risk of renal impairment. Similarly, HOFV has come under scrutiny after the OSCILLATE trial, which showed a trend toward increased mortality with early initiation of HFOV (D). Though the data are conflicted in regard to the utility of neuromuscular blockade, there is some evidence to suggest that cisatracurium may decrease the number of ventilator and ICU days, as well as potentially provide a mortality benefit (E).

References: Bein T, Grasso S, Moerer O, et al. The standard of care of patients with ARDS: ventilatory settings and rescue therapies for refractory hypoxemia. *Intensive Care Med*. 2016;42(5):699–711.

Ferguson ND, Fan E, Camporota L, et al. The Berlin definition of ARDS: an expanded rationale, justification, and supplementary material. *Intensive Care Med*. 2012;38(10):1573–1582.

Ferguson ND, Cook DJ, Guyatt GH, et al. High-frequency oscillation in early acute respiratory distress syndrome. *N Engl J Med*. 2013;368(9):795–805.

18. C. Pulmonary artery rupture is one of the most dreaded complications of pulmonary artery catheter placement. The most common etiologies are a balloon that is inflated too distal into the pulmonary system or too much force is used to obtain a wedge pressure. Most of the time, the rupture of the artery is heralded by an initial small volume hemoptysis as the injury is initially contained within a pseudoaneurysm. In suspected cases, the balloon should be left inflated and the patient taken for catheter-based angiography. By leaving the catheter in place, this allows for an immediate route of access for angiography. Additionally, the balloon may stop further bleeding (B). Overinflation of the balloon or repeated attempts at placement have the potential to worsen the initial injury and should be avoided (A, E). Open repair in the operating room is technically possible, but exposure of the pulmonary artery branch responsible is a morbid procedure and time consuming (D). Embolization of the pseudoaneurysm before full rupture is the preferred treatment modality.

19. B. The patient's new-onset irregular, narrow complex tachycardia is likely atrial fibrillation with a rapid ventricular response. While it is reasonable to attempt medical cardioversion in a stable patient, conversion to unstable tachycardia requires immediate electronic synchronized cardioversion (as outlined in ACLS). The "synchronization" refers to delivering a low energy shock at the peak of the QRS complex. This explains why there is a brief pause between pressing the shock button and delivery of the shock. The theoretical benefit of synchronized cardioversion is avoidance of the shock during cardiac repolarization, which may precipitate ventricular fibrillation. In contrast, unsynchronized cardioversion, also known as defibrillation, delivers a high-energy shock as soon as the button is pressed. This is reserved for pulseless ventricular tachycardia/fibrillation in which any delay in shock delivery leads to poorer outcomes (A, C). Amiodarone should be used with caution if a patient has paroxysmal atrial fibrillation or the chronicity is unknown because this can potentially chemically convert the patient to a sinus rhythm and embolize any clot that has formed (D). Adenosine is typically reserved for monomorphic narrow complex tachycardia consistent with supraventricular tachycardia (E).

20. D. The essential management of the septic patient includes early recognition, broad-spectrum IV antibiotics, pressors (norepinephrine first, then vasopressin), and fluid resuscitation. There is a notable absence of large randomized, controlled trials demonstrating improved survival of adjunctive treatment options aside from the above essentials. Sepsis is an inflammatory cascade that is triggered by injury or bacterial invasion in an attempt to control the noxious stimuli. The location and type of pathogen or injury are irrelevant and do not influence outcomes or survival. The core problem of septic shock is the poor utilization of oxygen, not a lack of perfusion. Blood delivery (and perfusion to end organs) is not significantly impaired and as such maintaining the hemoglobin above a certain threshold provides little benefit (A, B). Inflammatory mediators chiefly impair mitochondrial oxidation by inhibiting pyruvate dehydrogenase and cytochrome oxidase and thus destroy the cell's ability to produce its energy currency, adenosine triphosphate (ATP) (this is termed cytopathic hypoxemia). Additionally, whole oxygen body consumption is actually increased in early septic shock as inflammatory mediators induce production of toxic oxygen free radicals (respiratory burst) in an attempt to break down bacterial cell membranes, denature proteins, and destroy DNA (C). Although endogenous antioxidants are plentiful in homeostasis and prevent free radicals from causing havoc on normal functioning cells, the septic patient has an exaggerated, large, and widespread production of free radicals that exceed endogenous antioxidant protection; this is known as oxidant stress. Additionally, inflammatory mediators induce production of nitrous oxide resulting in systemic vascular dilation and high cardiac output (from increased heart rate). However, due to the increased stress put on the cardiovascular system, cardiac output begins to fall late in untreated septic shock and portends a poor prognosis. The systemic venodilation leaves the majority of the intravascular volume dormant in the venous system, which is the basis of why fluid resuscitation is essential early in septic shock. However, a large positive fluid balance should be avoided as it is associated with increased mortality. And lastly, although there is a systemic vascular dilation, there is relative splanchnic vasoconstriction resulting in gut ischemia and mucosal injury. This allows for enteric pathogen translocation and additional subsequent inflammatory mediators resulting in further splanchnic vasoconstriction and mucosal injury; this self-sustaining process of continued inflammation is known as the "motor" of multiorgan failure (E).

References: Abraham E, Singer M. Mechanisms of sepsis-induced organ dysfunction. *Crit Care Med.* 2007;35(10):2408–2416.

Babior BM. The respiratory burst of phagocytes. *J Clin Invest.* 1984;73(3):599–601.

Meakins JL, Marshall JC. The gastrointestinal tract: the "motor" of MOF. *Arch Surg.*1986;121(2):197–201.

21. C. The first step in the management of oliguria is often a fluid challenge; the hypovolemic patient will respond with a correspondent increase in urine output. In a septic patient (as in this case), oliguria is a result of intrinsic renal dysfunction secondary to widespread inflammation and thus a fluid bolus is unlikely to result in improved urine output. In the surgical ICU, the emphasis is placed on "preventative" critical care management, when appropriate (e.g., gastrointestinal [GI] prophylaxis to prevent ulcers). In this case, this translates into providing RRT before the overt presence of renal dysfunction: acidosis, hyperkalemia, volume overload, and azotemia. RRT is provided by either HD or CRRT in patients with acute kidney injury and/or renal failure. Both can be started using a nontunneled multilumen dialysis catheter (D). HD allows for rapid fluid and solute removal in a 4- to 5-hour time period, which can result in hypotension during dialysis. In contrast, CRRT works continuously with a slower unloading of fluid and solutes; this slow but continuous filtration allows for a larger overall amount of fluid removed. The primary modality for RRT in the septic patient is CRRT because HD is relatively contraindicated in hypotensive patients requiring pressors owing to the large fluid shifts that can occur with HD (A). Additionally, since septic shock is largely a result of widespread inflammatory mediators, CRRT can be used in an ultrafiltration mode to lower plasma concentrations of inflammatory mediators and thus decrease the risk of multiorgan failure. The less porous interface used in the filtration membrane of HD is inferior to CRRT in removing inflammatory mediators (B). However, this benefit is theoretically lost if CRRT is not employed early in the course of septic shock before widespread multiorgan damage and/or failure. Until recently, the timing of CRRT was up for debate because there were no large randomized studies demonstrating improved survival. However, in 2016, the ELAIN trial published in JAMA was the first large randomized controlled trial demonstrating improved 90-day mortality (39% versus 54%) with the initiation of early CRRT (defined as within 8 hours of acute kidney injury onset). The duration of renal replacement therapy and length of hospital stay (but not ICU stay) were significantly shorter in the early group versus the delayed group (E). However, there was no difference in the rate of requirement of RRT after day 90 between the two groups. Patients with an increased level of IL-8 had an increased risk of RRT dependence after hospital discharge.

References: Honore PM, Jamez J, Wauthier M, et al. Prospective evaluation of short-term, high-volume isovolemic hemofiltration on the hemodynamic course and outcome in patients with intractable circulatory failure resulting from septic shock. *Crit Care Med.* 2000;28(11):3581–3587.

Zarbock A, Kellum JA, Schmidt C, et al. Effect of early vs delayed initiation of renal replacement therapy on mortality in critically ill patients with acute kidney injury: the ELAIN randomized clinical trial. *JAMA.* 2016;315(20):2190–2199.

22. E. As with all trauma patients, the primary survey begins with checking airway and breathing. The patient is exhibiting signs of a tension pneumothorax with evidence of hypotension, tracheal deviation, and decreased breath sounds over the right hemithorax. Tension pneumothorax is a clinical diagnosis and does not require radiographic confirmation before instituting therapy (B). Treatment options include needle thoracostomy first followed by chest tube insertion (D). Intubation and application of positive pressure ventilation should not occur before decompressing a tension pneumothorax because this will worsen the tension physiology and further impede preload and cardiac output (C). If the patient continues to decompensate after tube thoracostomy, intubation can be considered. Resuscitative thoracotomy or tracheostomy is not indicated in this patient (A).

23. B. Hemorrhagic shock is a form of hypovolemic shock and the most common cause of shock in trauma patients. In response to hypovolemia, the sympathetic and cardiovascular systems increase the heart rate, myocardial contractility, and SVR to maintain blood pressure. This response occurs secondary to an increase in norepinephrine secretion and a decrease in vagal tone. The cardiovascular system also redistributes blood flow to the brain, heart, and kidneys and shunts it away from the skin, muscle, and gastrointestinal tract. The kidneys respond to hemorrhagic shock by increasing reabsorption of sodium and water, which results in a small volume of concentrated urine. When a patient is adequately resuscitated, the first sign is an improvement in urine output (A, C–E). There are 4 classes of hemorrhagic shock: Class 1 (up to 750 cc or <15% of total blood volume loss) does not have any hemodynamic changes; Class 2 (750–1500 cc or 15%–30%) can have tachycardia, decreased pulse pressure, and typically normal blood pressure; Class 3 (1500–2000 cc or 30%–40%) can have tachycardia, decreased pulse pressure, and decreased blood pressure; Class 4 (>2000 cc or >40%) can have tachycardia, decreased pulse pressure, and significantly decreased blood pressure, which may be incompatible with life.

24. C. Sepsis produces high-output cardiac failure with elevated cardiac index. If this goes untreated, the cardiac index will eventually decrease. SVR is decreased due to toxins that produce vasodilation (B). This is reflected in a low systemic blood pressure. Central venous pressures are low from the loss of intravascular volume due to increased capillary permeability (A). Wedge pressures are generally unaffected (D). SvO2 will be high because the tissues are unable to extract oxygen from the blood for consumption (E).

25. A. Magnesium depletion is a common problem in hospitalized patients, particularly in the intensive care unit. The kidney is primarily responsible for magnesium homeostasis through regulation by calcium/magnesium receptors on renal tubular cells that sense serum magnesium levels. Hypomagnesemia results from a variety of causes ranging from poor intake (starvation, alcoholism, prolonged administration of IV fluids, and total parenteral nutrition with inadequate supplementation of magnesium), increased renal excretion (alcohol, most diuretics, and amphotericin B), gastrointestinal losses (diarrhea), malabsorption, acute pancreatitis, diabetic ketoacidosis, and primary aldosteronism. Magnesium depletion is characterized by neuromuscular and central nervous system hyperactivity, and symptoms are similar to those of calcium deficiency. Signs include hyperactive reflexes, muscle tremors, and tetany with a positive Chvostek sign. Severe deficiencies can lead to delirium and seizures. Electrocardiographic changes including prolonged QT and PR intervals, ST-segment depression, flattening or inversion of P waves, torsade de pointes, and arrhythmias can also be seen (B–E). When hypokalemia or hypocalcemia coexists with hypomagnesemia, magnesium should be aggressively replaced to assist in restoring potassium or calcium homeostasis.

26. C. Treatment of hypermagnesemia includes withholding exogenous sources of magnesium, correcting volume deficits, and correcting acidosis if present. To manage acute symptoms, calcium chloride should be administered to antagonize the cardiovascular effects (C). If elevated levels or symptoms persist, dialysis is indicated (E). Insulin, dextrose, and dialysis are typically used in the treatment of hyperkalemia (A, B, D).

27. C. PEEP increases intrathoracic pressure, which may result in a decreased cardiac output via decreased preload, particularly in patients who are hypovolemic (B). PEEP does not decrease lung water, reduce vascular permeability, or hasten the resolution of pulmonary edema. PEEP may shift some edema fluid from the alveolar to the extraalveolar interstitial space, but PEEP does not reduce the overall degree of pulmonary edema (E). PEEP is often an effective way of increasing arterial oxygen content by increasing FRC through the recruitment of collapsed or atelectatic alveoli in patients who have decreased lung compliance, thereby improving SaO2. PEEP does not affect PCO2 nor does it alter cardiac contractility (A). PEEP can improve cardiac output by reducing left ventricular (LV) afterload and is a useful adjunct in patients with CHF exacerbations (D). It is important to keep in mind, however, that changing the PEEP will not have an immediate effect on oxygenation because it takes time to increase the FRC.

28. E. Although rare, the incidence of bacterial contamination of infused blood is higher than the incidence of viral infection transmission and can be acquired as a result of environmental contamination (collection bags or contaminated water baths) or from the donor's skin, blood, or phlebotomist's skin. Gram-negative organisms, especially *Yersinia enterocolitica* and *Pseudomonas* species, which are capable of growth at 4°C (39.2°F), are the most common cause (A–D). Gram-positive organisms are more frequently encountered as platelet contaminants. Clinical manifestations include fever, chills, abdominal cramps, vomiting, and diarrhea. There may be hemorrhagic manifestations and increased bleeding. If the diagnosis is suspected, the transfusion should be discontinued and resuscitative efforts initiated. Blood should be cultured and a workup for a transfusion reaction should be performed. Emergency treatment includes oxygen, adrenergic blocking agents, and the administration of broad-spectrum antibiotics.

References: Mullins R. Shock, electrolytes, and fluid. In: Townsend CM, Jr, Beauchamp RD, Evers BM, Mattox KL, eds. Sabiston textbook of surgery: *the biological basis of modern surgical practice.* 17th ed. Philadelphia: W.B. Saunders; 2004:67–112.

Peitzman A. Shock, electrolytes and fluid. In: Brunicardi FC, Andersen DK, Billiar TR, et al., eds. Schwartz's principles of surgery. 8th ed. New York: McGraw-Hill; 2005:85–108.

29. A. Intraabdominal hypertension is defined as a sustained increase in intraabdominal pressures greater than 12 mmHg. The increased pressure may be acute, subacute, or chronic. Abdominal compartment syndrome (ACS) is defined as sustained intraabdominal pressures greater than 20 mmHg associated with new organ dysfunction. ACS occurs in patients who have sustained multiple traumas, severe burns, or retroperitoneal injuries; have undergone an operation for massive intraabdominal infection; or have undergone a complicated, prolonged abdominal operation. Massive IV fluid resuscitation with resultant third spacing of fluid and marked bowel wall edema places patients at high risk of the development of this complication. The symptoms and signs include progressive abdominal distention, increasing peak airway pressure, decreased cardiac output, and oliguria. These complications are the result of the abdominal pressure decreasing venous return from the inferior vena cava and renal veins and from decreased pulmonary compliance. Renal failure, severe pulmonary compromise, and intracranial hypertension can eventually develop in patients. Intraabdominal pressures transduced from the bladder can be readily measured by instilling 25 mL of saline into the aspiration port of a Foley catheter with the drainage tube clamped. An 18-gauge needle attached to a pressure transducer may then be inserted into the aspiration port at which point the system should be zeroed at the level of the midaxillary line. A pressure of greater than 20 mmHg with evidence of physiologic compromise as manifested by renal, respiratory, or neurologic compromise is considered diagnostic. Treatment consists of opening the abdomen or paracentesis in select cases.

30. D. Patients with underlying cardiac disease are at increased risk of arrhythmias, seeming to be more sensitive to hypoxia, hypercarbia, and electrolyte abnormalities than patients without heart disease. VT is a serious wide-complex tachycardia that warrants immediate treatment because it may progress to unstable ventricular rhythms. Management of VT is dependent on the stability of the patient. For those without hypotension, altered mental status, signs of shock, chest pain, or acute heart failure, pharmacologic treatment with antiarrhythmic infusions is indicated. Amiodarone is the drug of choice, although procainamide and sotalol are also acceptable provided that the QT interval is not prolonged (B). If the patient exhibits altered mental status and/or hypotension, immediate synchronized cardioversion is indicated with an initial recommended dose of 100 J (D). Consideration should be given to the administration of sedation or analgesia before cardioversion, if possible. Defibrillaton and epinephrine are indicated in pulseless VT (A, C). Diltiazem is useful in atrial tachycardia but has no place in VT (F). Most importantly, a search for and correction of any reversible causes should be undertaken.

31. B. All are consequences of acute kidney injury; however, hyperkalemia is generally the most immediately life-threatening complication and can predispose the patient to ventricular tachycardia and fibrillation (A, C–E).

32. D. Hepatorenal syndrome is a functional renal problem that likely results from relative hypovolemia, splanchnic and peripheral arterial vasodilation, and intense vasoconstriction of the renal circulation (B, C). The syndrome is probably the final consequence of extreme underfilling of the arterial circulation secondary to arterial vasodilation in the splanchnic vascular bed. It is characterized by azotemia, oliguria, very low urinary sodium (<10 mEq/day), and a high urine osmolarity. The prognosis is poor. Type I is mainly associated with acute liver failure or alcoholic cirrhosis, but it can develop in any other form of liver failure. It is characterized by rapid deterioration of renal function, with a marked increase in serum creatinine and blood urea nitrogen over a short period of time (E). The optimal treatment is liver transplantation, but the patients may not receive the transplant in time. Hyponatremia and hyperkalemia are typical. Type II is a more stable form (A). The decrease in the glomerular filtration rate and the increase in creatinine are moderate. It occurs mostly in patients with a relatively preserved hepatic function. In one study, a combination of midodrine, an α-agonist, and octreotide improved 30-day survival.

Reference: Ginès P, Guevara M, Arroyo V, Rodés J. Hepatorenal syndrome. *Lancet*. 2003;362(9398):1819–1827.

33. B. The presentation is consistent with neurogenic shock. Findings suggestive of neurogenic shock include hypotension with relative bradycardia, warm, well-perfused extremities reflecting loss of sympathetic tone, evidence of a high spinal cord injury, and priapism (sustained erection due to unopposed parasympathetic stimulation). In a patient with a high cervical spine injury and evidence of hypercarbic or ventilatory failure, the first step is to secure an airway. The phrenic nerve is supplied by the C3 to C5 nerve roots. Thus, patients with an injury above C5 will routinely require ventilatory support. After the airway is secured and ventilation is adequate, fluid resuscitation and restoration of intravascular volume will often improve perfusion in neurogenic shock. Most patients with neurogenic shock will respond to the restoration of intravascular volume alone, with satisfactory improvement in perfusion and resolution of hypotension. It is always important to rule out hypovolemia due to hemorrhage in the trauma setting. In addition, one must always be aware that in the presence of spinal cord injury, one cannot rely on the abdominal examination. Thus, an abdominal and pelvic CT scan would be indicated to rule out visceral injury. If the patient does not respond to fluids, administration of vasoconstrictors will improve peripheral vascular tone, decrease vascular capacitance, and increase venous return but should only be considered once hypovolemia is excluded as the cause of the hypotension and the diagnosis of neurogenic shock is established (A, C–E). Restoration of blood pressure and circulatory perfusion is also important to improve perfusion to the spinal cord, prevent progressive spinal cord ischemia, and minimize secondary cord injury.

Trauma 16

NAVEEN BALAN, CAITLYN BRASCHI, AND DENNIS KIM

ABSITE 99th Percentile High-Yields

I. Traumatic Brain Injury (TBI)
   A. Subdural hematoma (SDH): craniectomy if, >10 mm in size or >5 mm midline shift; more consistent with nonaccidental trauma
   B. Epidural hematoma (EDH): craniectomy if >15 mm in size or >5 mm midline shift
   C. Massive subarachnoid hemorrhage: CTA head to evaluate for ruptured aneurysm or arteriovenous malformation
   D. Start VTE chemoprophylaxis 48 hours from most recent stable CT; low-molecular weight heparin preferred in TBI

II. Spinal Cord Injury (SCI)
   A. Unstable spine injury: disruption of 2/3 of the longitudinal spinal columns (requires surgery)
   B. High SCI (above T6), concern for neurogenic shock acutely (hypotension, vasodilation with warm skin, bradycardia, or inappropriately normal heart rate for trauma setting); long term concern (months later) for autonomic dysreflexia with bradycardia, diaphoresis, and uncontrolled hypertension

Injury	Location	Mechanism	Management
Hangman's fracture (bilateral pedicles)	Cervical	Hyperextension of the neck, caused by hanging, diving	Traction and external immobilization (Halo) vs spinal fusion
Dens fracture	C2 (odontoid process)	Hyperextension of the neck, falls in the elderly	Type I is above the base and considered a stable fracture. Type II (which extends to the base of dens) is unstable and need surgical fixation. Type III fractures extend into the C2 vertebral body—these tend to have a better healing rate than type II and rarely require surgery.
Chance fracture (horizontal disruption of all columns)	Thoracolumbar	Flexion-distraction injury from rapid deceleration during blunt trauma	Orthotic brace for low-grade injury, surgery if neurologic deficits or ligamentous injury; also higher risk of hollow viscous injury

III. Neck Trauma

A. Screening for blunt cerebrovascular injury (carotid or vertebral artery): use expanded Denver criteria

Risk factors for BCVI	Signs/symptoms of BCVI
LeFort II/III or mandible fracture	Pulsatile bleeding from neck or nasal/oral cavity
Complex skull fracture or basilar skull fracture	Carotid bruit
Traumatic brain injury (GCS <6)	Expanding hematoma
Cervical spine injury (subluxation, ligamentous injury, transverse foramen fracture, vertebral body fracture, any C1-C3 fracture	Focal neurologic deficit: hemiparesis, Horner syndrome (ptosis, miosis, anhidrosis)
Near hanging with anoxic brain injury	Stroke on CT HEAD or MRI BRAIN
Clothesline injury with neck seat belt sign	Neurologic deficit not explained by CT HEAD
Scalp degloving	

B. Esophagus (dysphagia, drooling, odynophagia, pneumomediastinum): start with water-soluble contrast study; only 1% of pneumomediastinum after blunt trauma have an esophageal injury, most cases are from air dissecting along pulmonary vasculature in pneumothorax (Macklin effect)
   1. Small, contained injury: NPO with broad-spectrum antibiotics (including antifungal)
   2. Free-perforation injury, stable: enlarge defect to easily view mucosal injury extent, close in 2 layers, and use muscle flap (strap muscle, intercostal muscle) to buttress repair
   3. Devitalization or >2 cm segmental loss: esophagectomy, wide drainage, and reconstruction if stable or diversion with esophagostomy (spit fistula) if unstable
   4. Surgical access: if cervical esophagus use left neck incision, if upper 2/3 of esophagus use right posterolateral thoracotomy, if distal 1/3 esophagus use left posterolateral thoracotomy
C. Tracheal injury: debride, repair with primary closure in one layer (two layers could lead to stenosis) using absorbable suture and buttress with strap muscles
D. Surgical airway: cricothyroidotomy preferred over tracheostomy; children (age <12- years) avoid surgical cricothyroidotomy (risk of subglottic stenosis) and consider needle cricothyroidotomy with jet-needle insufflation

IV. Thoracic Trauma

A. Cardiac injuries
   1. Blunt cardiac injury (BCI) screening
      a) ECG, troponin in all patients suspected of sustaining BCI (normal rules out injury)
      b) Any abnormality on EKG or elevated troponin: admit for cardiac monitoring
      c) Hemodynamic instability or new persistent arrhythmia: obtain ECHO
B. Rib fractures are the most common blunt thoracic trauma injury
   1. Medical management: aggressive pulmonary toilet, multimodal pain control, serratus anterior, paravertebral, or intercostal nerve block or epidural (latter improves mortality in elderly)
   2. Rib plating: indicated in patients with severe flail chest either causing respiratory distress (usually hypoventilation) or failure to extubate; compared to nonop management, rib fixation increases spirometry volumes, increases hospital costs, and decreases pneumonia rate, however, it does not decrease mortality rate or narcotic requirements
C. Diaphragmatic injury: repair after life-threatening injuries is managed, transabdominal approach favored over transthoracic to evaluate bowel, use nonabsorbable permanent suture; if penetrating trauma to left thoracoabdominal area in an asymptomatic patient, observe for 8 hours for evidence of peritonitis, if none, then perform diagnostic laparoscopy to rule out diaphragm injury

V. Abdominal Trauma

A. Pancreas injuries (most commonly after penetrating trauma)
   1. No ductal involvement (grades I–II): wide drainage
   2. Distal injury with ductal involvement (grade III): distal pancreatectomy with splenic preservation (if hemodynamically stable)

3. Pancreatic head transection or massive disruption (grades IV–V): with drainage or damage control operation, consider staged Whipple
4. If duct involvement is unclear intraoperatively, consider intraoperative cholangiogram or perform wide drainage with postoperative ERCP/MRCP

B. Duodenal injuries
1. Hematoma (grade I): trial nonoperative (NPO, TPN) for 2 weeks, exploration if nonop fails
2. Lacerations (II–IV) of < 50% circumference: favor two-layer primary repair
3. Lacerations (II–IV) of >50% circumference: segmental resection with primary anastomosis for all segments except D2

C. Colorectal injuries
1. Colon and intraperitoneal rectal:
   a) Nondestructive (<50% circumference): debridement and primary repair
   b) Destructive (>50% circumference): segmental resection with 1° anastomosis if stable, segmental resection left in discontinuity with planned 2nd look operation if unstable
2. Extraperitoneal rectum: proximal diversion alone (no presacral drainage or washout)

VI. Retroperitoneal hematomas

A. Zone I: explore all hematomas
B. Zone II: selective exploration for expanding hematoma (blunt or penetrating)
C. Zone III: explore penetrating, do not explore blunt

VII. Orthopedic and Neurovascular Injury Patterns

Fracture/Injury	Associated neurovascular injury	Complication/deficit
Anterior (more common) shoulder dislocation	Axillary nerve injury	Weak shoulder abduction
Posterior shoulder dislocation (e.g., seizures)	Axillary artery injury	
Humeral shaft fracture	Radial nerve palsy	Wrist-drop
Supracondylar humerus fracture	Brachial artery injury	Forearm compartment syndrome, Volkmann ischemic contracture
Colles fracture (distal radius)	Median nerve compression	Pain, paresthesias in digits 1–3 ½
Scaphoid fracture		Snuffbox tenderness, avascular necrosis; often normal initial XR
Posterior (more common) hip dislocation (adducted and internally rotated)	Sciatic nerve injury (peroneal branch)	
Posterior knee dislocation	Popliteal artery injury	
Fibula head fracture (or prolonged lithotomy)	Peroneal nerve injury	Foot drop

Exposure/maneuver	Location
Right posterolateral thoracotomy	Mid esophagus
Left posterolateral thoracotomy	Distal esophagus, descending aorta (distal to left subclavian takeoff)
Left anterolateral thoracotomy	Left distal subclavian artery
Median sternotomy	Ascending and arch of aorta, innominate artery, bilateral common carotid artery, superior vena cava, proximal right and left subclavian artery
Left infraclavicular incision	Left mid-subclavian artery
Kocher maneuver	Head of pancreas, SMV, SMA
Left medial visceral rotation (Mattox maneuver)	Aorta, celiac trunk, SMA, left renal artery, common iliac arteries
Right medial visceral rotation (Cattell-Braasch maneuver)	Inferior vena cava, right renal vessels, common iliac veins
Pringle maneuver	Control intrahepatic liver hemorrhage, max clamping 30–60 min

VIII. Acute Compartment Syndrome (ACS)

    A. Risk factors: open fractures > closed fractures, crush injuries, young, male, long bone fracture (e.g., tibia, radius), high voltage burns, >6 hours ischemia with reperfusion, combined arterial/venous injury

    B. Diagnosis: high clinical suspicion, compartment pressure >30 mmHg, delta P (compartment pressure/diastolic pressure) <30 mmHg

    C. Upper extremity:

        1. Forearm compartments: lateral (mobile wad), dorsal extensor, volar (contains median and ulnar nerves)

        2. Fasciotomy: S-shaped volar incision (often includes carpal tunnel if needed), linear dorsal incision (3 cm distal to lateral epicondyle toward the midline of the wrist)

    D. Lower extremity:

        1. Thigh compartments: anterior, posterior, medial

        2. Leg compartments: anterior (most common site ACS—sensory deficit of first web space secondary to deep peroneal nerve in this compartment), lateral, superficial posterior and deep posterior

            a) Fasciotomy—Two incision, four compartment technique: Medial incision 1 to 2 cm medial to tibia (take soleus off tibial periosteum; posterior compartments), Lateral incision along anterior margin of fibula (anterior and lateral compartments; risk of injury to superficial peroneal nerve—most common) (Figs. 16.1–16.3).

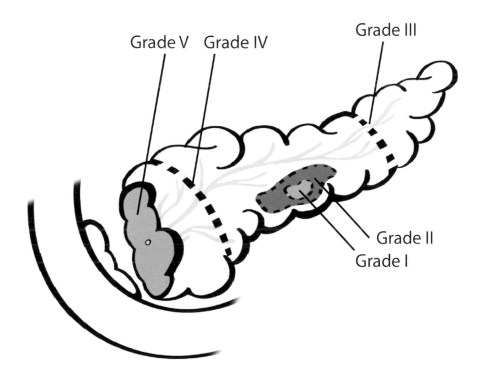

Grade I	Minor contusion or superficial laceration without duct involvement
Grade II	Major contusion or superficial laceration without duct involvement
Grade III	Distal transection or parenchymal injury *with* duct involvement
Grade IV	Proximal transection or parenchymal injury
Grade V	Major disruption of the pancreatic head

Fig. 16.1 Pancreatic Injury Grades.

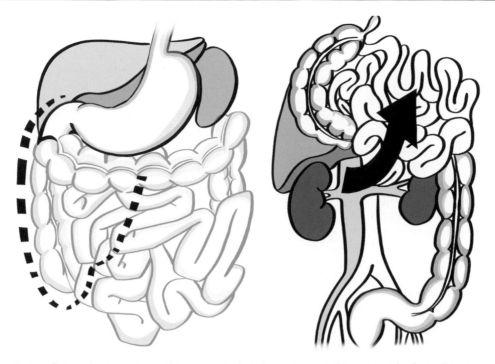

The Cattell-Braasch manuever provides exposure to the inferior vena cava, iliac veins, and right renal artery and vein. Also known as right medial rotation, the steps include mobilizing the duodenum and right colon, and incising the line of fusion of the small bowel mesentery and posterior peritoneum to the ligament of treitz to lift the colon, small bowel, and pancreas out of the abdomen.

Fig. 16.2 The Cattell-Braasch Maneuver.

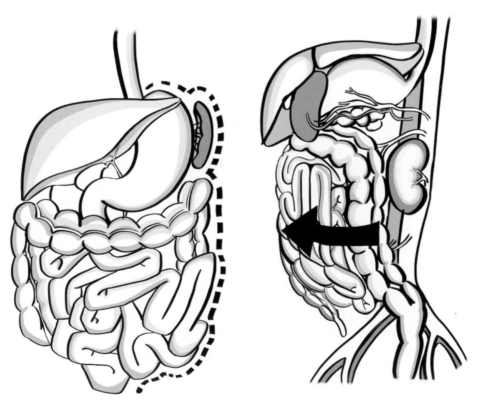

The Mattox manuever, also known as left medial visceral rotation, permits exploration of aortic, iliac, and pelvic vessel injuries. The steps include incising the parietal peritoneum at the White Line of Toldt from the sigmoid colon to the splenic flexure. The spleen, tail of the pancreas, and stomach are reflected medially to gain access to these vessels. When necessary, the kidney is also reflected medially (not pictured).

Fig. 16.3 The Mattox Maneuver.

Questions

1. A 23-year-old male presents to the emergency department with a left parasternal stab wound. His heart rate is 110 beats per minute and blood pressure is 130/70 mmHg. FAST shows a pericardial effusion. What is the next best step?
   A. Formal echocardiogram
   B. Subxiphoid pericardial window
   C. Left anterolateral thoracotomy
   D. Median sternotomy
   E. Pericardiocentesis

2. A 36-year-old male presents with right upper quadrant pain, jaundice, and melena. He was recently discharged for a blunt hepatic injury following a high-speed motor vehicle with injuries that included a liver injury that was managed nonoperatively. His heart rate is 120 beats per minute, blood pressure is 80/60 mmHg. IV fluids and blood transfusion are given with repeat blood pressure of 90/70 mmHg and heart rate of 110 beats per minute. He is afebrile. Laboratory values include a hematocrit of 24%, a normal white blood cell count, total bilirubin of 3.5 mg/dl, and alkaline phosphatase of 400 IU/L. What is the next best step?
   A. Endoscopic retrograde cholangiopancreaticography (ERCP)
   B. Angioembolization
   C. Abdominal ultrasound
   D. Endoscopy
   E. CT abdomen with IV contrast

3. A 25-year-old man presents with a gunshot wound (GSW) to the buttocks. Abdominal examination is unremarkable, and the patient is hemodynamically stable. Proctoscopy reveals blood and stool in the distal rectal vault, but an injury cannot be identified. Computed tomography (CT) scan of the abdomen and pelvis with rectal contrast is unremarkable. Which of the following is the best management option?
   A. IV antibiotics with close observation
   B. A proximal diverting colostomy
   C. Exploratory laparotomy with primary closure of rectal injury, diverting colostomy, distal rectal irrigation, and presacral drainage
   D. Presacral drainage and IV antibiotics
   E. Abdominal perineal resection

4. A 29-year-old male presents to the ED following a high-speed MVC. He complains of neck pain and he is neurologically intact on examination. Head CT is negative. He undergoes CT imaging which reveals an isolated C2 lateral mass fracture. CT angiography of the neck is significant for a small pseudoaneurysm of the left vertebral artery. What is the most appropriate management of this lesion?
   A. Initiate antithrombotic therapy with unfractionated heparin and repeat imaging in 7 days
   B. Endovascular stent placement
   C. Operative exploration
   D. Observation
   E. Thrombin injection

5. A 23-year-old woman with no medical history presents to the ED following a head-on motor vehicle crash at 45 mph. Her heart rate is 98 beats per minute, blood pressure is 112/72 mmHg, and SpO$_2$ is 98% on room air. Pan-CT shows isolated anterior pneumomediastinum. She denies symptoms. What is the next best step?
   A. Esophagoscopy, laryngoscopy, bronchoscopy
   B. Observation
   C. Bilateral tube thoracostomy
   D. CT thorax, abdomen with oral contrast
   E. Water-soluble swallow study

6. Which of the following orthopedic injuries is correctly paired with its commonly associated neurovascular finding?
   A. Supracondylar humerus fracture: Volkmann ischemic contracture
   B. Distal radius fracture: claw-hand deformity
   C. Posterior hip dislocation: obturator nerve injury
   D. Posterior shoulder dislocation: axillary nerve injury
   E. Scaphoid fracture: wrist drop

7. A 45-year-old male presents after blunt trauma to the neck. He is hemodynamically stable without respiratory distress. He is afebrile without leukocytosis and denies odynophagia. CT shows only subcutaneous emphysema. Bronchoscopy demonstrates a 3-cm laceration in the cervical trachea. The surrounding tissue is viable. What is the best next step in management?

   A. Antibiotics, voice rest, and repeat bronchoscopy
   B. Primary repair with permanent suture
   C. Primary repair with absorbable suture in one layer
   D. Primary repair with absorbable suture in two layers
   E. Tracheostomy through the laceration and closure of remaining injured trachea

8. A 45-year-old man presents with second- and third-degree burns to the anterior surface of both arms and entire right leg. He also has superficial burns to both hands. What is his estimated total body surface area (TBSA) burned?

   A. 25%
   B. 27%
   C. 29%
   D. 36%
   E. 38%

9. A 22-year-old male presents to the emergency department (ED) after a gunshot wound (GSW) to the abdomen. He is hypotensive. Which of the following intravenous (IV) routes is the most appropriate way to deliver rapid fluid resuscitation to this patient?

   A. 18-gauge peripheral catheter
   B. 20-gauge peripheral catheter
   C. 6-French femoral vein central line catheter
   D. 7-French subclavian vein central line catheter
   E. 7-French internal jugular vein central line catheter

10. Which of the following is the leading cause of death in the trauma patient reaching the hospital alive?

    A. Head injury
    B. Hemorrhagic shock
    C. Multiorgan failure
    D. Sepsis
    E. Cardiac injury

11. A 35-year-old male is taken to the ED after being stabbed in the right abdomen. He complains of minimal abdominal pain with no rebound or guarding. During local wound exploration (LWE), it appears that the anterior fascia is not violated. His vital signs are normal. Which of the following is the most appropriate management?

    A. Admission for 24-hour observation
    B. Discharge after 6 hours if abdominal exam does not change
    C. Computed tomography (CT) scan of the abdomen and pelvis
    D. Focused assessment with sonography for trauma (FAST)
    E. Discharge home

12. A 45-year-old male is brought to the ED after a GSW to the right leg. He is hypotensive in the ED, with a large amount of blood loss at the scene. Massive transfusion protocol is initiated. Following interposition vein graft for a superficial femoral artery transection, he is admitted to the ICU for observation. The following morning he is found to be oliguric, has rising peak airway pressures, and has a distended abdomen. Which of the following would be expected in this patient?

    A. Increased pulmonary compliance
    B. Increased functional reserve capacity (FRC)
    C. Decreased pulmonary vascular resistance
    D. Increased pulmonary capillary wedge pressure
    E. Increased venous return

13. Which of the following is true with regards to burn injury?

    A. Superficial partial-thickness burns do not have blistering
    B. Full-thickness third-degree burns can involve underlying fascia
    C. Deep partial-thickness burns have a loss of hair follicles
    D. Deep partial-thickness burns often heal spontaneously
    E. Superficial partial-thickness burns are not painful

14. Which of the following is correct regarding common topical antimicrobials used in burn care?

    A. Mafenide acetate leads to a respiratory alkalosis
    B. Silver sulfadiazine has broad coverage against *Pseudomonas*
    C. Silver nitrate can be used in patients with a sulfa allergy
    D. Mafenide acetate is not effective in patients with eschars
    E. Silver sulfadiazine can lead to electrolyte abnormalities

15. Which of the following is an indication to transfer a patient to a burn center?
    A. 45-year-old female with first-degree burns 30% TBSA
    B. 10-year-old female with third-degree burns 4% TBSA
    C. 21-year-old male with a chemical burn to the right hand
    D. 30-year-old female with second-degree burns 18% TBSA
    E. 71-year-old female with second-degree burns 8% TBSA

16. A 28-year-old male with morbid obesity arrives at the ED after suffering an electrical shock. He was working on his car at the time of injury. He has a burn mark on his hand and his forearm appears swollen. Which of the following is true regarding this patient?
    A. The source of the shock was likely a direct current
    B. Renal failure is the main cause of death in those who survive the initial injury
    C. He likely had repetitive, tetanic muscle contractions at the time of electrocution
    D. His body habitus will likely protect him from deep thermal injury
    E. Red urine on admission is suggestive of bladder injury

17. A 36-year-old alcoholic female arrives at the ED during a winter storm with a frostbite to the right arm and hand. She passed out in a park with her arm exposed on a freezing metallic bench. Her right hand has several areas of what appear to be hemorrhagic bullae. It has been 7 hours since she was brought to the ED. Which of the following is true regarding this patient?
    A. She likely has a second-degree frostbite
    B. She should receive early debridement of obviously necrotic tissue
    C. She will likely respond favorably to tissue plasminogen activator (tPA) treatment
    D. Reperfusion injury is an important contributor to the damage seen with her injury
    E. Rewarming in warm water should be done gradually

18. A 33-year-old alcoholic patient presents to the ED after a high-speed MVC. She appears to be inebriated and combative and is promptly intubated. Computed tomography (CT) demonstrates a Chance fracture at L1, and free fluid in the abdomen, but no evidence of solid organ injury. Vitals are normal and stable. The next step in management is:
    A. Magnetic resonance imaging (MRI) of the spine
    B. Admission to the ICU for close monitoring
    C. Exploratory laparotomy
    D. FAST scan
    E. Repeat CT scan of the abdomen in 6 hours

19. A 42-year-old female presents to the ED with abdominal pain after an MVC. CT scan shows contrast extravasation in the spleen with a significant hemoperitoneum. Heart rate is presently 120 beats per minute and blood pressure (BP) is 90/70 mmHg. Hemoglobin is 7.1 g/dL. She is a Jehovah's Witness and refuses blood transfusions. Which of the following is the most appropriate next step in management?
    A. Document refusal of blood products and administer normal saline to keep BP above 100 mmHg
    B. Document refusal of blood products and perform a splenectomy
    C. Document refusal of blood products and perform angiography with embolization
    D. Document refusal of blood products and consult the hospital ethics committee
    E. Administer 2 units of packed red blood cells given life-threatening situation and perform splenectomy

20. A 29-year-old male arrives at the ED after a high-speed MVC with a Glasgow Coma Scale (GCS) of 4. He has a cervical collar that was placed by emergency medical services (EMS). He is intubated and taken for a CT scan, which demonstrates a large subdural hemorrhage and diffuse punctate hemorrhage with no evidence of cervical spine injury. He is admitted to the ICU. With regard to the management of the cervical collar, which of the following is recommended?
    A. Remove immediately
    B. MRI cervical spine (c-spine) and remove the cervical collar if there are no injuries identified
    C. Continue cervical collar until the patient can be clinically evaluated
    D. Exchange the cervical collar placed by EMS with a soft-collar
    E. Exchange the cervical collar placed by EMS with a soft-collar and order MRI c-spine

21. Which of the following is true regarding pneumothorax in the trauma patient?
    A. A small asymptomatic pneumothorax identified on CT scan will resolve within 24 hours using 100% inspired supplemental oxygen
    B. A small asymptomatic pneumothorax should be managed with a tube thoracostomy if the patient is to undergo general anesthesia
    C. A small asymptomatic pneumothorax in a ventilated patient in the ICU, discovered on rereview of admission CT, should be managed with a tube thoracostomy
    D. A persistent air leak identified on postinjury day 3 is best managed with VATS
    E. Penetrating injuries leading to pneumothorax have concomitant hemothorax less than half of the time

22. A 31-year-old female with obesity presents to the ED after a large refrigerator fell on her. She is complaining of severe pain in her hips. Her hemoglobin is 7.9 g/dL. Her heart rate is 128 beats per minute, and her systolic blood pressure is 105 mmHg. She has no evidence of extremity injuries, and distal pulses are normal. She has an unstable pelvis, so a pelvic binder is applied. Massive transfusion protocol is initiated. She is rushed to the angiography suite and undergoes embolization, then stabilizes. The following day, her CK levels rise to 40,000 and her urine turns red-tinged. The most likely source is the muscles of her:
    A. Thighs
    B. Buttocks
    C. Abdominal wall
    D. Arms
    E. Calves

23. A 46-year-old woman presents to the ED hemodynamically stable after a high-speed MVC. A CT scan of the abdomen and pelvis reveals a right perinephric hematoma with a deep laceration in the inferior aspect of the renal parenchyma with some localized urine extravasation within the collecting system. Management consists of:
    A. Observation
    B. Right nephrectomy
    C. Attempt at partial nephrectomy
    D. Attempt at renal salvage with suture repair of the parenchyma
    E. Nephrostomy tube

24. A 28-year-old male presents to the ED 2 days after being involved in a bar fight where he punched another patron in the mouth. His right hand appears to have a soft-tissue infection. Which of the following is the most likely pathogen?
    A. *Treponema pallidum*
    B. *Prevotella* spp.
    C. Hepatitis C
    D. *Propionibacterium* spp.
    E. *Bacteroides*

25. A 45-year-old male arrives at the ED with a GSW to the head. He has declined organ donation on his driver's license registration which is several years old. He is declared to be brain dead the following morning. His parents and sister fly in from out of state. His sister has end-stage renal disease and would like to receive her brother's kidney because she states he was tested "and found to be a match." His parents are saddened by their son's passing but agree that their daughter should receive the kidney and that their son would have wanted this. The treating physician should:
    A. Arrange for organ harvesting and coordinate with a transplant surgeon to perform the kidney transplant
    B. Contact an organ donation service to facilitate a discussion with the family
    C. Remove the patient from ventilator support
    D. Administer a lethal dose of morphine sulfate
    E. Consult the hospital ethics committee

26. A 45-year-old male presents to the ED following a high-speed MVC with evidence of severe facial fractures and bilateral lower extremity deformities. Paramedics report a significant amount of blood in his airway, and the patient's respirations are being assisted with bag-valve mask ventilation. On exam, the patient is hemodynamically stable with an O2 saturation of 85% on a nonrebreather mask and GCS is 7. Attempts at rapid sequence intubation are unsuccessful because of the inability to visualize the airway as a result of ongoing bleeding. Attempts at bagging become more difficult. Which of the following is the next best step in management?
    A. Needle cricothyroidotomy
    B. Nasotracheal intubation
    C. Surgical cricothyroidotomy
    D. Fiberoptic bronchoscopic-assisted intubation
    E. Apneic oxygenation

27. A 36-year-old male is transferred from another hospital to the ED after a high-speed head-on MVC with significant front-end damage to the vehicle. The accident occurred over 4 hours ago. On arrival, the patient is complaining of left-sided chest and abdominal pain. His systolic blood pressure is 80 mm Hg and heart rate is 120 beats per minute. Breath sounds are present and equal bilaterally. Abdominal exam reveals significant tenderness to palpation. Plain film of the chest shows a widened mediastinum (10 cm) without hemothorax. Pelvic x-ray is normal. FAST is positive for free fluid in the abdomen. Following a 1-L crystalloid bolus and 2 units of blood, the patient's blood pressure and heart rate are unchanged. Which of the following is the most appropriate next step in management?

    A. Administer a bolus of tranexamic acid (TXA) and continue infusion on the way to the OR for an exploratory laparotomy
    B. CT scan of the chest, abdomen, and pelvis
    C. Take the patient to the OR for an exploratory laparotomy without administration of TXA
    D. Transthoracic echocardiography
    E. Intraoperative thoracic angiogram for possible endovascular repair of thoracic aorta followed by exploratory laparotomy

28. A 22-year-old man sustains a GSW to the right leg below the knee. Vital signs are within normal limits. Physical exam reveals a single GSW to the lateral leg with minimal swelling and no obvious deformity. Pulse exam reveals diminished pedal pulses on the right in comparison to the left. Which of the following is the most appropriate next step in management?

    A. CT angiogram
    B. OR and angiogram
    C. Administration of IV papaverine
    D. Formal angiogram
    E. Arterial-pressure index (API)

29. A 60-year-old male presents to the ED following an MVC in which he was a restrained passenger. The initial systolic blood pressure was 90 mm Hg but improves to 110 mm Hg after 1 L of normal saline. Abdominal exam reveals mild diffuse tenderness without peritonitis. CT of the abdomen reveals an isolated grade III splenic injury with active extravasation and a low-volume hemoperitoneum. Hemoglobin is stable at 12 g/dL. Which of the following is the best next step in management?

    A. Laparotomy with splenectomy
    B. Laparotomy with attempt at splenorrhaphy
    C. Angiography with embolization
    D. Serial abdominal examinations and hematocrits in the ICU
    E. Laparoscopic splenectomy

30. An 18-year-old male is brought to the ED following a motorcycle crash. He is hemodynamically stable and complains of severe pelvic pain. Examination reveals blood at the urethral meatus, scrotal ecchymosis, and a scrotal hematoma. A pelvic x-ray confirms the presence of a pelvic fracture. Which of the following is the most appropriate next step in diagnosis?

    A. Insertion of a Foley catheter
    B. CT abdomen with IV contrast
    C. Retrograde urethrogram (RUG)
    D. Cystogram
    E. Intravenous pyelogram

31. A 28-year-old man sustains a GSW to the right supraclavicular area with no exit wound. On arrival, his systolic blood pressure is 60 mmHg and he is confused and combative. E-fast demonstrates bilateral lung sliding and there is no evidence of active hemorrhage. Which of the following is the best next step in the management?

    A. Immediate endotracheal intubation
    B. Right tube thoracostomy
    C. Transfuse blood
    D. Resuscitative (ED) thoracotomy
    E. Insert resuscitative endovascular balloon occlusion of aorta (REBOA)

32. A 30-year-old man sustains a GSW to the left mid-neck. On arrival at the ED, his systolic blood pressure is 80 mmHg, heart rate is 120 beats per minute, and his GCS is 8. There is a moderate, but nonexpanding hematoma in the neck with no active bleeding or bruit. An airway is immediately established, and blood is given with repeat systolic blood pressure of 90 mmHg. The next most appropriate step in management is:

    A. Head CT scan
    B. CT angiography of the neck
    C. Standard four-vessel arteriography
    D. Surgical neck exploration
    E. Triple endoscopy

33. Which of the following is the best indication for resuscitative (ED) thoracotomy?

    A. Severe blunt abdominal and head trauma with sudden arrest in the ED
    B. Abdominal stab wound with no signs of life (SOL) in the field, cardiopulmonary resuscitation (CPR) en route
    C. Blunt trauma with loss of pulse in the field, CPR en route
    D. Stab wound to chest with agonal breathing on transport, no pulse in ED
    E. GSW to abdomen with asystole as presenting rhythm and no pericardial tamponade on FAST

34. An 11-month-old boy presents to the ED with hypotension after being involved in an MVC. He has obvious deformities of both legs below his knees. Numerous attempts are made to establish venous access at the antecubital fossa without success. The best option for establishing access for fluid administration would be:
    A. Internal jugular central line
    B. Distal saphenous vein cutdown
    C. Femoral vein central line
    D. Intraosseous (IO) cannulation of the proximal tibia
    E. IO cannulation of the distal femur

35. Which of the following is true regarding the pregnant trauma patient?
    A. Blood volume increases proportionally less than red blood cell volume
    B. A pregnant patient tends to have a mild respiratory acidosis
    C. Use of radiographs is unsafe for the fetus in the third trimester
    D. The 2,3-diphosphoglycerate level is increased
    E. The glomerular filtration rate decreases

36. A 30-year-old man sustains a GSW to the right chest. His blood pressure in the emergency department is 70/40 mmHg. A chest tube is placed in the right chest with 500 mL of initial output. A follow-up chest radiograph reveals a complete whiteout of the right lung. The patient is taken to the operating room and a right thoracotomy is performed. On evaluation of the right lung, there is a through-and-through injury to the right lower lobe that appears to have an active air leak and ongoing bleeding. Surgical management should consist of:
    A. Formal right lower lobectomy
    B. Pneumonectomy
    C. Closure of both the anterior and posterior parenchymal defects with interrupted sutures
    D. Pulmonary tractotomy
    E. Ligation of the right lower lobe pulmonary artery

37. Which of the following is true regarding flail chest?
    A. The initial chest radiograph provides a useful predictor of subsequent pulmonary insufficiency
    B. Respiratory failure is primarily caused by the paradoxical motion of the chest wall
    C. Operative chest wall stabilization in patients without pulmonary contusion may shorten the length of intubation
    D. Aggressive fluid resuscitation is an important management adjunct
    E. Once the diagnosis is established, the patient should be intubated

38. Which of the following is true regarding blunt cardiac injury (BCI)?
    A. Creatine kinase-myocardial bound (CK-MB) enzyme determination lacks sensitivity
    B. It commonly results in serious ventricular arrhythmias
    C. It usually results in traumatic thrombosis of a coronary artery branch
    D. Presence of a sternal fracture predicts the presence of BCI
    E. It should be suspected in patients with transient sinus tachycardia

39. Which of the following surgical maneuvers is most correct to access the corresponding blood vessel?
    A. Left-sided medial visceral rotation or Mattox maneuver for the mid inferior vena cava (IVC)
    B. Transection of the neck of the pancreas for the superior mesenteric artery
    C. Right-sided medial visceral rotation or Cattell maneuver for the suprarenal aorta
    D. Kocher maneuver for the celiac axis
    E. Division of the right common iliac artery for the distal vena cava and common iliac vein bifurcation

40. In the setting of trauma, ligation is best tolerated for which of the following vessels?
    A. Right renal vein
    B. Left renal vein
    C. Brachial artery
    D. Popliteal artery
    E. Suprarenal IVC

41. Which of the following is true regarding extremity compartment syndrome?
    A. The soleus muscle must be detached from the tibia to decompress the deep posterior compartment of the lower leg
    B. A compartment pressure greater than 40 mmHg is necessary to establish the diagnosis
    C. The lateral compartment is the most commonly affected lower leg compartment
    D. An early sign of anterior compartment involvement of the lower leg is numbness on the plantar aspect of the foot
    E. It does not occur in the buttocks

42. A 17-year-old boy is brought to the ED after being involved in a high-speed motorcycle collision. He is hypotensive with a systolic pressure of 60 mmHg. A FAST scan is positive. At laparotomy, he is found to have a large amount of bleeding from behind the liver. Temporary application of a Pringle maneuver does not control the bleeding. However, laparotomy packs are placed, and the bleeding appears to slow down. The systolic blood pressure increases to 110 mmHg after aggressive resuscitation. The patient's pH is 7.06 and his temperature is 34°C. The next best step in management is:
    A. Obtain control of the IVC above and below the liver
    B. Perform a median sternotomy for atriocaval shunt placement
    C. Damage control closure and transport to ICU
    D. Damage control closure and transport to interventional radiology (IR) suite for hepatic embolization
    E. Obtain control of aorta at the diaphragmatic hiatus

43. A 55-year-old man is brought into the ED after a high-speed MVC. The patient is hemodynamically stable. Gross hematuria is present. CT cystography reveals air in the bladder and an accumulation of contrast in the right paracolic gutter. Which of the following is the best management option?
    A. Foley catheter drainage
    B. Suprapubic cystostomy tube placement
    C. Open repair of the intraperitoneal bladder injury with absorbable sutures
    D. Obtaining a formal cystogram
    E. Open repair of the intraperitoneal bladder injury with silk sutures

44. A 30-year-old man sustains a GSW to the abdomen and presents to the ED with a systolic blood pressure of 60 mmHg. Emergent laparotomy reveals a 2-L hemoperitoneum with an injury to the IVC and right iliac vein. Both injuries are successfully repaired. Further exploration demonstrates a distal right ureteral injury below the level of the iliac vessels with a 3-cm defect. After 10 units of blood products, the patient's blood pressure is 80/60 mmHg, his heart rate is 110 beats per minute, and his temperature is 96°F. Which of the following is the best management option?
    A. Proximal and distal ligation of the ureter
    B. Ureteroureterostomy
    C. Transureteroureterostomy
    D. Psoas hitch
    E. Ureteroneocystostomy

45. After a motor vehicle accident, a 17-year-old girl with blunt abdominal trauma is found to have free fluid on abdominal CT without evidence of liver or spleen injury. She is hemodynamically stable. Her abdomen is diffusely tender. She is taken to the operating room. At surgery, she is found to have a 75% luminal circumference injury to the first portion of the duodenum. Surgical management consists of:
    A. Pyloric exclusion
    B. Duodenal diverticulization
    C. Primary duodenal repair
    D. Whipple resection
    E. Resection with duodenoduodenostomy

46. A 29-year-old man presents with a GSW to the right upper quadrant. On physical examination, the patient has a tender abdomen. At surgery, the patient is found to have a 500-mL hemoperitoneum with a through-and-through injury to the right lobe of the liver that is no longer actively bleeding. Further management would consist of:
    A. Closing the injury with a liver suture
    B. Packing the injury with omentum
    C. Application of a fibrin sealant
    D. No further management
    E. Drainage with a Penrose drain

47. A 20-year-old man with morbid obesity sustains a GSW to the abdomen. His blood pressure is 110/70 mmHg and heart rate is 100 beats per minute. At surgery, he is found to have a blast injury to the sigmoid colon involving 75% of the circumference of the bowel, with a moderate amount of fecal contamination. Hemodynamics, temperature, and base deficit are normal. Which of the following is the best option?
    A. Sigmoid colectomy with primary anastomosis with a diverting ileostomy
    B. Primary repair of the sigmoid colon
    C. Sigmoid colectomy with primary anastomosis
    D. Primary repair of the sigmoid colon with exteriorization of the repair
    E. Sigmoid colectomy with a proximal colostomy and oversewing of the rectal stump

48. A 46-year-old female is brought into the emergency department following a motorcycle crash. There is an open right tibia fracture. Plain radiographs of the chest and pelvis are normal. Heart rate is 110 beats per minute, blood pressure is 110/70 mmHg, and her SpO$_2$ is 99% on room air. CT imaging shows a small right pneumothorax. Orthopedic surgery is planning to take the patient to the operating room to place an external fixator. What is the best management for the pneumothorax?

    A. Right tube thoracostomy with 28 French chest tube
    B. Small pigtail catheter chest tube
    C. Careful intraoperative monitoring of end-tidal CO$_2$
    D. Repeat chest CT after orthopedic surgery
    E. Needle decompression

49. A 40-year-old man with a history of heavy alcohol use is admitted to the hospital after being hit by a car. The patient underwent pelvic fixation, intraperitoneal bladder repair, and splenectomy 4 days ago. On rounds, his vitals are normal, his abdomen is very distended, and there is increased output from his intraabdominal drain. Labs are as follows: Serum creatinine 1.5 mg/dL, serum albumin 3.0 g/dL, drain fluid creatinine 1.6 mg/dL, drain fluid albumin 1.5 g/dL, and drain fluid WBC 200. What is the most likely diagnosis?

    A. Hepatic ascites
    B. Urine leak
    C. Abdominal compartment syndrome
    D. Pancreatic leak
    E. Bacterial peritonitis

Answers

1. B. A parasternal penetrating injury with evidence of pericardial effusion in a trauma patient is concerning for hemopericardium with underlying cardiac injury. The patient being young makes this even more concerning as a chronic pericardial effusion would be highly unlikely. In recent years, there has been a shift toward the selective management of hemopericardium. Performing a median sternotomy or thoracotomy in all penetrating trauma patients with pericardial effusion leads to an unacceptably high nontherapeutic rate which may be as high as 38% (C, D). Additionally, a randomized controlled trial in stable patients demonstrated that penetrating thoracic trauma patients with a positive pericardial window after a 24-hour observation period can safely be managed with just irrigation and no additional surgery. However, in the case of obstructive shock (tachycardia, narrowed pulse pressure, lethargy, hypotension), performing a median sternotomy would be the appropriate intervention. There is no role for pericardiocentesis in trauma (E). A formal echocardiogram would be useful in the case of the stable patient with an equivocal FAST or to screen for pseudoaneurysms after cardiac repair (A). Left anterolateral thoracotomy would be the procedure of choice if the patient had presented as a traumatic arrest to rapidly resuscitate the patient (C). Median sternotomy provides the best exposure to repair cardiac injuries.

2. B. Hemobilia is characterized by the triad of upper GI bleeding (melena), jaundice, and right upper quadrant pain which may occur days to weeks after liver injury. The right hepatic artery is often involved, and the underlying lesion is an arterial pseudoaneurysm which forms a fistulous connection with the biliary tree. In a stable patient, workup would include a CT scan with IV contrast to look for a blush. But in an unstable patient with high suspicion, the next best step is angioembolization which can be both diagnostic and therapeutic (D). Biloma is another complication of traumatic liver injury if a bile duct is disrupted and has an ongoing leak. This can be demonstrated with an abdominal ultrasound and initially managed with percutaneous drainage and possibly ERCP (A, C). Another complication of liver trauma is hepatic necrosis and/or abscess. Injured or necrotic liver parenchyma can incite a massive inflammatory response and these patients often have a high fever and leukocytosis without GI bleed. This complication should be worked up with a CT abdomen with IV contrast (E).

3. B. The management of a rectal injury depends on whether it is intra- or extraperitoneal, the degree of tissue destruction, and the hemodynamic status of the patient. As a general rule, intraperitoneal injuries can be repaired primarily (they are treated like a colon injury). If it is an extraperitoneal injury, there are two basic options: primary repair of the injury or a diverting colostomy. The decision of whether to do primary repair relates to its accessibility. Proximal extraperitoneal injuries can be repaired primarily. In general, when primary repair of the extraperitoneal injury is performed, diversion

via a colostomy is not necessary (C). In addition, by exposing the extraperitoneal injury to the peritoneal cavity, it effectively renders it an intraperitoneal injury; thus, presacral drainage would not be indicated (D). If the extraperitoneal injury cannot be identified and repaired, a proximal diverting colostomy has been shown to be effective in allowing the injury to heal itself. Distal irrigation of the rectum and routine drainage of the presacral space are not necessary and may even contribute to forcing fecal material out from a rectal laceration. In particular, if the injury is to the anterior rectum, the drainage will be ineffective. Abdominoperineal resection would not be indicated (E). IV antibiotics alone are not appropriate (A). A CT scan is not reliable enough to rule out a distal rectal injury. As such, the finding of blood on proctoscopy is enough of an indication of an injury to proceed with stool diversion.

References: Bosarge PL, Como JJ, Fox N, et al. Management of penetrating extraperitoneal rectal injuries: an Eastern Association for the Surgery of Trauma practice management guideline. *J Trauma Acute Care Surg.* 2016;80(3):546–551.

Demetriades D, Murray JA, Chan L, et al. Penetrating colon injuries requiring resection: diversion or primary anastomosis? An AAST prospective multicenter study. *J Trauma.* 2001;50(5):765–775.

Gonzalez RP, Falimirski ME, Holevar MR. The role of presacral drainage in the management of penetrating rectal injuries. *J Trauma.* 1998;45(4):656–661.

4. A. Blunt cerebrovascular injury (BCVI) is the collective term for blunt injury to the carotid and vertebral arteries. These injuries are associated with significant morbidity and mortality following trauma, specifically related to risk of stroke. BCVI is graded using the Biffl classification. Grade I refers to intimal irregularity with <25% luminal narrowing, grade II is a dissection or intramural hematoma with >25% luminal narrowing, grade III is a pseudoaneurysm, grade IV a complete occlusion and Grade V is a transection with active extravasation. Most grade I–II injuries should be treated with antithrombotic therapy, either unfractionated heparin or antiplatelet agents (B–E). Antithrombotic therapy reduces the risk of stroke and reduces morality and therefore should be initiated as soon as safe. Repeat imaging is often recommended in 7 to 10 days to monitor for progression of these lesions.

Reference: Kim DY, Biffl W, Bokhari F, et al. Evaluation and management of blunt cerebrovascular injury: a practice management guideline from the Eastern Association for the Surgery of Trauma. *J Trauma Acute Care Surg.* 2020;88(6):875–887.

5. B. Asymptomatic pneumomediastinum following blunt chest trauma is most often benign. Associated aerodigestive injuries are rare, occurring in less than 1% of cases. Additional oral contrast studies have been shown to have no added benefit to identifying esophageal injuries in the absence of high-risk findings such as pleural effusion or dysphagia (D, E). Thoracostomy tubes are not indicated in this patient as there is no evidence of hemothorax or pneumothorax (C). An associated hemothorax, as well as air in all mediastinal compartments or specifically posterior compartment pneumomediastinum, are features that have been associated with an increase in mortality. These features may prompt additional workup. Panendoscopy with esophagoscopy, laryngoscopy, and bronchoscopy may be considered for select patients with penetrating neck injury (A).

References: Lee WS, Chong VE, Victorino GP. Computed tomographic findings and mortality in patients with pneumomediastinum from blunt trauma. *JAMA Surg.* 2015;150(8):757–762.

Matthees NG, Mankin JA, Trahan AM, et al. Pneumomediastinum in blunt trauma: if aerodigestive injury is not seen on CT, invasive workup is not indicated. *Am J Surg.* 2019;217(6):1047–1050.

Muckart DJJ, Hardcastle TC, Skinner DL. Pneumomediastinum and pneumopericardium following blunt thoracic trauma: much ado about nothing? *Eur J Trauma Emerg Surg.* 2019;45(5):927–931.

6. A. Supracondylar humerus fractures often occur in children who fall onto an outstretched arm. The classic finding is a patient with a "pink and pulseless" hand that may improve with closed reduction of the fracture. Vascular intervention versus watchful waiting is debated in these cases; however, the most common recommendation is to attempt reduction first and strongly consider surgical intervention of the brachial artery if the vascular exam does not improve after reduction. Volkmann ischemic contracture develops in the setting of ischemia or compartment syndrome which is manifested by a complex deformity of the wrist and hand. Claw hand develops after an injury to the distal ulnar nerve (B) which can be seen in lacerations or sports-related injuries. In the ulnar claw hand, the 4th and 5th fingers cannot be extended. Posterior hip dislocations are commonly associated with sciatic nerve injuries (C). Anterior shoulder dislocations are associated with axillary nerve injuries which can be detected by a "military patch" anesthesia over the deltoid (D). Chronic anterior shoulder dislocations should not be reduced secondary to the risk of axillary artery injury. Wrist drop is seen secondary to radial nerve injury and this is commonly in the setting of a humeral shaft fracture (E).

Reference: Delniotis I, Ktenidis K. The pulseless supracondylar humeral fracture: our experience and a 1-year follow-up. *J Trauma Acute Care Surg.* 2018;85(4):711–716.

7. A. Blunt trauma patients with small (<4 cm) tracheal lacerations with viable surrounding tissue that are hemodynamically stable without any concerning findings suggestive of concurrent esophageal trauma (fever, leukocytosis, odynophagia, dysphagia) can safely be managed nonoperatively with antibiotics, voice rest, PPI therapy, and repeat bronchoscopy in 24 to 48 hours. Large (≥4 cm) tracheal injuries in blunt trauma patients should be repaired. In the setting of isolated tracheal injuries in the neck requiring operative repair, a collar incision is appropriate. Primary repair can be attempted for wounds that are well-apposed after debridement of devitalized edges. Permanent suture should not be used in tracheal repair as it can serve as a nidus for infection (B–D). Additionally, a two-layer closure has a high chance or tracheal stenosis and so a one-layer closure with absorbable suture is most appropriate. Buttressing the repair with muscle (i.e., hyoid or sternocleidomastoid) is commonly performed. A tracheostomy is rarely needed but if indicated, it should be placed one ring-space below the injury (E).

Reference: Fernandez LG, Norwood SH, Berne JD. Tracheal, laryngeal, and oropharyngeal injuries. In: Asensio J, Trunkey D, eds.

Current therapy of trauma and surgical critical care. 2nd ed. Elsevier; 2016:192–204.

8. B. Estimated TSBA burned is useful to determine appropriate fluid resuscitation volumes. Each upper extremity accounts for 9% of the TBSA (anterior surface would be half that or 4.5%), each lower extremity accounts for 18%, the anterior and posterior trunk each accounts for 18%, the head and neck account for 9%, hands are 1% each, and the perineum accounts for 1%. First-degree burns are not included. For this patient, the anterior surface of both arms accounts for 9%, the entire leg is 18%, and the hands are not counted (first-degree burns), totaling 27% (A, C–E). The most widely used approach to fluid resuscitation in a burn patient is the Parkland formula: 4 mL/kg for each percentage of TBSA burned over the first 24 hours, with one-half of that amount administered in the first 8 hours and the remaining half over the next 16 hours. For children, some use a modified Parkland formula with 6 mL/kg. Keep in mind that Ringer lactate is the fluid of choice. Normal saline in such large volumes will lead to hyperchloremic metabolic acidosis. The most important endpoint of resuscitation is adequate urine output (0.5–1 cc/kg/hr).

9. A. In the emergent setting, the fastest way to gain vascular access is by a peripheral catheter, often at the median antecubital fossa, because this will typically accommodate a large bore IV and is easy to cannulate. Short-wide catheters are used to maximize volume flow for rapid resuscitation. The rate of fluid flow is proportional to the cross-sectional area of the catheter and inversely proportional to the fourth power of its radius. As such, an 18-gauge catheter is preferred over a 20-gauge catheter since the 18-gauge catheter has a larger diameter (B). Central vein catheterization is not the preferred mode of vascular access in the immediate trauma setting because it is time consuming and has a high rate of complications. These complications are exacerbated by the urgency of the line placement, central veins often being collapsed due to hypovolemia, and suboptimal use of sterile technique. Central line-associated bloodstream infections alone have a mortality rate as high as 20%. A short but large central vein cordis will allow for a faster route for infusion but is not appropriate in the initial trauma setting for the aforementioned reasons (C–E).

Reference: Mermel LA, Allon M, Bouza E, et al. Clinical practice guidelines for the diagnosis and management of intravascular catheter-related infection: 2009 Update by the Infectious Diseases Society of America. *Clin Infect Dis.* 2009;49(1):1–45.

10. A. Trauma is the leading cause of death for individuals over the age of 45 years in the United States. Although all the listed choices are causes of death in the trauma patient, traumatic brain injury (TBI) is the single largest contributor accounting for nearly half of all trauma deaths and is the most common cause of death in trauma patients reaching the hospital alive (B–E). Hemorrhagic shock is the most common cause of death in trauma patients within the first hour. An important component to the management of TBI is the prevention of secondary injury to the brain by avoiding hypotension and hypoxia.

References: Baker CC, Oppenheimer L, Stephens B, Lewis FR, Trunkey DD. Epidemiology of trauma deaths. *Am J Surg.* 1980;140(1):144–150.

National Center for Injury Prevention and Control. *Traumatic brain injury in the United States: a report to Congress.* Centers for Disease Control and Prevention, US Department of Health & Human Services; 1999.

11. E. The anterior abdomen is bounded by the nipples, groin crease, and anterior axillary lines. Stab wounds to this area are divided into thirds; one-third do not penetrate the peritoneal cavity, one-third penetrate the peritoneal cavity but don't cause significant intraabdominal injury, and one-third penetrate the peritoneal cavity causing significant intraabdominal injury. Immediate exploratory laparotomy is mandated in the hemodynamically unstable patient or in the presence of diffuse peritonitis. In a hemodynamically stable patient without peritonitis, the surgeon has several options to choose from. These include admission for serial abdominal exams, CT scan, FAST scan (which has a lower sensitivity than CT but is quick and inexpensive), and LWE (C, D). The main advantage of LWE is that if the study is negative (anterior fascia has not been penetrated), the patient can be discharged from the ED. If LWE is positive, it does not mean the peritoneum has been violated. Taking all positive LWE patients to the operating room (OR) will result in a high negative laparotomy rate. As such several options exist: proceed to CT scan, admission for serial abdominal exams, or diagnostic laparoscopy. The decision of which to perform depends on the institution (A, B).

References: Cothren CC, Moore EE, Warren FA, Kashuk JL, Biffl WL, Johnson JL. Local wound exploration remains a valuable triage tool for the evaluation of anterior abdominal stab wounds. *Am J Surg.* 2009;198(2):223–226.

Shanmuganathan K, Mirvis S, Chiu W. Penetrating torso trauma: triple-contrast helical CT in peritoneal violation and organ injury-a prospective study in 200 patients. *Radiology.* 2004;231(3):775–784.

12. D. This patient has received a large volume of fluid resuscitation that led to abdominal compartment syndrome, which presents with the triad of oliguria, rise in peak airway pressures, and increased intraabdominal pressure. Bladder pressure (as measured via an indwelling Foley) is used as a surrogate to determine abdominal pressure. Intraabdominal hypertension has somewhat arbitrarily been defined as a sustained intraabdominal pressure greater than or equal to 12 mmHg. End-organ damage typically occurs with pressures greater than 20 mmHg. As the pressure in the abdomen increases, the diaphragm's ability to contract is compromised, and this subsequently lessens pulmonary compliance and FRC (A, B). This translates to an increased intrathoracic pressure resulting in decreased venous return, increased pulmonary vascular resistance, and increased pulmonary capillary wedge pressure (C, E). Treatment is to perform a decompressive laparotomy, leaving the abdomen open (though covered with a protective bag).

Reference: Papavramidis TS, Marinis AD, Pliakos I, Kesisoglou I, Papavramidou N. Abdominal compartment syndrome—Intraabdominal hypertension: defining, diagnosing, and managing. *J Emerg Trauma Shock.* 2011;4(2):279–291.

13. C. Burn injuries are classified into five categories with second-degree burns having two subclassifications. First-degree, or superficial, burns only involve the epidermis with red skin, no blisters, and pain. Sunburns are considered first-degree burns. Second-degree burns are divided into two categories: (1) Superficial partial-thickness burns are characterized by blistering, pain, blanching, and intact hair follicles, are limited to the dermal layer, and do not typically require any skin grafting. (2) Deep partial-thickness burns are characterized by blistering, are less sensitive (sometimes painless) and nonblanchable, and involve loss of hair follicles (A, E). Since the hair follicles offer the regenerative capacity for the skin, deep partial-thickness burns will not heal spontaneously and will often require intervention such as skin grafting (D). Third-degree burns are considered full-thickness because they involve all the layers of the skin and are characterized by a white leathery appearance. Fourth-degree burns are also considered full thickness but also involve either underlying muscle, fascia, or bone and typically lead to disfigurement (B).

Reference: Tiwari VK. Burn wound: how it differs from other wounds? *Indian J Plast Surg.* 2012;45(2):364–373.

14. C. Prophylactic use of IV antibiotics should be discouraged in the burn patient because this will breed multidrug-resistant organisms. However, several topical ointments are available that are used widely in burn care to prevent bacterial colonization. Silver sulfadiazine is considered a broad-spectrum agent, but it has poor coverage for *Pseudomonas*, has poor eschar penetration, and can lead to neutropenia and thrombocytopenia (B). It should be avoided in patients with a sulfa allergy. An advantage is its painless application. Silver nitrate, also considered a broad-spectrum agent, does not work against *Pseudomonas*, and its application is painful. It has poor eschar penetration, causes tissue discoloration, and can lead to severe electrolyte derangements (depletes Na+, K+, and Cl–) (E). It can be used in patients with a sulfa allergy. Bacitracin and neomycin have a painless application, limited eschar penetration, and poor gram-negative coverage. Mafenide acetate (Sulfamylon) is considered a broad-spectrum agent including activity against *Pseudomonas* and *Enterococcus* spp. and has good eschar penetration (D). Since it is a carbonic anhydrase inhibitor it can lead to hyperchloremic metabolic acidosis, and thus its use should be limited to small areas of full-thickness burns (A).

Reference: Dai T, Huang YY, Sharma SK, Hashmi JT, Kurup DB, Hamblin MR. Topical antimicrobials for burn wound infections. *Recent Pat Antiinfect Drug Discov.* 2010;5(2):124–151.

15. C. The American College of Surgeons and American Burn Association have set guidelines as to which patients should be transferred to a burn center. These patients have been demonstrated to have improved outcomes and survival when treated in a nationally recognized burn center that can approach the burn patient with a multidisciplinary approach. Indications for transfer are as follows: (1) second- or third-degree burns greater than 20% TBSA in patients age 10 to 50 years old; (2) second- or third-degree burns greater than 10% TBSA in patients younger than 10 years or older than 50 years; (3) third-degree burns greater than 5% TBSA in any age; (4) any second- or third-degree burn to hands, feet, face, eyes, genitalia, perineum, or skin over major joints; (5) any electrical or chemical burn; and (6) any concomitant inhalation injury or multiple trauma. From the available answer choices, the only patient that has an indication for transfer to a burn center is the 21-year-old male with both a hand burn and a chemical burn (A, B, D, E). First-degree burns do not need referral.

References: American College of Surgeons. *Resources for optimal care of the injured patient*; 1993:64.

Hospital and prehospital resources for optimal care of patients with burn injury: guidelines for development and operation of burn centers. American Burn Association. *J Burn Care Rehabil.* 1990;11(2):98–104.

16. A. Electrical shock requires the expertise of a burn center, and all patients should be transferred as soon as they are stable. The two types of electrical currents are alternating and direct. An alternating current will lead to repetitive, tetanic muscle contractions (C). An example of this is a city worker who gets electrocuted on a power line that emits an alternating current. Since flexor muscle tone is generally stronger than extensor muscle tone, patients will often grip the source of electricity leading to a prolonged exposure. In contrast, direct current electrocution will often result in a single, large muscle contraction that will throw the patient several feet away from the source. A car battery has a direct current, so this patient likely suffered a direct current electrocution. Adipose tissue has a high resistance to electricity, which will result in an increased tissue temperature and subsequent coagulation; thus, patients with obesity will have a higher amount of deep thermal burns (D). The main cause of death in the early post electrocution period is cardiac arrhythmias (B). Other immediate complications of electrocution injury include posterior shoulder dislocation and spinal cord injury. Long-term, patients are at increased risk of cataracts, polyneuritis, and ototoxicity. The skin burn mark with an electrical injury can vastly underestimate the severity of the burn. Often there is severe injury to the underlying muscle and connective tissue despite a relatively minor outer skin burn. As such, these patients are susceptible to rhabdomyolysis, which would be suggested by the presence of red urine. Thus, creatine kinase (CK) levels should routinely be sent (E). These patients should be admitted, placed on cardiac monitoring, and resuscitated with IV fluids to maintain high urine output.

Reference: Wesner ML, Hickie J. Long-term sequelae of electrical injury. *Can Fam Physician.* 2013;59(9):935–939.

17. D. Frostbite can occur when tissue is exposed to temperatures below −2°C or 28°F. The severity of the injury increases proportionally to the duration of exposure. Frostbites are classified as follows: (1) First degree are hyperemic without necrosis and characterized by a yellow plaque; (2) second degree have superficial vesicles with hyperemia and partial-thickness necrosis; (3) third-degree have hemorrhagic bullae and full-thickness necrosis; and (4) fourth degree are characterized by frank gangrene with involvement of underlying muscle and bone (A). Treatment begins with rewarming the extremity in a warm water bath between 40 and 42°C. It should be done rapidly (E). Because tissue viability will often take weeks to determine, early debridement and/or amputation should be avoided (B). Tissue freezing and reperfusion both contribute to the tissue damage seen in frostbite burns. Crystallization of the extracellular space leads to an increased extracellular oncotic pressure resulting in cellular dehydration and impaired intracellular metabolism. An inflammatory response ensues ultimately leading to thrombosis, tissue ischemia, and endothelial injury. Reperfusion injury occurs when blood flow is restored, and

it is for this reason that tPA has had an emerging role in the management of frostbite burns. Thrombolytic therapy will limit microvascular thrombosis and prevent reperfusion injury. Predictors of poor response to tPA include warm ischemia time longer than 6 hours, more than 24 hours of cold exposure, and multiple freeze-thaw cycles. Because this patient has had a warm ischemia time of 7 hours, she is ineligible for tPA treatment (C). Patients that are deemed appropriate candidates for tPA therapy should continue until there is evidence of tissue reperfusion, 48 hours have passed, or the treating team feels there is no further therapeutic gain from continued infusion.

Reference: Gross EA, Moore JC. Using thrombolytics in frostbite injury. *J Emerg Trauma Shock.* 2012;5(3):267–271.

18. C. Chance fractures are also called seat-belt fractures. In children, they occur when the child is only wearing a lap belt. They are flexion-distraction type injuries of the spine. There is a significant association with intraabdominal injuries (most commonly hollow viscus and pancreas). Recent reports using large-scale trauma registry data suggest that the rate of intraabdominal injury is close to 33% (previously reported much higher). The presence of a Chance fracture is in and of itself not an indication for a laparotomy. However, the patient presented has an unreliable abdominal examination. In addition, the presence of free fluid on CT, in the absence of a solid organ injury, should raise the suspicion of a hollow viscus injury. As such laparotomy is indicated. In an alert and oriented, nonventilated patient, serial abdominal examination would be the initial management (in spite of the free fluid) (B). MRI of the spine will be helpful to determine spinal cord impingement, but this will need to be performed after exploratory laparotomy (A). Until then, the patient should remain in strict spine precautions. Repeat imaging alone is not appropriate if there is concern for a hollow-viscous injury (D, E).

References: Neugebauer H, Wallenboeck E, Hungerford M. Seventy cases of injuries of the small intestine caused by blunt abdominal trauma: a retrospective study from 1970 to 1994. *J Trauma.* 1999;46(1):116–121.

Tyroch AH, McGuire EL, McLean SF, et al. The association between Chance fractures and intra-abdominal injuries revisited: a multicenter review. *Am Surg.* 2005;71(5):434–438.

19. B. Adult Jehovah's Witnesses have the right to refuse blood products, even in lifesaving situations. Anemia does not render the patient incapable of making an informed decision and giving blood products against the patient's wishes is a violation of her autonomy, and the physician may be reprimanded by the American Medical Association (E). The patient should still continue to receive the care she would otherwise get if she did consent to blood transfusion (A). With the relative hemodynamic instability (tachycardia and hypotension), contrast extravasation in the spleen, anemia, and hemoperitoneum, there is little margin for error, so the patient should undergo a splenectomy. The physician should document the patient's refusal of blood products in the electronic medical record because this places her at higher risk for death given her present anemia. Angiography with embolization is considered an appropriate option for hemodynamically stable patients with contrast extravasation (C). In a true emergency setting, there is no time to consult the ethics committee (D).

20. A. In the trauma patient, c-spine clearance is accomplished using the National Emergency X-Radiography Utilization Study (NEXUS) criteria. Patients that have any one of the NEXUS criteria should continue with spinal precautions until a CT scan of the c-spine is performed. The NEXUS criteria can be remembered by the "NSAID" mnemonic: Neurologic deficit, Spinal (cervical) tenderness, Altered mental status, Intoxicated, or Distracting injury. Patients with a negative CT c-spine can then be clinically cleared and the c-collar may be removed. This is not possible in an obtunded or intubated patient. If the patient is only expected to be obtunded or intubated for a short period of time (e.g., combative drunk patient), it is reasonable to keep the c-collar on and assess the c-spine once the patient is awake. This patient has extensive traumatic brain injury and is likely going to be intubated for a prolonged period of time. Prolonged application of a hard cervical collar appears to compress the jugular veins, causing venous outflow obstruction, and thus increasing intracranial pressure (ICP). The collar also creates a nociceptive stimulus, which might also contribute to elevated ICP; therefore, keeping the c-collar on for a prolonged period of time increases the risk for complications (C). Previously, this patient would have received an MRI c-spine and if no injuries were identified, the c-collar would then be removed. However, the Eastern Association for the Surgery of Trauma (EAST) has recently recommended that in an obtunded adult blunt trauma patient, the c-collar should be removed after a negative CT c-spine alone. MRI c-spine may no longer have a role in the obtunded trauma patient as it has been demonstrated that it may lead to a higher complication rate and longer ICU stay as occult injuries that are not clinically relevant may be identified and acted upon (B). There are no studies showing improved outcomes in switching to a soft-collar (D, E).

Reference: Patel MB, Humble SS, Cullinane DC, et al. Cervical spine collar clearance in the obtunded adult blunt trauma patient: a systematic review and practice management guideline from the Eastern Association for the Surgery of Trauma. *J Trauma Acute Care Surg.* 2015;78(2):430–441.

21. D. Pneumothorax is a common complication of both penetrating and blunt trauma. It is a clinical diagnosis that can be made during the primary survey. Patients with decreased breath sounds, trachea deviation, and hypotension should be suspected of having a tension pneumothorax and should have needle decompression or tube thoracostomy performed immediately. In equivocal cases, imaging can be helpful. Occult pneumothorax is one that is not seen on the initial radiograph but may be demonstrated on CT. Pneumothorax as a result of penetrating trauma has a concomitant hemothorax up to 80% of the time (E). Small pneumothoraces identified on CT can be observed if the patient is stable. Normally, 1.25% of the pneumothorax volume is absorbed in 24 hours. Additionally, the use of 100% inspired supplemental oxygen is controversial because it can result in oxygen toxicity (A). EAST recommends that an occult pneumothorax can be safely observed in a stable patient undergoing general anesthesia. This recommendation was based on two prospective randomized studies that supported the notion that occult pneumothoraces will likely not progress regardless of the presence of positive pressure ventilation (B). Similarly, an occult pneumothorax can be observed in a ventilated patient that remains asymptomatic (C). EAST also recommends that persistent air leaks on postinjury day 3 should be further evaluated with VATS because this can be suggestive of underlying bronchial injury or bronchopleural fistula.

References: Mowery NT, Gunter OL, Collier BR, et al. Practice management guidelines for management of hemothorax and occult pneumothorax. *J Trauma.* 2011;70(2):510–518.

Sharma A, Jindal P. Principles of diagnosis and management of traumatic pneumothorax. *J Emerg Trauma Shock.* 2008;1(1):34–41.

22. B. The patient described has evidence of muscle ischemia/necrosis and has developed rhabdomyolysis as evidenced by the rise in CK. Rhabdomyolysis can present with CK levels of 10,000 to 20,0000 u/L; no other condition can cause such an extreme rise in CK (normal is 45–260 u/L). Rhabdomyolysis can occur in any setting that causes ischemia to the muscles (such as hypotension after trauma), or from prolonged pressure on muscle compartments during surgery. It is likely exacerbated by obesity and improper padding on the OR or procedure table. The ischemia/reperfusion cycle that ensues places the patient at risk of developing compartment syndrome. A small study of patients with obesity undergoing Roux-en-Y bypass found that body mass index (BMI) was an independent risk factor for the development of postoperative rhabdomyolysis. In a patient positioned in the supine position, the muscles that would most likely be compressed are the gluteal ones. In addition, pelvic embolization, as performed for trauma or endovascular abdominal aortic aneurysm (AAA) repair, is a known risk for developing buttock claudication. Rarely, it is associated with devastating pelvic ischemia and/or buttock ischemia/necrosis (A, C–E). So in this patient, in addition to aggressive fluid hydration, it would be imperative to roll the patient over to inspect the buttock muscles.

References: Benevides ML, Nochi Júnior RJ. Rhabdomyolysis secondary to gluteal compartment syndrome after bariatric surgery: case report. *Rev Bras Anestesiol.* 2006;56(4):408–412.

Yasumura K, Ikegami K, Kamohara T, Nohara Y. High incidence of ischemic necrosis of the gluteal muscle after transcatheter angiographic embolization for severe pelvic fracture. *J Trauma.* 2005;58(5):985–990.

23. A. Kidney injuries are graded from I to V, with grade I being a contusion or subcapsular, nonexpanding hematoma and grade V a completely shattered kidney or an avulsion of the renal hilum. Grade I and II injuries are considered minor, grade III injuries are deep lacerations that do not involve the collecting system, whereas grade IV injuries are lacerations extending into the collecting system or an injury to the main renal artery. The vast majority of blunt renal injuries (approximately 90%) can be managed nonoperatively. The injury described in this patient would be a grade IV and, in a stable patient, can be managed nonoperatively (B–D). Grade IV injury from blunt trauma can be managed nonoperatively provided the patient is hemodynamically stable. Most urinary extravasation resolves. If it persists, or if the patient demonstrates evidence of sepsis, it should be treated using a combination of endourologic and percutaneous techniques (such as a percutaneous nephrostomy) (E). The decision to explore a zone II or perinephric retroperitoneal hematoma at the time of operation and in the absence of preoperative imaging has classically been based on the mechanism of injury and hemodynamic status of the patient. Following blunt trauma and in the absence of hemodynamic instability or a rapidly expanding or pulsatile perinephric hematoma, these perinephric hematomas should not be explored. Following penetrating trauma and in the absence of preoperative imaging to assist in the identification of a renal injury, the presence of a perinephric retroperitoneal hematoma mandates exploration. If indicated, nephrectomy should be preceded by palpation for a contralateral kidney. Surgery is indicated for vascular or renal pedicle injuries or in a completely shattered kidney.

References: Kuan JK, Wright JL, Nathens AB, Rivara FP, Wessells H, American Association for the Surgery of Trauma. American Association for the Surgery of Trauma Organ Injury Scale for kidney injuries predicts nephrectomy, dialysis, and death in patients with blunt injury and nephrectomy for penetrating injuries. *J Trauma.* 2006;60(2):351–356.

Tinkoff G, Esposito TJ, Reed J, et al. American Association for the Surgery of Trauma Organ Injury Scale I: spleen, liver, and kidney, validation based on the National Trauma Data Bank. *J Am Coll Surg.* 2008;207(5):646–655.

24. B. A patient who has punched another person in the mouth is at risk for a human bite wound. The most common organism found isolated in wounds from infected human bites is *Streptococcus* followed by *Staphylococcus.* Other common organisms include *Eikenella, Fusobacterium, Prevotella,* and *Porphyromonas. T. pallidum* is the organism that causes syphilis and has been reported to be transmitted by a human bite, but this is rare (A). *Propionibacterium* and *Bacteroides* are anaerobic organisms and are unlikely to be transmitted from a human bite (D, E). Hepatitis C is the leading cause of death from liver disease in the United States and the most common etiology leading to liver transplantation. However, transmission from infected persons is rare (C). Hepatitis B is more likely to be transmitted from a human bite.

References: Stevens DL, Bisno AL, Chambers HF, et al. Practice guidelines for the diagnosis and management of skin and soft tissue infections: 2014 update by the Infectious Diseases Society of America. *Clin Infect Dis.* 2014;59(2):e10–e52.

Talan DA, Abrahamian FM, Moran GJ, et al. Clinical presentation and bacteriologic analysis of infected human bites in patients presenting to emergency departments. *Clin Infect Dis.* 2003;37(11):1481–1489.

25. B. Brain death is diagnosed by a standardized set of tests including electroencephalography, nucleotide brain scan, apnea test, and clinical assessment including brain stem reflexes. Brain death is both a medical and legal determination of death. It is appropriate to support a brain-dead patient using a ventilator for a limited period of time. This will help the patient's family come to terms with their loss and will help coordinate possible organ donation. This should always be facilitated by an organ donation service and not by the physician. If the patient is not registered for or against organ donation, the decision regarding organ donation should be guided by the standard of substituted judgment. This involves a family member or close friend making the decision based on the known wishes or preferences of the patient at the time of death. However, this should never be refereed by the physician. If a query for organ donation is initiated from a family member, a third-party service should be made available to the family to facilitate a discussion. Any inconsistencies of the patient's wishes regarding organ

donation should be properly investigated by an organ donation service (A, C). Administering a lethal dose of morphine sulfate, or euthanasia, is only practiced in certain states and requires an awake patient to consent (D). Consulting the hospital ethics committee would not be appropriate in this situation (E).

Reference: Emanuel EJ, Emanuel LL. Proxy decision making for incompetent patients: an ethical and empirical analysis. *JAMA.* 1992;267(15):2067–2071.

26. C. In the uncommon scenario in which a patient "cannot be intubated nor ventilated," a surgical cricothyroidotomy should be immediately undertaken. This is performed using an 11 blade via a transverse or vertical incision of the skin directly over the cricothyroid membrane followed by a transverse incision through the cricothyroid membrane. A vertical incision is preferred on the skin and subcutaneous tissue to avoid injuring the anterior jugular veins. The airway should be dilated using one's finger allowing for insertion of an appropriately sized endotracheal or tracheostomy tube (6 French or smaller). Needle cricothyroidotomy is traditionally reserved for children under the age of 12 years old because a surgical or open cricothyroidotomy in this population may result in subglottic stenosis (A). In the absence of a percutaneous needle cricothyroidotomy kit, a high-jet insufflator is typically required to permit temporary oxygenation of patients in whom a needle cricothyroidotomy has been performed. Nasotracheal intubation requires that a patient is spontaneously breathing and is contraindicated in a patient with severe maxillofacial fractures or in those with the potential for a cribriform plate fracture (B). Due to the significant amount of bleeding, fiberoptic bronchoscopy is unlikely to be of benefit in this situation (D). Issues related to setup, equipment, and availability also limit the use of this modality in emergent trauma situations. Apneic oxygenation is a technique of providing supplemental high-flow oxygenation via nasal cannula in addition to standard preoxygenation techniques. This adjunct may decrease the incidence of desaturation in patients undergoing intubation but is not a replacement for a definitive airway (E).

Reference: American College of Surgeons Committee on Trauma. *Advanced trauma life support program for doctors.* 9th ed. American College of Surgeons; 2012.

27. C. This patient is hemodynamically unstable with a positive abdominal FAST following blunt trauma. In general, patients in hemorrhagic shock are classified as responders, transient responders, and nonresponders on the basis of whether or not their vital signs improve following a fluid challenge. Transient and nonresponders should be considered to have ongoing blood loss until proven otherwise. Given these findings, the patient should be taken to the operating room for an exploratory laparotomy (B, E). The CRASH-2 trial demonstrated that the early administration of TXA (antifibrinolytic agent) in blunt trauma reduced all-cause mortality. The benefit of TXA is best seen if given within the first hour of trauma and nonexistent after three hours. In fact, TXA given after three hours may increase mortality secondary to bleeding (A). The finding of chest pain, a widened mediastinum, in conjunction with the high-speed deceleration injury is concerning for blunt aortic injury.

Management of traumatic blunt aortic injury typically begins with blood pressure and pain control. Management depends on injury grade (E). However, it is more that the source of the patient's hemodynamic instability (with the positive FAST scan) is bleeding in the abdomen. A transthoracic echocardiogram may provide information regarding cardiac function and volume status, but it is not indicated given the patient's ongoing hemodynamic instability (D). Due the patient's ongoing shock and nonresponsiveness to a crystalloid challenge, transfusion of blood products in conjunction with hemorrhage control, should be initiated.

References: American College of Surgeons Committee on Trauma. *Advanced trauma life support program for doctors.* 9th ed. American College of Surgeons; 2012.

CRASH-2 Trial Collaborators, Shakur H, Roberts I, et al. Effects of tranexamic acid on death, vascular occlusive events, and blood transfusion in trauma patients with significant haemorrhage (CRASH-2): a randomised, placebo-controlled trial. Lancet. 2010;376(9734):23–32.

Demetriades D, Velmahos GC, Scalea TM, et al. Blunt traumatic thoracic aortic injuries: early or delayed repair–results of an American Association for the Surgery of Trauma prospective study. *J Trauma.* 2009;66(4):967–973.

Henry DA, Carless PA, Moxey AJ, et al. Anti-fibrinolytic use for minimising perioperative allogeneic blood transfusion. *Cochrane Database Syst Rev.* 2007;(4):CD001886.

28. E. Penetrating extremity trauma may be accompanied by hard or soft signs of vascular injury. Hard signs including shock, pulsatile bleeding, expanding or pulsatile hematoma, palpable thrill or bruit, or absent distal pulses warrant immediate operative exploration (B). Soft signs are findings on the physical exam that are suggestive of a potential vascular injury and require further diagnostic testing. Soft signs include diminished pulse, proximity of wounds to vessels, hematomas, and reports of significant blood loss. Given the absence of a hard sign, this patient is stable to undergo further diagnostic workup and does not require an immediate operation. Ankle-brachial index (ABI) is both sensitive and specific for lower extremity vascular injuries. In comparison to CT angiography or formal angiography, ABI does not require ionizing radiation or the administration of contrast (A, D). ABI less than 0.9 is suggestive of vascular injury and prompts a CT angiography. Significant vascular injury can be excluded with a negative predictive value of 99% when ABI is >0.9. An alternative to ABI is API and is used in the same way. API is the arterial pressure just distal to the injury compared to the uninvolved contralateral extremity. Although arterial vasospasm may occur following proximity trauma, this diagnosis is usually one of exclusion and does not warrant immediate treatment with papaverine (C).

References: Feliciano DV, Moore EE, West MA, et al. Western Trauma Association critical decisions in trauma: evaluation and management of peripheral vascular injury, part II. *J Trauma Acute Care Surg.* 2013;75(3):391–397.

Feliciano DV, Moore FA, Moore EE, et al. Evaluation and management of peripheral vascular injury. Part 1. Western Trauma Association/critical decisions in trauma. *J Trauma.* 2011;70(6):1551–1556.

Johansen K, Lynch K, Paun M, Copass M. Non-invasive vascular tests reliably exclude occult arterial trauma in injured extremities. *J Trauma.* 1991;31(4):515–522.

29. C. Nonoperative management (NOM) of solid organ injuries is a well-accepted treatment modality. Several criteria should be considered when selecting patients for NOM

of splenic injuries. Patients should have no other indications for laparotomy on the basis of physical exam findings (peritonitis or hemorrhagic shock) or the results of other diagnostic tests (free air on CT scan of the abdomen) and should be evaluable (absence of a complete high spinal cord injury or intoxication). The presence of a traumatic brain injury does not preclude NOM, nor does older age. An increasing volume of hemoperitoneum is associated with higher failure rates of NOM as is an increasing American Association for the Surgery of Trauma (AAST) grade of injury. Angiography with embolization should be considered for patients with AAST injury grade of greater than III, presence of a contrast blush, moderate hemoperitoneum, evidence of ongoing splenic bleeding (requiring >2 units of packed red blood cells [PRBCs]), presence of a pseudoaneurysm or suspected arteriovenous fistula provided that they are hemodynamically stable. Serial abdominal exams and trending the hematocrit would be inappropriate in the presence of active extravasation of contrast (D). If angioembolization is not available, laparoscopic and open splenectomy are both reasonable options in hemodynamically stable patients that meet the above indications for surgery (A, E), whereas in the unstable patient or with diffuse peritonitis, open splenectomy is recommended. Once in the operating room, attempts at splenic preservation via splenorrhaphy are reasonable in hemodynamically stable patients (B).

Reference: Stassen NA, Bhullar I, Cheng JD, et al. Selective nonoperative management of blunt splenic injury: an Eastern Association for the Surgery of Trauma practice management guideline. *J Trauma Acute Care Surg.* 2012;73(5 Suppl 4):S294–S300.

30. C. The physical exam findings are concerning for the presence of a urethral injury. The most common location is at the prostatic urethra. Genitourinary injuries may occur in up to 15% of patients with pelvic fractures. Head injury is the most common associated injury seen in patients with pelvic fractures. Clinical suspicion of a urethral injury warrants the performance of a RUG to identify the presence and location of a urethral injury. Blind insertion of a Foley catheter is contraindicated in this patient (A). CT abdomen with IV contrast is helpful for identifying injuries to the kidneys and delayed acquisition images may also aid in the identification of ureteral or bladder injuries (B). A CT cystogram accurately diagnoses both extraperitoneal and intraperitoneal bladder injuries (D). Intravenous pyelogram is used to identify renal injuries and is rarely performed (E). Management of urethral injuries depends on the location and severity of injury, as well as presence of associated injuries, and surgical expertise.

Reference: Johnsen NV, Dmochowski RR, Mock S, Reynolds WS, Milam DF, Kaufman MR. Primary endoscopic realignment of urethral disruption injuries—A double-edged sword? *J Urol.* 2015;194(4):1022–1026.

31. C. Although A, B, C (Airway, with cervical spine precautions; Breathing; Circulation with hemorrhage control) has always been the recommended sequence in trauma patients, recent recommendations are shifting to C, A, B in those with penetrating injuries who are severely hypotensive, as the combination of rapid-sequence intubation and positive pressure ventilation can worsen hypotension and lead to cardiac arrest (A). Thus, blood products would be the preferred first step, followed by immediate transport to the operating room. Some medical centers are now providing initial resuscitation with whole blood for the trauma patient in shock. Given the location of the injury (zone I of the neck), one should have a high suspicion for a right subclavian or innominate artery injury. Once in the operating room (if possible), the patient is prepped and draped prior to intubation. REBOA (E) is utilized for control of vascular injuries below the diaphragm. Proximal control of such an injury on the right via an open approach is best achieved by a median sternotomy. If the same injury were present on the left, proximal control of the left subclavian artery is best achieved via a left anterolateral thoracotomy. Endovascular balloon occlusion is another option. If blood is exsanguinating through the bullet hole, manual compression in this area is ineffective. Temporary tamponade can be achieved via insertion and inflation of a Foley balloon directly into the wound, permitting rapid transportation to the operating room. Thoracostomy is indicated for pneumothorax or hemothorax seen on radiograph imaging or after primary survey suggestive of these conditions (B). The above patient has not had a cardiopulmonary arrest, nor does he meet any indication for ED thoracotomy (D).

References: American College of Surgeons Committee on Trauma. *Advanced trauma life support program for doctors.* 9th ed. American College of Surgeons; 2012.

Demetriades D, Chahwan S, Gomez H, et al. Penetrating injuries to the subclavian and axillary vessels. *J Am Coll Surg.* 1999;188(3):290–295.

32. D. With penetrating neck trauma, there is concern that bleeding may rapidly compress the trachea. As such, the first step in the management algorithm is to establish an airway, particularly in the presence of an expanding hematoma or depressed level of consciousness. If the patient has a "hard sign" of a vascular injury, such as a rapidly expanding or pulsatile hematoma, visible exsanguination, palpable thrill or audible bruit, or dense neurologic deficit (such as this patient with GCS 8), the patient should then be transported directly to the OR. If the patient is hemodynamic unstable, without hard signs, the presumption should be that the patient exsanguinated in the field. Thus, shock is another indication for immediate surgical exploration (this patient has a low BP as well). Conversely, in the absence of hard signs, the next step would be to obtain CT arteriography of the neck vessels. This historically has been achieved with formal arteriography, because of the ease and rapidity of its use (B, C). In addition, an assessment for injuries to the aerodigestive tract (triple endoscopy and/or esophagography) and cervical spine needs to be performed (E). As a general guide, repairing a carotid artery injury in a patient with a neurologic deficit is recommended as it may result in improved neurologic function, whereas carotid ligation typically does not. Repair can be achieved by primary suturing, resection with a primary reanastomosis, or interposition graft placement (saphenous vein or polytetrafluoroethylene) (A).

33. D. Resuscitative thoracotomy is a potentially lifesaving procedure. Indications and guidelines continue to evolve. There are many articles in the literature on the topic, with variable findings and recommendations. However, several overarching themes consistently permeate these studies. Outcomes are better for those with SOL than those without, penetrating trauma than blunt, chest trauma than abdominal, isolated injury than multiple injuries, without head injury than with, short duration

of CPR than long duration, and stab wounds than GSW (A–C, E). Thus, the best scenario for resuscitative thoracotomy would be an isolated stab wound to the chest, with SOL (survival from pooled data is 21%). Such a patient is much more likely to have arrested due to cardiac tamponade and therefore has not suffered exsanguinating hemorrhage. Conversely, at the other extreme, for blunt trauma without SOL, survival was only 0.7%. The following are considered SOL: agonal respirations, cardiac electrical activity, palpable pulse, measurable blood pressure, spontaneous movement, or pupillary reactivity. Thus, the benefit of resuscitative thoracotomy for SOL and penetrating chest trauma is clear. Less compelling but still potentially beneficial indications would be penetrating chest trauma without SOL, penetrating extrathoracic injury with or without SOL, and blunt trauma with SOL. There is no benefit for blunt trauma with no SOL. For those that survive, a surprising majority survive with favorable neurologic outcomes.

References: Burlew CC, Moore EE, Moore FA, et al. Western Trauma Association critical decisions in trauma: resuscitative thoracotomy: resuscitative thoracotomy. *J Trauma Acute Care Surg.* 2012;73(6):1359–1363.

Seamon MJ, Haut ER, Van Arendonk K, et al. An evidence-based approach to patient selection for emergency department thoracotomy: a practice management guideline from the Eastern Association for the Surgery of Trauma. *J Trauma Acute Care Surg.* 2015;79(1):159–173.

34. E. The preferred access for young children and infants following trauma is via the peripheral percutaneous route (antecubital fossa or saphenous vein at the ankle). After two unsuccessful attempts, consideration should be given to IO infusion via a bone marrow needle (18 gauge in infants, 15 gauge in young children). IO cannulation of the proximal tibia provides good short-term access for resuscitation because it targets the noncollapsible veins of the medullary sinus. The optimal site of insertion is the anteromedial tibia 2 to 3 cm below the tibial tuberosity, ensuring to angle away from the growth plates. This can be performed using a bone marrow needle or an IO vascular access system such as the EZ-IO®. Once the patient has been resuscitated, follow-up attempts at peripheral access should be made. If a patient has obvious deformities in the tibiae (as in this patient), the next location for IO cannulation would be the distal femur just above the femoral condyles (D). In adults, there has been a shift in recent years, and sternal IO access is now considered the preferred initial site for cannulation (thinner cortex and abundant red bone marrow) followed by the tibia. The proximal humerus is an additional option in adults. It is also important to note that serum electrolytes, blood gases, and type and cross can all be performed using blood from interosseous access. A distal saphenous vein cutdown is another option in children ages 1 to 6 years, but in a child younger than 1 year of age, it would be challenging and not appropriate in the setting of obvious leg deformity (B). In hypovolemic pediatric patients younger than 6 years of age, percutaneous femoral vein cannulation is another alternative but is associated with an increased risk of venous thrombosis and would be much more challenging in a child younger than 1 year (C). Subclavian and internal jugular central lines would be too difficult to perform in the trauma setting in such a small child and would be associated with an increased risk of iatrogenic injury (A). The interosseous cannula should be removed expeditiously (within 24 hours) because of the potential risk of infectious complications including osteomyelitis. Extremity compartment syndrome is another potential complication of IO infusion.

References: Cullen PM. Intraosseous cannulation in children. Anaesth Intensive Care Med, 2012; 13:28–30.

Pasley J, Miller CHT, DuBose JJ, et al. Intraosseous infusion rates under high pressure: a cadaveric comparison of anatomic sites. *J Trauma Acute Care Surg.* 2015;78(2):295–299.

35. D. Both blood volume and red cell volume increase in the pregnant patient, but blood volume increases more than red cell volume. Blood volume increases by approximately 50% as term approaches, whereas red cell volume increases by approximately 30%, resulting in a functional hemodilution and resultant physiologic anemia of pregnancy (A). Thus, pregnant patients are less likely to manifest signs of blood loss such as tachycardia and hypotension, and if such signs are present, they are indicative of an even more severe blood loss than in the nonpregnant patient (on the order of 1500–2000 mL of blood loss). The pregnant patient has an increased tidal volume and minute ventilation, designed to increase oxygen release to the fetus. This results in a mild respiratory alkalosis, with a PCO_2 in the 27 to 32 range (B). Oxygen consumption is increased, and functional residual capacity is decreased. In addition, the 2,3-diphosphoglycerate level is increased to enhance the release of oxygen to the fetus. However, these physiologic changes result in less pulmonary reserve in an acutely ill pregnant patient. The use of radiographs is thought to be safe for the fetus after the 20th week of gestation (C). The glomerular filtration rate increases, resulting in a decrease in serum creatinine (E). Other important aspects to be aware of are that the gravid uterus can compress the IVC, resulting in decreased venous return. Therefore, the pregnant patient should be placed in the left lateral position at approximately 15 degrees. Pregnant patients are more prone to aspiration, so early NG tube decompression is important. Finally, the progressive stretching of the peritoneum leads to desensitization so that a pregnant patient is less likely to demonstrate peritoneal signs.

Reference: Shah AJ, Kilcline BA. Trauma in pregnancy. *Emerg Med Clin North Am.* 2003;21(3):615–629.

36. D. In the past, the injury described would have been dealt with by performing a formal lobectomy (A). However, pulmonary tractotomy is now used as a less aggressive alternative. The technique involves using a linear stapling device to insert directly into the injured bullet tract. Two hemostatic staple lines are created, and the lung is divided in between. This allows direct access to the bleeding vessels within the parenchyma as well as any leaking bronchi. Bleeding vessels can then be oversewn with a polypropylene monofilament (C). Lobectomy is a better choice for a completely devascularized or destroyed lobe. A pneumonectomy is rarely indicated and, in the trauma setting, is associated with an 80% mortality rate (B). Similarly, ligation of a lobar pulmonary artery has a high rate of morbidity (E).

References: Cothren C, Moore EE, Biffl WL, et al. Lung-sparing techniques are associated with improved outcome compared with anatomic resection for severe lung injuries. *J Trauma.* 2002;53(3):483–487.

Kim DY, Coimbra R. Thoracic damage control. In: Di Saverio S, Tugnoli G, Catena F, Ansaloni L, Naidoo N, eds. *Trauma surgery: volume 2: thoracic and abdominal Trauma.* Springer Milan; 2014:35–46.

37. C. Flail chest occurs when two or more ribs are fractured in at least two locations. Paradoxical movement of this free-floating segment of chest wall is typically not sufficient alone to compromise ventilation (B). Rather, pain and splinting, in conjunction with underlying pulmonary contusions, may result in hypoxemia and hypercarbia due to shunting and ineffective ventilation, respectively. Most patients can be managed without intubation (E). Respiratory failure often does not occur immediately, and frequent reevaluation is warranted. The initial chest radiograph usually underestimates the degree of pulmonary contusion, and the lesion tends to evolve with time and with fluid resuscitation (A). Intravenous fluid administration should be limited as overzealous resuscitation may result in blossoming of pulmonary contusions (D). The most important aspect of treatment of flail chest is pain control. Standard approaches include the use of patient-controlled analgesia and oral pain medications and the placement of continuous epidural catheters. Although the treatment of flail chest has historically been nonoperative, recent literature indicates that internal fixation of the chest wall in select patients without pulmonary contusion decreases intubation time, decreases mortality, shortens duration of mechanical ventilation as well as hospital stay, decreases complications, and improves cosmetic and functional results. In the presence of a pulmonary contusion, however, internal fixation may not be as beneficial. Eastern Association for the Surgery of Trauma (EAST) guidelines recommend ORIF in adults with flail chest after blunt trauma. Situations in which internal fixation should be considered include flail chest in patients who are already undergoing thoracotomy for an intrathoracic injury, flail chest without pulmonary contusion, noticeable paradoxical movement of a chest wall segment while a patient is being weaned from the respirator, and severe deformity of the chest wall.

References: Kasotakis G, Hasenboehler EA, Streib EW, et al. Operative fixation of rib fractures after blunt trauma: a practice management guideline from the Eastern Association for the Surgery of Trauma. *J Trauma Acute Care Surg.* 2017;82(3):618–626.

Leinicke JA, Elmore L, Freeman BD, Colditz GA. Operative management of rib fractures in the setting of flail chest: a systematic review and meta-analysis. *Ann Surg.* 2013;258(6):914–921.

Voggenreiter G, Neudeck F, Aufmkolk M, Obertacke U, Schmit-Neuerburg KP. Operative chest wall stabilization in flail chest–outcomes of patients with or without pulmonary contusion. *J Am Coll Surg.* 1998;187(2):130–138.

38. A. BCI should be suspected in anyone with severe blunt chest trauma. Attempts to identify a BCI and stratify severity on the basis of CK-MB, nuclear scans, and echocardiography have not been successful because these modalities lack sensitivity. ECG is the most commonly recommended tool for the initial diagnosis of BCI. The presence of a sternal fracture is not a marker for BCI (D). A normal screening ECG has a negative predictive value of 95% (E). Addition of a normal cardiac troponin increases the negative predictive value to 100%. If a stable patient has an abnormal cardiac troponin level or ECG, he/she should be admitted for observation to a monitored bed. However, troponin level does not correlate with risk of cardiac complications in BCI. If the patient is unstable, an emergent echocardiogram should be performed. If a tamponade is seen, emergent sternotomy should be performed for suspected cardiac rupture. Very rarely, BCI can lead to coronary artery thrombosis, valvular disruption, or septal disruption (C). In an unstable patient with BCI without an anatomic abnormality on echocardiography, invasive blood pressure monitoring with pressor support should be instituted. Most patients with a diagnosis of myocardial contusion have a benign course, with very few developing arrhythmias or heart failure (B).

References: Clancy K, Velopulos C, Bilaniuk JW, et al. Screening for blunt cardiac injury: an Eastern Association for the Surgery of Trauma practice management guideline. *J Trauma Acute Care Surg.* 2012;73(5 Suppl 4):S301–S306.

Velmahos GC, Karaiskakis M, Salim A, et al. Normal electrocardiography and serum troponin I levels preclude the presence of clinically significant blunt cardiac injury. *J Trauma.* 2003;54(1):45–50.

39. E. The Cattell maneuver involves a right medial visceral rotation of the cecum and ascending colon. It is achieved by incising the peritoneal reflection at the white line of Toldt. It is useful for exposing right retroperitoneal structures, such as the IVC and the right ureter (C). Further cephalad, mobilization and medial rotation of the duodenum (Kocher maneuver) additionally assists in exposing the suprarenal IVC below the liver. The Kocher maneuver is not useful for exposing the celiac axis (D). This is best done by combining a Mattox maneuver with a division of the left crus of the diaphragm and dividing the celiac plexus (A). The Mattox maneuver consists of a left medial rotation of the descending colon (again at the line of Toldt), spleen, and/or kidney toward the midline. Exposure of injuries to the distal IVC and iliac vein bifurcations can be exceedingly difficult. On occasion, division of the right common iliac artery is needed to expose and repair an injury of this area. A primary repair of the iliac artery can then be performed. On rare occasions, with massive bleeding, the junction of the superior mesenteric vein (not artery), splenic, and portal veins may need to be exposed by division of the neck of the pancreas (B).

References: Asensio JA, Chahwan S, Hanpeter D, et al. Operative management and outcome of 302 abdominal vascular injuries. *Am J Surg.* 2000;180(6):528–533.

Hoyt DB, Coimbra R, Potenza BM, Rappold JF. Anatomic exposures for vascular injuries. *Surg Clin North Am.* 2001;81(6):1299–1330.

40. B. Most veins can be safely ligated in the setting of traumatic injury. However, certain veins are less likely to tolerate ligation well. These include the superior vena cava (because it may result in an acute superior vena cava syndrome), the renal veins close to the renal parenchyma (because there is then inadequate outflow for the kidney), the IVC above the renal veins (because it will impair outflow to both kidneys), or just at the diaphragm (because this will cause an acute Budd-Chiari syndrome), and the portal vein (because it supplies 75% of the blood to the liver) (A, E). An exception to the aforementioned is ligation of the left renal vein close to the IVC is well tolerated because drainage can occur via the adrenal, gonadal, and iliolumbar veins. This is sometimes performed during open abdominal aortic aneurysm repair. The portal vein has been ligated successfully, provided adequate fluid is administered to compensate for the dramatic but transient edema that occurs in the bowel, but ligation seems to be associated with a higher mortality rate than repair.

Ligation of the IVC below the renal veins is better tolerated than the suprarenal IVC; however, marked leg swelling may develop and may require fasciotomies. Ligation of the superior mesenteric vein is also fairly well tolerated and better tolerated than portal vein ligation, although again it is preferable to repair the superior mesenteric vein if the patient is stable and it is technically feasible because there is similarly marked bowel edema and risk of bowel infarction as with portal vein repair. Arteries for which repair should always be attempted include the innominate, brachial, superior mesenteric, proper hepatic, iliac, femoral, and popliteal arteries and the aorta (C, D). If definitive repair is precluded due to hemodynamic instability or if a damage control approach is deemed appropriate, perfusion or flow may be maintained via a temporary intravascular shunt. In the forearm, either the radial or ulnar artery can be ligated, provided the other vessel is palpable. Similarly, in the lower leg, at least one of the two palpable vessels (anterior or posterior tibial artery) should be salvaged. Because of the excellent collateralization around the shoulder, ligation of the subclavian artery is well tolerated. In fact, the artery is often occluded during stent-grafting of thoracic aneurysms or aortic transection.

Reference: Rich NM, Mattox KL, Hirshberg A. *Vascular trauma.* 2nd ed. Elsevier Science; 2004.

41. A. Extremity compartment syndrome can occur anywhere in the extremities, including the buttocks, shoulders, and hands (E). The mechanisms of compartment syndrome are numerous and can be divided into extrinsic and intrinsic causes. Extrinsic causes include constriction by a cast, tight circumferential dressings, or eschar from a burn. Intrinsic causes are divided into bleeding, edema, and exogenous fluid. Bleeding is usually due to trauma but can also be seen after relatively minor injuries in patients with an underlying coagulopathy or those receiving anticoagulants. Edema of the compartment is the largest and broadest category. It is most often seen after reperfusion of an ischemic limb, from either an arterial embolus or thrombosis or trauma. Ischemia/reperfusion is also seen in a person with a drug overdose or an alcoholic who falls asleep on the limb, in patients with profound shock in whom diffuse muscle ischemia with subsequent reperfusion develops, and after massive iliofemoral deep venous thrombosis. Finally, inadvertent infusion of IV fluid into the subcutaneous tissue can lead to compartment syndrome. Diagnosis of compartment syndrome begins by having a high clinical index of suspicion and knowing the clinical scenarios in which it occurs. The most common features are severe pain in the limb typically out of proportion to the physical exam, pain on passive motion of the limb, and tense edema with tenderness on palpation of the compartment. Distal arterial pulses typically remain palpable with compartment syndrome. The anterior compartment of the leg is usually the first compartment to be involved in the lower extremity (C). The deep peroneal nerve runs within it so numbness in the first web space of the toe is one of the early findings (D). Once the diagnosis is suspected, confirmation is sought by doing direct pressure measurements of the individual compartments. If the pressures are increased more than 30 mmHg in any of the compartments, then strong consideration should be given to performing a four-compartment fasciotomy. The use of an absolute value has been questioned because the perfusion pressure necessary for oxygenation is partly dependent on the patients' blood pressure and, therefore, could lead to unnecessary fasciotomies (B). The use of differential pressure (Δp = diastolic blood pressure—intracompartmental pressure), with a proposed threshold of 30 mmHg, has been proposed to be of greater diagnostic value. It is also important to remember that there is no absolute pressure level that rules compartment syndrome in or out. The measurements should be used in conjunction with the patient's clinical examination. The deep posterior compartment is the one that is most commonly inadequately decompressed. Because this compartment contains the tibial nerve, missing this compartment can have devastating consequences. The soleus muscle must be detached from the tibia to decompress the deep posterior compartment. Buttock compartment syndrome has been described in patients with obesity after prolonged anesthesia as well.

Reference: von Keudell AG, Weaver MJ, Appleton PT, et al. Diagnosis and treatment of acute extremity compartment syndrome. *Lancet.* 2015;386(10000):1299–1310.

42. C. The management of liver injuries has undergone a major evolution in the past 25 years, from routine laparotomy in the past to the current application of selective nonoperative management in hemodynamically stable patients, liberal use of angiographic embolization, and operative management with selective packing and damage control when the patient is cold and coagulopathic. In a patient who has sustained blunt trauma and is hemodynamically stable, a CT scan with IV contrast should be performed. If a contrast blush is seen in the liver, the patient should be taken to angiography for embolization, provided there are no other injuries that require operative intervention. Conversely, if the patient is hemodynamically unstable (as in this patient), the patient should be taken to the operating room and undergo packing of all four quadrants to obtain temporary hemostasis while anesthesia attempts to "catch up" or adequately resuscitate the patient. Strong consideration should be given to activating the institutional massive transfusion protocol in addition to administering tranexamic acid. Given that this patient had continued bleeding despite application of a Pringle maneuver, he has likely sustained an injury to the retrohepatic IVC or hepatic veins. If the bleeding is controlled with packing and, in addition, the patient is cold (temperature <34 °C), coagulopathic, and with a refractory acidosis (as in this patient), the best option would be to perform a damage control operation and transfer the patient to the ICU for resuscitation (A, B, D, E). If, conversely, the bleeding is not controlled, the next step would be to rapidly take down the hepatic ligaments including the ligamentum teres, falciform ligament, triangular ligament, and the right coronary ligament, and perform a Kocher maneuver. This allows better direct compression with packing in the retrohepatic space. A decision must then be made as to whether to attempt repair of a retrohepatic IVC injury. This decision depends on the experience of the surgeon, the clinical status of the patient, and whether bleeding is controlled. If bleeding has now stopped with packing, one option is to take the patient back to the ICU to resuscitate and rewarm. If bleeding persists, total vascular exclusion of the liver is now possible because control of the IVC just below the diaphragm and just inferior to the liver can be performed, combined with the Pringle maneuver. Alternatively, an atriocaval (Schrock) shunt could be placed or venovenous bypass initiated.

References: Asensio JA, Demetriades D, Chahwan S, et al. Approach to the management of complex hepatic injuries. *J Trauma.* 2000;48(1):66–69.

Kozar RA, Feliciano DV, Moore EE, et al. Western Trauma Association/critical decisions in trauma: operative management of adult blunt hepatic trauma. *J Trauma.* 2011;71(1):1–5.

43. C. The majority of bladder injuries occur following a blunt mechanism of injury, and over 80% of patients with a bladder rupture will have a concomitant pelvic fracture. Bladder injuries are classified as extraperitoneal, intraperitoneal, or combined, with extraperitoneal injuries being the most common (as many as 70%). Extraperitoneal bladder injuries often result from perforation due to adjacent pelvic bony fragments or spicules, whereas intraperitoneal injuries typically occur due to a sudden increase in pressure when a full bladder sustains a direct blow (i.e., MVC following binge-drinking). These injuries usually result in large tears involving the dome of the bladder. Hematuria in the presence of a pelvic fracture should increase the suspicion for a bladder injury. If blood is visible at the urethral meatus, then a Foley catheter should not be inserted until a retrograde urethrogram is performed to rule out a urethral injury (A). Otherwise, in the presence of hematuria, the diagnosis of a bladder injury can usually be made by stress cystography. This may be performed using a standard radiographic or CT technique. Advantages of CT cystography include the ability to assess other abdominal and pelvic injuries. Typically, 300 to 400 cc of iodinated contrast is instilled into the bladder via the Foley catheter, which is then clamped. When extravasation is seen, it is important to determine whether it is intraperitoneal, extraperitoneal, or both. Contrast above the peritoneal reflection is intraperitoneal (the paracolic gutter would be intraperitoneal). The management of an extraperitoneal rupture of the bladder is nonsurgical in most instances and consists of placing an 18- to 20-French or larger Foley catheter for 7 to 10 days followed by a repeat cystogram to ensure no further extravasation of contrast before catheter removal. Intraperitoneal injuries are managed operatively via a transabdominal approach. Before closure of the injury, palpation and visualization of the interior of the bladder should be performed to ensure absence of other injuries. Repair is undertaken using absorbable sutures. Silk suture is inappropriate because permanent sutures in the bladder will increase the risk of ongoing bladder mucosal irritation and are lithogenic (E). A suprapubic cystostomy is generally not required in the absence of very large wounds or the presence of significant devitalized tissue (B). If CT cystography is equivocal, a formal cystogram should be obtained; it is otherwise unnecessary (D).

Reference: Myers JB, Taylor MB, Brant WO, et al. Process improvement in trauma: traumatic bladder injuries and compliance with recommended imaging evaluation. *J Trauma Acute Care Surg.* 2013;74(1):264–269.

44. A. Ureteral injuries are relatively uncommon and most often occur following penetrating trauma. Surgical management is dictated by the patient's hemodynamics, as well as level of injury (upper, middle, or lower third), degree of ureteral loss, and status of surrounding tissues. Ureteral repairs following trauma are usually repaired over a stent. For upper and middle third urethral injuries that have a small ureteral segment missing (<2 cm), a primary repair can often be done. Reimplantation to the bladder (ureteroneocystostomy) is preferred for small segment injuries of the lower third as it is technically easier to perform compared with primary repair (E). For larger ureteral injuries involving the upper or middle ureter, the ideal repair entails debriding devitalized tissue, spatulating the two ends, and performing an end-to-end anastomosis over a double J stent (ureteroureterostomy) using an absorbable monofilament (B). Some mobilization of the ureter is feasible, but mobilization risks interrupting the blood supply that runs just adjacent to the ureter. As such, the dissection should be maintained approximately 1 cm away from the ureter so as not to disrupt its blood supply. A good guide to the viability of the two ends of the ureter is whether the cut edges are bleeding. Lower ureteral injuries may require reimplantation of the ureter into the bladder if there is not enough distal ureter for a primary anastomosis. When a large segment of ureter has been injured and primary reanastomosis is not possible, several options are available. A psoas hitch involves mobilization of the bladder, which is then sutured to the iliopsoas fascia above the iliac vessels, to perform tension-free reimplantation of the ureter (D). If a tension-free repair cannot be achieved following mobilization of the bladder, a Boari or bladder flap may be considered. More complex techniques include anastomosing the ureter to the contralateral ureter (transureteroureterostomy), ileal-ureteral replacement, and renal autotransplantation (C). In this patient, however, with massive blood loss and hemodynamic instability, a damage control approach should be used. There are two options. The first is to simply ligate the ureter proximally and distally followed by placement of a percutaneous nephrostomy once the patient is stabilized. The patient can later be taken back for a more elective repair of the ureter. The other option is to perform a temporary cutaneous ureterostomy over a single J stent, placing a tie around the ureter and stent and then bringing the stent up to the level of the skin. Given the location of the injury and the length of injured ureter, the patient would eventually likely need a psoas hitch or other more complex repairs.

Reference: Smith TG 3rd, Coburn M. Damage control maneuvers for urologic trauma. *Urol Clin North Am.* 2013;40(3):343–350.

45. E. The current trend in the management of severe duodenal injuries is "less is better." Management of duodenal injuries depends on location, extent of injury, associated pancreatic injury, and clinical status of the patient. Duodenal injuries are graded from I to V, with grade I being a hematoma or partial-thickness injury and grade V being a massive disruption of the pancreaticoduodenal complex or complete duodenal devascularization. If a simple duodenal hematoma is recognized preoperatively, it can be managed without surgery, with nasogastric decompression and parenteral nutrition. If it is found intraoperatively, it is left alone if small (<2 cm). If it is a large hematoma (involving >50% of the lumen), it is recommended to incise the serosa, drain the hematoma, and then reclose the serosa. The majority of full-thickness lacerations of the duodenum can be repaired primarily in a transverse fashion to avoid narrowing the lumen, with or without placement of an overlying omental patch (C). Conversely, if the injury involves more than 50% of

the luminal circumference, then resection is often required. If such an injury is in the first, third, or fourth portion of the duodenum, then resection with duodenoduodenostomy (as in this patient) or duodenojejunostomy may need to be performed. Segmental resection of the second part is challenging because of the presence of the ampulla of Vater and the common blood supply with the pancreas, which make the mobilization difficult. In this situation or if a tension-free anastomosis is not possible, a Roux-en-Y duodenojejunostomy may be indicated. Alternatively, a direct Roux-en-Y loop anastomosed over the duodenal defect may be considered. Pyloric exclusion should be considered in rare cases with tenuous repairs (A). Duodenal diverticulization is not commonly performed (B). A Whipple resection can be considered for a subsequent surgery in patients with grade V or complexed combined pancreatic and duodenal injuries (D).

46. D. Various techniques may be employed to control bleeding from the liver. The simplest method of controlling bleeding from the liver is the application of manual compression with or without the use of topical hemostatic agents such as microfibrillar collagen, oxidized cellulose, and gelatin matrix thrombin sealants. If these are unsuccessful, a Pringle maneuver should be performed. Ongoing bleeding following occlusion of the porta hepatis suggests the potential for a hepatic vein or retrohepatic IVC injury. In addition to packing, several other hemostatic maneuvers can be used in patients with severe parenchymal injury. Liver sutures can be placed, using a chromic suture with a blunt-tipped needle. This is best used for relatively superficial lacerations. Another option is to perform a hepatotomy via a finger fracture technique to access the bleeding site to directly suture it. However, profuse bleeding from a small hole in the liver presents a more difficult dilemma because bleeding may be emanating from the center of the liver, and a hepatotomy may not be feasible. In this circumstance, one novel approach that has been well described is to fashion a balloon tamponade catheter. A catheter with side holes is placed through a Penrose drain, and a tie is placed on either end of the Penrose drain (E). The catheter is advanced into the bullet wound, and air with or without contrast is insufflated into the catheter, effectively inflating the Penrose drain and creating a tamponade effect. In this case, however, because the bleeding has stopped, there is no role for any additional treatment (A–C). Placing liver stitches is unnecessary and does increase the risk of causing liver necrosis. Packing the injury with omentum is useful in large stellate lesions, but hemostasis is better achieved in that setting with packing. The use of drains is controversial. For smaller wounds, drains are not recommended. For larger injuries, closed suction drainage is used by some surgeons. In general, open drains should not be employed because of a potentially increased risk of infection.

Reference: Kozar RA, Feliciano DV, Moore EE, et al. Western Trauma Association/critical decisions in trauma: operative management of adult blunt hepatic trauma. *J Trauma.* 2011;71(1):1–5.

47. C. Increasingly, colon injuries are being treated with either primary repair, if feasible, or resection with a primary anastomosis (A, B, D, E). This approach applies to both right- and left-sided colon injuries. Primary repair is used when less than 50% of the circumference of the bowel is involved, whereas resection is recommended for larger wounds. Once a resection is performed, a decision must be made as to whether to perform a primary reanastomosis or a colostomy. The primary contraindication to attempting a primary reanastomosis is hemodynamic instability. In these situations, damage control surgery should be performed and the decision to reanastamose or create a colostomy can be made at a subsequent operation when the patient has stabilized and been fully resuscitated. Factors associated with intraabdominal complications in patients with severe colon injuries undergoing resection include severe fecal contamination, transfusion of 4 or more units of blood in the first 24 hours, and administration of single-agent antibiotics. The use of vasopressors at the time of repair may also be associated with anastomotic leaks, whereas the method of performing the anastomosis (handsewn versus stapled) has not been shown to effect leak rates. Another important consideration is obesity. Morbid obesity makes the creation of a stoma difficult, predisposes the stoma to the development of ischemia, and, if this occurs, increases the risk of the development of a necrotizing soft-tissue infection. It also makes the subsequent colostomy takedown more challenging. As such, strong consideration should be given in patients with obesity to a primary reanastomosis.

References: Demetriades D, Murray JA, Chan LS, et al. Handsewn versus stapled anastomosis in penetrating colon injuries requiring resection: a multicenter study. *J Trauma.* 2002;52(1):117–121.

Naumann DN, Bhangu A, Kelly M, Bowley DM. Stapled versus handsewn intestinal anastomosis in emergency laparotomy: a systemic review and meta-analysis. *Surgery.* 2015;157(4):609–618.

48. C. An occult pneumothorax is defined as one that is not detected on a chest x-ray but is found on CT scan. It is reasonable to closely observe patients with occult pneumothoraces if they are not showing signs of respiratory distress or hemodynamic instability. These patients should be managed with serial chest x-rays (D). Without oxygen supplementation, a pneumothorax will resolve at a rate of 1% per day. Some studies suggest that oxygen therapy may accelerate resolution, but whether this helps with an occult pneumothorax is debatable. Although there is concern about an occult

pneumothorax worsening in patients undergoing positive pressure ventilation (urgent or elective surgery with general anesthesia) most studies indicate that patients can safely be observed without a chest tube (A, B). In recent years, there has been a shift toward the use of small-bore chest tubes as several reports have suggested no difference in outcomes between large and smaller bore chest tubes (A, D). Needle decompression is still considered the first-line intervention for patients with a tension pneumothorax (E).

Reference: Mowery NT, Gunter OL, Collier BR, et al. Practice management guidelines for management of hemothorax and occult pneumothorax. *J Trauma.* 2011;70(2):510–518.

49. A. This patient has multiple conditions that could lead to the development of ascites. His heavy alcohol use could lead to cirrhosis and hepatic ascites or spontaneous bacterial peritonitis. His recent bladder repair and splenectomy raise suspicion for a urinoma or pancreatic injury. In this case, correctly interpreting the labs is necessary to determine the etiology of the ascites. The serum ascites albumin gradient (SAAG) is calculated with the equation: SAAG = serum albumin—ascites albumin. A SAAG <1.1 occurs with conditions where the oncotic pressure of the ascites is elevated, which draws fluid into the peritoneal space. A SAAG>1.1 is usually associated with high hydrostatic pressure pushing fluid into the peritoneal space, but can also be associated with urine leak (urine should not contain albumin). In this case, the SAAG is >1.1 (3.0–1.5 = 1.5). A pancreatic leak would have a SAAG <1.1 and an amylase 3× the serum amylase (D). Primary bacterial peritonitis is associated with a SAAG >1.1, however, fluid neutrophil count is ≥250 in bacterial peritonitis (E). Urine leak would have a SAAG >1.1, but fluid creatinine would be much higher than serum creatinine (B). Patients with abdominal compartment syndrome have abdominal distention, oliguria, decreased lung compliance, and hypotension. This patient with normal vital signs does not have abdominal compartment syndrome (C).

Reference: Runyon BA, Montano AA, Akriviadis EA, et al. The serum-ascites albumin gradient is superior to the exudate-transudate concept in the differential diagnosis of ascites. *Ann Intern Med.* 1992;117(3):215–220.

Vascular—Arterial 17

AMANDA C. PURDY AND NINA M. BOWENS

ABSITE 99th Percentile High-Yields

I. Peripheral Arterial Disease (PAD)
   A. Normal ankle-brachial index (ABI) ranges from 1 to 1.2; ABI <0.9 suggests PAD; ABI ≤0.4 consistent with rest pain; diabetes and renal disease cause calcification of tibial vessels falsely elevating ABI
   B. Initial management of claudication is medical: walking program (most effective), smoking cessation, aspirin, statin
   C. Indications for surgical intervention: rest pain, tissue loss (non healing ulcer or gangrene), life-limiting claudication refractory to medical management (relative)
   D. Surgical options include open bypass and endovascular angioplasty +/− stent
   E. Considerations for lower extremity bypass:
      1. Need an adequate inflow artery, conduit, and distal target
      2. Best choice for conduit is ipsilateral autologous vein (greater saphenous) ≥3 mm diameter and no history of thrombosis
      3. Prosthetic grafts have acceptable patency rates only if distal target is above the knee
   F. Bypass graft failure:
      1. Early (<30 days), due to a technical error
      2. Intermediate (30 days to 2 years), due to intimal hyperplasia
      3. Late (>2 years), due to native disease (atherosclerosis)
   G. Monitor grafts with duplex scans (every 3 months initially, then annually) to detect stenoses

II. Acute Limb Ischemia (due to embolism, thrombosis, dissection, or trauma)
   A. Nerve dies first (within 4 hours), then muscle (within 6 hours)
   B. Presents with the 6 Ps: pain, pulselessness, pallor, poikilothermia, paresthesia, paralysis (paralysis occurs late and is indicative of poor prognosis)
   C. Initial management: IV fluids, IV heparin, place limb in dependent position
   D. Rutherford classification helps guide management; class 1 can sometimes be managed with heparin alone; class 2 a can attempt lytic therapy first; class 2b requires emergent surgical intervention; class 3 will not benefit from revascularization (needs amputation)
   E. Also perform fasciotomy if suspect limb ischemia for ≥6 hours
   F. Rutherford Classification of Acute Limb Ischemia

Category	Prognosis	Findings		Doppler	
		Sensory loss	**Muscle weakness**	**Arterial**	**Venous**
1 *Viable*	Not immediately threatened	None	None	Audible	Audible
2 a *Marginally Threatened*	Salvageable if promptly treated	None-Minimal (only in toes)	None	Inaudible	Audible
2b *Immediately Threatened*	Salvageable with immediate revascularization	Yes (more in toes)	Mild, Moderate	Inaudible	Audible
3 *Irreversible*	Major tissue loss or permanent nerve damage inevitable	Profound, complete anesthesia	Profound, complete paralysis	Inaudible	Inaudible

III. Carotid Stenosis (causes strokes or transient ischemic attacks from embolization of plaque)
   A. Symptomatic 70% to 99% carotid stenosis benefits the most from surgical intervention
   B. Carotid endarterectomy (CEA) is the preferred surgical option, but carotid artery stenting (CES) preferred in symptomatic patient with:
      1. Severe cardiac or lung disease
      2. Hostile neck: previous lateral neck dissection or radiation, contralateral vocal cord paralysis
      3. Extremely proximal or distal plaque (difficult to access with open surgery)
   C. If bilateral carotid arteries require surgical intervention, operate on symptomatic side first
   D. Nerve injuries after CEA: hypoglossal (can be under facial vein and tethered by artery to sternocleidomastoid, most common) (→tongue deviates towards the side of surgery), vagus [recurrent laryngeal nerve) (→hoarseness), marginal mandibular branch of the facial nerve (→ipsilateral mouth droop, traction injury), glossopharyngeal (→difficulty swallowing, rare, mostly with high dissections)
   E. Management of Carotid Stenosis

Symptoms	Degree of stenosis	Management
Symptomatic	70%–99%	CEA
	50%–69%	CEA (greater benefit in men)
	<50%	Medical management
Asymptomatic	80%–99%	CEA
	60%–79%	Controversial, consider CEA (greater benefit in men)
	<60%	Medical management

IV. Abdominal Aortic Aneurysm (AAA)
   A. Smoking has the greatest impact on development and growth of AAA; degeneration of the walls in AAA is due to increased matrix metalloproteinases and decreased elastic & smooth muscle fibers; more common in white than black men
   B. Aneurysm: a focal dilation of all arterial wall layers to >1.5× the diameter of the normal artery
   C. Men aged 65 to 75 who have ever smoked should have one-time ultrasound screening for AAA
   D. Indications to repair AAA: symptomatic, diameter of >5 cm in females, diameter of >5.5 cm in males, growth of >0.5 cm in 6 months or >1 cm in 1 year

E. Surgical options include open AAA repair and endovascular repair (EVAR)

F. Compared to open AAA repair, EVAR has a lower perioperative (30-day) mortality rate but similar long-term mortality

G. Complications of AAA repair:

1. MI is the most common cause of in-hospital death after AAA repair

2. Kidney injury: increased incidence if intraoperative hypotension or suprarenal aortic cross-clamp

3. Ischemic colitis: risk factors (coverage of the IMA or internal iliac, ruptured AAA, intraoperative hypotension; can present with abdominal pain and diarrhea (sometimes bloody); diagnose with flexible sigmoidoscopy; treat with antibiotics, NPO, and resuscitation, if patient deteriorates or develops peritonitis will require surgery

4. Aortoenteric fistula (after open or endovascular repair): upper GI bleed usually >6 months after surgery; due to infected graft that erodes into the duodenum; upper endoscopy (first step in workup) usually negative, CT shows fluid/air around aortic graft/sac; management is graft excision, close the duodenum, and revascularization either with in situ human aortic homograft, neoaortoiliac procedure (NAIS) or extra anatomic axillobifemoral bypass

V. Mesenteric Ischemia

A. Acute mesenteric ischemia (AMI) etiologies: embolism (to SMA, most common), thrombosis, low flow state (non occlusive), venous thrombosis

B. AMI presentation: writhing around complaining of severe abdominal pain, but not significantly tender on exam (pain out of proportion to physical exam); dx with CTA and have preop discussion regarding bowel viability, quality of life, and possible bowel resection

C. Surgery for AMI due to embolism: resect frankly necrotic bowel, open SMA embolectomy

1. Transverse arteriotomy proximal to the middle colic artery, then embolectomy

2. If any bowel with questionable viability: do not resect, leave abdomen open, plan for 2nd look within 24 to 48 hours

D. Chronic mesenteric ischemia (CMI) from atherosclerosis of the celiac, superior mesenteric, and/or inferior mesenteric arteries.

E. CMI presentation: severe abdominal pain about 30 to 60 minutes after eating, often leading to "food fear" (intestinal angina) and weight loss

F. First-line treatment for CMI is angioplasty and stenting; if bypass is required in high-risk or sick patient, perform retrograde mesenteric bypass from common iliac artery or infrarenal aorta to avoid supraceliac clamping

G. Aggressive fluid resuscitation should be used with caution in non occlusive mesenteric ischemia in the setting of decompensated congestive heart failure, use direct intraarterial papaverine instead

H. Venous thrombosis usually treated with anticoagulation (unless peritonitis); need hypercoagulable workup

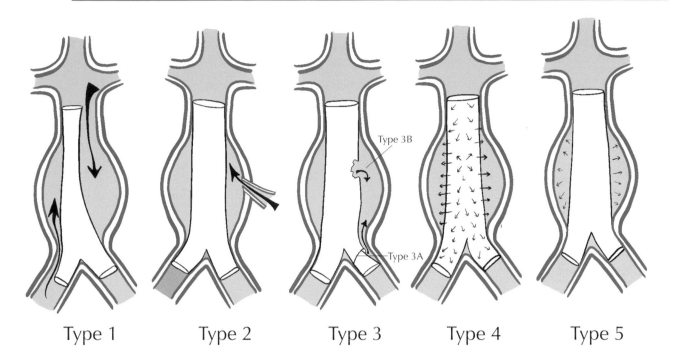

Type 1   Type 2   Type 3   Type 4   Type 5

Endoleaks occur when blood flows back into the aneurysm sac after endovascular aneurysm repair. A **Type 1** endoleak occurs if the proximal or distal end of the stent is not apposed to the vessel wall. Type 1 endoleaks should be repaired prior to leaving the OR if identified intraoperatively. **Type 2** endoleaks (the most common type of endoleak) occur when a vertebral artery or the IMA supplies retrograde blood flow to the aneurysm sac, causing it to expand. **Type 3a** endoleaks occur if there is disruption between components of the graft, and **Type 3b** endoleaks occur if there is a tear or hole in the graft. **Type 4** endoleaks result from the porous nature of specific graft materials that allow blood to extravasate into the sac. Type 5 leaks are poorly understood but thought to be due to enndotension. **Type 5** endoleaks occur when the aneurysm continues to expand without a clear source.

Fig. 17.1 Types of Endoleaks

QUESTIONS

1. A 25-year-old woman presents to the trauma bay after a motor vehicle accident. A pan-CT scan is negative for any acute injuries but does show an incidental focal dilation of the mid-splenic artery to a diameter of 2.5 cm. The best management of this finding is:
   A. No further management is necessary
   B. Elective splenectomy
   C. Elective coil embolization
   D. Open repair with vein interposition graft
   E. Surveillance with repeat imaging in 6 months

2. A 40-year-old woman with refractory hypertension undergoes further workup. Her plasma and urine metanephrines are normal, aldosterone to renin ratio is <20, cortisol is normal, and creatinine is 1.2. CT of the abdomen shows no adrenal lesions, and renal arteries have a "string-of-beads" appearance. How should this be managed?
   A. Aspirin and statin
   B. Corticosteroids
   C. Percutaneous angioplasty
   D. Percutaneous angioplasty and stent
   E. Open bypass

3. Occlusion of a reverse saphenous vein femoral-to-popliteal artery bypass 3 weeks after surgery is most often due to:
   A. Myointimal hyperplasia
   B. Progressive atherosclerosis
   C. Hypercoagulable state
   D. Technical error
   E. Persistent valve

4. A 65-year-old man presents with a 4-hour history of sudden onset of left leg pain. He has no pulses in his left femoral artery or distally. The calf is tender to palpation. The foot is cool and pale with diminished capillary refill. He has diminished extension of his left great toe as well as a sensory loss of his toes. On the unaffected side, the femoral, popliteal, and distal pulses are normal. ECG shows an irregularly irregular rhythm. After administration of heparin, the next step in management would be:
   A. Diagnostic arteriography
   B. Thrombolytic therapy
   C. Transfemoral embolectomy
   D. Echocardiogram
   E. Below-knee popliteal embolectomy

5. A 60-year-old woman presents with sudden onset of acute abdominal pain. On examination, the patient is writhing because of severe pain, yet the abdomen is only mildly tender, without guarding or rebound. The cardiac examination reveals an irregularly irregular rhythm. She denies a history of abdominal pain. The serum lactate level is elevated. Serum amylase is slightly elevated. Plain abdominal radiographs are negative. A computed tomography (CT) scan of the abdomen reveals diffuse edema of the small bowel wall. The next step in the management would be:
   A. Thrombolytic therapy
   B. Arteriography
   C. Intravenous heparin
   D. Exploratory laparotomy
   E. Duplex ultrasound scan

6. A 45-year-old man presents with a 2-week history of vague, diffuse abdominal pain and distention. He reports that his mother and grandmother both had leg blood clots. On examination, he has mild diffuse tenderness without guarding or rebound. A CT scan reveals thickened loops of small bowel and failure of opacification of the superior mesenteric vein. The best management approach would consist of:
   A. Catheter-directed thrombolytic therapy
   B. Intravenous (IV) heparin followed by 3 months of rivaroxaban
   C. IV heparin followed by lifelong apixaban
   D. Arteriography with papaverine infusion
   E. Immediate operative exploration

7. Claudication symptoms are most improved with the use of:
   A. Pentoxifylline
   B. Aspirin
   C. Cilostazol
   D. Clopidogrel
   E. Coumadin (warfarin)

8. Four days after a left femoral-to-popliteal arterial bypass with ipsilateral reverse saphenous vein, the patient reports swelling in the left leg. This most likely indicates:
   A. Deep venous thrombosis
   B. Reperfusion edema
   C. Decreased venous return from saphenous vein harvest
   D. Cellulitis
   E. Lymphatic disruption

9. A 65-year-old man with a history of a coronary artery bypass graft 2 years earlier presents with recurrent chest pain. He describes the pain as substernal and radiating to his jaw. He works as a carpenter and also states that his left arm tires out easily with use. Blood pressure in the right arm is 150/90 mmHg and 100/60 mmHg in the left arm. Relief of his chest pain is likely best achieved with:
   A. Redo coronary artery bypass graft
   B. Coronary stenting
   C. Increasing the dose of nitrates
   D. Subclavian artery stenting
   E. Increasing beta-blocker dose

10. Which of the following is most appropriate in the surgical management of bowel ischemia due to an embolus to the superior mesenteric artery (SMA)?
   A. Intraoperative angiography
   B. Planned second-look laparotomy
   C. Dopamine
   D. Longitudinal arteriotomy of SMA
   E. Resection of bowel with questionable viability

11. At surgery for suspected acute mesenteric ischemia, almost the entire small bowel as well as the right colon appears ischemic. However, the proximal jejunum, duodenum, and left colon appear healthy. The most likely etiology of these findings is:
   A. Thrombosis of the SMA
   B. Embolus to the SMA
   C. Superior mesenteric vein thrombosis
   D. Portal vein thrombosis
   E. Nonocclusive mesenteric ischemia

12. Which of the following is true regarding the timing and/or indications for carotid endarterectomy (CEA) in a patient with a stroke?
   A. CEA is indicated even if a patient has complete hemiplegia
   B. CEA is best performed within 6 to 8 weeks of the stroke
   C. CEA is best performed 3 months after the stroke
   D. CEA should be performed urgently
   E. CEA is best performed within 2 weeks of the stroke

13. According to the Asymptomatic Carotid Atherosclerosis Study (ACAS), which of the following is true regarding CEA for asymptomatic internal carotid artery (ICA) stenosis?
   A. CEA reduces the 5-year risk of stroke and death from 20% to 10% in patients with high-grade stenosis
   B. It is beneficial, provided the perioperative stroke and death rates are 9% or less
   C. The ACAS trial used both aspirin and a lipid-lowering agent in the medical arm of the trial
   D. It is indicated for patients with ICA stenosis ranging from 50% to 100%
   E. There is less benefit in women

14. Which of the following would provide the greatest benefit from CEA?

Symptom	Percentage ICA stenosis
A. Asymptomatic	Right 90%
B. Right eye amaurosis fugax	Left 60%
C. Right arm/leg transient ischemia attack	Right 80%
D. Left eye amaurosis fugax	Left 80%
E. Right arm/leg paresis	Left 45%

15. Thirty minutes after arriving in the recovery room after a right CEA, the patient develops left hemiparesis. The most appropriate next step would be:
   A. Immediate operative reexploration of the carotid artery
   B. Tissue plasminogen activator (tPA) infusion
   C. Cerebral angiography
   D. Carotid duplex ultrasound scan
   E. Head computed tomography (CT)

16. Following a right CEA, a 65-year-old male develops a severe 10/10 right frontal headache followed by a seizure. There are no focal neurologic deficits. Which of the following is true regarding this condition?
   A. It typically presents within 24 hours of surgery
   B. It is usually self-limited
   C. Postoperative hypertension is a risk factor
   D. Vasodilators are useful in the treatment
   E. The patient will likely need a return to the operating room

17. A 25-year-old woman presents with several episodes of dizziness, syncope, upper extremity claudication, and an elevated erythrocyte sedimentation rate. On examination, she has no radial, brachial, or carotid pulses. Her blood pressure is 70/50 mmHg in her right arm and 60/40 mmHg in her left. Magnetic resonance angiography reveals occlusion of both subclavian arteries as well as high-grade stenosis of both common carotid arteries at their mid portion. Which of the following is true about this condition?
    A. Methotrexate is not helpful
    B. Transluminal angioplasty is the treatment of choice
    C. Surgery should be performed urgently
    D. The disease can involve the pulmonary and coronary arteries
    E. Antihypertensive agents are contraindicated

18. A 40-year-old woman presents to the emergency department after a motor vehicle accident with a mandible fracture. She is neurologically intact. She is otherwise hemodynamically stable, alert, and oriented. A CT scan of the head and neck is negative for an intracranial bleed but demonstrates an intimal injury of the right internal carotid artery. She is hemodynamically stable and will not require operative intervention for the mandible fracture. Which of the following is true about this injury?
    A. Aspirin is the treatment of choice
    B. Associated Horner syndrome is extremely rare
    C. The injured carotid artery should be stented
    D. Complete healing of the carotid artery is rare
    E. Urgent surgical intervention is indicated

19. A 60-year-old man presents with a right arm and leg hemiparesis that has persisted for 1 hour. He has a history of a left modified radical neck dissection and neck irradiation for cancer 10 years previously. CT angiography reveals a 75% stenosis of the left internal carotid artery just distal to the bifurcation. Which of the following is recommended as the definitive management?
    A. Aspirin
    B. Aspirin and clopidogrel
    C. Carotid endarterectomy
    D. Resection of the diseased carotid artery with an interposition graft
    E. Carotid stenting with a cerebral protection device

20. Four months after CEA, a duplex ultrasound scan reveals recurrent 70% ICA stenosis. The patient reports no symptoms. Optimal management would consist of:
    A. Repeat CEA
    B. Carotid stenting
    C. Observation
    D. Interposition saphenous vein bypass
    E. Interposition polytetrafluoroethylene bypass

21. A 35-year-old woman presents to the emergency department with right-sided headache, right eye ptosis, and sudden onset of left arm and leg weakness that lasts 1 hour and then resolves spontaneously. There is no history of trauma. Duplex ultrasound scan of the right carotid artery reveals a complete occlusion of the ICA. CT angiography confirms a tapering of the ICA with occlusion approximately 2 to 3 cm distal to the bifurcation. Management consists of:
    A. CEA
    B. Lytic therapy with tissue plasminogen activator
    C. Carotid stenting
    D. Anticoagulation
    E. Fogarty embolectomy

22. Thromboangiitis obliterans (Buerger disease) is characterized by:
    A. Frequent coronary artery involvement
    B. Frequent involvement of aortoiliac arterial segments
    C. Disease limited to pedal arteries
    D. Successful treatment with saphenous vein bypass
    E. Corkscrew collaterals

23. Which of the following is true regarding noninvasive hemodynamic assessment?
    A. In normal resting subjects in the supine position, the ankle pressure can be lower than that of the arm
    B. There is poor correlation between ankle-brachial index (ABI) and severity of symptoms
    C. End-stage renal failure can cause a false elevation of the ABI
    D. In diabetic patients, toe pressures are usually falsely elevated
    E. In diabetic patients, transcutaneous oximetry is unreliable

24. Which of the following is true regarding the use of thrombolytic therapy for arterial limb ischemia?
    A. It can safely be used in patients within a week of cataract surgery
    B. Bleeding risk correlates with fibrinogen levels
    C. It is useful in patients with a profound motor deficit in the ischemic limb
    D. It is highly effective regardless of the length of duration of symptoms
    E. It can safely be used for as long as 72 hours

25. A relatively healthy 60-year-old diabetic male patient presents with gangrene of his right great toe. The patient has normal femoral and popliteal pulses but no distal pulses. His ABI is 0.5. An angiography reveals patent iliac, femoral, and popliteal arteries with a long-segment occlusion of the trifurcation vessels with reconstitution of the anterior tibial artery just above the ankle and runoff into the dorsalis pedis artery. Bilateral saphenous veins are 4 mm in diameter on ultrasound. Which of the following is the best option?
    A. Common femoral-to-anterior tibial bypass with ipsilateral saphenous vein
    B. Common femoral-to-anterior tibial bypass with contralateral saphenous vein
    C. Popliteal-to-anterior tibial bypass with ipsilateral greater saphenous vein
    D. Endovascular stenting of anterior tibial artery
    E. Great toe amputation only

26. A 32-year-old woman notes that her hands become cold and painful when exposed to cold temperatures. The hand changes in color from pale to cyanotic to red. Her medical history is negative, and vascular pulse examination is normal. Arterial noninvasive studies reveal a marked decrease in digital blood pressure with exposure to cold temperatures. Symptoms persist despite wearing gloves and avoidance of cold exposure. The next step in management is:
    A. Upper extremity sympathectomy
    B. Prostaglandins
    C. Fluoxetine
    D. Arteriography
    E. Diltiazem

27. Which of the following is true regarding femoral pseudoaneurysms that occur after arteriography?
    A. Ultrasound compression is the procedure of choice
    B. Ultrasound compression is usually successful even if the patient is receiving anticoagulation therapy
    C. Surgical repair typically requires interposition vein grafting
    D. It can be managed with ultrasound-guided direct thrombin injection
    E. A trial of observation is contraindicated because of the high risk of bleeding

28. One day after open abdominal aortic aneurysm (AAA) repair, watery diarrhea and abdominal distention develop in the patient. On examination, the patient has mild lower left quadrant tenderness without guarding. WBC count is 14,000 cells/μL. Which of the following is appropriate for this patient?
    A. Proctosigmoidoscopy
    B. CT angiography
    C. Exploratory laparotomy
    D. Diagnostic laparoscopy
    E. Transfemoral arteriography

29. A 69-year-old man presents to the emergency department (ED) with sudden onset of left flank and back pain, abdominal tenderness, a blood pressure of 100/60 mmHg, heart rate of 100, and a tender pulsatile midline abdominal mass. He is awake and alert. Which of the following is recommended next?
    A. A 2-liter bolus of normal saline
    B. A CT scan of the abdomen and pelvis
    C. Bedside ultrasound
    D. Immediate transport to operating room
    E. Endotracheal intubation in the ED

30. Which of the following is true regarding popliteal artery aneurysms?
    A. Observation is recommended for an asymptomatic 3-cm popliteal aneurysm
    B. An asymptomatic aneurysm with intraluminal thrombus should be repaired only when it is larger than 2 cm in size
    C. Bypassing the aneurysm with saphenous vein with interval ligation is the standard operative approach
    D. An endovascular stent graft is not recommended for popliteal aneurysms
    E. A posterior approach to the aneurysm is not technically feasible

31. One year after open AAA repair, a patient presents to the emergency department vomiting blood. Vital signs are stable. CT scan shows some standing and a small pocket of air around the aortic graft. Which of the following is true regarding this condition?
    A. Inflammatory changes around the graft are common 1 year after surgery
    B. Arteriography is useful in establishing the diagnosis
    C. A tagged nuclear white blood cell scan is unlikely to aid in the diagnosis
    D. Upper endoscopy will have a high sensitivity for establishing the diagnosis
    E. In situ placement of an aortic homograft will likely be needed

32. The threshold for elective repair of an asymptomatic common iliac aneurysm is greater than:
    A. 2.0 cm
    B. 2.5 cm
    C. 3.5 cm
    D. 4.0 cm
    E. 4.5 cm

33. The most common symptom of a popliteal aneurysm is:
    A. Rupture
    B. Thrombosis
    C. Distal embolization
    D. Adjacent nerve compression
    E. Adjacent venous compression

34. Which of the following is true regarding AAA repair?
    A. The appropriate AAA diameter threshold for elective repair for men and women is the same
    B. In low operative risk patients, the AAA diameter threshold for endovascular aneurysm repair (EVAR) is lower than that for open repair
    C. Women have higher perioperative mortality rates for both EVAR and open AAA repair as compared with men
    D. Careful surveillance of AAA up to 6.0 cm is safe
    E. In a high–cardiac risk patient with a 5.0-cm AAA, the EVAR approach should be used rather than delaying surgery

35. The most common endoleak after an EVAR is type:
    A. I
    B. II
    C. III
    D. IV
    E. V

36. A 61-year-old male with end-stage renal disease (ESRD) presents with a cold, painful right leg of 2-hour duration. He has an irregular heart rate on exam. CT angiography confirms an occlusion of the common femoral artery. He is appropriately treated with a heparin drip and surgical embolectomy with symptom resolution. Symptoms recur 4 days later, and the pulses disappear. He is taken back for a repeat embolectomy, at which time a whitish-appearing clot is removed. Which of the following is true regarding this condition?
    A. He should receive bivalirudin
    B. tPA would have been a good alternative to reexploration
    C. He likely has antithrombin-III deficiency
    D. He should receive lepirudin
    E. He should receive argatroban

ANSWERS

1. C. This patient was incidentally found to have a splenic artery aneurysm, the most common visceral artery aneurysm. The major concern is rupture. Patients with ruptured splenic artery aneurysms classically present with the "double rupture phenomenon," where they experience acute abdominal pain at first without hypotension while blood pools in the lesser sac. Then, once the lesser sac ruptures through the foramen of Winslow freely into the peritoneal cavity, the patient develops distention and hemorrhagic shock. The most common management of splenic artery aneurysms is coil embolization. The indications for intervention include rupture, symptoms, diameter >3 cm in patients with low surgical risk, and any size in women of childbearing age. Coil embolization is appropriate for proximal and mid-portion aneurysms as the spleen continues to be perfused by the short-gastric arteries avoiding splenic infarction. For distal-third aneurysms, resection with splenectomy is usually performed (B). Open repair with vein interposition graft has largely fallen out of favor (D). Because this patient is a woman of childbearing age, it would be inappropriate to proceed with conservative management and surveillance (A, E). Patients found to have a splenic artery aneurysm without indication for repair should be followed with annual CT angiogram or ultrasound. Women are at highest risk for splenic artery aneurysm rupture during the 3rd trimester of pregnancy.

Reference: Chaer RA, Abularrage CJ, Coleman DM, et al. The Society for Vascular Surgery clinical practice guidelines on the management of visceral aneurysms. *J Vasc Surg.* 2020;72(1 S):3 S–39 S.

2. C. This patient has fibromuscular dysplasia (FMD). Renal artery stenosis is a cause of secondary hypertension and can be due to atherosclerosis or FMD. FMD is an idiopathic disease of the musculature of the arterial walls leading to stenosis of small and medium-sized arteries and is most common in women from 30 to 60 years old. The most commonly involved arteries are the renal, carotid, and vertebral arteries. The "string-of-beads" appearance is a classic imaging finding seen in FMD. FMD is noninflammatory and there is no role for steroids (B). Patients with renal artery stenosis due to atherosclerosis should receive aspirin and statin; most are managed medically. A renal stent may be considered in the case of refractory hypertension or flash pulmonary edema (A, D). On the other hand, patients with renal artery stenosis due to FMD are most appropriately treated with percutaneous angioplasty, as stents have a high rate of fracture when used for FMD renal disease. Open bypass is more invasive and has similar success as angioplasty (E).

Reference: Gornik HL, Persu A, Adlam D, et al. First international consensus on the diagnosis and management of fibromuscular dysplasia. *J Hypertens.* 2019;37(2):229–252.

3. D. Early failure (within 30 days) after surgery generally indicates a technical error. Technical errors include anastomotic stenosis, a kink or twist within the graft, poor choice of proximal or distal target, and inadequate-caliber saphenous vein. Intermediate failures, from 30 days to 2 years after

bypass, are generally caused by myointimal hyperplasia (A). Late graft failures (beyond 2 years) are caused by progression of atherosclerotic occlusive disease, either within the inflow or outflow vessels (B). A persistent valve would be a potential problem with an in situ vein bypass (not with a reverse vein), in which case valves are intentionally cut with a valvulotome (E). Young patients may have a more aggressive form of atherosclerotic disease (virulent disease), and some have postulated that this may be secondary to an underlying hypercoagulable state (C).

Reference: McCready RA, Vincent AE, Schwartz RW, Hyde GL, Mattingly SS, Griffen WO Jr. Atherosclerosis in the young: a virulent disease. *Surgery.* 1984;96(5):863–869.

4. C. In an acutely ischemic limb, in addition to the neurovascular exam of the ischemic limb, the most important aspects of the physical examination are the cardiac exam and the neurovascular examination of the nonischemic limb. If the nonischemic limb has normal pulses and no other evidence of chronic ischemia (e.g., hair loss, thin dry skin), then the ischemia is most likely embolic in nature. Finding an irregularly irregular rhythm would further confirm that the heart is the most likely source of the clot due to atrial fibrillation. With an absent femoral pulse, the embolus has likely lodged in the common femoral artery. Because the patient described has class 2b ischemia (immediately threatened), heparin should be started, and revascularization should be performed without delay (E). In class 1 ischemia (not threatened; no sensory or motor loss), there is no immediate urgency to going to the operating room. Heparin should be started. It is then useful to obtain imaging to confirm the diagnosis. This can be achieved via an arterial duplex scan or CT angiogram, which has replaced diagnostic arteriography as the gold standard (A). An advantage of CT over angiogram is that it may detect etiologies of acute ischemia that would otherwise be unsuspected, such as an aortic dissection or aneurysm, and one can image the chest and abdomen for possible pathology. Following diagnosis, if the patient is not immediately threatened, they may undergo definitive treatment via thrombolytic therapy or open embolectomy (B, C). Native arterial occlusions due to cardiac embolization tend to respond less favorably to thrombolytic therapy. Thus, open embolectomy is preferred by some. For the patient in the vignette, a transfemoral approach is optimal because it can be done with the patient under local anesthesia and allows selective embolectomy down the superficial femoral and profunda femoral arteries. The below-knee popliteal artery approach to embolectomy is reserved for situations in which the patient has normal femoral and popliteal pulses and the embolus is lodged in the tibial vessels (E). However, such an approach is technically more difficult. If the limb is not immediately threatened, distal clots are better managed by lytic therapy as the tPA can be directed via catheter directly into the involved vessel. Echocardiogram would eventually be useful to look for a cardiac source of thrombus, but it would not be of immediate help in the management (D). With the advent of hybrid operating rooms, patients with more advanced ischemia (class 2) can be taken directly to the operating room where a diagnostic angiography followed by immediate intervention can be achieved.

Reference: Results of a prospective randomized trial evaluating surgery versus thrombolysis for ischemia of the lower extremity. The STILE trial: The STILE investigators (appendix A). *Ann Surg.* 1994;220(3):251–268.

5. C. This patient's history and CT scan findings are most consistent with acute mesenteric ischemia. Acute mesenteric ischemia can be divided into four major causes. Embolization from a cardiac source is the most common cause (30%–50% of cases), is seen most often in the setting of atrial fibrillation and is the likely etiology in the patient presented. The finding of an irregularly irregular heart rhythm suggests an arterial embolism from atrial fibrillation. The most common site of mesenteric embolization is the superior mesenteric artery (SMA) (due to its angle from the aorta). The embolus typically occludes the SMA just distal to the middle colic artery. These patients often have sparing of the proximal jejunum and transverse colon because the middle colic artery remains patent. Celiac artery embolization is rare, given its take-off at a right angle to the aorta. The inferior mesenteric artery orifice is so small that a cardiac thrombus rarely lodges inside. Mesenteric arterial thrombosis is usually due to underlying mesenteric artery atherosclerosis. In this situation, the patient will typically have a long-standing history of pain after eating, fear of eating, and weight loss, and the physical examination will reveal evidence of diffuse atherosclerosis and bruits. Mesenteric venous thrombosis is a third etiology and is most often seen in patients with hypercoagulable states. The acute venous occlusion leads to massive bowel edema with secondary arterial insufficiency from bowel wall distention. Patients with mesenteric venous thrombosis tend to present in a less dramatic fashion, often with days or weeks of abdominal pain. Finally, nonocclusive mesenteric ischemia results from shock that creates hypoperfusion of the bowel, such as with cardiac failure or severe hypovolemia. The classic findings in acute mesenteric ischemia are the sudden onset of severe pain out of proportion to the physical examination findings. Elevated serum lactate levels should raise the suspicion of ischemic bowel, but they are not sensitive enough to detect early bowel ischemia. A plain abdominal radiograph is often unremarkable, although it may demonstrate evidence of edema in the small bowel wall. If the patient has peritoneal signs on abdominal examination, this will indicate that the bowel has already been infarcted. In the absence of peritonitis and because the differential diagnosis is extensive, CT provides the greatest diagnostic yield initially (E). However, CT scan may not be diagnostic because it may not necessarily demonstrate opacification in the mesenteric veins or arteries (depending on the timing of contrast). The first step in the management is the administration of IV heparin. Following heparin, for an embolus, immediate surgery offers the best chance of treatment and would involve an SMA embolectomy (D). If the history were suggestive of underlying mesenteric atherosclerosis (longstanding postprandial abdominal pain and weight loss) with thrombosis, arteriography would be helpful because the management would involve an arterial bypass or stenting (B). If the CT scan revealed a thrombus in a mesenteric vein, definitive treatment would be heparin alone, provided there is no peritonitis. For nonocclusive

ischemia, correcting the underlying shock is the initial management. Catheter directed papaverine may also be useful. There are some case reports in which mesenteric emboli have been successfully managed with lytic therapy, but this is not the standard approach and is not the best option for elevated lactate suggesting a compromised bowel (A).

6. C. Mesenteric venous thrombosis accounts for approximately 10% to 15% of cases of mesenteric ischemia. It tends to have a slow, insidious onset, as in this case. Risk factors for mesenteric venous occlusion include hypercoagulable states such as factor V Leiden, antithrombin III deficiency, and protein C and S deficiency, as well as liver disease with portal hypertension, pancreatitis, and any intraperitoneal inflammatory conditions. Venous thrombosis is less dramatic than arterial occlusion. Abdominal pain is vague, and tenderness is mild or equivocal. CT may demonstrate a thickened bowel wall with delayed passage of IV contrast agent into the portal system and a lack of opacification of the portal or superior mesenteric vein. If the diagnosis is established from the CT scan, further diagnostic tests are unnecessary. Another useful diagnostic modality is duplex ultrasound scanning. Arteriography may demonstrate venous congestion and a lack of prompt filling of the portal system (D). If the patient is manifesting peritoneal signs, operative exploration is indicated (E). However, in the absence of peritonitis, therapy should consist of fluid hydration, hemodynamic support, anticoagulation with heparin, and serial examination. If peritonitis subsequently develops, exploratory laparotomy is appropriate to assess bowel viability with segmental bowel resection. Surgical thrombectomy of the venous system is not likely to be successful. Fibrinolytic therapy has been used increasingly, but is not yet the standard treatment of choice, and is ideal when symptoms are of short duration (A). Following heparin, warfarin or a novel oral anticoagulant, such as apixaban or rivaroxaban, is recommended for 3 to 6 months if the hypercoagulable state is provoked or temporary (B). Lifelong warfarin or NOAC is recommended if the venous thrombosis is unprovoked or associated with a permanent thrombophilic state. The family history of venous thrombosis in this patient is highly suggestive of an inherited hypercoagulability and would warrant lifelong anticoagulation. Additionally, any mesenteric arterial embolism requires lifelong anticoagulation.

Reference: Kumar S, Sarr MG, Kamath PS. Mesenteric venous thrombosis. *N Engl J Med.* 2001;345(23):1683–1688.

7. C. Cilostazol has a number of functions including inhibiting platelet aggregation and smooth muscle proliferation, increasing vasodilation, and lowering high-density lipoprotein and triglyceride levels. Cilostazol has been shown to significantly increase walking distance by 50% to 67% in patients with claudication in several randomized trials and results in improvement in physical functioning and quality of life. This drug is contraindicated in patients with congestive heart failure. This drug is more effective than pentoxifylline in the treatment of claudication (A). Pentoxifylline is a methylxanthine derivative that has hemorrheologic properties. Two meta analyses showed that it improves walking distance, but in some more recent randomized studies, it proved to be no better than placebo. Pentoxifylline improves symptoms of claudication by increasing red blood cell flexibility and reducing blood viscosity. Antiplatelet medications such as aspirin are used in the treatment of peripheral vascular disease and for cardiac and stroke prevention but do not appear to improve walking distance (B). Aspirin has been found to reduce the vascular death rate by approximately 25% in patients with any manifestation of atherosclerotic disease (e.g., coronary, peripheral). Clopidogrel is effective in reducing overall acute cardiovascular events, especially in patients with lower extremity occlusive disease, but is much more expensive (D). It does not seem to directly improve walking distance. Pure vasodilators have not been efficacious in the treatment of peripheral vascular disease because most patients with such occlusive disease already exhibit marked vasodilation. Anticoagulants also have not been shown to alter the course of peripheral atherosclerosis (E).

Reference: Money SR, Herd JA, Isaacsohn JL, et al. Effect of cilostazol on walking distances in patients with intermittent claudication caused by peripheral vascular disease. *J Vasc Surg.* 1998;27(2):267–274.

8. E. Leg edema after femoral-to-popliteal arterial bypass is common. In most instances, it is due to lymphatic disruption. This disruption occurs at both the groin and popliteal incisions as well as from harvesting of the saphenous vein. Deep venous thrombosis can occur after this procedure but is relatively uncommon (A). Reperfusion edema may be associated with compartment syndrome and can present with the Ps (pain, pallor, paralysis, paresthesia, and poikilothermia) (B). It is more likely to present after revascularization due to acute limb ischemia. The saphenous veins are part of the superficial venous system, which contributes a minority of the venous drainage in the leg, so swelling secondary to venous congestion is not expected after a saphenous vein harvest (C). Cellulitis would present with erythema, pain, warmth, and possible systemic signs such as fever or leukocytosis (D).

Reference: AbuRahma AF, Woodruff BA, Lucente FC. Edema after femoropopliteal bypass surgery: lymphatic and venous theories of causation. *J Vasc Surg.* 1990;11(3):461–467.

9. D. The patient's history and examination are most consistent with symptoms of coronary-subclavian steal syndrome. Most patients with a coronary artery bypass graft have undergone a left internal mammary artery-to-left anterior descending graft. In the setting of subclavian artery stenosis or occlusion proximal to the take-off of the internal mammary artery, arm exercise leads to vasodilation of the arm vessels and lower resistance. Blood will travel through the path of least resistance and flow in a reverse fashion from the left anterior descending artery into the left internal mammary artery and toward the arm, leading to the development of angina. The differential blood pressure in the arms is the clue, as is the left arm claudication. Treatment involves relieving the subclavian artery obstruction. This can be done by subclavian artery stenting but on occasion requires a carotid-to-subclavian artery bypass (A). Since the problem is not related to underlying cardiac disease, carotid stenting, increasing beta-blocker dose, or increasing dose of nitrates will not resolve the patient's chest pain with exercise (B, C, E).

Reference: Bryan F, Allen R, Lumsden A. Coronary subclavian steal syndrome: report of 5 cases. *Ann Vasc Surg.* 1995;9(1):115–122.

10. B. Initial management of patients with acute mesenteric ischemia includes fluid resuscitation and systemic anticoagulation with heparin sulfate to prevent further thrombus propagation. Significant metabolic acidosis should be corrected with sodium bicarbonate. A central venous catheter, peripheral arterial catheter, and Foley catheter should be placed for fluid resuscitation and hemodynamic status monitoring. Appropriate antibiotics are given before surgical exploration. The operative management of acute mesenteric ischemia is dictated by the cause of the occlusion. For an SMA embolus, exposure of the SMA is obtained via rotation of the small bowel to the right and by sharply dissecting the ligament of Treitz. The SMA will be found at the root of the mesentery. The primary goal in the surgical treatment of embolic mesenteric ischemia is to restore arterial perfusion with removal of the embolus from the vessel. This is done by performing a Fogarty embolectomy using a transverse arteriotomy (longitudinal arteriotomy will cause stenosis upon closure) (D). It is important to avoid resecting bowel until perfusion has been restored; that way, bowel viability can be better established. After restoration of SMA flow, an assessment of the intestinal viability is made, and nonviable bowel is resected. Because the amount of bowel resected can be extensive and this places the patient at risk of short bowel syndrome, bowel that is of borderline viability should be left in place with a planned second-look procedure performed 24 to 48 hours later to reassess whether additional bowel resection is needed (E). Low-dose dopamine leads to vasodilatation of mesenteric arteries; however, its benefits are unclear (C). Intraoperative angiography will not provide any additional information that would assist in the surgical management of SMA embolus (A).

11. B. The most common cause of mesenteric ischemia is a cardiac embolus to the SMA. The SMA provides blood to the bowel from the ligament of Treitz to the mid transverse colon. Cardiac embolus tends to lodge just past the SMA origin at a point where the artery begins to narrow, which is just beyond the first jejunal branches. These patients often have sparing of the proximal jejunum and transverse colon because the middle colic artery remains patent. Thrombosis of the SMA, conversely, is usually caused by underlying atherosclerotic disease that occurs at the SMA origin and would thus not spare the proximal jejunum (A). Mesenteric venous thrombosis and nonocclusive mesenteric ischemia would more likely cause patchy areas of ischemia (C–E).

Reference: Eldrup-Jorgensen J, Hawkins RE, Bredenberg CE. Abdominal vascular catastrophes. *Surg Clin North Am.* 1997;77(6):1305–1320.

12. E. The timing of CEA after a stroke is controversial. A delay in surgery increases the risk of recurrent stroke. The risk is highest within the first month. Conversely, operating too early (within 24 hours) creates a potential risk of a reperfusion injury, particularly if a large infarction is present on computed tomography (CT) and if hypertension cannot be controlled postoperatively. Intracranial bleeding is thought to occur because of altered autoregulation and hyperperfusion of ischemic tissue. In the North American Symptomatic Carotid Endarterectomy Trial (NASCET), however, postoperative intracranial hemorrhage occurred in only 0.2% of patients. Until recently, CEA was routinely delayed for 4 to

6 weeks after a stroke. Subsequent analysis of the NASCET showed that patients with a stable, nondisabling acute stroke, a normal CT scan, and a normal level of consciousness can safely undergo CEA shortly after the diagnosis is made, the symptoms have stabilized, and preoperative risk assessment is complete. Thus, the operation is not urgent (D). Delaying the surgery for 6 weeks or more eliminates much of the benefit of CEA because the risk of recurrent stroke is greatest early on (B, C). Current treatment guidelines from the American Academy of Neurology and from the American Stroke Association/American Heart Association recommend that CEA for patients with nondisabling strokes should preferably be performed within 2 weeks of the primary stroke. Patients with a large stroke on CT scan or those with a midline shift may be at higher risk of reperfusion injury, particularly if they have a depressed level of consciousness. Operation should be delayed until these patients improve and plateau in their clinical recovery, which is usually in the range of 4 to 6 weeks. If the stroke is completely disabling (A), there remains little if any motor cortex to protect from future stroke, so CEA is not indicated. Thus, patients with severe neurologic deficits, without meaningful recovery or with marked alteration of consciousness, are not candidates for CEA because the goal of CEA is to prevent further damage to the ipsilateral motor cortex.

References: Henderson RD, Eliasziw M, Fox AJ, Rothwell PM, Barnett HJ. Angiographically defined collateral circulation and risk of stroke in patients with severe carotid artery stenosis. North American Symptomatic Carotid Endarterectomy Trial (NASCET) Group. *Stroke*. 2000;31(1):128–132.

North American Symptomatic Carotid Endarterectomy Trial Collaborators, Barnett HJM, Taylor DW, et al. Beneficial effect of carotid endarterectomy in symptomatic patients with high-grade carotid stenosis. *N Engl J Med*. 1991;325(7):445–453.

Sacco RL, Adams R, Albers G, et al. Guidelines for prevention of stroke in patients with ischemic stroke or transient ischemic attack: a statement for healthcare professionals from the American Heart Association/American Stroke Association Council on Stroke: co-sponsored by the Council on Cardiovascular Radiology and Intervention: the American Academy of Neurology affirms the value of this guideline. *Circ*. 2006;113(10):e409–e449.

13. E. The ACAS randomized patients with asymptomatic carotid artery stenosis of 60% to 99% to either CEA and aspirin or aspirin alone (C). The study was interrupted because of a significant benefit identified in patients undergoing CEA. A relative reduction in stroke rate by 50%, from 11% to 5% at 5 years, was observed in patients undergoing CEA (A). The Asymptomatic Carotid Surgery Trial confirmed the ACAS findings that in patients with 60% to 99% stenosis, the net 5-year risk was 6.4% for all strokes or death in patients undergoing CEA, versus 11.8% in those not undergoing surgery. This was a net absolute gain of 5.4% (relative risk reduction, 46%). The trial also showed that patients who underwent CEA were much less likely to have a fatal or disabling stroke (3.5% in the surgery group versus 6.1% in the no-surgery group). The studies have found that there is less or no benefit in women (E). The greatest benefit was in men younger than 75 years of age. CEA for asymptomatic stenosis will only benefit the group as a whole if the combined stroke and death rate is less than 3% (B). Keeping this combined endpoint low is dependent on both patient risk and surgeon skill (C). There is no benefit to CEA once the ICA

is completely occluded (100%) (D). There is no further flow in the artery, thus the embolic risk is eliminated. The benefit of aggressive medical management (including antiplatelet agents) is that it can also be protective from coronary events. The biggest limitation of ACAS is that it did not include the use of a statin, which, in addition to its lipid-lowering response, also has pleiotropic effects such as plaque stability, which may prove to be a more important contributor in preventing the progression to stroke in carotid disease. The Aggressive Medical Treatment Evaluation for Asymptomatic Carotid Artery Stenosis (AMTEC) trial attempted to compare modern medical management with CEA, but the study was prematurely terminated and the results are not yet available. Newer studies are needed to determine if modern medical therapy continues to be inferior to surgical intervention in patients with carotid disease. Some authors have suggested that we shift away from using decreased luminal caliber as our primary determinant of choosing which asymptomatic patients to offer surgery. Newer methods of identifying high-risk patients such as those with plaque ulceration and instability should be studied to either replace or supplement existing societal guidelines.

References: Endarterectomy for asymptomatic carotid artery stenosis. Executive Committee for the Asymptomatic Carotid Atherosclerosis Study. *JAMA*. 1995;273(18):1421–1428.

Halliday A, Mansfield A, Marro J, et al. Prevention of disabling and fatal strokes by successful carotid endarterectomy in patients without recent neurological symptoms: randomised controlled trial. *Lancet*. 2004;363(9420):1491–1502.

Kolos I, Loukianov M, Dupik N, Boytsov S, Deev A. Optimal medical treatment versus carotid endarterectomy: the rationale and design of the Aggressive Medical Treatment Evaluation for Asymptomatic Carotid Artery Stenosis (AMTEC) study. *Int J Stroke*. 2015;10(2):269–274.

Weyer GW, Davis AM. Screening for asymptomatic carotid artery stenosis. *JAMA*. 2015;313(2):192–193.

14. D. The first NASCET study found that CEA was of benefit for symptomatic severe ICA stenosis (70%–99%). A symptomatic carotid artery stenosis was defined as a nondisabling stroke, a hemispheric transient ischemic attack, or a retinal symptom (amaurosis fugax). Life-table estimates of the cumulative risk of any ipsilateral stroke at 2 years were 26% in the aspirin group and 9% in the aspirin and CEA group. In the second NASCET study, there was no benefit for symptomatic patients with less than 50% stenosis (E). For symptomatic patients with stenosis from 50% to 69%, there was a very modest benefit: 5-year risk of ipsilateral stroke was 15.7% in the CEA group and 22.2% in the medical group (P = 0.04). The benefit was greatest in men, in those with hemispheric symptoms (as opposed to retinal ones), and with recent stroke. Women appeared to have less risk of stroke and also had higher perioperative mortality than men. ACAS demonstrated the benefit of CEA compared with aspirin for asymptomatic ICA stenosis of 60% to 99%. However, the benefit is much less than for symptomatic high-grade stenosis. Thus in this question, choice A would be beneficial but of less benefit than choice D (symptomatic). Choice B would be of no benefit because the stenosis is moderate, and the symptoms are on the wrong side (retinal is ipsilateral). In choice C, the symptoms are also on the wrong side with respect to the stenosis.

15. A. New neurologic deficits that present within the first 12 hours of operation are almost always the result of thromboembolic phenomena stemming from the CEA site. Possibilities include the development of thrombus on the endarterectomized arterial surface, a residual intimal flap in the ICA leading to occlusion, or a residual flap in the external carotid artery (ECA) leading to ECA thrombosis and retrograde embolization of the clot into the ICA. Immediate heparinization and exploration are indicated without the need for confirmatory arteriography or noninvasive tests. On reexploring the wound, the ECA and ICA should be palpated for the presence of a pulse. If there is no pulse, this indicates thrombosis, and initial on-table arteriography is not necessary. The artery should be reopened and inspected to look for a cause of the thrombosis. Before closing the arteriotomy, care should be taken to ensure that there is good back-bleeding from the ICA. Fogarty balloon embolectomy of the cephalad ICA should be avoided because this can lead to a carotid-cavernous sinus fistula. The arteriotomy should then be reclosed with a patch. On-table arteriography should then be performed to ensure that the distal ICA is patent and to determine whether there is an embolus in the middle cerebral artery. If an embolus is present in the intracranial carotid or middle cerebral artery, local infusion of a lytic agent should be considered (B). If on reopening the wound, an excellent pulse is present in the ICA and ECA, with normal signals on hand-held Doppler ultrasonography, on-table arteriography is performed (C, D). If arteriography reveals an intimal flap or irregular mural thrombus at the endarterectomy site, then reopening of the vessel is indicated. Neurologic deficits that develop 12 to 24 hours after the operation are usually due to thromboembolic phenomena stemming from the CEA site but may also be caused by a postoperative hyperperfusion syndrome. These latter conditions may be worsened by immediate heparinization and reexploration. Therefore, deficits occurring 12 to 24 hours after the operation should be promptly investigated with head CT and CT arteriography (E).

16. C. The incidence of hyperperfusion syndrome after a CEA is reportedly 0.3% to 1%. It is thought to occur as a result of impaired autoregulation of cerebral blood flow and does not need to be taken back to the OR (E). The thought is that longstanding, severe carotid stenosis leads to hypoperfusion, leading to a compensatory dilation of cerebral vessels distal to the stenosis as part of the normal autoregulatory response to maintain adequate cerebral blood flow. After CEA restores normal pressure, however, autoregulation is impaired and does not immediately adjust to the sudden increase in blood flow. Risk factors associated with cerebral hyperperfusion include recent stroke, surgery for very tight ICA stenosis, concomitant contralateral ICA occlusion, evidence of chronic ipsilateral hypoperfusion, staged bilateral CEA performed within 2 months of each other, and poorly controlled pre- and postoperative hypertension. Pathologic changes range from mild cerebral edema and petechial hemorrhage to severe intracerebral hemorrhage and death, particularly if not promptly treated (B). The syndrome is heralded by an ipsilateral frontal headache, most commonly occurring at a median of the fifth postoperative day (A). By that time, the patient is already at home. Thus, it is imperative to warn patients of this rare syndrome and ideally have the patient check his or

her blood pressure daily for the first week postoperatively. The headache may be followed by focal motor seizures that are often difficult to control. Management consists of controlling blood pressure, ideally with a beta-blocker, with the avoidance of vasodilators (as these may increase cerebral blood flow), and use of antiseizure medications (D).

Reference: Schroeder T, Sillesen H, Sørensen O, Engell HC. Cerebral hyperperfusion following carotid endarterectomy. *J Neurosurg.* 1987;66(6):824–829.

17. D. This patient has Takayasu arteritis, an inflammatory disease of the aorta and its branches, as well as the coronary and pulmonary arteries (A–C, E). It occurs most commonly in young women, with a median age of 25 years. The clinical course has been described as beginning with constitutional symptoms such as fever and malaise. However, a National Institutes of Health study showed that only one-third of patients recall such symptoms. Characteristic clinical features include hypertension, retinopathy, aortic regurgitation, cerebrovascular symptoms, angina, congestive heart failure, abdominal pain or gastrointestinal bleeding, pulmonary hypertension, and extremity claudication. The gold standard for diagnosis is arterial imaging, with the demonstration of occlusive disease in the subclavian arteries. Unlike atherosclerosis, which tends to affect the origin of these vessels, Takayasu arteritis affects the midportions of these arteries. Characteristic signs and symptoms include pulselessness or blood pressure differential in the arms, upper or lower extremity claudication, syncope, amaurosis fugax, blurred vision, and palpitations. Treatment initially consists of steroid therapy with the addition of cytotoxic agents used in patients who do not achieve remission. Carotidynia, which is pain along inflamed arteries, is pathognomonic for Takayasu arteritis. Surgical treatment with arterial bypass is only performed in advanced states and in situations in which the patient does not respond to medical therapy. It should ideally be performed when the disease is not active. Because the disease causes transmural arterial inflammation with concentric fibrosis, there is no role for endarterectomy, and angioplasty has not been met with good results.

18. A. The most common mechanisms of blunt carotid injury include motor vehicle accidents, fist fights, hanging, and intraoral trauma. However, it has also been reported with relatively minor trauma, such as after chiropractic manipulation of the neck and forceful sneezing. Biffl et al. have graded blunt carotid injury as follows: grade I: luminal irregularity or dissection with less than 25% luminal narrowing; grade II: dissection or intramural hematoma with greater than or equal 25% luminal narrowing; grade III: pseudoaneurysm; grade IV: occlusion; grade V: transection with free extravasation. Horner syndrome (oculosympathetic paresis) is common with this injury and is thought to be related to the involvement of the internal part of the pericarotid sympathetic plexus (B). The decision to perform surgery is based on (1) injury severity, (2) presence or absence of symptoms, and (3) surgical accessibility of the lesion (C). In general, there is little role for surgical intervention in patients with grade I or II blunt carotid injury as in this patient (E). Antiplatelet therapy with aspirin is the best treatment option. However, some trauma centers chose to use subtherapeutic heparin initially in case patients may require a surgery. Minor (intimal) injuries tend to heal themselves (D). Pseudoaneurysms typically do not and are a relative indication for surgery if accessible in the neck.

References: Biffl WL, Moore EE, Offner PJ, Brega KE, Franciose RJ, Burch JM. Blunt carotid arterial injuries: implications of a new grading scale. *J Trauma*. 1999;47(5):845–853.

Bromberg WJ, Collier BC, Diebel LN, et al. Blunt cerebrovascular injury practice management guidelines: the Eastern Association for the Surgery of Trauma. *J Trauma*. 2010;68(2):471–477.

19. E. The patient has a symptomatic high-grade carotid stenosis, and, as such, an intervention is indicated. With the history of radiation therapy and neck dissection, the patient has what is termed a "hostile neck." This increases the risk of carotid endarterectomy, in terms of cranial nerve injury and wound healing. The previous neck dissection results in a paucity of tissue coverage between the skin and the carotid artery. This can lead to the catastrophic complication of carotid blow out. The best alternative in this patient would be to perform carotid stenting with a cerebral protection device (A–D). Patients with asymptomatic ICA stenosis in the 50% to 69% range should be started on medical therapy with an antiplatelet agent (for all patients), antihypertensive agent (if they have hypertension), and the use of a high-intensity statin irrespective of lipid levels (due to the pleiotropic effect of plaque stabalization).

Reference: Harrod-Kim P, Kadkhodayan Y, Derdeyn CP, Cross DT 3rd, Moran CJ. Outcomes of carotid angioplasty and stenting for radiation-associated stenosis. *AJNR Am J Neuroradiol*. 2005;26(7):1781–1788.

20. C. Recurrent carotid stenosis can occur after CEA. The risk of more than 50% restenosis is 5.8%, 9.9%, 13.9%, and 23.4% at 1, 3, 5, and 10 years, respectively. However, severe (>80%) stenosis develops in only 2.1% of patients. Early (within 4 weeks) restenosis is usually due to a technical error. Recurrent carotid stenosis occurring beyond 1 month but within the first 2 years after CEA is usually secondary to myointimal hyperplasia. This type of stenosis tends to have a benign course (the lesion is smooth and less prone to embolization), with a low risk of recurrent stroke. In addition, reoperative CEA carries a higher risk of cranial nerve injury (7.3% rate of permanent injury in one series) (A). The patient is asymptomatic. If the patient had a symptomatic recurrence, the best option would be carotid stenting (B, D–E). When the recurrent stenosis develops 2 or more years after CEA, recurrent atherosclerosis is the usual cause.

21. D. Sudden occlusion of the ICA in a young patient is highly suggestive of a spontaneous dissection. This is further supported by the tapered occlusion seen on imaging (described as "flame-shaped"). On the other hand, occlusion due to atherosclerosis typically occurs flush with the common carotid, and in older patients ICA dissection may occur either spontaneously or after trauma. Cervical artery dissection is a significant cause of stroke in patients younger than 40 years. Common presenting symptoms of ICA dissection are headache, transient ischemic attack and/or stroke, and Horner syndrome (ptosis, miosis, anhydrosis). Risk factors for dissection include history of infection (syphilis), smoking, Ehlers-Danlos syndrome type IV, cystic medial necrosis, Marfan syndrome, family history, oral contraceptives, and atherosclerosis. In a young female, fibromuscular dysplasia

would be high on the differential. The diagnosis is made by duplex scan and/or CT angiography. Duplex scan may be diagnostic, if it demonstrates a membrane within the lumen, consistent with a dissection. The most likely mechanism of acute dissection is an intimal tear followed by an acute intimal dissection, which produces luminal occlusion due to secondary thrombosis. The occlusion angiographically is typically 2 to 3 cm beyond the bifurcation. Autopsy studies have shown a sharply demarcated transition between the normal carotid artery and the dissected segment. Treatment is with anticoagulation and, in most cases, results in complete resolution within a few months. Stenting may be an option in symptomatic patients in the absence of occlusion (C). CEA, Fogarty embolectomy, or lytic therapy is not appropriate for a spontaneous dissection (A, B, E).

22. E. Thromboangiitis obliterans (Buerger disease) is a progressive nonatherosclerotic segmental inflammatory disease that most often affects small- to medium-sized arteries, veins, and nerves of the upper and lower extremities (C). The typical age at onset is 20 to 50 years, and the disorder is more common in men who smoke. The disease also affects the veins, and specifically the upper extremities may be affected by a migratory superficial thrombophlebitis. Patients initially present with foot, leg, arm, or hand claudication. Progression of the disease leads to ischemic rest pain and ulcerations of the toes, feet, and fingers. Characteristic angiographic findings may show disease confinement to the distal circulation, usually infrapopliteal and distal to the brachial artery. The occlusions are segmental and show skip lesions with extensive collateralization, the so-called corkscrew collaterals. The diagnosis is difficult to establish and is a diagnosis of exclusion because there are no pathognomonic features. As such, the disease can be confused with chronic embolization and other diseases. Several criteria have been established to confirm the diagnosis: age younger than 45 years; current (or recent) smoker; distal extremity ischemia (claudication, pain at rest, ischemic ulcers, gangrene); exclusion of autoimmune diseases, hypercoagulable states, and diabetes mellitus; exclusion of a proximal source of emboli by echocardiography and arteriography; and characteristic arteriographic findings in the involved limbs. The aortoiliac segments are typically spared, as are the coronary arteries (A, B). The mainstay of treatment revolves around smoking cessation. In patients who are able to abstain, disease remission is impressive and amputation avoidance is increased. The role of surgical intervention is minimal because there is usually no acceptable target vessel for bypass (D). Sympathectomy may result in mild improvement of symptoms.

Reference: Olin JW. Thromboangiitis obliterans (Buerger's disease). *N Engl J Med*. 2000;343(12):864–869.

23. C. The ABI normally varies between 1 and 1.2 because the ankle pressure in the supine position can be as much as 20% higher than in the arm (A). Peripheral arterial disease has been defined as a value less than 0.9 and indicates some degree of stenosis. Patients with claudication typically have an ABI between 0.5 and 0.7, and those with rest pain have an ABI less than 0.4 (B). Patients with diabetes and end-stage renal disease are at risk of developing calcification of the arterial medial layer, known as medial calcinosis, or

Mönckeberg arteriosclerosis. This process makes blood vessels rigid and difficult to compress, causing falsely increased pressure readings. The process tends to affect tibial vessels primarily and spares digital vessels in the toes. As such, toe pressures are more reliable, as are other measures of distal perfusion such as transmetatarsal pulse volume recordings and transcutaneous oximetry (D, E).

Reference: Belkin M, Whittemore A, Donaldson M, et al. Peripheral arterial occlusive disease. In: Townsend CM, Jr, Beauchamp RD, Evers BM, Mattox KL, eds. *Sabiston textbook of surgery: the biological basis of modern surgical practice.* 17th ed. Philadelphia: W.B. Saunders; 2004:1992.

24. B. Absolute contraindications to thrombolytic therapy include recent stroke or transient ischemic attack, active or recent bleeding, and significant coagulopathy. Relative contraindications include patients with recent major surgery (within 2 weeks, and greatest with recent neurosurgery or eye surgery), recent trauma, uncontrolled hypertension, intracranial tumors, and pregnancy (A). Thrombolytic therapy is most effective in patients with ischemia of less than 2 weeks' duration (D). The risk of bleeding with thrombolytic therapy is increased with the longer duration of therapy and with decreasing fibrinogen levels. In most series, thrombolytic therapy is used for as long as 48 hours, at which point the bleeding risk increases significantly (E). The causes of acute limb ischemia can be divided into embolic and thrombotic. The heart is the most common source of emboli leading to acute ischemia, most often in the setting of atrial fibrillation. Other cardiac sources include mural thrombus after an acute myocardial infarction, valvular disease, and atrial myxoma. Other sources of emboli include arterial aneurysms and atherosclerotic plaques. Thrombosis is most often caused by underlying atherosclerosis in the peripheral arteries, and these patients typically have a history of claudication. The severity of acute limb ischemia is based primarily on the motor and sensory examination. Patients should be placed in four categories: class 1 (nonthreatened) has normal motor and sensory function; class 2 (threatened) includes 2 a—sensory deficit only and 2b—(immediately threatened) both motor and sensory deficit; and class 3 indicates irreversible complete motor and sensory loss. In addition, consideration should be given to the duration of ischemia. As a general rule, patients with class 1 ischemia can be treated with multiple options, a trial of heparin alone, thrombolytic therapy, or operative embolectomy/bypass. Patients with class 2 ischemia need prompt restoration of blood flow, so heparin alone is not acceptable. With class 2b ischemia, the threat of limb loss is more immediate. Since thrombolytic therapy may require more than 24 to 48 hours to restore flow, class 2b ischemia (motor and sensory deficit) is a relative contraindication to thrombolysis (C). Such a patient should be taken to the operating room. Category 3 ischemia is considered irreversible and requires amputation. Irreversible ischemia is confirmed by an absence of arterial or venous Doppler signals, duration of ischemia of more than 6 to 8 hours, presence of mottling of the skin, absence of capillary refill, and complete anesthesia and paralysis.

References: Norgren L, Hiatt WR, Dormandy JA, et al. Inter-society consensus for the management of peripheral arterial disease (TASC II). *J Vasc Surg.* 2007;45 Suppl S:S5–S67.

Semba CP, Murphy TP, Bakal CW, Calis KA, Matalon TA. Thrombolytic therapy with use of alteplase (rt-PA) in peripheral arterial

occlusive disease: review of the clinical literature. The Advisory Panel. *J Vasc Interv Radiol.* 2000;11(2):149–161.

Results of a prospective randomized trial evaluating surgery versus thrombolysis for ischemia of the lower extremity. The STILE trial: The STILE investigators (appendix A). *Ann Surg.* 1994;220(3):251–268.

25. C. The ipsilateral greater saphenous vein is the conduit of choice for lower extremity distal bypass for peripheral arterial disease (contralateral vein for trauma). An ideal conduit should be a minimum of 3 mm (but ideally 4 mm). When the greater saphenous vein is not available, options include the lesser saphenous and cephalic veins. Ectopic veins (i.e., lesser saphenous, arm veins) are generally inferior to a single-segment saphenous vein, although they are still superior to the performance of synthetic grafts. A composite graft, which is a vein graft sewn to a polytetrafluoroethylene graft, has a patency rate similar to that of a prosthetic graft and tends to develop neointimal hyperplasia. The bypass should be as short as possible (proximal inflow from the most distal normal artery (in this case, popliteal), and distal outflow to where the artery reconstitutes most proximally (in this case, above the ankle). Options A and B are suboptimal because it involves a longer bypass than is necessary given the patent femoral artery and normal popliteal pulse and harvesting contralateral vein. Endovascular approaches (such as angioplasty) are options but are less durable, particularly in the presence of a long segment of occlusion. However, in a relatively healthy patient, with a good saphenous vein and good runoff into the foot, a bypass is likely the better option (D). Amputation of the toe is unlikely to heal in the absence of a palpable pedal pulse and such a low ABI (E).

Reference: Gentile AT, Lee RW, Moneta GL, Taylor LM, Edwards JM, Porter JM. Results of bypass to the popliteal and tibial arteries with alternative sources of autogenous vein. *J Vasc Surg.* 1996;23(2):272–279.

26. E. This is Raynaud disease. First described in 1862 by Maurice Raynaud, the term Raynaud disease applies to a heterogeneous symptom array associated with peripheral vasospasm, more commonly occurring in the upper extremities. The characteristically intermittent vasospasm classically follows exposure to various stimuli, including cold temperatures, tobacco, or emotional stress. Formerly, a distinction was made between Raynaud disease and the Raynaud phenomenon for describing a benign disease occurring in isolation or a more severe disease secondary to another underlying disorder, respectively. However, collagen vascular disorders develop in many patients at some point after the onset of vasospastic symptoms; the rate of progression to a connective tissue disorder ranges from 11% to 65% in reported series. Characteristic color changes occur in response to the arteriolar vasospasm, ranging from intense pallor to cyanosis to redness as the vasospasm occurs. The digital vessels then relax, eventually leading to reactive hyperemia. The majority of patients are women younger than 40 years of age. As many as 70% to 90% of reported patients are women, although many patients with only mild symptoms may never present for treatment. Geographic regions located in cooler, damp climates such as the Pacific Northwest and Scandinavian countries have a higher reported prevalence of the disease. Certain occupational groups, such as those that use vibrating tools, may be more predisposed to Raynaud disease or digital ischemia. The exact pathophysiologic mechanism behind the development of such severe vasospasm remains elusive, and much attention has focused on increased levels of α2-adrenergic receptors and their hypersensitivity in patients with Raynaud disease, as well as abnormalities in the thermoregulatory response, which is governed by the sympathetic nervous system. There is no cure for Raynaud disease; thus, all treatments mainly palliate symptoms and decrease the severity and perhaps frequency of attacks. Conservative measures predominate, including the wearing of gloves, use of electric or chemically activated hand warmers, avoiding occupational exposure to vibratory tools, abstinence from tobacco, and relocating to a warmer, drier climate. The majority (90%) of patients will respond to avoidance of cold and other stimuli. The remaining 10% of patients with more persistent or severe syndromes can be treated with a variety of vasodilatory drugs, albeit with only a 30% to 60% response rate. Calcium channel blocking agents such as diltiazem and nifedipine are the drugs of choice. The selective serotonin reuptake inhibitor fluoxetine has been shown to reduce the frequency and duration of vasospastic episodes but is not the first-line treatment (C). Intravenous infusions of prostaglandins have been reserved for nonresponders with severe symptoms (B). Upper extremity sympathectomy may provide relief in 60% to 70% of patients; however, the results are short-lived, with a gradual recurrence of symptoms in 60% within 10 years (A). Cervical sympathectomy has fallen out of favor and has been replaced by localized digital sympathectomy using microsurgery. This involves stripping the adventitia of digital arteries and thus removing sympathetic fibers. A cold stimulation test or nail fold capillaroscopy may be used to confirm the diagnosis of Raynaud disease, but there is no role for arteriography (D).

27. D. Pseudoaneurysms can manifest with pain, a pulsatile mass, and/or compression of adjacent structures. Large, expanding, painful pseudoaneurysms are at significant risk of rupture and should be repaired urgently. Smaller, stable pseudoaneurysms may be observed (E). Duplex ultrasonography has been the diagnostic procedure of choice because it helps define size, morphology, and location. Pseudoaneurysms less than 2 cm in diameter have a higher likelihood of spontaneous thrombosis with compression therapy, whereas larger ones and those in patients receiving anticoagulation therapy are likely to persist. However, given the reported high failure rates with ultrasound compression (A, B), ultrasonography-guided thrombin injection is the best treatment option and is the treatment of choice. Surgery is reserved for infected or rapidly expanding pseudoaneurysms (C).

Reference: Wixon CL, Philpott JM, Bogey WM Jr, Powell CS. Duplex-directed thrombin injection as a method to treat femoral artery pseudoaneurysms. *J Am Coll Surg.* 1998;187(4):464–466.

28. A. Colonic ischemia is a recognized complication after AAA repair, whether open or endovascular. It occurs in approximately 1% to 3% of cases. It is thought to be due to either ligation of the inferior mesenteric artery (IMA) or ligation or exclusion of internal iliac arteries. The most common presentations include an unexpectedly early return of bowel function manifested by diarrhea, left lower quadrant pain, abdominal distention, persistent leukocytosis, elevated white blood cell count, and lactic acidosis. Diagnosis is confirmed by flexible proctosigmoidoscopy, which reveals a friable mucosa. Proctosigmoidoscopy may not be able to accurately distinguish partial ischemia from full-thickness necrosis. Initial management is medical and consists of nasogastric tube decompression, IV hydration, placing the patient on NPO, and broad-spectrum antibiotics. Full-thickness necrosis of the colon should be suspected in patients with evidence of peritonitis or unremitting acidosis. In such cases, laparotomy with colonic resection and colostomy is indicated (C, D). The mortality rate after emergent colectomy approaches 50%. Arteriography would not typically be helpful because the usual cause is an intended ligation or exclusion of an internal iliac artery or IMA (B, E).

Reference: Becquemin JP, Majewski M, Fermani N, et al. Colon ischemia following abdominal aortic aneurysm repair in the era of endovascular abdominal aortic repair. *J Vasc Surg.* 2008;47(2):258–263.

29. B. The presentation is consistent with a ruptured AAA. If the patient was hemodynamically unstable, he should be taken directly to the operating room (D). If the patient is relatively stable (as in this case), a CT scan is preferred to confirm the presence of a ruptured AAA and determine feasibility of endovascular repair, provided there is a coordinated multidisciplinary ruptured aneurysm team that has immediate endovascular capabilities. Although most surgeons would approach a ruptured AAA via the endovascular approach, recent Cochrane analysis demonstrated no difference in 30-day mortality for patients with ruptured AAA that were treated with an endovascular approach compared to an open approach. Although ultrasonography is useful for determining the presence of an AAA, it is not accurate for determining the presence of a retroperitoneal rupture (C). Ultrasonography would be reasonable to perform in this patient was unstable, and no pulsatile mass could be felt on physical examination, so as to confirm that an aneurysm was present. Once in the operating room, the patient should be prepped and draped before anesthesia induction because the anesthesia may induce a precipitous decrease in blood pressure (E). Because of the large retroperitoneal hematoma that is typically found, proximal control is best achieved by clamping the aorta at the diaphragm. Most surgeons would recommend a policy of "permissive hypotension" en route to the operating room. Excessive fluid administration and elevation of the blood pressure may further exacerbate bleeding (A).

References: Badger SA, Harkin DW, Blair PH, Ellis PK, Kee F, Forster R. Endovascular repair or open repair for ruptured abdominal aortic aneurysm: a Cochrane systematic review. *BMJ Open.* 2016;6(2):e008391.

Lee WA, Hirneise CM, Tayyarah M, Huber TS, Seeger JM. Impact of endovascular repair on early outcomes of ruptured abdominal aortic aneurysms. *J Vasc Surg.* 2004;40(2):211–215.

Van Der Vliet JA, Van Aalst DL, Schultze Kool LJ. Hypotensive hemostasis (permissive hypotension) for ruptured abdominal aortic aneurysm: are we really in control? *Vascular.* 2007;15(4):197–200.

30. C. Popliteal aneurysms are the most common peripheral artery aneurysms (overall, aortic and iliac aneurysms are more common). They can be suspected on physical examination. They are bilateral in 50% of patients. Patients who are found to have a popliteal aneurysm should undergo screening for an AAA because 30% will have a concomitant AAA. The most frequent complication of popliteal aneurysms is leg ischemia due to thrombosis and embolization from the aneurysm. Guidelines for repair are controversial. Some authors recommend repair for all popliteal aneurysms. Most would agree that indications for repair are (1) all aneurysms larger than 2 cm, (2) aneurysms with intraluminal thrombus, regardless of size, or (3) those that are symptomatic or have evidence of previous embolization (A, B). Diagnosis is made by duplex ultrasonography, which can measure the aneurysm size and detect the presence of thrombus. Arteriography assists in operative planning but should not be used for diagnosis because it does not detect the thrombus nor accurately measure the size. The surgical approach to the popliteal artery is either via the medial approach or the posterior approach (E). The posterior approach is ideal if the aneurysm is just behind the knee joint. Magnetic resonance imaging and CT angiography can be used as alternatives for operative planning. The standard operative approach involves bypassing the aneurysm with saphenous vein and interval ligation of the popliteal artery. With this approach, the aneurysm sac is not opened, and as such, there is a small risk of continued aneurysm expansion and compression of adjacent structures. Formal endoaneurysmorrhaphy, as is done with an open AAA repair, is another alternative. In the setting of acute thrombosis, lytic therapy is the initial treatment of choice. Endovascular stent grafting is another option, especially if no suitable vein is available in a high risk patient, but this may have a lower primary patency (D).

References: Ascher E, Markevich N, Schutzer RW, Kallakuri S, Jacob T, Hingorani AP. Small popliteal artery aneurysms: are they clinically significant? *J Vasc Surg*. 2003;37(4):755–760.

Lowell RC, Gloviczki P, Hallett JW Jr, et al. Popliteal artery aneurysms: the risk of nonoperative management. *Ann Vasc Surg*. 1994;8(1):14–23.

31. E. A patient with an upper gastrointestinal bleed and a history of aortic surgery should be presumed to have an aortoenteric fistula until proven otherwise. The treatment algorithm depends on the hemodynamic stability of the patient. If the patient is unable to be stabilized due to massive hemorrhage, the patient should be taken emergently to the operating room, even if a diagnosis has not yet been established. Oftentimes, the patient will have a so-called herald bleed, after which the bleeding may temporarily stop, allowing a workup for an aortoenteric fistula. The diagnosis can be difficult to establish. Upper endoscopy is negative surprisingly often and has a low sensitivity but should be the first step in the workup. Duodenal graft erosion typically occurs at the fourth portion of the duodenum, and findings may be subtle, such as mild mucosal erosion. CT scan is highly useful, as in the presence of an aortoenteric fistula will likely demonstrate perigraft fluid, air, or inflammation, indicative of a graft infection (though less likely contrast extravasation). Fluid and inflammatory changes around a graft would be abnormal findings beyond 6 weeks after surgery (A). If the CT scan findings are negative, a nuclear-tagged white blood cell scan may be useful for establishing a graft infection (C). Arteriography is of limited benefit for the diagnosis of vascular graft infections but can be useful in preoperative planning (B). In some instances, no source of an upper gastrointestinal

bleed is found, and thus one must empirically proceed to graft excision (D). The classic operative management consisted of obtaining proximal aortic control of the aorta at the diaphragm, graft excision, closure of the aortic stump in two layers, closure of the duodenum, placing omentum in the area of the aortic stump closure, followed by an extra anatomic axillobifemoral bypass. Recently, the more accepted treatment is excision of the aortic graft and in situ placement of a human aortic homograft.

Reference: Berger P, Moll FL. Aortic graft infections: is there still a role for axillobifemoral reconstruction? *Semin Vasc Surg*. 2011;24(4):205–210.

32. C. Common iliac aneurysms are usually diagnosed incidentally. In most cases, they are found in association with an aortic aneurysm. Rare presentation includes the development of a fistula with the adjacent iliac vein or compression of the iliac vein. The natural history of common iliac aneurysms is less well defined. In a recent study, the expansion rate of common iliac aneurysms was 0.29 cm per year, and hypertension predicted faster expansion. Because no rupture of a common iliac aneurysm smaller than 3.8 cm was observed, the recommended threshold for elective repair of asymptomatic patients was larger than 3.5 cm (A, B, D, E). Treatment options include open surgical replacement with prosthetic graft or endovascular stent grafting. In patients with suitable anatomy, namely, the presence of proximal and distal landing zones, stent grafting has become the treatment of choice. Endovascular repair is associated with fewer complications overall but poses a higher risk of creating buttock claudication due to occlusion of the internal iliac artery.

Reference: Huang Y, Gloviczki P, Duncan AA, et al. Common iliac artery aneurysm: expansion rate and results of open surgical and endovascular repair. *J Vasc Surg*. 2008;47(6):1203–1210.

33. B. Popliteal aneurysms rarely rupture (A). Most commonly, they cause acute or chronic ischemia. In most series, the most common symptom is thrombosis, in as many as 49%, followed by distal embolization. As the aneurysm continues to grow, less commonly, it can compress adjacent structures, such as the popliteal vein (D, E). Chronic embolization can lead to occlusions of the infrapopliteal vessels and can complicate revascularization (C). If they present with acute ischemia, thrombolysis is the intervention of choice, followed by operative repair. Recently, endovascular stent grafting has been used, although long-term patency data are still lacking.

References: Dorigo W, Pulli R, Turini F. Acute leg ischemia from thrombosed popliteal artery aneurysms: role of preoperative thrombolysis. *Eur J Vasc Endovasc Surg*. 2002;23(3):251–254.

Shortell CK, DeWeese JA, Ouriel K, Green RM. Popliteal artery aneurysms: a 25-year surgical experience. *J Vasc Surg*. 1991;14(6):771–776.

34. C. Recent studies have shown that AAAs as large as 5.5 cm in diameter can be safely observed (D). Another recent randomized study indicated that although the perioperative mortality rate of EVAR is lower than that of open repair, long-term mortality is the same (C). Women have been shown to have higher perioperative mortality rates than men with either EVAR or open repair. EVAR should not lower the size threshold for repair in a high-cardiac risk patient if the AAA has not yet reached the 5.5-cm threshold (B). Following are the guidelines for treatment of AAAs as reported by a subcommittee of the Joint Council of the American Association for Vascular Surgery and Society for Vascular Surgery:

1. The arbitrary setting of a single-threshold diameter for elective AAA repair that is applicable to all patients is not appropriate because the decision for repair must be individualized in each case.

2. Randomized trials have shown that the risk of rupture of small AAAs is quite low and that a policy of careful surveillance of those with a diameter of as large as 5.5 cm is safe, unless there is rapid expansion (>1 cm/yr) or symptoms develop. However, early surgery is comparable to surveillance with later surgery, so patient preference is important, especially for AAAs 4.5 to 5.5 cm in diameter.

3. Based on the best available current evidence, a diameter of 5.5 cm appears to be an appropriate threshold for repair in an average patient. However, subsets of younger, low-risk patients with a long projected life expectancy may prefer early repair. If the surgeon's personal documented operative mortality rate is low, repair may be indicated at smaller sizes if that is the patient's preference.

4. For women or for AAAs with a greater than average rupture risk, 4.5 to 5 cm is an appropriate threshold for elective repair (A).

5. For high-risk patients, delay in repair until the diameter is larger is warranted, especially if endovascular aortic repair is not possible (E).

6. In view of its uncertain long-term durability and effectiveness as well as the increased surveillance burden, EVAR is most appropriate for patients at increased risk of conventional open aneurysm repair. EVAR may be the preferred treatment method if anatomy is appropriate for older high-risk patients, those with a hostile abdomen, or other clinical circumstances likely to increase the risk of conventional open repair.

7. Use of EVAR in patients with unsuitable anatomy markedly increases the risk of adverse outcomes, the need for conversion to open repair, or AAA rupture.

8. At present, there does not seem to be any justification that EVAR should change the accepted size threshold for intervention in most patients.

9. In choosing between open repair and EVAR, patient preference is of great importance. It is essential that the patients be well informed to make such choices.

References: Brewster DC, Cronenwett JL, Hallett JW Jr, et al. Guidelines for the treatment of abdominal aortic aneurysms. Report of a subcommittee of the Joint Council of the American Association for Vascular Surgery and Society for Vascular Surgery. *J Vasc Surg.* 2003;37(5):1106–1117.

Mureebe L, Egorova N, McKinsey JF, Kent KC. Gender trends in the repair of ruptured abdominal aortic aneurysms and outcomes. *J Vasc Surg.* 2010;51(4 Suppl):9 S–13 S.

35. B. Endoleak is a common complication after EVAR that can lead to aneurysm enlargement and even rupture. Endoleaks occur in as many as 40% of patients after EVAR. Most endoleaks are found in the immediate postoperative period, but late endoleaks also develop. For this reason, routine lifelong postoperative surveillance with CT scanning is recommended. New endoleaks have been identified as late as 7 years after EVAR. Endoleaks are classified into five major types (types I–V) based on the source of communication between the circulation and the aneurysm sac. The most common type of leak after endovascular repair is a type II leak, which results from retrograde filling of the aneurysm sac from the lumbar arteries or the IMA. Management of type II leaks is controversial and is based on whether the aneurysm is enlarging or stable. Options include coil embolization of the vessel, laparoscopic ligation, or observation. Type I leaks occur at the stent–graft attachment sites (either at the aorta or at the iliac arteries) (A); type III leaks occur at a stent–stent interface and are also known as modular disassociations (C); type IV leaks are directly through the graft and are due to graft material porosity (D). They usually heal spontaneously. The most dangerous type of leak is a proximal type I leak because there is a failure to achieve a proximal seal, leading to continued filling of the aneurysm sac at systemic pressures. Type I leaks require immediate treatment when discovered, typically by deploying another stent or, if unsuccessful, by open surgical conversion. Type III endoleaks represent a true mechanical failure of the endograft and require repair with an additional endograft to eliminate systemic flow and pressure in the aneurysm. Type V leak is also referred to as endotension. This can be considered idiopathic because the aneurysmal sac may appear to be enlarging without any evidence of a leak site on imaging (E).

Reference: Corriere MA, Feurer ID, Becker SY, et al. Endoleak following endovascular abdominal aortic aneurysm repair: implications for duration of screening. *Ann Surg.* 2004;239(6):800–807.

36. E. This patient most likely has an arterial thrombus secondary to heparin-induced thrombocytopenia thrombosis (HITT). The classic laboratory finding is a decrease in the platelet count of more than 50%. Although thrombocytopenia usually increases the risk of bleeding, HITT is paradoxically known to cause a hypercoagulable state; it is the second most common acquired hypercoagulable state (smoking is the most common). There are two types of HITT with type II being more common and responsible for the clinical syndrome. HITT type II is caused by antibodies to platelet-factor 4 and heparin sulfate resulting in a prothrombotic state (will appear as a white clot). It typically occurs 3 to 5 days after starting heparin. If this is suspected, heparin should be discontinued, and the patient should be started on a direct thrombin inhibitor. Argatroban is the recommended agent for patients with HITT and renal impairment. Lepirudin and bivalirudin both undergo renal excretion and should be avoided in patients with ESRD (A, D). The patient initially had acute limb ischemia secondary to cardiac emboli from atrial fibrillation. His symptoms resolved with initiation of heparin so it is unlikely that he has underlying antithrombin III deficiency (C). More studies are needed to evaluate the role of tPA in HITT (B).

References: Guzzi LM, McCollum DA, Hursting MJ. Effect of renal function on argatroban therapy in heparin-induced thrombocytopenia. *J Thromb Thrombolysis.* 2006;22(3):169–176.

Visentin GP, Ford SE, Scott JP, Aster RH. Antibodies from patients with heparin-induced thrombocytopenia/thrombosis are specific for platelet factor 4 complexed with heparin or bound to endothelial cells. *J Clin Invest.* 1994;93(1):81–88.

Vascular—Venous *18*

AMANDA C. PURDY AND JOHN McCALLUM

ABSITE 99th Percentile High-Yields

I. Deep Vein Thrombosis (DVT) and Pulmonary Embolism (PE)
   A. Can be provoked (known inciting event, such as recent surgery, malignancy) or unprovoked
   B. Most common inherited prothrombotic disorder: Factor-V Leiden mutation (unable to breakdown Factor-V); higher incidence on left side (May-Thurner syndrome)
   C. Catheter-associated upper extremity DVTs—determine if catheter is required, if it is, can keep catheter and start therapeutic anticoagulation; if not required, start anticoagulation and remove catheter in 3 to 5 days; in both cases, continue anticoagulation for 3 to 6 months
   D. Malignancy-associated DVT/PE best treated with low-molecular-weight heparin (not warfarin)

Situation	Duration of anticoagulation
Provoked DVT/PE without associated malignancy	3 months
Provoked DVT/PE in association with malignancy	Indefinite
Unprovoked DVT/PE in patient with low-moderate bleeding risk	Indefinite
Unprovoked DVT/PE in patient with high bleeding risk	3 months
DVT/PE pregnant woman	3 months OR 6 weeks after delivery (whichever is longer)
Superficial thrombophlebitis of legs	4–6 weeks of fondaparinux

   E. Phlegmasia alba dolens
      1. Caused by massive DVT, deep venous channels are affected while sparing collateral veins and therefore maintaining some degree of venous return; patients have pale blanching of extremity (milky color), edema, and discomfort
      2. Treatment is immediate anticoagulation and leg elevation; may progress to cerulea dolens
   F. Phlegmasia cerulea dolens
      1. Venous outflow of the entire lower extremity is affected; persistent venous obstruction eventually inhibits arterial inflow
      2. Patients present with pain, swelling, and a blue discoloration (cyanosis) of the extremity; pedal pulses may be diminished
      3. In addition to anticoagulation, catheter-directed thrombolysis is also recommended (unless >2 weeks duration)
   G. Paget-Schroetter syndrome (effort thrombosis of axillary or subclavian vein)
      1. Thrombosis of the axillary and/or subclavian veins
      2. Often seen in athletes who overuse the affected extremity, leading to recurrent vein compression

3. Often related to thoracic outlet syndrome, with compression of the subclavian vein in the costoclavicular space (between the 1st rib and the clavicle)
4. Diagnosed with duplex ultrasound or venogram
5. Treat with anticoagulation; if moderate-severe symptoms of <2 weeks duration can consider catheter-directed thrombolysis; after acute treatment of the DVT, proceed with 1st rib resection to prevent recurrence

H. PE
1. Signs: shortness of breath, pleuritic chest pain, tachycardia, increased respiratory rate, hypoxemic respiratory alkalosis
2. Chest radiograph usually normal, most common EKG finding is sinus tachycardia
3. Best diagnosis is CT angiogram of the chest
4. Treatment considerations:
   a) Most treated with anticoagulation
   b) Massive PE (defined as PE + hypotension): treat with systemic thrombolysis (if no contraindication)
      (1) If thrombolysis fails or patient has a contraindication to systemic thrombolysis: catheter-assisted thrombus removal
      (2) If catheter-assisted thrombus removal fails: surgical pulmonary embolectomy

II. Chronic Venous Disease
   A. Can have insufficiency in superficial, deep, and/or perforator veins
   B. Symptoms: painful varicose veins, leg swelling, and medial malleolar ulcers
   C. Hyperpigmentation in venous insufficiency caused by breakdown of extravascular RBC & subcutaneous scar tissue (liposclerosis)
   D. Diagnosis: duplex ultrasound (specifically for valve incompetence); reflux (incompetence) is diagnosed if the ultrasound shows retrograde flow of >1 second in the femoral or popliteal veins, or >0.5 second in the saphenous, tibial, deep femoral, or perforator veins; also, duplex ultrasound scan to rule out DVT
   E. Mainstay of treatment of venous insufficiency is compression therapy
   F. If compression fails, can consider surgical intervention if incompetence/reflux is in superficial or perforator veins:
      1. For superficial veins (greater or small saphenous veins) or perforator veins—treat with endovenous ablation
      2. If have concomitant symptomatic varicose veins: treat underlying venous incompetence AND can also perform sclerotherapy or stab phlebectomy of superficial varicose veins
      3. Complication of saphenous vein ablation: thrombus at saphenofemoral junction (potential risk for DVT), start ASA
      4. Telangiectasias (spider veins): not always associated with reflux—if no reflux compression and ablation will not help; treatment is cosmetic: includes injection sclerotherapy or transdermal laser therapy

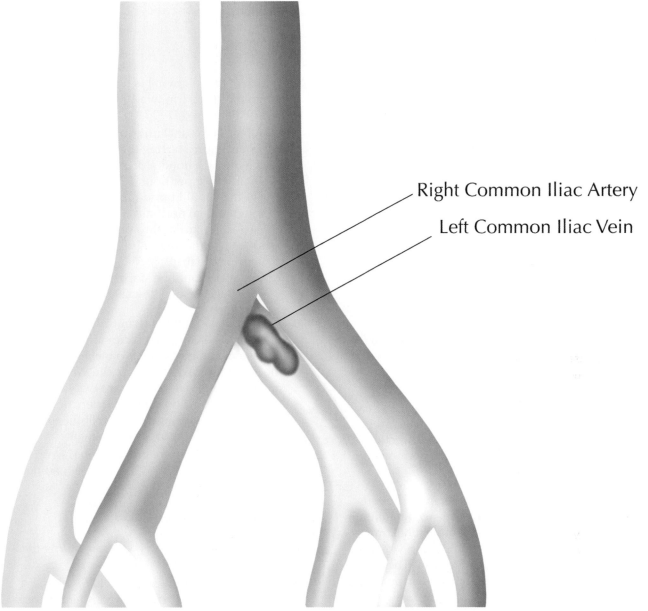

Right Common Iliac Artery

Left Common Iliac Vein

Fig. 18.1 May-Thurner Syndrome

Questions

1. Which of the following is the most common risk factor for spontaneous venous thromboembolism?
   A. Antithrombin III deficiency
   B. Factor V Leiden
   C. Protein C deficiency
   D. Protein S deficiency
   E. Antiphospholipid syndrome

2. A 60-year-old male presents with pain over his left mid-medial thigh. He had a similar event in his other thigh a month earlier. He has noted a decreased appetite. On exam the skin over the medial thigh is red, warm, and tender. He has no varicose veins, nor evidence of skin hyperpigmentation or leg swelling. Duplex scan shows an 8-cm segment of thrombosis of the mid saphenous vein, but no DVT. Which of the following is recommended?
   A. IV heparin followed by warfarin
   B. Warm compresses, nonsteroidal antiinflammatory drugs (NSAIDs), and a CT of the abdomen
   C. Ligation of the sapheno-femoral junction
   D. Fondaparinux and a CT of the abdomen
   E. Warm compresses and NSAIDs

3. A 25-year-old male college swimmer presents with sudden onset of right arm swelling and pain. A duplex ultrasound scan demonstrates thrombosis of the axillary-subclavian vein. The patient is started on IV heparin. The most important additional adjunctive therapy for this patient is:
   A. First rib resection
   B. Catheter-guided thrombolysis
   C. Lifelong anticoagulation
   D. Venous stenting
   E. Physical therapy

4. Which of the following is true regarding venous circulation?
   A. The perforating veins in the leg direct blood flow from deep to the superficial system
   B. The common iliac veins have valves
   C. In a healthy person, venous pressure increases with walking
   D. The greater saphenous vein joins the femoral vein to become the common femoral vein
   E. Muscle contraction plays no role in venous return

5. Which of the following is true regarding the initiation of heparin in a 100-kg patient with a newly diagnosed DVT?
   A. A bolus of 10,000 units of heparin should be given before starting the drip
   B. Following a bolus a drip should be started at 18 units/kg per hour
   C. Dosing should be adjusted using the international normalized ratio (INR)
   D. Activated partial thromboplastin time (aPTT) should be titrated to 100 to 120 seconds after starting the drip
   E. Heparin should be stopped if the platelet count decreases below 200,000

6. A 35-year-old female presents with left leg swelling. There are no precipitating factors. Ultrasound confirms a left iliofemoral DVT, and the patient is started on heparin. Workup reveals no evidence of risk factors for DVT, such as recent surgery, prolonged immobilization, nor any evidence of malignancy. Which of the following is most likely to be of long-term benefit?
   A. Low-molecular-weight heparin (LMWH)
   B. Long-term (>12 months) anticoagulation
   C. Lifelong compression stocking
   D. Right-to-left femoral vein bypass
   E. Venous thrombectomy

7. Which of the following is true regar ding the management of DVT?
   A. For patients with proximal DVT of the leg and no cancer history, direct Xa inhibitor is recommended over warfarin
   B. For a leg DVT in association with malignancy, warfarin is preferred over LMWH
   C. For incidentally discovered DVT, anticoagulation is unnecessary
   D. In patients with isolated distal (calf) DVT of the leg, anticoagulation therapy is superior to serial imaging
   E. In patients with a second episode of DVT, three months of anticoagulation is recommended

8. A 58-year-old male with newly diagnosed metastatic colon cancer presents to the ED with a swollen right leg and severe pain that started 1 day earlier. On exam, he has massive edema of the right leg that is tender to palpation. His foot appears blue. Duplex scan confirms a DVT. Which of the following is true about this condition?

   A. The risk of limb loss is low
   B. This occurs more commonly on the right side
   C. A pale, white foot carries a worse prognosis than a blue foot
   D. Associated hypotension is usually the result of sepsis
   E. Catheter-directed thrombolysis should be performed

9. Which of the following is the best indication for placement of an inferior vena cava (IVC) filter?

   A. A pregnant patient in the third trimester diagnosed with a new DVT
   B. A patient with severe pelvic fractures
   C. A patient with a large free-floating vena cava thrombus
   D. A recurrent DVT in a patient who is already therapeutic on warfarin
   E. Before planned thrombolysis of a new DVT

10. The most common electrocardiographic change after pulmonary embolism (PE) is:

    A. Atrial fibrillation
    B. Right bundle branch block
    C. Nonspecific ST and T wave changes
    D. S1, Q3, T3 pattern
    E. Sinus tachycardia

11. Trauma patients sustaining what type of injury are at highest risk of venous thromboembolism?

    A. Head trauma
    B. Femur fracture
    C. Pelvic fracture
    D. Splenectomy
    E. Spinal cord injury

12. A 45-year-old woman presents with a nonhealing ulcer at the medial malleolus associated with leg edema and hyperpigmentation but no signs of infection. First-line management consists of:

    A. Wet-to-dry dressings
    B. Split-thickness skin grafting
    C. Subfascial perforator ligation
    D. Local wound debridement followed by intravenous antibiotics
    E. Compression dressings

13. A 50-year-old male presents with a medial malleolar ulcer that has failed to heal with 4 weeks of compression dressings. He has large varicose veins in the lower leg, edema, and hyperpigmentation. There is no deep vein thrombosis (DVT) identified on duplex ultrasound. However, there is incompetence of the superficial, deep, and perforator systems. Which of the following is the best next step?

    A. Vein stripping of the greater saphenous vein
    B. Radiofrequency ablation (RFA) of the greater saphenous vein and ultrasound-guided perforator sclerotherapy
    C. RFA of the greater saphenous vein and compression stockings
    D. Continue with a 3-month course of compression dressing treatment
    E. Ultrasound-guided perforator vein sclerotherapy

14. A 44-year-old male presents to the emergency department (ED) with a temperature of 103°F. He is hypotensive despite a 2-L fluid bolus. He is prepped for a right internal jugular 9-French central venous line to start pressors while being worked up for an underlying cause. Following placement of the catheter, pulsatile bleeding is noted from the catheter. What is the best next step?

    A. Downsize to a smaller catheter in the ED, transfer the patient to the intensive care unit (ICU), and remove it in several hours
    B. Immediately remove the catheter and hold pressure for 10 to 15 minutes
    C. Immediately remove the catheter and get a duplex ultrasound study of the neck
    D. Remove the catheter under direct surgical exposure
    E. Transfer patient to the ICU, then remove, hold pressure, and place a suture in the skin

15. A 40-year-old woman presents with pain and tenderness at the site of a longstanding varicose vein in her calf. There is a palpable cord with surrounding erythema. Duplex scan shows localized thrombus within the varicose vein, and no DVT. Management consists of:

    A. Intravenous (IV) heparin sodium
    B. Subcutaneous low-molecular-weight heparin
    C. Warm compresses and nonsteroidal antiinflammatory drugs
    D. Ligation of saphenous vein at saphenofemoral junction
    E. IV antibiotics

Answers

1. B. The primary risk factors for spontaneous venous thromboembolism (VTE) as described by Virchow include stasis of blood flow, endothelial injury, and hypercoagulability. In cases of spontaneous VTE, hypercoagulability is the most important factor. Factors that contribute to hypercoagulability include factor V Leiden, prothrombin gene mutation, protein C and S deficiency, antithrombin III deficiency, elevated homocysteine levels, and antiphospholipid syndrome. In addition, nonacquired causes of VTE include smoking (most common), obesity, pregnancy, malignancy, and use of oral contraceptives. In surgical patients, the cause of VTE is multifactorial because postoperative stasis from prolonged bed rest and endothelial injury from trauma or recent surgery are significant factors. In trauma patients, spinal cord injury has the highest risk of VTE. Other risk factors for VTE include history of VTE, advanced age, and varicose veins. Factor V Leiden is the most common genetic defect associated with thrombophilia (A, C–E). Factor V Leiden is a single-point mutation in the gene that codes for coagulation factor V. It makes factor V resistant to inactivation by activated protein C (which is a natural anticoagulant protein). The mutation is transmitted in an autosomal dominant fashion and accounts for 92% of cases of anticoagulant protein resistance. The mutation is present in 4% to 6% of the general population and is associated with a sixfold increased risk of VTE in heterozygotes. In homozygotes, the risk is 80-fold. In patients with their first VTE, factor V Leiden was present in 15% to 20%. There is no standard guideline for the duration of anticoagulation therapy in patients with an acquired hypercoagulable state. It is believed an individualized approach should be taken to access each person's risk of a recurrent VTE and compare this to their relative risk of a bleeding event. Interestingly, in one study, the risk of recurrent VTE was similar among carriers of the factor V Leiden gene compared with those without this mutation, suggesting that they do not need longer anticoagulation than the standard recommendation for a first-time event.

References: Bauer KA. Duration of anticoagulation: applying the guidelines and beyond. *Hematology Am Soc Hematol Educ Program*. 2010;2010(1):210–215.

Mazza JJ. Hypercoagulability and venous thromboembolism: a review. WMJ. 2004;103(2):41–49.

2. D. Unprovoked SVT, and in particular, recurrent unprovoked SVT, and more specifically recurrent, unprovoked SVT in different limbs (superficial migratory thrombophlebitis) should prompt concern for hypercoagulability and, in particular, malignancy. Superficial migratory thrombophlebitis is particularly associated with pancreatic cancer (Trousseau sign) and, to a lesser degree, stomach and lung cancer. Thus, treatment should include a targeted workup for malignancy (that should be tailored to findings on history, review of systems, and physical exam) (B, C–E). Given the decreased appetite, suspicion for GI cancer should be high and a CT scan appropriate. SVT within the saphenous vein in the upper thigh, within 3 cm of the saphenofemoral junction, and those with long segments (>5 cm) have an increased risk of propagating into the deep system and thus benefit from anticoagulation (A). A recent study comparing fondaparinux with placebo demonstrated a decrease in DVT, recurrent thrombophlebitis, and clot progression with fondaparinux.

References: Chengelis DL, Bendick PJ, Glover JL, Brown OW, Ranval TJ. Progression of superficial venous thrombosis to deep vein thrombosis. *J Vasc Surg*. 1996;24(5):745–749.

Decousus H, Prandoni P, Mismetti P, et al. Fondaparinux for the treatment of superficial-vein thrombosis in the legs. *N Engl J Med*. 2010;363(13):1222–1232.

3. A. Paget-Schroetter syndrome, also known as effort-induced thrombosis, is a spontaneous thrombosis of the axillary-subclavian vein. It is thought to be, in most instances, a manifestation of thoracic outlet syndrome, whereby a hypertrophied or aberrant muscle compresses the axillary-subclavian vein as it passes between the first rib and the clavicle. It tends to develop in young, active patients after vigorous activity (swimming, pitching, weightlifting), although it can also occur spontaneously. It usually presents in men more often than women. Secondary axillary/subclavian vein thrombosis can also present in those with mediastinal tumors, congestive heart failure (CHF), and nephrotic syndrome. Diagnosis is best established via duplex ultrasonography. The patient should be promptly started on IV heparin. The most important adjunctive measure to prevent recurrence and long-term swelling is thoracic outlet decompression via first rib resection. The timing is controversial but is not time sensitive. Systemic thrombolysis is not indicated. However, the journal CHEST recommends catheter-directed thrombolysis for this condition if the patient has moderate-severe symptoms and presents with less than 2 weeks of symptoms. The benefit of catheter-directed thrombolysis in this situation is a decreased risk of postthrombotic syndrome (B). A follow-up venogram is frequently obtained to identify any correctable anatomic abnormalities. Stenting a residual stenosis in this area without decompressing the thoracic outlet is contraindicated because the ongoing compression will invariably crush the stent and cause further venous damage, making any further intervention even more difficult. Residual venous stenoses can be treated with angioplasty, although some authors recommend doing this after the first rib resection. A recent metaanalysis demonstrated a significant improvement in symptoms in those that received a first rib resection compared to those that did not. More than 40% of patients in the control group needed to have a rib resection due to recurrent symptoms. In an active athlete, and in particular one who performs repetitive movements with the arm overhead (which by itself can compress the vein), first rib resection is the best option (C–E).

References: Angle N, Gelabert HA, Farooq MM, et al. Safety and efficacy of early surgical decompression of the thoracic outlet for Paget-Schroetter syndrome. *Ann Vasc Surg*. 2001;15(1):37–42.

Lee WA, Hill BB, Harris EJ Jr, Semba CP, Olcott C IV. Surgical intervention is not required for all patients with subclavian vein thrombosis. *J Vasc Surg*. 2000;32(1):57–67.

Machleder HI. Evaluation of a new treatment strategy for Paget-Schroetter syndrome: spontaneous thrombosis of the axillary-subclavian vein. *J Vasc Surg*. 1993;17(2):305–315.

Urschel HC Jr, Razzuk MA. Paget-Schroetter syndrome: what is the best management? *Ann Thorac Surg.* 2000;69(6):1663–1668.

Lugo J, Tanious A, Armstrong P, et al. Acute Paget-Schroetter syndrome: does the first rib routinely need to be removed after thrombolysis? *Ann Vasc Surg.* 2015;29(6):1073–1077.

4. D. The lower extremity veins are divided into superficial, perforating, and deep veins. The superficial venous system consists of the greater saphenous and lesser saphenous veins. The deep veins follow the course of major arteries. Paired veins parallel the anterior and posterior tibial and peroneal arteries and join to form the popliteal vein. The popliteal vein becomes the femoral vein as it passes through the adductor hiatus. In the proximal thigh, the greater saphenous vein joins with the femoral vein to become the common femoral vein. Multiple perforating veins traverse the deep fascia to connect the superficial and deep venous systems. The most important perforators are the Cockett and Boyd perforators. The Cockett perforators drain the lower part of the leg medially, whereas the Boyd perforators connect the greater saphenous vein to the deep vein higher up in the medial lower leg, approximately 10 cm below the knee. Blood flows from the superficial to the deep venous system (A). Incompetence of these perforators is a major contributor to the development of venous stasis and ulceration. There are no valves in the portal vein, superior vena cava, inferior vena cava (IVC), or common iliac vein (B). The calf muscles serve an important function in augmenting venous return by acting as a pump to return blood to the heart (E). For this reason, patients who are bedridden are prone to venous stasis. Venous pressure drops dramatically with walking because of the action of the calf muscles but increases in patients with venous obstruction because this leads to persistent stasis that muscle contraction cannot overcome (C). This is why compression stockings are recommended for these patients as an adjunct to normal venous return.

5. B. If a heparin drip is started, a bolus of 80 units/kg (8000 units for the above patient) should first be given followed by the continued infusion of heparin at 18 units/kg per hour (A). In patients with DVT, the aPTT needs to be drawn every 6 to 12 hours with a goal rate of 60 to 90 seconds (D). INR is checked in patients on warfarin (C). Heparin can potentially lead to heparin-induced thrombocytopenia (HIT). This usually happens 5 days or more after the initiation of heparin and will present as a 50% drop in platelet count (E).

Reference: Hirsh J, Bauer KA, Donati MB, Gould M, Samama MM, Weitz JI. Parenteral anticoagulants: American college of chest physicians evidence-based clinical practice guidelines (8th edition). *Chest.* 2008;133(6 Suppl):141S–159S.

6. B. DVT and pulmonary embolism (PE) affect up to 900,000 people per year in the United States, and their incidence increases with age. When a patient presents with a DVT, always try to determine which part of the Virchow triad (stasis, vascular injury, and hypercoagulability) can explain the event. This will serve as a reminder to perform a careful history and physical examination to assess risk factors for DVT. In most cases, the causes are multifactorial. The duration and type of anticoagulation depend on whether the DVT is provoked (i.e., malignancy, recent surgery, prolonged immobilization) or unprovoked, what the provoking factor is, and on the location (proximal or distal leg) of the DVT. Proximal (iliofemoral) DVTs are more likely to lead to massive swelling and long-term sequelae of postphlebitic syndrome. As such, more consideration should be given to the type of anticoagulant, the duration, use of thrombolytics, and mechanical thromboembolectomy as compared with distal DVT. LMWH is not as efficacious for proximal DVT (A). For a proximal (iliofemoral) DVT, that is unprovoked (no clear contributing factors), the recommendation is for long-term (>12 months) anticoagulation. The benefit of compression stockings to prevent postphlebitic syndrome is controversial (C). Most authors recommend 2 years of compression; lifelong compression has no benefit, has poor patient compliance, and is associated with significant costs of renewing expensive stockings every 6 months. A right-to-left femoral vein bypass (with right leg saphenous vein) is rarely performed and would be a last resort for chronic venous stasis that is unresponsive to endovascular options (D). Thrombolytic therapy is an option for select patients with severe iliofemoral DVT, particularly if they present with phlegmasia. Venous thrombectomy is reserved for patients with phlegmasia who have failed thrombolytic therapy (E).

Reference: Heffner JE. Update of antithrombotic guidelines: medical professionalism and the funnel of knowledge. *Chest.* 2016;149(2):293–294.

7. A. The American College of Chest Physicians released updated guidelines in 2016 for the management of DVTs. One major change is that patients with proximal DVT of the leg and no cancer history should now be treated with a direct Xa inhibitor (dabigatran, rivaroxaban, apixaban, or edoxaban) over warfarin. Additionally, initial parenteral anticoagulation with a heparin drip is not required when using rivaroxaban and apixaban. However, a heparin drip should be started before administering dabigatran or edoxaban and overlapped with warfarin therapy. Several reports have shown the superiority of these novel oral anticoagulants (NOACS). Additionally, idarucizumab is now available as a reversal agent for dabigatran allowing NOACs to be more commonly prescribed. In patients with a cancer history and proximal DVT of the leg, LMWH is recommended over warfarin and direct Xa inhibitors (B). This is unchanged from the prior guidelines. In patients with a proximal DVT of the leg provoked by surgery, 3 months of anticoagulation therapy is recommended over a longer time-limited period (6, 9, 12, or 24 months). This recommendation applies to patients with both low and high bleeding risks. The management of isolated calf DVT remains controversial. Anticoagulation is recommended for those with severe leg symptoms or those with risk factors for propagation. In patients with an isolated distal DVT of the leg and without severe symptoms or risk factors for extension, serial imaging of the deep veins for 2 weeks is recommended over anticoagulation therapy (D). There is no consensus on the duration of therapy for patients with a second episode of DVT because this depends on the presence of reversible risk factors, underlying cause, malignancy, life expectancy, and the burden of therapy. However, most surgeons would recommend at least 1 year of anticoagulation therapy for patients with a second episode of DVT and lifelong anticoagulation for patients with more than two episodes of DVT (E). Incidentally discovered DVTs should be treated with anticoagulation (C).

References: Connors JM. Antidote for factor Xa anticoagulants. N Engl J Med. 2015;373(25):2471–2472.

Heffner JE. Update of antithrombotic guidelines: medical professionalism and the funnel of knowledge. *Chest.* 2016;149(2):293–294.

8. E. Massive iliofemoral DVT can lead to impaired arterial blood flow due to massive swelling. Early on, the limb turns pale and is referred to as phlegmasia alba (white) dolens. In a subgroup of patients, this may progress to impending gangrene phlegmasia cerulea (blue) dolens as in the patient described. When the majority of the deep venous channels are burdened with clots, the relatively smaller superficial venous channels are tasked with draining the entire leg. Patients develop a tender, pale, and edematous extremity. This is known as "milk-leg" since the pale extremity appears whitish (alba). As the disease progresses and the superficial venous channels are also affected, the entire venous drainage of the leg is compromised, causing massive edema in the leg. As the swelling continues, arterial malperfusion ensues, leading to severe ischemia (blue extremity), risking limb loss (C). DVT and as an extension, phlegmasia, both occur more commonly on the left. This is a result of the left iliac vein frequently being compressed by the right iliac artery (known as May-Thurner syndrome) (B). Underlying malignancy is the most common risk factor identified for phlegmasia. The fastest and safest method of confirming the diagnosis is with duplex ultrasound. CT angiography is not required unless history, exam, and ultrasound findings are equivocal. Initial treatment is similar to that for an acute DVT, with some qualifiers. More emphasis should be placed on leg elevation. Due to fluid sequestration, patients may present with hypovolemic shock and thus may need massive volume resuscitation (D). The risks of limb loss, pulmonary embolism, postphlebitic syndrome, and mortality are all high (A). As such, thrombolytic therapy has emerged as the treatment of choice.

Reference: Chinsakchai K, Ten Duis K, Moll FL, de Borst GJ. Trends in management of phlegmasia cerulea dolens. *Vasc Endovascular Surg.* 2011;45(1):5–14.

9. D. Enthusiasm for the aggressive use of IVC filters is diminishing. Filters left in place for long periods of time can lead to complications, including migration of the filter, fracturing of the legs of the filter, vena cava perforation, and the increased risk of a recurrent DVT. In a prospective randomized study of patients with DVT, the routine addition of an IVC filter did not improve mortality compared with heparin and warfarin alone. Additionally, PREPIC 2 trial has also demonstrated an increase number of recurrent PEs in the filter group compared to the anticoagulation only group (3% versus 1.5%). Thus, the majority of IVC filters are now retrievable and should optimally be removed within 9 to 12 weeks. Consensus opinion from most societies is that the strongest indication for an IVC filter placement is a patient who develops a venous thromboembolic event (VTE [DVT or PE]) who has a contraindication to anticoagulation (such as active gastrointestinal bleeding). Other indications are a new VTE that develops in a patient who is already receiving therapeutic anticoagulation, or a patient with a VTE who is already receiving anticoagulation and in whom a major hemorrhage develops (B, C–E). Relative indications include prophylaxis in high-risk populations (severe head, pelvic, or spinal cord trauma), massive PE treated with thrombolysis or

thrombectomy (to prevent further decompensation), and the presence of a large free-floating thrombus in the IVC. Pregnant patients diagnosed with a new DVT should be started on anticoagulation with low-molecular-weight heparin for the remainder of the pregnancy and up to 6 weeks postpartum (A). Warfarin should be avoided since it is teratogenic.

References: Decousus H, Leizorovicz A, Parent F, et al. A clinical trial of vena caval filters in the prevention of pulmonary embolism in patients with proximal deep-vein thrombosis. *N Engl J Med.* 1998;338(7):409–416.

Millward SF, Oliva VL, Bell SD, et al. Günther tulip retrievable vena cava filter: Results from the Registry of the Canadian Interventional Radiology Association. *J Vasc Interv Radiol.* 2001;12(9):1053–1058.

Rajasekhar A. Inferior vena cava filters: current best practices. *J Thromb Thrombolysis.* 2015;39(3):315–327.

10. E. The most common finding on electrocardiography after a PE is sinus tachycardia (present in almost half of patients) (A–D). A heart rate greater than 100 beats per minute with associated tachypnea in the setting of suspected PE should further raise concern. The classic finding on an electrocardiogram is the S1, Q3, T3 pattern, which consists of a prominent S wave in lead I and a Q wave and inverted T wave in lead III. This electrocardiographic finding indicates right ventricular strain from a large PE, but it is not commonly present. A large PE will lead to an enlargement of the right ventricle causing the interventricular septum to deviate to the left. The right bundle branch stretches, leading to a right bundle branch block.

11. E. The increased risk of the development of VTE in surgical patients is multifactorial. Patients will have a period of activated coagulation, transient depression of fibrinolysis, and temporary immobilization. In addition, many patients may have a central venous catheter in place and have concomitant cardiac disease, malignancy, or intrinsic hypercoagulable states, all of which increase a patient's chance of a VTE. Trauma patients, in particular, have a high risk of VTE. In trauma patients, spinal cord injury (odds ratio, 8.33) and fracture of the femur or tibia (odds ratio, 4.82) were the injuries with the greatest risk of VTE (A–D). In one large prospective study, other risk factors in trauma patients on multivariate analysis included older age, blood transfusion, and need for surgery.

Reference: Geerts WH, Code KI, Jay RM, Chen E, Szalai JP. A prospective study of venous thromboembolism after major trauma. *N Engl J Med.* 1994;331(24):1601–1606.

12. E. This patient has classic signs of chronic venous insufficiency. Venous stasis ulcers are classically located at the medial malleolus. The precise cause of venous stasis ulcers is unclear but seems to be multifactorial. The increased venous pressure from incompetent valves results in an impedance of capillary flow, which leads to leukocyte trapping. These leukocytes release oxygen free radicals and proteolytic enzymes that lead to local inflammation. The increased venous pressure also leads to the leakage of proteins such as fibrinogen, which act as a barricade to oxygen and growth factors necessary for wound healing. First-line therapy for the treatment of venous stasis ulcers is compression therapy (A–D). The workup for this patient should include a duplex ultrasound scan of the venous system, specifically looking for valvular incompetence of the deep, superficial, and perforating veins.

A popular and effective compression bandage is the Unna boot, which contains zinc oxide, glycerin, gelatin, and calamine lotion. The boot should be wrapped starting at the foot, up to just below the knee. It can remain in place for as long as a week. It should not be used in the setting of an active infection of the ulcer. In this situation, debridement and antibiotics will be needed first.

13. C. A spectrum of chronic venous disorders, from varicose veins to venous stasis ulcers, afflicts 20% to 25% of the population. The underlying etiology is incompetence of the venous valves in either the deep, superficial (saphenous), or perforator veins. Patients with chronic venous disease are classified and treated based on the severity of their disease. The CEAP (clinical, etiologic, anatomic, and pathophysiologic) classification is used worldwide to standardize this evaluation. It is important when discussing treatment with a patient that he or she understands that this is an incurable disease and that the goal of intervention is to minimize symptoms and prevent recurrence. In general, superficial incompetence is dealt with first. In a patient with a nonhealing wound that has incompetent valves in all three venous systems, (superficial, perforator, and deep) and is unresponsive to compression therapy, the superficial venous incompetence is addressed first by obliterating the saphenous vein along with compression therapy. This can be done via saphenous vein stripping, foam sclerotherapy, or RFA. A recent randomized study demonstrated equal results with all three approaches. That being said, RFA is generally preferred and is the current recommendation of the American Venous Forum, due to its less invasive nature as compared with stripping (A–E). Freedom of reflux has been seen in 93% of patients at 2 years after ablation therapy. Primary venous insufficiency is a recognized risk factor for the development of DVT, and it is important to rule this out before intervention to minimize treatment failure. If treating the superficial system is not successful, the next step is to treat the perforator incompetence. This is done via ultrasound-guided sclerotherapy. There is no surgical treatment that is reliably effective for deep system incompetence. A recent randomized study confirmed the benefit of early ablation of the saphenous vein to promote wound healing, as opposed to a longer (6 month) trial of compression therapy.

References: Gohel MS, Heatley F, Liu X, et al. A randomized trial of early endovenous ablation in venous ulceration. *N Engl J Med.* 2018;378(22):2105–2114.

Meissner MH. What is effective care for varicose veins? *Phlebology.* 2016;31(1 Suppl):80–87.

O'Donnell TF Jr, Passman MA, Marston WA, et al. Management of venous leg ulcers: clinical practice guidelines of the Society for Vascular Surgery and the American Venous Forum. *J Vasc Surg.* 2014;60(2 Suppl):3S–59S.

14. D. The right internal jugular vein is the preferred option for central line placement because it is easily accessible and has a lower risk of pneumothorax compared to a subclavian line. It also has a straight course into the right atrium. In 70% of individuals, the internal jugular vein lies anterolateral to the carotid artery. However, in some cases, it may lie directly anterior or posterior to the carotid artery, increasing the risk of a carotid artery cannulation. If the carotid artery is entered with the probe needle (as evidenced by pulsatile bleeding), the needle should be immediately removed and pressure should be held for 10 minutes. If the artery is cannulated with a dilator or catheter, then the catheter should not be removed blindly. This could lead to a potential airway-threatening hemorrhage. It is safer to remove the catheter in the operating room via direct surgical exposure, followed by suture repair of the artery (A–C, E).

Reference: Kron I, Ailawadi G. Cardiovascular monitoring and support. In: Fischer JE, ed. *Fischer's mastery of surgery.* 6th ed. Lippincott Williams & Wilkins; 2011:45–66.

15. C. The patient has superficial venous thrombosis (SVT) or thrombophlebitis. This entity is essentially a clotted surface vein. A palpable cord is suggestive of the diagnosis, as are accompanying pain and erythema. There are a few pitfalls in the diagnosis and management of SVT. Patients with SVT may have a concomitant DVT (5%–40%); thus, a duplex ultrasound scan of the venous system is essential. Second, SVT can easily be misdiagnosed as cellulitis, in which case antibiotics may be inappropriately prescribed and a duplex ultrasound scan not obtained. SVT is generally best managed with warm compresses and NSAIDs. IV antibiotics are reserved for septic thrombophlebitis, which is typically associated with an intravenous line (E). Systemic anticoagulation is reserved for a SVT that is near the deep system (A, B). If anticoagulation is contraindicated, ligation of the saphenous vein at the saphenofemoral junction is indicated for a saphenous vein SVT (D). Varicose veins cause stasis and thus predispose to SVT.

Vascular—Access 19

LUIS FELIPE CABRERA VARGAS, MARK ARCHIE, AND CHRISTIAN DE VIRGILIO

ABSITE 99th Percentile High-Yields

I. Vascular access for hemodialysis (HD) in Patients with End-Stage Renal Disease (ESRD)
   A. Catheters
      1. Temporary noncuffed, nontunneled dialysis catheter
      2. Permanent (cuffed) or tunneled-dialysis catheter (TDC)
   B. Autogenous surgical access (arteriovenous fistula [AVF])
      1. Preferred locations
         a) Upper > lower extremities; distal > proximal
         b) Nondominant > dominant arm
         c) Cephalic > basilic > brachial veins > femoral vein of the thigh
      2. End-to-side preferred to side-to-side anastomosis
   C. Nonautogenous surgical access (arteriovenous graft [AVG])
      1. Material: prosthetic (PTFE), biologic (bovine, human cryopreserved veins)
      2. Locations: upper arm, forearm, thigh

II. Comparing Vascular Access for HD

Catheters	AVF	AVG
1. Ideal for short-term hemodialysis, or as a bridging tool (AVF, graft or kidney transplantation)	1. Best overall option for long-term hemodialysis	1. Ideal for patients who are not candidates for AVF
2. Best avoided for long-term use	2. Advantages: lower risk of infection and thrombosis, highest long-term patency (70%–80% at 1 year), greatest blood flow volume during dialysis, lowest need for reinterventions	2. Advantages: widely available, short wait time to access (does not need to mature), if thrombose relatively easy to declot.
3. To reduce infection, often coated with antibiotics, silver, or heparin (reduces bacterial trapping)	3. Disadvantages: require at least 6 weeks to mature, some never work	3. Disadvantages: lower long-term patency (about 50% at 1 year), higher thrombosis rates (due to intimal hyperplasia), higher infection rate (vs AVF)
4. Advantages: immediate use, easily removed if infected		
5. Disadvantages: highest incidence of 1 year mortality, thrombotic complications, central vein stenosis, and bacterial infections		

III. Surgical Planning
   A. Age (elderly may be less suitable for AVF), hand-dominance (prefer nondominant arm), comorbid conditions (diabetics may develop severe radial/ulnar artery atherosclerosis), presence of pacemaker (leads to stenoses of proximal veins)
   B. Duplex ultrasound vein and artery mapping
      1. Veins (with soft tourniquet in place)
         a) Cephalic, basilic, brachial; assess patency and size (ideally > 3 mm)
      2. Arteries
         a) Brachial, radial, ulnar; assess size (ideally > 2 mm); severe medical calcification may be unclampable, look for flow limiting plaque

C. Fistula first initiative (order of preference): radio-cephalic (Cimino) > brachio-cephalic > brachio-basilic (may require 2 stages, first construction, second superficialization) > AVG

D. For distal fistulas from radial or ulnar arteries, assess arterial dominance of the hand with Allen test

IV. Complications
  A. Excessive bleeding from dialysis puncture site
    1. Need to rule out stenosis of outflow vein or central venous system (high venous pressure)
    2. Rule out use of anticoagulants
  B. Aneurysm of AVF (may be due to repeat needle trauma or central stenosis)
    1. Most are benign and can be observed
    2. Repair if rapidly expanding, overlying skin thinning, skin ulceration, or excessive bleeding
    3. Prior to repair, rule out stenosis of outflow vein or central venous system as cause
  C. Pseudoaneurysm of AVG (due to repeat needle trauma or infection)
    1. Small or uninfected ones can be observed
      a) Repair if large
    2. Resect AVG if infected
  D. Thrombosis
  E. Steal
    1. Stage I: asymptomatic retrograde diastolic flow (US finding alone)
    2. Stage II: pain on exertion and/or during HD
    3. Stage III: pain at rest
    4. Stage IV: ulceration/necrosis/gangrene
  F. Ischemic monomelic neuropathy (IMN)
  G. High-output cardiac failure

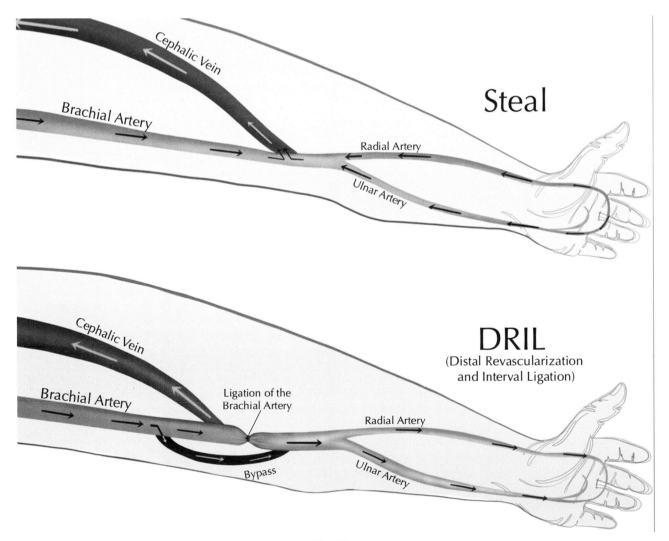

Fig. 19.1

V. Surgical Treatments of Steal Syndrome

Access Ligation	Banding Procedure	MILLER Procedure (Minimally Invasive Limited Ligation Endoluminal-Assisted Revision)	PAI Procedure (Proximalization of the Arterial Inflow)	DRIL Procedure (Distal Revascularization with Interval Ligation)	RUDI Procedure (Revision Using Distal Inflow)	RUPI Procedure (Revision Using Proximal Inflow)
Complete resolution of steal syndrome Loss of the vascular access Con: need new AVF with new risk of developing steal syndrome	Reduction of the access flow for high flow-associated steal syndrome Best results if intraoperative flow measurements are used Con: banding a low-flow vascular access will lead to inefficient dialysis and thrombosis	Banding of the vascular access with a nonresorbable suture guided with a 4–5 mm dilatation balloon Controlled reduction in the vessel diameter Only for high flow-associated steal syndrome	Enhances access flow Ideal for low flow-associated steal syndrome	Cons: complex surgery Longer operative time Need to harvest suitable vein Hand perfusion reliant on a bypass graft	Ideal for brachial AV access patients with high flow-induced steal or cardiac failure Creates bypass from distal artery to fistula (while ligating original anastomosis)	Uses smaller caliber graft to increase resistance

Questions

1. A 63-year-old man with end-stage renal disease on dialysis via a left upper arm arteriovenous graft (AVG) presents to the emergency department with what he describes as "pulsatile bleeding" from the area of where dialysis was performed the day before. He states the bleeding stopped after wrapping his arm. On physical exam, his temperature is 100.5°C and his heart rate is 100. The AVG has a thrill. Overlying the AVG, at the site of the bleed, there is a small black eschar with a small aneurysmal swelling. His white blood cell (WBC) count is $12,000 \times 10^3/mm^3$ and a duplex ultrasound demonstrates a pseudoaneurysm at the site of eschar. What is the next best step in management?
   A. Discharge the patient with oral antibiotics
   B. Admit the patient for intravenous (IV) antibiotics
   C. Obtain a fistulogram
   D. Take patient to the operating room for graft excision
   E. Place a covered stent across the pseudoaneurysm

2. A 45-year-old female returns to the emergency department 8 hours after having undergone a left upper arm arteriovenous graft (AVG) complaining of severe forearm pain. On examination, the forearm is soft and supple. The hand appears to be pink, with a normal temperature, and a 1+ radial pulse. There is a good thrill in the graft. She has both motor and sensory deficits in the hand in both the median and ulnar nerve distributions. The next step in the management is:
   A. Distal revascularization with interval ligation
   B. Observation
   C. Ligation of the graft
   D. Obtain nerve conduction studies
   E. Forearm fasciotomy

3. A 65-year-old female with end-stage renal disease presents with recurrent episodes of congestive heart failure. She is currently dialyzed via a left arm brachiocephalic arteriovenous fistula (AVF). Upon compression of the fistula, her heart rate decreases from 80 to 60 beats per minute, and blood pressure increases from 120/70 to 140/80 mm-Hg. Which of the following is true about this condition?
   A. The fistula should be ligated
   B. It is unlikely that the fistula is contributing to the patient's heart failure

   C. Plicating the fistula may help prevent another episode of heart failure
   D. She should undergo a distal revascularization and interval ligation
   E. The fistula should be converted to a graft

4. A 65-year-old woman undergoes creation of an upper arm arteriovenous (AV) graft for hemodialysis in the left arm using a 6-mm polytetrafluoroethylene graft. Three weeks later, the patient reports marked coolness, pallor, and numbness in the hand as well as pain in the hand at rest. Motor exam is normal. On examination, there is no palpable pulse at the radial artery and only a monophasic Doppler signal. Upon graft compression, a pulse becomes palpable and the signal becomes biphasic. Which of the following is the best management option?
   A. Distal revascularization and interval ligation of the brachial artery
   B. Ligation of the AV graft and placing the upper arm graft in same arm
   C. Ligation of the AV graft and placing the fistula in the dominant arm
   D. Banding of the AV graft adjacent to the arterial anastomosis
   E. Banding of the AV graft adjacent to the venous anastomosis

5. A 45-year-old male develops progressive end-stage renal disease secondary to severe hypertension. His glomerular filtration rate is 19 mL/min, and dialysis is anticipated within the next 6 months. He is right-handed and appears to have good veins in both arms and normal pulses. Which of the following is the best management plan for dialysis access?
   A. Delay access until about a month before anticipated dialysis
   B. Proceed with left radiocephalic AVF (Cimino fistula)
   C. Proceed with left brachiocephalic AVF
   D. Proceed with left brachiobasilic AVF
   E. Proceed with right radiocephalic AVF

6. A 45-year-old female with end-stage renal disease presents with recent onset of headaches, hoarseness of her voice, and bilateral arm swelling for 2 days. She has a history of multiple procedures in both arms and legs for hemodialysis access. Most recently, she underwent an arteriovenous graft (AVG) in her right upper arm 2 weeks earlier. On examination her neck appears to be engorged and her face swollen. There are numerous visible veins on her chest wall. Which of the following is the best management option?

A. Ligation of the AVG

B. Plication of the AVG

C. Attempt venoplasty of superior vena cava (SVC)

D. Place stent in SVC

E. Move AVG to right arm

7. A 45-year-old male with long-standing diabetes and progressive end-stage renal failure presents to the emergency department (ED) with progressive shortness of breath, vague abdominal pain, and marked leg edema. Laboratory values are remarkable for metabolic acidosis and azotemia but a normal white blood cell count. Dialysis is urgently needed. Dialysis access would be best instituted via:

A. Right internal jugular vein tunneled, cuffed catheter

B. Right internal jugular vein nontunneled, uncuffed catheter

C. Left internal jugular vein, tunneled, cuffed catheter

D. Right subclavian vein uncuffed, nontunneled catheter

E. Right femoral vein cuffed tunneled catheter

8. A left internal jugular vein central line is placed. Fifteen minutes later, the patient is hypotensive. Distended neck veins are noted. Breath sounds are clear bilaterally. What is the most likely cause of the patient's hypotension?

A. Perforated right atrium

B. Perforated subclavian vein

C. Perforated subclavian artery

D. Tension pneumothorax

E. Perforated right ventricle

9. A 50-year-old male with longstanding history of hemodialysis via a left brachiocephalic arteriovenous fistula (AVF) presents with an aneurysm within the midportion of the AVF. He reports that there has recently been excessive bleeding when the needles have been pulled out. On physical examination, the aneurysm is about 3 cm in size. The overlying skin appears supple, without ulceration. The next step in the management consists of:

A. Fistulogram

B. Resection/plication of the aneurysm

C. Replacement of fistula with an AV graft

D. Ligation of the fistula

E. Observation

10. In comparing the three modalities used for hemodialysis (central venous catheter [permacath], arteriovenous [AV] graft, and AV fistula), which of the following is true?

A. They are equal in terms of 1-year patient mortality

B. The primary patency for AV fistula and AV graft is similar

C. The secondary patency for AV fistula and AV graft is similar

D. Time to maturation for AV fistulas and grafts is similar

E. A permacath is the best dialysis option in the elderly

11. An intubated patient in the OR develops an air embolism after central venous catheter insertion. Which of the following murmurs are associated with this condition?

A. Austin-Flint murmur

B. Carey Coombs murmur

C. Means-Lerman scratch murmur

D. Still murmur

E. Millwheel murmur

Answers

1. D. This patient has a pseudoaneurysm of his AVG that appears to be infected, given his fever and elevated WBC. This requires excision of his graft. Though the bleeding has stopped, an infected pseudoaneurysm is inherently unstable and will likely bleed again, which could be catastrophic. Thus, antibiotics alone would not be adequate (A, B). A fistulogram is also not indicated as the graft is infected (C). For a large, noninfected pseudoaneurysm, a covered stent is a potential treatment option (E).

Reference: Mudoni A, Cornacchiari M, Gallieni M, et al. Aneurysms and pseudoaneurysms in dialysis access. *Clin Kidney J.* 2015;8(4):363–367.

2. C. This patient has findings of ischemic monomelic neuropathy (IMN), a rare complication after vascular access surgery. The incidence of this complication is less than 1% and is more common in female and diabetic patients. IMN results in pain, numbness (in fingers), paresthesia, and motor weakness (intrinsic hand muscles) usually shortly after surgery. It can be distinguished from steal syndrome by its faster onset and mild or absent signs of clinical ischemia. The pathophysiology of IMN is poorly understood but is thought to be caused by a loss of blood flow from distal nerve tissue leading to distal neuropathies. IMN is a clinical diagnosis and electromyography and nerve conduction studies are only needed when the clinical neurologic exam is equivocal (D). The recommended treatment for IMN is ligation of the newly created access, which may lead to resolution of neuropathy in some patients (B,C). Distal revascularization and interval ligation(DRIL) can be utilized in steal syndrome, but not in IMN (A). This patient should not undergo forearm fasciotomy, as she has a soft and supple forearm, making compartment syndrome very unlikely (E).

References: Datta S, Mahal S, Govindarajan R. Ischemic monomelic neuropathy after arteriovenous fistula surgery: clinical features, electrodiagnostic findings, and treatment. *Cureus.* 2019;11(7):e5191.

Thimmisetty RK, Pedavally S, Rossi NF, Fernandes JAM, Fixley J. Ischemic monomelic neuropathy: diagnosis, pathophysiology, and management. *Kidney Int Rep.* 2017;2(1):76–79.

3. C. Blood flow through an AVF is essentially a left-to-right shunt, and a portion of the cardiac output is stolen by the fistula (B). Although there is no change in peripheral oxygen consumption after fistula placement, there is a drop in peripheral vascular resistance (PVR). Consequently, a compensatory increase in cardiac output occurs. The increase in venous return increases cardiac preload and causes rises in atrial natriuretic peptide (ANP) and brain natriuretic peptide (BNP). The decrease in afterload results in a decrease in aldosterone and renin levels. This subsequently leads to a decrease in afterload as well as suppression of the renin-aldosterone-angiotensin system, which promotes natriuresis. Compressing the fistula increases PVR and afterload, leading to a decrease in pulse rate and an increase in blood pressure (Nicoladoni-Branham sign). Patients with higher fistula flow will exhibit greater hemodynamic changes with fistula occlusion. Objectively, the minimum fistula flow rate required to support hemodialysis is greater than 400 to 500 cc/min. However, when the flow rate exceeds 2000 cc/min or 30% of the cardiac output, there is a risk of high-output cardiac failure. These patients, and those with clinically evident episodes of cardiac failure, should undergo intervention aimed at reducing flow rates. Surgical plication (narrowing the vein just beyond the anastomosis to the artery by suturing or banding) reduces the flow rate and can partially reverse the hemodynamic changes and prevent future episodes of heart failure. If heart failure continues to occur after an appropriate reduction in flow rates, eventual ligation of the fistula is indicated (A). Distal revascularization and interval ligation (DRIL) is used to treat steal syndrome, causing ischemic steal syndrome distal to the fistula. The procedure increases resistance to the fistula and decreases resistance to the distal extremity but may not effectively reduce fistula flow in the setting of cardiac failure (D). Converting a native fistula to a graft would not help because the large diameter of a graft would maintain high flow rates (E).

References: MacRae JM, Levin A, Belenkie I. The cardiovascular effects of arteriovenous fistulas in chronic kidney disease: a cause for concern?: cardiovascular effects of arteriovenous fistulas. *Semin Dial.* 2006;19(5):349–352.

High arteriovenous (AV) access flow and cardiac complications. NKF Task Force on Cardiovascular Disease, *America Journal of Kidney Disease*, 32(5).

4. A. A patient presenting with marked coolness, pallor, pain at rest, and hand numbness following an AV graft should be suspected of having steal syndrome. Ischemic steal syndrome occurs in approximately 2% to 4% of patients undergoing AV access for hemodialysis. Risk factors for steal syndrome include females, diabetes, age >60, and use of the brachial artery. Proximal fistulas have a higher risk of developing steal syndrome, while distal wrist fistulas (Cimino fistulas) have a very low risk. AV grafts also have a greater risk of steal compared with native AV fistulas (B). This is likely due to the fact that the large diameter of the graft creates a low-resistance bed. In addition, steal secondary to grafts tends to occur early after the access placement, whereas steal after native AV fistulas has a bimodal distribution, with some presenting early and others late after the native vein has undergone dilation with lowered resistance. Some degree of physiologic steal occurs in every patient with an AV fistula, but only a small minority manifests severe symptoms. The steal syndrome is caused by a diversion of blood flow from the anastomosed artery to the low-resistance vein. In addition, the low-resistance venous anastomosis leads to blood flowing in a retrograde fashion from the distal circulation into the fistula. Mild steal can be managed conservatively with exercise. More severe symptoms require intervention. Although ligation of the AV graft would have a great chance of resolving the steal syndrome, the patient will require a new access and will again be at risk of developing steal (C). Several options exist for the management. The most effective treatment that maintains fistula function is distal revascularization and interval ligation. The disadvantage of this procedure is that it requires creating a new bypass, usually with a saphenous vein, from the native artery proximal to the AV graft to the artery distal to it, with interval ligation of the native artery just proximal to the distal anastomosis. Banding or plicating of the AV graft, adjacent to the arterial anastomosis, serves to increase the resistance in the graft and reduce steal. The primary disadvantage of this approach (for grafts) is that inadequate banding leads to persistent steal, and excessive banding causes graft thrombosis (fistulas less likely to thrombose) (D, E). Banding or plication is a more attractive option for steal in an autologous AV fistula, such as a brachial artery cephalic vein fistula, because the vein is more resistant to thrombosis. This is not yet the standard approach, however.

References: Walz P, Ladowski JS, Hines A. Distal revascularization and interval ligation (DRIL) procedure for the treatment of ischemic steal syndrome after arm arteriovenous fistula. *Ann Vasc Surg.* 2007;21(4):468–473.

Yaghoubian A, de Virgilio C. Plication as primary treatment of steal syndrome in arteriovenous fistulas. *Ann Vasc Surg.* 2009;23(1):103–107.

Yu SH, Cook PR, Canty TG, McGinn RF, Taft PM, Hye RJ. Hemodialysis-related steal syndrome: predictive factors and response to treatment with the distal revascularization-interval ligation procedure. *Ann Vasc Surg.* 2008;22(2):210–214.

5. B. When permanent hemodialysis access is needed, the nondominant arm (E) should be considered first in order to mitigate the effects of potentially devastating complications, including severe steal syndrome, limb ischemia, ischemic monomelic neuropathy, and nerve injury. Once the side is determined, the type of AVF must be considered. Radiocephalic fistulas should generally be placed first (assuming adequate artery and vein) because subsequent thrombosis will not preclude the placement of a brachiocephalic or brachiobasilic fistula more proximally in the arm. Additionally, radiocephalic fistulas may cause dilation of the proximal arm veins, allowing higher success rates of more proximal fistulas in the future. Radiocephalic fistulas also rarely require a second-stage superficialization or transposition procedure because the forearm cephalic vein is close enough to the skin to be used upon maturation. If radiocephalic is not possible or has failed, a brachiocephalic should be considered next (C). Brachiocephalic fistulas allow fistulas to form on the dorsal surface of the upper arm and allow easier cannulation and use during hemodialysis. Further, depending on body habitus, brachiocephalic fistulas may also not require a second stage to superficialize the fistula close to the skin. The third choice for autogenous fistula is the brachiobasilic fistula. Since the basilic vein is deep, it requires superficialization of the vein. Many surgeons perform this in two stages so as to allow the vein to mature before superficialization (D). Maturation of a fistula typically requires at least 6 weeks and may require additional interventions. Waiting until 1 month before dialysis will result in placement of a temporary dialysis catheter, which carries high mortality risks (A). Despite the advantages, the radiocephalic fistula has a higher early failure or nonmaturation rate and may not be a good option in diabetics due to medial calcinosis within the radial artery. Further, when a patient is already hemodialysis dependent via tunneled catheter, there is ongoing debate about whether the ability to rapidly cannulate a graft (~2 weeks) shifts the preferences toward initial graft placement rather than fistula first. A forearm loop graft also has the advantage of dilating the basilic and upper cephalic veins for future fistula creation.

References: Disbrow DE, Cull DL, Carsten CG 3rd, Yang SK, Johnson BL, Keahey GP. Comparison of arteriovenous fistulas and arteriovenous grafts in patients with favorable vascular anatomy and equivalent access to health care: is a reappraisal of the Fistula First Initiative indicated? *J Am Coll Surg.* 2013;216(4):679–685; discussion 685–686.

Hakaim AG, Nalbandian M, Scott T. Superior maturation and patency of primary brachiocephalic and transposed basilic vein arteriovenous fistulae in patients with diabetes. *J Vasc Surg.* 1998;27(1):154–157.

[No authors listed]. NKF-K/DOQI clinical practice guidelines for vascular access. *Am J Kidney Dis.* 2006;48(Suppl. 1):S227–S409.

6. D. The patient is presenting with superior vena cava (SVC) syndrome with bilateral arm, neck, and face swelling and hoarseness of the voice. The patient likely has a preexisting central vein stenosis (in the SVC). A high proportion of patients with end-stage renal disease have central vein stenosis (25%–40%) due to prior central venous access. These stenoses are often asymptomatic, and if SVC syndrome does develop, it is usually insidious in onset. However, placement of an upper arm AVG access creates a sudden, massive increase in venous return that cannot be accommodated by the stenosis, leading to abrupt venous congestion (E). Central venous stenosis complicates hemodialysis access because it impairs venous fistula outflow and can reduce flow rates and reduce the likelihood of maturation in fistulas. Further, when access is placed ipsilateral to a stenotic lesion, there is a high likelihood of symptoms due to the increased venous congestion combined with high venous resistance. Arteriovenous grafts are more likely to cause symptoms than fistulas, and upper arm access is more likely to cause symptoms than forearm access. When central stenosis is suspected, either from history or symptoms, a central venogram should be performed to diagnose the lesion. Concomitant endovascular venoplasty is a reasonable option and has a high rate of success. However, first-line treatment is now endovascular stenting of the SVC (C). This is appropriate for both benign and malignant cases of SVC syndrome. Ligation or plication of the graft is not indicated because this destroys the access and does not address the underlying pathology (A, B). Open SVC repair via sternotomy for a benign lesion is overly invasive and unnecessary given the high initial success rates of endovascular treatment.

References: Jones RG, Willis AP, Jones C, McCafferty IJ, Riley PL. Long-term results of stent-graft placement to treat central venous stenosis and occlusion in hemodialysis patients with arteriovenous fistulas. *J Vasc Interv Radiol.* 2011;22(9):1240–1245.

Rizvi AZ, Kalra M, Bjarnason H, Bower TC, Schleck C, Gloviczki P. Benign superior vena cava syndrome: stenting is now the first line of treatment. *J Vasc Surg.* 2008;47(2):372–380.

Trerotola SO, Kothari S, Sammarco TE, Chittams JL. Central venous stenosis is more often symptomatic in hemodialysis patients with grafts compared with fistulas. *J Vasc Interv Radiol.* 2015;26(2):240–246.

7. A. When hemodialysis is urgently needed, temporary rapid vascular access must be established with a catheter that will support high flow (generally >400 cc/min) via 2 lumens. If long-term dialysis is anticipated, as in this patient, a tunneled, cuffed hemodialysis catheter, or permacath, is preferred (B) and placed into a central vein and exits the skin at least 10 cm away via a subcutaneous tract. Tunneled catheters are ready to use immediately and are less prone to infection than a nontunneled, noncuffed catheter (Quinton catheter). Quinton catheters are preferred in patients needing urgent dialysis for a short term, or for those with sepsis (as they are removed rapidly). The right internal jugular vein is the first choice because it is the most direct route to the right atrium. Left-sided placement is less preferable because it jeopardizes venous patency for future permanent access in the left arm (as most patients are right-hand dominant). Left-sided catheters also result in lower catheter blood flow rates and increase the risk of stenosis/thrombosis due to the longer and more tortuous length of contact with central vein side-wall (C). The subclavian position is associated with higher rates of complications (D), namely central vein stenosis and pneumothorax, and in some studies has a higher risk of infection when compared with internal jugular catheters. The femoral position carries the highest risk of infection, which is a significant cause of mortality in patients with temporary access catheters (E). Femoral lines may compromise a future kidney transplant because it may lead to proximal iliac vein stenosis/thrombosis.

Reference: [No authors listed]. NKF-K/DOQI clinical practice guidelines for vascular access. *Am J Kidney Dis.* 2006;48(Suppl. 1): S227–S409.

8. A. Clinical signs of cardiac tamponade include hypotension, distended neck veins, and muffled or distant heart sounds (Beck triad). This patient exhibits two of these signs after an invasive procedure of the chest and likely developed cardiac tamponade as a result of perforation of the right atrium. Tamponade caused by central venous catheter placement is a known complication resulting from puncture by the wire, introducer, or the catheter itself. Perforation of the right atrium more often occurs because it has a thinner wall compared to the right ventricle (E). Placing the catheter tip at the right tracheobronchial angle helps avoid placing the catheter tip in the right atrium. A perforated subclavian artery or vein would likely lead to hemothorax rather than pericardial tamponade (B, C). A tension pneumothorax is a known complication of line placement and may result in hypotension and distended neck veins, but breath sounds would not be clear bilaterally (D).

References: Barton JJ, Vanecko R, Gross M. Perforation of right atrium and resultant cardiac tamponade: a complication of catheterization to measure central venous pressure. *Obstet Gynecol.* 1968;32(4):556–560.

Darling JC, Newell SJ, Mohamdee O, Uzun O, Cullinane CJ, Dear PR. Central venous catheter tip in the right atrium: a risk factor for neonatal cardiac tamponade. *J Perinatol.* 2001;21(7):461–464.

Hunt R, Hunter TB. Cardiac tamponade and death from perforation of the right atrium by a central venous catheter. *AJR Am J Roentgenol.* 1988;151(6):1250.

9. A. AVF can eventually undergo aneurysmal degeneration over time, and intervention is required to prevent rupture and exsanguination (E). High outflow resistance is a common cause of aneurysm formation and must be ruled out by a fistulogram. Repeated needle cannulation can cause stenosis, resulting in higher pressures distal to the lesion and subsequent aneurysm formation. Alternatively, repeated needle cannulation can also lead to aneurysmal degeneration of the vein at the stick site. Therefore, cannulation must be avoided in areas undergoing aneurysmal change. A fistulogram is diagnostic of the stenotic lesion and potentially therapeutic via venoplasty with or without stent placement. Further, the fistulogram will also help distinguish between a true and

pseudo aneurysm. If no lesion is seen on the fistulogram, a central venogram should be performed to rule out a central stenosis as a cause of high outflow pressures. After treatment of the venous stenoses, bleeding may resolve because the abnormally high pressures within the fistula return to normal. Thinned/atrophic skin, translucent skin, ulceration, suspected infection, intraluminal thrombus, high-output cardiac failure, steal syndrome, or spontaneous bleeding from the fistula prompts consideration for revision by resection and plication or reanastomosis with a healthy vein (B). The size of the aneurysm is not an indicator for revision. If no healthy vein is available, graft implantation is an option (C). If outflow cannot be salvaged, the access may require ligation (D).

Reference: Cronenwett JL, Wayne Johnston K. *Rutherford's vascular surgery.* 7th ed. New York, NY: Saunders/Elsevier; 2010.

10. C. Fistulas are superior to grafts, which are superior to catheters in terms of patient survival, mainly because of the infection risks of prosthetic material (A–E). Diabetics have an exaggerated increase in mortality due to their depressed immune systems. Interestingly, despite the risk of high-output cardiac failure associated with fistula and graft, patients with tunneled catheters also have the highest risk of cardiac-related mortality. When comparing patency, fistulas are known to have higher primary patency (intervention-free patency of 85% at 1 year, 50% at 5 years) compared to grafts (60% at 1 year, 10% at 5 years) (B). However, fistulas have a higher rate of primary failure (nonmaturation or early thrombosis) of up to 40%. Furthermore, when comparing secondary patency (patency with interventions to maintain or reestablish flow), fistulas and grafts are similar. Grafts do not require maturation because their lumen diameter does not change (D). However, healing time of at least 10 days must be observed after graft placement before cannulation to avoid massive pseudoaneurysm formation. Fistulas require at least 6 weeks for maturation, during which time the outflow vein undergoes remodeling secondary to increased flow resulting in an increase in diameter and further increase in flow. Fistulas are deemed mature if they meet the rule of sixes: at 6 weeks, they must be 6 mm in diameter, less than 6 mm from skin surface, support 600 mL/min flow (although a minimum of 400 mL/min is adequate), and have a 6-inch straight segment for use.

References: [No authors listed]. NKF-K/DOQI clinical practice guidelines for vascular access. *Am J Kidney Dis.* 2006;48(Suppl. 1): S227–S409.

Lok CE, Sontrop JM, Tomlinson G, et al. Cumulative patency of contemporary fistulas versus grafts (2000–2010). *Clin J Am Soc Nephrol.* 2013;8(5):810–818.

11. E. Intubated patients with an air embolus may have an abrupt increase in end-tidal CO_2 followed by a decrease in end-tidal CO_2 and hypotension, and auscultation may reveal a "millwheel" murmur. This is often described as a loud churning sound. An Austin-Flint murmur is associated with aortic insufficiency and is a mid-diastolic rumble heard best at the apex (A). Carey Coombs murmur is also a mid-diastolic rumble that is associated with rheumatic fever (B). Means-Lerman scratch murmur sounds similar to a pericardial rub and may be heard in patients with hyperthyroidism (C). Still murmur is associated with a small ventral septal defect and is described as a vibratory systolic ejection rumble (D).

Transplant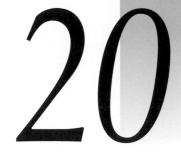

JOSEPH HADAYA, AREG GRIGORIAN, AND CHRISTIAN DE VIRGILIO

ABSITE 99th Percentile High-Yields

I. Type of Transplant Rejection
  A. Hyperacute: occurs in minutes to hours after transplantation (type-2 hypersensitivity)
    1. Due to the presence of preformed or natural antibodies against major blood group (ABO) or HLA antigen (sensitization from prior transplants, pregnancy, transfusions)
    2. Complement and coagulation cascade is activated causing graft thrombosis and ischemia
    3. Requires prompt removal of transplanted organ
    4. Kidney, heart, pancreas, and lung allografts all are susceptible to hyperacute rejection; however, liver grafts resist this process, so ABO compatibility is not essential for liver transplantation
  B. Acute: occurs in days to months
    1. Caused by cellular (macrophages and T-lymphocytes) or humoral (antibody-mediated) response and typically requires biopsy for diagnosis
    2. Treated with immunosuppressants, steroids, antithymocyte globulin
  C. Chronic: occurs in months to years (major cause of graft failure and mortality)
    1. Caused by cellular (cytotoxic T-lymphocyte, helper T cell) and antibody-mediated reactions
    2. Gradual process resulting in fibrosis and progressive graft dysfunction
    3. Treated by increasing immunosuppression, though usually requires retransplantation

II. Liver Transplantation
  A. Indications: end-stage liver disease secondary to alcohol (most common, replaced hepatitis C), nonalcoholic steatohepatitis, primary hepatic malignancy, cholangiocarcinoma, fulminant hepatic failure; most common indication in pediatrics: biliary atresia
    1. Milan criteria for hepatocellular carcinoma: single tumor less than 5 cm OR 3 tumors less than 3 cm each
  B. Model for end-stage liver disease (MELD): utilizes creatinine, INR, bilirubin, and sodium
    1. Originally developed for risk assessment for TIPS, now accepted as the score to prioritize organ allocation for liver transplantation
    2. Score is 0–40; MELD > 15 is indication for liver transplant
    3. Considered a superior scoring system to Childs-Pugh because all parameters are objective
  C. Operative considerations: for living donors, right lobe is utilized in adults, left lateral lobe utilized in children (size comparable)
  D. Postoperative complications
    1. Infection is the most common cause of death, accounting for over 50% of mortality
    2. Bile leak: most common complication, 10% and 30% incidence, may present with abdominal pain, bilious drainage, fever; early and large-volume leaks managed surgically, late or small volume leaks, or strictures, can be managed by biliary stenting or drainage
    3. Hepatic artery thrombosis: most common vascular complication, high mortality and graft loss rate (>50%)

a) Early thrombosis presents with transaminitis, hepatic failure, bile leak (due to breakdown of biliary anastomosis), or primary nonfunction
b) Late thrombosis presents as biliary stricture and/or abscesses
c) Doppler ultrasound first-line, may be confirmed with angiography, CT scan, or surgical exploration
d) If identified early (<24 hours), consider thrombectomy and revascularization, but may require retransplantation

4. Portal vein thrombosis (PVT): rare, early presents as abdominal pain, late presents as ascites and gastrointestinal bleed, can result in severe injury or graft loss, treated with thrombectomy if detected early; complete or partial recanalization of PVT is associated with better survival rates and, therefore, anticoagulation is recommended in all patients
   a) If fever and rising leukocytosis, consider pylephlebitis (infected thrombosis); add IV antibiotics

III. Kidney Transplantation
   A. Indications: Should be referred for transplantation evaluation when estimated GFR <30 or when on chronic dialysis
   B. Operation: graft placed in iliac fossa, extraperitoneal (close to bladder and avoids possible peritoneal contamination); most common arterial and venous anastomoses to external iliac artery and vein; order of anastomoses: vein first, artery second, ureter third
   C. Complications: urine output surrogate for graft function
      1. Oliguria: most common cause of delayed graft function is acute tubular necrosis, presents with gradual decline in urine output, first step with all cases of postop oliguria is to check for kinking of the foley catheter followed by Doppler ultrasound to rule out renal arterial occlusion
      2. Urine leak: common, presents with fever, pain, swelling, oliguria; evaluate with ultrasound and aspiration of fluid (compare fluid creatinine to serum level) or nuclear renography
      3. Lymphocele: most common cause of fluid around the transplanted kidney; often asymptomatic and found incidentally; can present with pain; if significant compression of ureter, can reduce urine output and elevate creatinine levels
      4. Renal artery stenosis: presents as graft dysfunction, diagnosed on ultrasound as flow acceleration at level of stenosis, can be treated with angioplasty and stent
      5. Arterial thrombosis: rare (<1%), acutely presents as low or no urine output, evaluate with ultrasound; if graft thrombosed, kidney salvage possible if segmental vessels involved and successful thrombectomy, otherwise may need graft nephrectomy.
   D. Living donor: improved posttransplant outcomes, lower delayed graft dysfunction rates, reduced wait times and time spent on dialysis
   E. Simultaneous pancreas and kidney (SPK) transplant or pancreas after kidney (PAK) considered for those with end-stage renal disease and diabetes mellitus; improves glucose control, diabetic complications (nephropathy, neuropathy, gastroparesis, retinopathy), and quality of life

IV. Most Common Posttransplant Malignancies
   A. Most common skin cancer: squamous cell carcinoma
   B. Kaposi sarcoma: caused by HHV-8, typically presents as cutaneous lesions on legs or mucosal lesions, treated by reducing immunosuppression
   C. Posttransplant lymphoproliferative disorder: proliferation of monoclonal B-cells, result of Epstein-Barr virus (EBV), check serology; more commonly develops in children; usually presents with vague abdominal pain or obstructive symptoms
      1. First-line treatment is to reduce the immunosuppressive regimen; second-line is rituximab (anti-CD20 monoclonal antibody); this can be followed by adding on chemotherapeutic regimens; surgery does not play a role

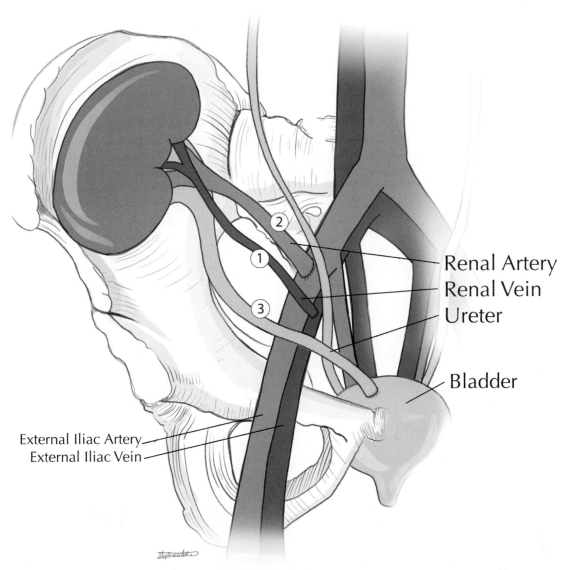

Renal Artery
Renal Vein
Ureter

Bladder

External Iliac Artery
External Iliac Vein

In kidney transplantation, the kidney is traditional placed in the pelvis and anastamoses are created between the renal vein and the external iliac vein first, the renal artery and the external iliac artery second, and then finally the ureter is sewn to the bladder. The right hemipelvis is depicted in this illustration. In living kidney donors, the left kidney is typically preferred due to implantation advantages since the left renal vein is longer than the right renal vein.

Fig. 20.1 Order of Anastomosis in Kidney Transplantation.

Questions

1. A 45-year-old female undergoes orthotopic liver transplantation for end-stage liver disease secondary to hepatitis C. Eighteen hours after surgery, she remains intubated and sedated, has required 1 unit of packed red blood cells since surgery, and a norepinephrine drip to keep her mean arterial pressure >65 mmHg. Her transaminases have doubled since return from the operating room and her total bilirubin level remains at 10 mg/dL. There is minimal output from her surgical drains. What is the next best step?
   A. Immediate reexploration and listing for retransplantation
   B. Repeat complete blood count, liver function tests, and prothrombin time/INR in 4 hours
   C. Ultrasound and doppler study of graft
   D. CT scan of abdomen and pelvis with IV contrast
   E. Fluid resuscitation and broad-spectrum antibiotics

2. A 41-year-old male with end-stage renal disease secondary to diabetes is undergoing routine renal ultrasound 1 month after kidney transplantation. He has a 4-cm fluid collection next to the donor kidney. He has no complaints and he is making adequate urine. Which of the following is the best next step?
   A. Observation
   B. Ultrasound-guided aspiration for culture and creatinine
   C. CT scan
   D. Internal drainage in the OR
   E. External pigtail catheter drainage

3. Which of the following is true regarding posttransplant lymphoproliferative disorder (PTLD)?
   A. It is usually of monoclonal T-cell origin
   B. It occurs more commonly following renal transplantation compared to heart transplantation
   C. The risk of developing PTLD is lowest in the first year following transplant
   D. Epstein-Barr virus (EBV)-negative patients are at a lower risk than EBV-positive patients
   E. Cytomegalovirus (CMV)-negative patients are at higher risk once they seroconvert following transplant

4. A 39-year-old female is undergoing kidney transplant. Shortly after performing the arterial anastomosis, the surgeon notes that the donor kidney appears soft, flabby, mottled, and edematous. The patient's heart rate is 136 beats per minute and blood pressure is 90/60 mm-Hg. Which of the following is true?
   A. This is a T-cell mediated response
   B. The patient should be started on pressors and the operation completed
   C. The donor kidney should be immediately removed without further workup
   D. Lymphokines are involved in this process
   E. This complication occurs more commonly in liver transplants than with kidney transplants

5. A 46-year-old male with end-stage renal disease secondary to diabetes arrives at clinic to discuss his placement in the kidney transplant list. His panel reactive antibody (PRA) score is 85%. He had a failed kidney transplant 5 years ago. Which of the following is true?
   A. He has a low risk of rejection
   B. Given his high PRA, he will be given priority on the transplant list
   C. He will lose points in the kidney allocation algorithm because he had a previous kidney transplant
   D. He will experience a shorter wait time compared to a similar patient with a lower PRA
   E. PRA is calculated using nationally pooled data

6. Which of the following patients with hepatocellular carcinoma is eligible for liver transplantation?
   A. Single 3-cm tumor in segment 2 with regional lymphadenopathy
   B. Single 6-cm tumor in segment 4 with no regional lymphadenopathy
   C. Single 2-cm tumor in segment 5 with vascular invasion
   D. 1-cm, 2-cm, and 2.5-cm tumors in segments 3 and 4 with no evidence of lymphadenopathy
   E. 1-cm and 3.5-cm tumors both in segment 4 with no lymphadenopathy or distant disease

7. The most clinically important viral infection in transplant recipients is:
   A. Varicella-zoster
   B. Cytomegalovirus (CMV)
   C. Epstein-Barr virus
   D. Hepatitis C virus
   E. Herpes simplex

8. Which of the following is the best indication for pancreas transplantation in type 1 diabetes?
   A. A 45-year-old male with stage 2 chronic kidney disease and recurrent episodes of marked hyperglycemia
   B. A 66-year-old female with end-stage renal disease who underwent kidney transplantation 10 years ago
   C. A 41-year-old male with severe anxiety associated with insulin therapy, refractory gastroparesis, and recurrent episodes of marked hyperglycemia
   D. A 38-year-old female that was recently hospitalized for metabolic complications associated with diabetes
   E. A 51-year-old male with stage 3 chronic kidney disease and recurrent episodes of marked hyperglycemia

9. Which of the following poses the highest risk of death in a patient awaiting renal transplantation?
   A. Chronic obstructive pulmonary disease (COPD)
   B. Cerebrovascular accident
   C. Smoker
   D. Black race
   E. Congestive heart failure

10. Which of the following is true regarding kidney transplant donation?
   A. The most common cause of death postoperatively for kidney donors is acute renal failure
   B. The most common postoperative complication for kidney donors is acute tubular necrosis
   C. Donors must prove to have a glomerular filtration rate (GFR) greater than 80 mL/min to be considered as appropriate candidates
   D. The serum creatinine will be persistently higher following kidney donation
   E. The rate of live kidney donation has increased in the past 10 years

11. A 35-year-old brain dead trauma victim is being considered for kidney donation. Which of the following donor conditions would be a contraindication to kidney donation?
   A. History of arm melanoma status post wide local resection 10 years ago
   B. History of lymphoma as a child
   C. Current urinary tract infection
   D. Recent hospitalization for meningococcemia, now with negative blood cultures
   E. Open cholecystectomy 4 months ago

12. A 45-year-old male arrives at clinic 1 year after liver transplantation. He would like to discuss his recent laboratory studies and the health of his liver. Which of the following is the best measure of the function of his liver?
   A. Aspartate aminotransferase (AST)
   B. Alanine transaminase (ALT)
   C. Total bilirubin
   D. Serum albumin
   E. International normalized ratio (INR)

13. A 42-year-old male with end-stage renal disease secondary to glomerulonephritis has been matched with a deceased donor kidney and arrives at the hospital for transplantation. Which of the following is a guiding principle in this surgery?
   A. The right peritoneum is the preferred initial implant site
   B. The left retroperitoneum is the preferred initial implant site
   C. Baseline biopsy of the donor kidney should be obtained at the conclusion of the case
   D. The native kidney should not be removed
   E. The renal artery should be anastomosed to the internal iliac artery

14. A 28-year-old female with end-stage renal disease secondary to lupus nephritis undergoes a living-related donor kidney transplant and is making appropriate urine at the conclusion of the case. On postoperative day 2, the surgical intern finds that her urine output has dropped from 180 cc the previous hour to only 4 cc in the last hour. The indwelling Foley is flushing well. Which of the following is the most appropriate next step in management?
   A. Take patient to the operating room (OR)
   B. Ultrasound
   C. Magnetic resonance angiography (MRA)
   D. Computed topography (CT)
   E. Urinalysis

Answers

1. C. Within 12 hours of liver transplantation and graft reperfusion, a patient's hemodynamic status, urine output, and coagulopathy should all begin to improve. Laboratory tests, including INR and transaminases, may follow with a slight delay. A lack of improvement in a patient's clinical status or significant worsening of transaminases, bilirubin levels, or INR, should prompt a clinician to assess for a major vascular/biliary complication or primary nonfunction. In this particular case, a doubling of transaminases and persistent vasopressor requirement is concerning for a major vascular complication, most commonly hepatic artery thrombosis. A large biliary leak, while possible, is less likely with minimal output from the patient's surgical drains. An ultrasound and doppler study of the graft can confirm the diagnosis without requiring cross-sectional imaging (C, D). Hepatic artery thrombosis, if detected early, can be treated with thrombectomy and revision of the arterial anastomosis and may result in graft salvage. However, many cases require retransplantation (A). While less common, portal vein thrombosis may present similarly and, if found early, may be treated with thrombectomy to salvage the graft. Fluid resuscitation, broad-spectrum antibiotics, and repeating laboratory tests will delay treatment of the underlying condition in this case (B, E).

Reference: Mourad MM, Liossis C, Gunson BK, et al. Etiology and management of hepatic artery thrombosis after adult liver transplantation: etiology and management of hepatic artery thrombosis. *Liver Transpl.* 2014;20(6):713–723.

2. A. Patients who have undergone kidney transplantation commonly have fluid collections around the donor kidney. This is frequently an asymptomatic finding and is incidentally discovered during routine imaging studies, often in the first year. If the fluid collection is small (<5 cm), it is unlikely to cause any symptoms, and the patient can initially be observed with no additional studies required (C). Possible etiologies include lymphocele, seroma, urine leak, and hematoma. The most common cause is lymphocele, which occurs secondary to severed lymphatic vessels during surgery. This is a self-limited complication and will resolve with time. With larger fluid collections, patients may develop oliguria (extrinsic compression of the ureter), graft failure (extrinsic compression of renal artery or vein), or infection. Symptomatic fluid collections will need to be treated with image-guided drainage or surgical drainage (E). In recurrent cases, a peritoneal window allowing internal drainage can be performed (D). Additionally, the fluid creatinine level should be compared to the serum level (B). This will help determine if the patient has a urine leak. In this case, the patient may need to receive a renal stent or nephrostomy tube and, rarely, ureteral reconstruction in the OR.

Reference: Fuller TF, Kang SM, Hirose R, Feng S, Stock PG, Freise CE. Management of lymphoceles after renal transplantation: laparoscopic versus open drainage. *J Urol.* 2003;169(6):2022–2025.

3. E. PTLD is the second most common cancer affecting patients with solid organ transplants, with the majority occurring in the first year (C). The most common cancer is squamous cell carcinoma of the skin, with most occurring about 8 years after the transplant. The most common type of PTLD is of monoclonal B-cell origin (A). It occurs more commonly in heart and lung transplants compared to liver and renal transplants (B). Early diagnosis requires a high index of suspicion because it can present with nonspecific symptoms including fevers (most common), lymphadenopathy, night sweats, and weight loss. Declining graft function can also be a presenting symptom. Diagnosis begins with checking serum EBV viral load, although EBV-negative patients can also develop PTLD. In fact, EBV-negative patients are at higher risk than EBV-positive patients (D). Additionally, CMV-negative patients are at increased risk once they seroconvert following transplant.

References: Opelz G, Henderson R. Incidence of non-Hodgkin lymphoma in kidney and heart transplant recipients. *Lancet.* 1993;342(8886–8887):1514–1516.

Walker RC, Paya CV, Marshall WF, et al. Pretransplantation seronegative Epstein-Barr virus status is the primary risk factor for posttransplantation lymphoproliferative disorder in adult heart, lung, and other solid organ transplantations. *J Heart Lung Transplant.* 1995;14(2):214–221.

Walker RC, Marshall WF, Strickler JG, et al. Pretransplantation assessment of the risk of lymphoproliferative disorder. *Clin Infect Dis.* 1995;20(5):1346–1353.

4. C. This patient is experiencing hyperacute rejection. This will present with the donor kidney appearing soft, flabby, mottled, and edematous and can progress to widespread interstitial hemorrhage and necrosis. This occurs within minutes to hours after the arterial anastomosis and is mediated by preformed recipient antibodies to donor HLA antigens (A). The antibodies bind to the graft endothelium and ensue a cascade of events resulting in tissue necrosis. This is an uncommon complication, but renal grafts are more commonly affected. For reasons that are unclear, liver transplants are largely resistant to hyperacute rejection, but it is thought to be related to the enormous size of the liver and its ability to absorb circulating antibodies (E). The only treatment for hyperacute rejection is immediate removal of the donor kidney because this can result in hemodynamic instability, multiorgan failure, and death if left untreated (B). This is particularly important in a patient who is already hypotensive. Acute rejection is a T-cell-mediated response with activated monocytes secreting soluble mediators including lymphokines IL-1 and IL-2 (D). This typically occurs 1 to 2 months after the transplant and should be confirmed with a renal biopsy. Patients will present with oliguria and/or rising creatinine. Treatment involves high-dose steroids. Chronic graft rejection is a poorly understood process that can occur years after having a well-functioning donor graft. Immunosuppression is largely ineffective in these cases.

References: Bhowmik DM, Dinda AK, Mahanta P, Agarwal SK. The evolution of the Banff classification schema for diagnosing renal allograft rejection and its implications for clinicians. *Indian J Nephrol.* 2010;20(1):2–8.

Gordon RD, Iwatsuki S, Esquivel CO, Tzakis A, Todo S, Starzl TE. Liver transplantation across ABO blood groups. *Surgery.* 1986;100(2):342–348.

Ramsey G, Wolford J, Boczkowski DJ, Cornell FW, Larson P, Starzl TE. The Lewis blood group system in liver transplantation. *Transplant Proc.* 1987;19(6):4591–4594.

5. B. PRA is performed in all patients that are listed for a kidney transplant. This tests the patient's blood against blood from a panel of donors in the same geographic area (E). The panel serves as the HLA makeup of the potential organs available for donation for the recipient. Patients that have a high PRA are considered to be "highly sensitized" and will have a higher likelihood of rejection (A). Patients with a PRA greater than 80% will need to wait much longer to match with a compatible donor, so they are given additional points on the kidney allocation algorithm prioritizing them to the top of the list. However, even though their names come up frequently as potential matches for newly available kidneys, they are frequently incompatible, so their wait times are much longer than patients with lower PRAs (D). Having a previous kidney transplant likely contributed to his high PRA, but this in and of itself does not factor in the kidney allocation algorithm (C).

Reference: Hart A, Smith JM, Skeans MA, et al. OPTN/SRTR 2015 Annual Data Report: Kidney. *Am J Transplant.* 2017;17(Suppl. 1): 21–116.

6. D. Liver transplantation can be offered to patients with hepatocellular carcinoma and if appropriate candidates are selected, outcomes can be favorable. Mazzaferro and others demonstrated that patients with certain tumor characteristics that undergo liver transplantation can achieve a 4-year survival of 75%. This is now known as the Milan criteria and is used by UNOS to select appropriate candidates. Milan criteria are as follows: a single tumor 5 cm or smaller or up to three tumors with none larger than 3 cm, and no evidence of vascular invasion, regional lymphadenopathy, or distant disease (A–C, E). Tumors limited to a particular liver segment do not factor into selecting appropriate candidates.

Reference: Mazzaferro V, Regalia E, Doci R, et al. Liver transplantation for the treatment of small hepatocellular carcinomas in patients with cirrhosis. *N Engl J Med.* 1996;334(11):693–699.

7. B. CMV is a member of the herpesvirus family and is the most clinically significant viral infection in transplant recipients. In healthy, nonimmunosuppressed individuals, CMV is clinically silent or mild. In immunosuppressed transplant recipients, CMV is associated with increased mortality and graft loss. In one large study of liver transplant recipients, CMV infection was found to be an independent risk factor for graft failure. In a cardiac transplantation study, CMV-negative recipients of CMV-positive donor hearts had impaired distal epicardial endothelial function and an increased incidence of cardiovascular-related events and death during follow-up.

References: Burak KW, Kremers WK, Batts KP, et al. Impact of cytomegalovirus infection, year of transplantation, and donor age on outcomes after liver transplantation for hepatitis C. *Liver Transpl.* 2002;8(4):362–369.

Petrakopoulou P, Kübrich M, Pehlivanli S, et al. Cytomegalovirus infection in heart transplant recipients is associated with impaired endothelial function. *Circulation.* 2004;110(11 Suppl 1):II207–II212.

8. C. Pancreas transplantation has been shown to improve survival and quality of life in patients with type 1 diabetes.

It may halt progression of diabetes-related disease such as retinopathy and may even reverse disease including neuropathy and autonomic dysfunction. It does not lead to reversal of vascular disease secondary to diabetes. The American Diabetes Association has provided indications for pancreas transplantation: (1) diabetic patients with imminent or established end-stage renal disease who have had or plan to have a kidney transplant or (2) patients meeting all three of the following criteria: frequent episodes of metabolic complications related to diabetes (hypoglycemia, ketoacidosis, hyperglycemia), emotional problems with insulin therapy that are severe enough to be incapacitating, and consistent failure of insulin-based management to prevent complications. From the answer choices provided, the best indication is for the 41-year-old male with severe emotional problems associated with insulin therapy, refractory gastroparesis, and recurrent episodes of marked hyperglycemia (A, D, E). Pancreas transplantation should be avoided in patients older than 45 to 65 because these patients have poor graft and 5-year survival (B).

References: Robertson RP, Davis C, Larsen J, Stratta R, Sutherland DER, American Diabetes Association. Pancreas and islet transplantation in type 1 diabetes. *Diabetes Care.* 2006;29(4):935.

Siskind E, Maloney C, Akerman M, et al. An analysis of pancreas transplantation outcomes based on age groupings–an update of the UNOS database. *Clin Transplant.* 2014;28(9):990–994.

9. A. While it is true that the most common cause of death in patients with diabetes is cardiac-related, a history of coronary artery disease does not place patients at the highest risk for death while awaiting renal transplantation (E). This speaks to the prevalence of heart disease in this patient population. A large multivariable survival model analyzing over 160,000 patients demonstrated that COPD is the most significant factor independently associated with death among patients awaiting renal transplantation (adjusted hazard ratio of 1.31). This is followed by, in descending order, smoker status, nonambulatory status, coronary artery disease, peripheral vascular disease, congestive heart failure, cerebrovascular disease, and hypertension (B, C). Black patients awaiting kidney transplantation survive longer than white patients, but this reverses when black patients receive kidney transplantation (D). Additionally, COPD is the most significant risk factor associated with poor graft function and survival following a kidney transplant.

References: Kapur A, De Palma R. Mortality after myocardial infarction in patients with diabetes mellitus. *Heart.* 2007;93(12):1504–1506.

van Walraven C, Austin PC, Knoll G. Predicting potential survival benefit of renal transplantation in patients with chronic kidney disease. *CMAJ.* 2010;182(7):666–672.

10. C. As the incidence of diabetes and end-stage renal disease has steadily risen in the past several decades, the number of patients awaiting kidney transplantation has also been increasing. Due to a multidisciplinary approach and the concerted efforts of transplant groups such as the United Network for Organ Sharing (UNOS), the availability of deceased kidney donors has risen. However, the rate of live kidney donation has dropped in greater numbers, leaving a total deficit in the availability of kidney donors despite the increase in deceased donors (E). There are several societal guidelines to determine the candidacy of live kidney donors, and one prevailing requirement across all governing bodies is the requirement of a GFR greater than 80 mL/min confirmed with a nuclear test or 24-hour urine collection. The most common cause of death postoperatively for kidney donors is pulmonary emboli (A). The most common complication for kidney donors postoperatively is wound infection (B). Although the serum creatinine may be higher in the immediate postoperative period, it will eventually go back down and the baseline creatinine will remain the same or close to the baseline as the donor will continue to have one functioning kidney remaining (D).

References: Clinical Practice Guidelines for Living Kidney Donors. Kidney Disease Improving Global Outcomes; KDIGO, 2017.

Najarian JS, Chavers BM, McHugh LE, Matas AJ. 20 years or more of follow-up of living kidney donors. *Lancet*. 1992;340(8823):807–810.

Hart A, Smith JM, Skeans MA, et al. OPTN/SRTR 2015 Annual Data Report: Kidney. *Am J Transplant*. 2017;17(Suppl. 1):21–116.

11. A. Since the availability of kidney donors has been declining, establishing appropriate guidelines for diseased kidney donation is imperative to maximize the scarcity of available organs. Several absolute contraindications to organ donation exist, including patients with HIV (unless the recipient also has HIV), hepatitis (unless the recipient also has the same hepatitis type), cirrhosis, and active systemic infection with positive blood cultures. A previous hospitalization for systemic infection is not considered an absolute contraindication as long as the patient has proven to have negative blood cultures (D). Similarly, urosepsis would preclude organ donation, but a urinary tract infection in and of itself would not (C). A history of cholecystectomy in a patient without significant liver disease does not preclude organ donation (E). A history of cancer may preclude deceased donors from organ donation. Some exceptions can be made for patients with a remote history of low-grade visceral malignancy such as colorectal cancer or patients with less aggressive cancers such as basal cell carcinoma or childhood lymphomas. Similarly, low-grade primary CNS tumors do not pose a high risk of transmission (B). Melanoma in particular poses a risk for transmission even in patients with a remote history, so this will prevent the patient from being an eligible donor.

References: Birkeland SA, Storm HH. Risk for tumor and other disease transmission by transplantation: a population-based study of unrecognized malignancies and other diseases in organ donors. *Transplantation*. 2002;74(10):1409–1413.

Feng S, Buell JF, Cherikh WS, et al. Organ donors with positive viral serology or malignancy: risk of disease transmission by transplantation. *Transplantation*. Published online 2002;78:1657–1663.

12. E. A liver function test (LFT) measures the levels of AST, ALT, and alkaline phosphatase, but does not reflect the synthetic function of the liver; thus, LFT is a misnomer (A, B). The best test to determine the liver's function is the prothrombin time (PT), or INR. Albumin and PTT are also helpful (D). Total bilirubin is influenced by biliary tree obstruction, intrinsic hepatic disease, and hemolysis (C).

13. D. Kidney transplantation has led to improved survival and quality of life in patients with end-stage renal disease. It was first performed in France by Rene Kuss in 1951, and

the surgical approach originally described has changed very little in modern practice. The peritoneum is a poor choice for implantation because it poses a high risk of graft contamination and infection. The retroperitoneum and pelvic fossa are the preferred sites (A). Most surgeons prefer the right side because the iliac vessels are longer and more horizontal, allowing for a technically easier anastomosis (B). However, if there are any previous dissections or operations involving mesh (e.g., herniorrhaphy) on the right side, the left side can be chosen. Generally, it is preferable to perform the venous anastomosis before the arterial anastomosis to avoid vascular congestion of the kidney, followed finally by ureteral reconstruction. The external iliac vein and artery are the preferred targets for the anastomosis (E). This is because dissection of the internal iliac vessels is technically challenging, which increases operative time and subjects the patient to additional risks such as autonomic plexus injury (e.g., erectile dysfunction). The standard ureteral reconstruction is a ureteroneocystostomy because it avoids the deep dissection necessary for a ureteroureterostomy. The utility of obtaining a baseline biopsy is controversial at best. The argument against it is that it exposes the patient to a biopsy-induced vascular thrombosis, which can compromise the graft (C). It should be noted that the native kidney should remain in place because it can often continue to have a small role by secreting erythropoietin.

Reference: Zhao J, Gao Z, Wang K. The transplantation operation and its surgical complications. In: *Understanding the Complexities of Kidney Transplantation*. InTech; 2011.

14. B. Providing adequate fluid resuscitation following kidney transplantation is essential in preventing graft failure. Although there is no consensus on the optimal postoperative fluid regimen in kidney transplantation, the use of crystalloids should be the volume replacement of choice, and most transplant surgeons would agree to aim to achieve a urine output greater than 100 cc per hour. The most common cause of postoperative oliguria is acute tubular necrosis (ATN), which can be initially worked up with urinalysis (E). However, ATN will present with a gradual decrease in urine output and will frequently respond to a fluid bolus. A sudden drop in urine output or anuria is concerning for graft thrombosis. This could have catastrophic outcomes if not diagnosed early. In fact, it is considered the main cause of graft failure in the first year, with the majority occurring at 48 hours. It typically involves the renal vein, but the renal artery can also be affected. In any patient with a sudden decrease in urine output, the first step is to flush the Foley to ensure there is no kinking preventing urine flow. The next step is to perform a bedside ultrasound to look for vascular thrombosis. If this is identified, the next step is to go to the OR for surgical revascularization or intraarterial thrombolytic therapy (A). If ultrasound findings are equivocal, the next step is to perform an adjunct imaging study such as MRA, CT, or renal scintigraphy (C, D).

References: Ponticelli C, Moia M, Montagnino G. Renal allograft thrombosis. *Nephrol Dial Transplant*. 2009;24(5):1388–1393.

Schnuelle P, Johannes van der Woude F. Perioperative fluid management in renal transplantation: a narrative review of the literature. *Transpl Int*. 2006;19(12):947–959.

Thoracic Surgery

21

JORDAN M. ROOK AND SHONDA L. REVELS

ABSITE 99th Percentile High-Yields

I. Anatomy:
   A. Azygous vein: ascends along right thoracic vertebral column and drains into SVC
   B. Thoracic duct: Begins in abdomen at cisterna chyli (L1), traveling between azygous and aorta until T5, where it crosses right to left, draining into junction of the left subclavian and internal jugular vein
   C. Phrenic nerve: descends anterior to hilum; Vagus nerve: travels posterior to hilum
   D. Dual blood supply to lung:
      1. Alveoli: unoxygenated blood via pulmonary artery (low-pressure system)
      2. Bronchi: oxygenated blood via bronchial arteries; originate from thoracic aorta (most common), aortic arch, or intercostal arteries
   E. Cellular anatomy:
      1. Type 1 pneumocytes: gas exchange; Type 2 pneumocytes: surfactant

II. Preoperative Evaluation:
   A. No matter the surgery, mortality and morbidity increase if predicted postoperative FEV1<40%
   B. Preoperative FEV1 greater than 2 L—can tolerate pneumonectomy
   C. Preoperative FEV1 greater than 1.5 L—can tolerate lobectomy
   D. If concern with any of the above, obtain quantitative perfusion lung scan or SPECT/CT to determine how much diseased lung contributes to FEV1

III. Pathology:
   A. Bronchogenic cysts
      1. Rare congenital malformations of the tracheobronchial tree
      2. Many are asymptomatic and incidentally found on imaging
      3. Those with symptoms present during the second decade of life with coughing, wheezing, and pneumonia
      4. The standard of care is surgical excision by partial or total lobectomy
   B. Pleural effusion management:
      1. Simple (nonloculated): treat underlying cause, drain, pleurodesis if needed
      2. Hemothorax (retained): Video-assisted thoracoscopic surgery (VATS) washout; decortication if lung is trapped
      3. Empyema: requires complete drainage (difficult due to loculations) -> attempt fibrinolytic therapy (TPA and DNase) -> VATS or thoracotomy for decortication
   C. Chylothorax:
      1. Disruption of the thoracic duct (1.5–2.5 L/day)
      2. Causes: 50% trauma (includes iatrogenic) and 50% malignancy (most common is lymphoma)
      3. Dx: greater than 110 mg/dL of triglycerides with lymphocytic predominance. Positive Sudan red stain.
      4. Treatment: no-fat/low-fat medium-chain fatty acid diet, NPO +TPN, drainage, octreotide
         a) If fails: right VATS/thoracotomy and ligation of thoracic duct by surgery or endovascular embolization

D. Mediastinal tumors:
 1. Most common cause of lymphadenopathy: lymphoma
 2. Most common tumor in children: neurogenic tumors (posterior mediastinum)
 3. Most common germ cell tumor: teratoma (anterior mediastinum)
 4. Thymoma (anterior mediastinum): all require resection
E. Superior vena cava syndrome:
 1. Common causes: malignancy most common (#1 small cell; #2 lymphoma); also, stenosis related to prior central venous catheters or pacemaker wires
 2. Treatment:
   a) Malignancy: definitive chemoradiation, endovascular stenting if life-threatening venous hypertension (airway obstruction, cerebral edema)
   b) Venous stenosis: angioplasty and stent placement
F. Hemoptysis:
 1. Can "drown" with only 150 mL of blood; 90% due to high-pressure bronchial arteries
 2. Tx: establish airway with mainstem intubation of nonbleeding bronchus with bronchoscopy (rigid preferred to flexible), place patient in lateral decubitus (bleeding side down), bronchoscopy versus selective bronchial artery embolization

IV. Lung Cancer:
 A. Screening: 2020 guidelines recommend annual low-dose CT scan for adults aged 50 to 80 with at least a 20-pack year smoking history; must be current smokers or have quit within the past 15 years
  1. Nonsmall cell lung cancer: approximately 80% of all cancers; 3 types are adenocarcinoma (30%–50%) (peripheral location, nonsmokers), squamous cell (20%–35%), and large cell (4%–15%)
  2. Small cell (oat cell) carcinoma accounts for 20% of all lung cancer, occurs centrally near hilum, almost exclusively in smokers and not amenable to surgery, typically tx chemoradiation
 B. Solitary pulmonary nodule (SPN)
 C. Paraneoplastic syndromes:
  1. Squamous cell: hyperparathyroidism (PTHrP)
  2. Small cell: Cushing disease (ACTH) and SIADH

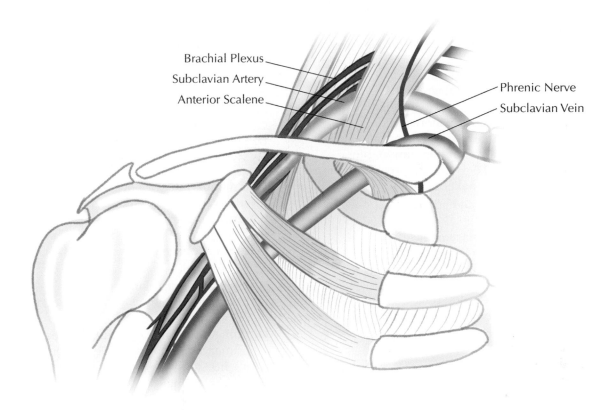

Thoracic outlet syndrome (TOS) can be divided into Arterial TOS, Venous TOS, and Neurogenic TOS. Arterial and neurogenic TOS typically occur when the brachial plexus or subclavian artery are compressed between the anterior and middle scalene muscles. Venous thoracic outlet syndrome, also known as Paget Schroetter syndrome or effort thrombosis, occurs when the subclavian vein is compressed between the clavicle and first rib.

Fig. 21.1 Anatomy of the Thoracic Outlet.

Questions

1. A 54-year-old male presents to clinic for surgical evaluation of his recently diagnosed T2N1M0 (Stage II) esophageal cancer. He is scheduled to undergo neoadjuvant chemoradiation and presents for surgical planning. His primary complaint is dysphagia limiting him to thin liquids. Albumin is 2.6 g/dL and prealbumin is 8 mg/dL. What is the next best step?
   A. Proceed with chemoradiation
   B. J tube placement
   C. Attempt PEG tube placement
   D. G-J tube placement
   E. TPN supplementation

2. A 63-year-old male is undergoing evaluation of a 4-cm left upper lobe mass. CT demonstrates a 1.1-cm suspicious para aortic (station 6) lymph node. What is your next best step?
   A. Cervical mediastinoscopy
   B. Anterior mediastinoscopy
   C. Endobronchial ultrasound
   D. Percutaneous core needle biopsy
   E. Esophageal ultrasound

3. A 43-year-old female is undergoing a workup of an incidentally discovered 3.8 cm mediastinal mass. CT demonstrates a small, well-circumscribed thymic mass without evidence of invasion into local structures. What is your next best step?
   A. Percutaneous image-guided biopsy
   B. Interval CT in 6 months
   C. Fine needle aspirate
   D. Thymectomy
   E. Referral to an oncologist

4. A 22-year-old male is sent to thoracic surgery clinic for evaluation of a bronchogenic cyst incidentally discovered on chest x-ray and confirmed on CT. He denies any symptoms. What is the best treatment?
   A. VATS lobectomy
   B. Cyst fenestration
   C. Observation
   D. 6-month interval CT
   E. Endobronchial ultrasound for sampling of cyst fluid

5. The most common cause of lung abscess is:
   A. Aspiration
   B. Bronchial obstruction by tumor
   C. Pneumococcal pneumonia
   D. Pneumocystis jiroveci pneumonia
   E. Mycobacterium tuberculosis pneumonia

6. Four months after prolonged intubation after a motor vehicle accident, a 40-year-old woman presents with stridor and dyspnea on exertion. Endoscopy reveals marked tracheal stenosis 4 cm in length. Management consists of:
   A. Laser ablation
   B. Bronchoscopic dilation
   C. Primary resection of all scarred segments with primary anastomosis
   D. Primary resection of all scarred segments, primary anastomosis, and temporary tracheostomy
   E. Metal stenting

7. Which of the following is true regarding Lambert-Eaton myasthenic syndrome?
   A. It is most often associated with squamous cell carcinoma of the lung
   B. 3,4-Diaminopyridine is not effective in treating symptoms
   C. Intravenous (IV) immunoglobulin is effective in treating symptoms
   D. Thymectomy is effective in patients in whom medical management fails
   E. Patients present with distal muscle weakness

8. A 65-year-old woman presents with a chronic nonproductive cough of 2 months duration. A chest radiograph reveals a 2-cm mass in the right upper lobe. A CT scan of the chest confirms the presence of the 2-cm mass corresponding to that found on the chest radiograph, which appears to be malignant, along with 5-mm nodes in the mediastinum. The next step in management would be:
   A. Positron emission tomography (PET) scan
   B. Abdominal CT
   C. Bone scan
   D. Mediastinoscopy
   E. Brain CT

9. A 24-year-old woman presents with recurrent episodes of right-sided pneumothorax requiring chest tube insertion. A diagnosis of a catamenial pneumothorax as the cause of recurrent pneumothorax in this patient would be supported by the finding of:
   A. Pneumocystis
   B. Endometriosis
   C. Cystic fibrosis
   D. Idiopathic pulmonary fibrosis
   E. Apical blebs

10. A 35-year-old male with diffuse axonal injury following a motorcycle collision is recovering in the surgical intensive care unit (ICU). He has been intubated for 3 weeks. This morning the patient developed an endotracheal air leak that persisted even with tube exchange and hyperinflation. His abdomen appears distended. Bronchoscopy is performed and demonstrates yellow-colored secretions in both main stem bronchi. Which of the following is true?
    A. The patient should be switched to low tidal volume ventilation
    B. Early conversion to tracheostomy decreases the risk for this complication
    C. Nasogastric tube increases the risk for this complication
    D. Low intracuff pressure contributes to the development of this complication
    E. CT scan of the abdomen should be performed

11. A 65-year-old man presents with anorexia, nausea, lethargy, and hyponatremia. A chest radiograph reveals a large right upper lobe mass. This most likely represents:
    A. Adenocarcinoma
    B. Small cell carcinoma
    C. Squamous cell carcinoma
    D. Carcinoid
    E. Bronchoalveolar carcinoma

12. Which of the following is true of thoracic anatomy?
    A. The left lung has three lobes
    B. The azygous vein runs along the left side draining into the subclavian vein
    C. The vagus nerve runs anterior to the lung hilum
    D. The sternocleidomastoid muscle is considered an accessory muscle to breathing
    E. The phrenic nerve runs posterior to the lung hilum

13. What happens to the partial pressure of arterial oxygen as blood flows from the pulmonary capillaries to the left atrium?
    A. Increase
    B. Decrease
    C. Stay the same
    D. Depends on cardiac output
    E. Depends on pulmonary vascular resistance

14. The most common primary chest wall malignancy is:
    A. Osteochondroma
    B. Chondrosarcoma
    C. Ewing sarcoma
    D. Plasmacytoma
    E. Primitive neuroectodermal tumors

15. A 60-year-old male presents to the emergency department (ED) with right arm swelling and pain. He has a 40-pack-per-year smoking history. He reports a 20-pound weight loss over the past 2 months. His exam is notable for pitting edema to the right upper extremity. Chest x-ray demonstrates a large mass in the right upper lobe. Which of the following is the best next step in treatment?
    A. Chemotherapy
    B. Chemotherapy and radiation
    C. Radiation therapy
    D. Endovascular stenting
    E. Thoracotomy

16. A 62-year-old male with esophageal cancer develops shortness of breath 3 days status post an esophagectomy after up-titration of his J-tube feeds. He is afebrile with a normal white blood cell (WBC) count. Chest x-ray demonstrates a large right-sided pleural effusion, and a chest tube is inserted evacuating one liter of milky white fluid. Fluid analysis demonstrates elevated triglycerides and an exudative effusion with a lymphocytic predominance. What is the next best step?
    A. NPO and TPN
    B. IR embolization of the thoracic duct
    C. VATS thoracic duct ligation
    D. Octreotide
    E. No fat, elemental tube feed regimen

17. A 45-year-old male presents to the ED with 200 mL of hemoptysis. He continues to expectorate blood and appears to be in respiratory distress. His blood pressure is 150/90 mmHg and his heart rate is 130 beats per minute with an SpO2 of 78% despite attempts at bedside suctioning. A chest radiograph reveals bilateral infiltrates. What is the next best step in management?
    A. Intubation with a double-lumen endotracheal tube
    B. Rigid bronchoscopy
    C. Bronchial artery embolization
    D. Pulmonary arteriography with selective embolization
    E. Flexible bronchoscopy

18. Which of the following is true regarding pulmonary sequestration?
    A. MRI is considered the diagnostic imaging of choice
    B. The most common presentation is recurrent pulmonary infection
    C. It typically communicates with the tracheobronchial tree
    D. Extra lobar pulmonary sequestration remains within the visceral pleura of the native lung
    E. The majority of asymptomatic cases can be observed

19. A 49-year-old male has a right-sided perihilar mass incidentally found on CT scan performed after a motor vehicle trauma 1 month ago. He has a 30-pack-per-year smoking history. He reports his clothes fit more loosely. On examination, he has purple striae on his abdomen and prominent fat on his posterior neck. PET/CT scan confirms a 4-cm irregular mass as well as an FDG avid hilar lymph node but no evidence of metastatic disease. Which of the following most likely represents this patient's definitive treatment?
    A. Radiation therapy alone
    B. Combination chemotherapy and radiation
    C. Neoadjuvant chemotherapy and resection
    D. Resection and adjuvant chemotherapy
    E. Chemotherapy

20. A rare but well-recognized complication of bronchial artery embolization performed for massive hemoptysis is:
    A. Esophageal necrosis
    B. Pulmonary infarction
    C. Paraparesis
    D. Vocal cord paralysis
    E. Tracheal necrosis

21. Which of the following is true regarding aortic stenosis (AS)?
    A. In low-risk patients with severe symptomatic AS, transcatheter aortic valve replacement is preferred
    B. The most common cause of AS is rheumatic fever
    C. Symptoms generally develop when the valve area is less than 2 cm²
    D. Swollen legs and elevated brain natriuretic peptide portend a poor prognosis
    E. Valve repair is preferred to valve replacement

22. Which of the following is true regarding intraaortic balloon pump (IABP)?
    A. It improves cardiac function in patients with cardiogenic shock due to aortic regurgitation
    B. It is beneficial in patients with aortic dissection
    C. It improves coronary blood flow during systole
    D. It is only beneficial in patients that have exhausted coronary autoregulation
    E. It is not indicated in acute myocardial infarction

23. A 50-year-old Central American man presents with a chronic cough and a draining sinus in his left chest wall. Examination of the drainage reveals sulfur granules. Which of the following is true regarding this condition?
    A. Surgical resection is indicated
    B. The organism involved is likely *Nocardia asteroids*
    C. The organism involved is an anaerobe
    D. Optimal treatment consists of trimethoprim-sulfamethoxazole
    E. Central nervous system involvement is common

24. A 45-year-old male with adenocarcinoma of the right lung presents to clinic to discuss surgical resection. Which of the following is the most important pulmonary function study to order for this patient?
    A. Arterial blood gas
    B. Forced expiratory volume 1 (FEV1)
    C. Total lung capacity
    D. Minute ventilation
    E. Diffusing capacity of the lung for carbon monoxide (DLCO)

25. The patient in question 24 undergoes pulmonary function testing for a planned lobectomy of the right lung and his FEV1 is 1.2 L. Which of the following is true?
    A. The patient is not a candidate for lobectomy
    B. Surgery can proceed as the plan is for a lobectomy
    C. A ventilation-perfusion (VQ) scan should be performed
    D. He should undergo respiratory muscle training with incentive spirometer
    E. Repeat testing should be performed following breathing treatment with albuterol

26. Which of the following statements is true regarding tracheal anatomy?
    A. The blood supply is predominantly from the superior thyroid arteries
    B. The rich collateral blood supply allows circumferential mobilization
    C. As much as 50% of the length of the trachea can be resected with a primary anastomosis following resection
    D. A tracheostomy tube is ideally placed through the first tracheal ring
    E. The first complete cartilaginous ring is the thyroid cartilage

27. Which of the following is considered a contraindication to surgical resection of a primary (nonsmall cell) carcinoma of the lung?
    A. Invasion of the chest wall
    B. A positive ipsilateral mediastinal lymph node
    C. A malignant pleural effusion
    D. Stage 3A disease
    E. Invasion of parietal pericardium

28. A 47-year-old woman presents to the ED with worsening fatigue and moderate dyspnea on exertion. She is a lifelong nonsmoker. A chest radiograph demonstrates a 3-cm nodule in the periphery of the left lung with a mild pleural effusion. She reports night sweats and a 20-pound weight loss in the past 3 months. Which of the following is the most likely diagnosis?
    A. Squamous cell carcinoma
    B. Adenocarcinoma
    C. Small cell carcinoma
    D. Bronchoalveolar
    E. Carcinoid

29. Rasmussen aneurysms form in association with:
    A. Aspergillosis
    B. Mucormycosis
    C. Cryptococcosis
    D. Tuberculosis
    E. Small cell lung cancer

30. Which one of the following statements is true regarding thymoma?
    A. The primary treatment modality is chemotherapy
    B. Malignancy is determined by mitotic activity
    C. The majority of patients with myasthenia gravis have an associated thymoma
    D. In patients with myasthenia gravis, thymectomy results are more favorable in those without a thymoma than those with one
    E. It is not associated with SVC syndrome

31. A woman who had an osteogenic sarcoma of the femur removed 2 years earlier now presents with two small lesions in the right lung and one small lesion in the left lung. A metastatic workup reveals no other abnormalities. The treatment of choice is:
    A. Bilateral wedge resections
    B. Chemotherapy
    C. Radiation therapy
    D. Immunotherapy with (bacille Calmette-Guérin) vaccine
    E. Observation

Answers

1. B. This patient presents with potentially curable esophageal cancer (stage 2). Any patient with stage 2 or greater disease should undergo neoadjuvant chemoradiation followed by esophagectomy. Based on symptoms and laboratory testing, this patient is malnourished due to dysphagia restricting adequate PO nutrition. To optimize surgical outcomes, it is vitally important to improve nutrition prior to proceeding with chemoradiation and esophagectomy (A). Enteral nutrition is preferred over parenteral nutrition (E). Enteral access should be established. Gastric conduits are preferred in reconstructing the intrathoracic esophagus. As such, all attempts should be made to avoid placement of a gastrostomy tube, which may irreparably damage the stomach and prevent future creation of a gastric conduit (C, D).

2. B. The patient in this question likely has a new diagnosis of lung cancer with concern for a para aortic lymph node metastasis. Aortopulmonary lymph node stations 5 and 6 are among the mediastinal N2 stations. With a biopsy positive for carcinoma, this patient would be no less than Stage 3A, indicating a need for downstaging with neoadjuvant chemoradiation. Cervical mediastinoscopy is the most widely used method of sampling mediastinal lymph nodes, stations 2L, 2R, 4L, 4R, and 7 (A). VATS, anterior mediastinotomy (Chamberlain procedure), or anterior mediastinoscopy (B) are reasonable methods to sample the aortopulmonary nodes, stations 5 and 6. VATS is additionally useful for stations 2, 4R, 8, and 9. Neither endobronchial ultrasound nor esophageal ultrasound offers access to the aortopulmonary lymph node stations (C, E). It is not advised to attempt percutaneous biopsy of mediastinal lymph nodes (D).

3. D. Surgical resection is the mainstay of therapy for all thymic masses. This patient has tumor characteristics that are reassuring for benign thymoma, including its size of less than 5 cm, absence of invasion into local structures, and well-defined capsule. Despite this, she should undergo resection to rule out malignancy and to prevent complications of unimpeded growth within the mediastinum. It would not be appropriate to observe with interval CT (B). Percutaneous image-guided biopsy would not affect management (A). Fine needle aspirate has no role in the diagnosis of thymoma (C). It would be premature to refer this patient to an oncologist (E). While half of patients with thymoma have concomitant myasthenia gravis, EMG would not be indicated nor help determine management.

4. A. Bronchogenic cysts are rare congenital malformations of the tracheobronchial tree. Typically, these patients present during the second decade of life with coughing, wheezing, and pneumonia. Many are asymptomatic and incidentally found on imaging. The standard of care for this condition is surgical excision by partial or total lobectomy. Even for asymptomatic patients, given concern for the development of symptoms due to airway compression or infection in addition to malignant potential, surgical excision is advised.

Thus, observation and conservative procedural management (B–E) are incorrect.

5. A. A lung abscess usually results from an aspiration event that causes a suppurative bacterial infection, leading to localized pulmonary parenchymal necrosis. These abscesses, known as primary lung abscesses, have similar risk factors as aspiration pneumonia, including history of alcohol abuse, poor dentition or gum disease, and seizure disorder or altered level of consciousness. Secondary lung abscesses, or those resulting from a preexisting condition, can result from bronchial obstruction by tumors, leading to postobstructive pneumonia and hematogenous spread via septic pulmonary emboli from infected indwelling catheters, prosthetic devices, or endocarditis. Various opportunistic infections (Nocardia, M. tuberculosis, etc.) can cause abscesses in the immunocompromised host (B–E).

Reference: Federman DD, Nabel EG, eds. *Infectious diseases: the clinician's guide to diagnosis, treatment, and prevention.* Decker Publishing; 2014.

6. C. Tracheal stenosis is most commonly due to trauma from prolonged endotracheal intubation or tracheostomy. The risk of stenosis is greater when tracheostomies are placed too high (through the first tracheal ring) or for cricothyroidotomies (the cricothyroid membrane marks the narrowest portion of the trachea). Patients with tracheal stenosis present with stridor and dyspnea on exertion, which can be confused with asthma, and usually present within 2 to 12 weeks after decannulation or extubation. The treatment of tracheal stenosis is resection and primary anastomosis. As much as 50% of the trachea (average length between 10 and 13 cm) can be resected in most adult patients using laryngeal release procedures. Most patients can be immediately extubated without tracheostomy placement (D). Laser ablation, dilation, and stenting are not definitive treatment options and are not indicated for circumferential scar formation or a stenotic segment greater than 1 cm (A, B, E).

Reference: George M, Lang F, Pasche P, Monnier P. Surgical management of laryngotracheal stenosis in adults. *Eur Arch Otorhinolaryngol.* 2005;262(8):609–615.

7. C. Lambert-Eaton or Eaton-Lambert myasthenic syndrome is a paraneoplastic syndrome associated with several malignancies, but in particular with small cell carcinoma. It presents with proximal muscle weakness and can be confused with myasthenia gravis (E). More than half (estimated to be as great as 84%) of patients have or will be discovered to have SCLC (A). The syndrome is thought to be caused by antibodies directed against presynaptic calcium channels in the neuromuscular junction that prevent the release of acetylcholine. Treatment is aimed at the underlying malignancy; however, medications shown to improve symptoms include 3,4-diaminopyridine, IV immunoglobulin, and steroids (B). Unlike in myasthenia gravis, neostigmine is not helpful and thymectomy is not effective (D).

Reference: Maddison P, Newsom-Davis J. Treatment for Lambert-Eaton myasthenic syndrome. *Cochrane Database Syst Rev.* 2005;(2):CD003279.

8. A. The recommended sequential workup for a potentially resectable lung cancer should begin with a CT scan of the chest, followed by a PET/CT scan. If the CT scan shows a mediastinal lymph node larger than 1 cm or if a mediastinal lymph node lights up on PET scan, mediastinoscopy is indicated (D). PET scanning has replaced multiorgan scanning in the search for distant metastases to the liver, adrenal glands, and bones (B, C, E). If PET scanning detects potential metastasis, it is important to obtain a tissue diagnosis before denying a possible resection.

References: Maddaus MA, Lukeitch JD. Chest wall, mediastinum, and pleura. In: Brunicardi FC, Andersen DK, Billiar TR, et al., eds. *Schwartz's principles of surgery.* 8th ed. New York: McGraw-Hill; 2005:545–610.

Silvestri GA, Tanoue LT, Margolis ML, Barker J, Detterbeck F, American College of Chest Physicians. The noninvasive staging of non-small cell lung cancer: the guidelines. *Chest.* 2003;123(1 Suppl):147S–156S.

9. B. Catamenial pneumothorax is an uncommon cause of pneumothorax in women that occurs around the time of menstruation. The exact etiology is unclear; however, it is associated with endometriosis and endometrial deposits on the pleura in most instances. The endometrial deposits lead to pleural irritation. Given that catamenial pneumothorax is difficult to diagnose prior to surgical intervention, it is often treated similarly to other spontaneous pneumothoraces with tube thoracostomy for a first episode. Similar to spontaneous pneumothorax, patients with recurrent pneumothorax should undergo VATS, blebectomy, and pleurodesis. At the same time, most clinicians suggest ligating all diaphragmatic perforations (which allows for the transfer of intraperitoneal endometrial cells to the thoracic cavity) and resecting visible endometrial implants. Treatment with hormonal suppressive therapy has been effective in preventing recurrent attacks. Apical blebs along with the other given choices are also possible etiologies of spontaneous pneumothorax but are less likely to be the cause in a patient diagnosed with catamenial pneumothorax (A, C–E).

10. C. This patient has developed a tracheoesophageal fistula (TEF) as a result of prolonged intubation. This is the most common cause of benign TEF, with an incidence of up to 3% in ventilated patients. Risk factors include high cuff pressure (single most important), high airway pressure, excessive tube motion, prolonged intubation, esophagitis, hypotension, steroids, and advanced age (D). If the endotracheal tube is placed against a rigid nasogastric tube in the esophagus, it can produce an ischemic necrosis, resulting in abnormal communication. TEF can also manifest after the patient has been extubated and will present with expectoration of food, deglutition followed by cough, and bronchopulmonary suppuration. In ventilated patients, TEF is suggested by persistent air leaks even with a hyperinflated cuff, abdominal distention (air entering the stomach through the TEF), and bronchial contamination with food and bile-colored (e.g., yellow) secretions. Bronchoscopy can often identify the TEF. Performing tracheostomy early has not been demonstrated in any large studies to prevent or decrease the development

of this complication (B). Low tidal volume ventilator management is preferred for adult respiratory distress syndrome (A). CT scan of the abdomen is not required (E).

Reference: Paraschiv M. Tracheoesophageal fistula–A complication of prolonged tracheal intubation. *J Med Life.* 2014;7(4):516–521.

11. B. This patient likely has small cell lung cancer with a paraneoplastic syndrome of inappropriate secretion of antidiuretic hormone (SIADH). This paraneoplastic syndrome develops in approximately 10% of patients with SCLC. Overall, 70% of paraneoplastic SIADH is due to SCLC. The diagnosis is made by a combination of hyponatremia, low serum osmolality, and high urine sodium and osmolality. In mild cases, treatment consists of free water restriction. In more severe cases, treatment consists of adding demeclocycline or a vasopressin-receptor antagonist such as tolvaptan. SIADH would be unusual with the other tumors listed (A, C–E). Hypercalcemia is associated with squamous cell carcinoma due to the production of parathyroid hormone (PTH)-related protein.

12. D. There are several key anatomic landmarks in the thorax that all surgeons must know. The right lung has three lobes, including the upper, middle, and lower lobes, while the left lung has two lobes, including the upper and lower lobes (A). The left lung also has the lingula, which is considered an extension of the upper lobe. The azygous vein runs along the right side, draining into the superior vena cava (B). The majority of breathing occurs by using the diaphragm, but accessory muscles can contribute up to 20% of the work of breathing. These include the sternocleidomastoid muscle, intercostal muscles, anterior scalene, and oblique muscles. The phrenic nerve runs anterior and the vagus nerve runs posterior to the lung hilum (C, E). Of note, the azygous vein is typically divided in infants during repair of esophageal atresia.

13. B. Deoxygenated blood leaves the right ventricle via the pulmonary arteries to receive oxygen in the lungs. The hemoglobin traveling in the pulmonary capillaries participates in air exchange in the alveolar sac. The newly oxygenated hemoglobin is then carried by the blood in the pulmonary veins to drain into the left atrium. Additionally, bronchial veins carrying deoxygenated blood used by the lung parenchyma also drain into the pulmonary veins and ultimately the left atrium. This results in blood in the left ventricle having a partial pressure of arterial oxygen that is 5 mmHg lower than that of blood in the pulmonary capillary (A, C). Cardiac output and pulmonary vascular resistance do not change the general flow of blood (D, E).

14. B. Chondrosarcomas are the most common primary malignancy of the chest wall (A, C–E). They usually arise anteriorly. They are typically low-grade malignancies and are slow-growing, so they are not very sensitive to chemotherapy or radiation. Treatment is radical resection. Those with unresectable disease or positive margins should be treated with radiation therapy. There is no role for adjuvant or neoadjuvant chemotherapy.

15. B. This patient likely has compression or invasion of his right subclavian vein and possibly brachial plexus due to a superior sulcus tumor (Pancoast tumor). Although not present in all patients, such as this one, the constellation of symptoms, including ipsilateral shoulder and arm pain and swelling, paresthesias, paresis, and Horner syndrome, is referred to as Pancoast syndrome. Nonsmall cell lung cancers account for up to 85% of Pancoast tumors. Small cell lung cancer is rarely associated with this syndrome. Currently, best practice for treatment of these malignancies is neoadjuvant chemotherapy and radiation followed by resection. In the previous century, surgery alone (E) as well as neoadjuvant radiation followed by surgery (C) were found to be less effective than neoadjuvant chemo-radiation. Chemotherapy alone is not the standard of care (A). The increasing instrumentation of central veins for dialysis access and pacemaker insertion has led to an increase in central vein stenosis and obstruction from scarring and fibrosis, for which endovascular intervention can be indicated (D). This patient's swelling is likely due to malignancy, and thus endovascular intervention is not indicated.

Reference: Kozower BD, Larner JM, Detterbeck FC, Jones DR. Special treatment issues in non-small cell lung cancer: diagnosis and management of lung cancer, 3rd ed: American College of Chest Physicians evidence-based clinical practice guidelines. *Chest.* 2013;143(5 Suppl):e369S–e399S.

16. E. Overall, approximately 50% of thoracic duct leaks are due to trauma, of which iatrogenic trauma is the most likely. The remainder are due to neoplastic obstruction (most common is lymphoma). The thoracic duct originates from the cisterna chyli located posterior to the abdominal aorta and ascends toward the thorax, entering the aortic hiatus at T-12 traveling to the right of the vertebral column. It crosses over to the left thorax at T5-6 and drains at the junction of the subclavian and internal jugular vein. Injury to the thoracic duct can result in pleural effusion secondary to chylothorax. Not all cases present with the white milky color suggestive of the diagnosis. Many patients present with bloody, yellow, or serosanguinous effusion. Pleural fluid analysis demonstrating chylomicrons and/or triglycerides is highly suggestive of chylothorax. Initial management of chylothorax is focused on minimizing lymphatic absorption of dietary fats. In the postsurgical patient, enteral nutrition is preferred to parenteral nutrition. With a J-tube in place, it is reasonable to change feeds to an elemental no-fat diet to minimize the production of chyle. If this fails, it is reasonable to consider NPO and TPN (A). Surgical intervention is reserved for persistent high-volume lymph leaks, defined as greater than 1 liter per day (B, C). Octreotide can be considered as a pharmacologic adjunct (D).

17. B. Up to 14% of people presenting with hemoptysis will have life-threatening hemoptysis, also known as massive hemoptysis (greater than 100 mL/hr or 500 mL/24 hr). The estimated anatomic dead space of the upper airways is 150 mL, a volume that can easily be overcome by bleeding despite coughing and mucociliary clearance. Sources of hemoptysis are variable but most commonly (up to 90% of cases) involve high-pressure bronchial arteries. Initial management should always follow standard resuscitation protocols, with ensuring a secure airway as the primary concern. This patient is unstable, with evidence of aspiration and hypoxia. As such, it would be premature to attempt interventional radiology

procedures (bronchial artery embolization or pulmonary artery catheterization and embolization) without first establishing a safe airway (C, D). Rigid bronchoscopy is the safest means to identify the source of bleeding, potentially treat the bleed and, most importantly, to establish an airway. In the event that bleeding is identified distal to the carina, rigid bronchoscopy allows for the effective intubation of the contralateral mainstem bronchus. If a rigid bronchoscope is unavailable, flexible bronchoscopy can be utilized, although these finer scopes offer less effective suctioning, which can be critical with significant hemorrhage (E). Intubation with a double-lumen tube, by itself, will not offer any therapeutic intervention to this patient (A). Furthermore, double-lumen endotracheal tubes sometimes preclude therapeutic bronchoscopic intervention given the smaller diameter of each lumen, as well as the possibility that these types of endotracheal tubes will obscure the source of bleeding. Once stable, this patient can be considered for thoracic aortogram and selective bronchial arterial embolization.

Reference: Kathuria H, Hollingsworth HM, Vilvendhan R, Reardon C. Management of life-threatening hemoptysis. *J Intensive Care.* 2020;8(1):23

18. B. Pulmonary sequestration is a rare anomaly of the lung that is classified into two types: intralobar and extralobar, with the former being more common. The key to the diagnosis is that they both have no connection to the tracheobronchial tree (C), with the intralobar type remaining within the visceral pleura of the native lung and the extralobar type enveloped in a separate pleural lining (D). They also have their own arterial supply, with the intralobar type most commonly receiving its blood supply from the thoracic aorta, while the extralobar type receives its supply from the abdominal aorta. For reasons that are unclear, the left side and lower lobes are more commonly involved. Men are more commonly affected in a 3:1 ratio. In the largest case series involving 2625 patients, the most common presentations were productive sputum, fever, and hemoptysis. The gold standard to confirm the diagnosis is pulmonary angiography, but CT angiography is considered the diagnostic imaging of choice because it is less invasive and has high sensitivity/specificity (A). Surgical resection (segmentectomy preferred over lobectomy) has been and remains the standard of care for most patients, given the potential for recurrent infections and massive hemoptysis (E). Of note, in recent years, as more adult cases are incidentally identified via cross-sectional imaging, nonoperative management is increasingly being considered for individuals with small asymptomatic lesions.

References: Alsumrain M, Ryu JH. Pulmonary sequestration in adults: a retrospective review of resected and unresected cases. *BMC Pulm Med.* 2018;18(1):97.

19. B. This patient most likely has small cell lung cancer complicated by ectopic Cushing syndrome due to the tumor's secretion of ACTH. This paraneoplastic syndrome is identified in 1% to 5% of small cell lung cancers. While pulmonary carcinoid can also cause ectopic Cushing syndrome, in a patient with a significant smoking history, small cell cancer is more likely. Small cell carcinoma of the lung (SCLC) accounts for 20% of all lung cancers and is defined by its aggressive course with a dismal 5-year survival of 5% to 10%. The term limited SCLC is given to patients with locoregional disease and offers the only hope for cure. For those with stage 1 disease (T1-2, N0) with no nodal disease, resection of the primary tumor and mediastinal sampling followed by adjuvant chemotherapy is indicated (D). There is no role for neoadjuvant chemotherapy (C). Most patients with limited SCLC will present with hilar or mediastinal lymph node involvement, such as this patient. In this case, definitive chemoradiation is indicated and presents the best chance for long-term survival. Overall, most patients present with extensive-stage disease defined as metastatic disease or extensive nodal involvement. These individuals are often excluded from radiation therapy given the toxicity induced by the wide radiation field. Most of these individuals will be managed definitively with chemotherapy (E).

References: Non-Small Cell Lung Cancer Treatment (PDQ)– Health Professional Version. National Cancer Institute. Updated January 19, 2021. https://www.cancer.gov/types/lung/hp/non-small-cell-lung-treatment-pdq

20. C. Bronchial artery embolization is an effective tool for treating patients with hemoptysis because most cases arise from the bronchial circulation rather than the pulmonary artery circulation. Embolization is highly effective in stopping the hemoptysis; however, recurrent bleeding will develop in as many as 50% of patients. In approximately 5% of patients, the blood supply to the spine (anterior spinal artery) may have a common origin with a bronchial artery, or the bronchial arteries themselves may contribute to the spinal blood supply. As such, the inadvertent embolization of the spinal artery can result in paralysis and has been estimated to occur in 1% to 4% of cases. The clinician must be aware of this rare but potentially devastating complication. Clinically apparent necrosis or infarction of the other structures is not well recognized (A, B, D, E). The most common overall complications are chest pain and transient dysphagia, which can occur in up to 30% of patients.

Reference: Kathuria H, Hollingsworth HM, Vilvendhan R, Reardon C. Management of life-threatening hemoptysis. *J Intensive Care.* 2020;8(1):23.

21. D. Aortic stenosis is most commonly due to senile calcific aortic valve disease and becomes symptomatic later in life. Since the advent of penicillin, rheumatic fever has become an uncommon etiology for this disease (B). The classic signs of aortic stenosis are angina, syncope, and congestive heart failure (CHF), which can present with swollen legs and elevated brain natriuretic peptide. Of these 3, CHF portends the worst prognosis, with median survival as low as 2 years. Patients do not have symptoms until the stenosis is severe, which occurs when the aortic valve area decreases below 1 cm^2 or the mean gradient increases above 40 mmHg (C). Aortic and pulmonary stenosis both present with a systolic murmur. Symptomatic patients who are appropriate surgical candidates should undergo aortic valve replacement. In high-risk patients (and some intermediate-risk patients) with severe symptomatic AS, transcatheter aortic valve replacement is preferred (A). Valve repair is preferred over valve replacement in patients with mitral valve disease (E).

Reference: Otto CM, Nishimura RA, Bonow RO, et al. 2020 ACC/AHA guideline for the management of patients with valvular heart disease: executive summary: a report of the American college of Cardiology/American Heart Association Joint Committee on clinical practice guidelines. *Circulation.* 2021;143(5):e35–e71.

22. D. IABP is being used more frequently in patients with low cardiac output states. The balloon is positioned in the descending thoracic aorta just distal to the left subclavian artery. The principal use of IABP is to augment coronary blood flow and, thus, myocardial oxygen supply. This is accomplished by the balloon deflating at systole, thereby reducing left ventricular afterload, and inflating at diastole, resulting in higher diastolic aortic pressure and higher coronary perfusion pressure. Coronary blood flow is improved during diastole (C). The three widely recognized indications for IABP include high-risk percutaneous coronary intervention, acute myocardial infarction, and cardiogenic shock (E). Its use outside of these clinical scenarios has led to less-than-ideal outcomes in several recent large, randomized trials, causing some to speculate if there is an added benefit in the use of IABP. The major limiting factor in these studies was poor patient selection. IABP only works by improving myocardial blood flow, which it can only do when coronary autoregulation is exhausted; otherwise, the increased coronary perfusion will be counteracted by the increased coronary vascular resistance, which under normal physiologic conditions works with high fidelity to guarantee constant myocardial blood flow over a wide range of aortic pressures. There are several absolute contraindications to IABP, including aortic regurgitation, because it can worsen the magnitude of regurgitation (A). Additionally, IABP should be avoided in patients with suspected aortic dissection (because it can extend into the false lumen) and used with caution in patients with abdominal aortic aneurysm (because it can result in rupture) (B).

Reference: van Nunen LX, Noc M, Kapur NK, Patel MR, Perera D, Pijls NHJ. Usefulness of intra-aortic balloon pump counterpulsation. *Am J Cardiol.* 2016;117(3):469–476.

23. C. Given the draining sinus and sulfur granules, the patient most likely has actinomycosis, a chronic disease usually caused by *Actinomyces israelii* that occurs most commonly in the head and neck region. Because of its rarity and chronicity, the diagnosis is often delayed and unrecognized. A key to the diagnosis is the finding of chronic sinuses with discharge of purulent material containing yellow-brown sulfur granules. The organisms enter the lungs via the oral cavity. The organisms are often not cultured out because they are anaerobes. Lung involvement can present with progressive pulmonary fibrosis. Central nervous system involvement is not common (E). Prolonged, high-dose penicillin is the treatment of choice (D). Surgery is generally not indicated; however, pulmonary actinomycosis can easily be confused with a lung cancer, prompting surgical intervention (A). *N. asteroides* is a gram-positive rod that mimics fungi microscopically because of its branched filamentous morphology and causes nocardiosis in immunocompromised patients (B). It is associated with pneumonia, endocarditis, and central nervous system abscess. The treatment is trimethoprim-sulfamethoxazole.

Reference: Hsieh MJ, Liu HP, Chang JP, Chang CH. Thoracic actinomycosis. *Chest.* 1993;104(2):366–370.

24. B. Pulmonary function studies are routinely performed when any resection greater than a wedge resection is planned. FEV1 is regarded as the best predictor of complications of lung resection in the initial assessment of patients. If the

FEV1 is greater than 80% of what is expected, the patient can tolerate a pneumonectomy. Typically, a preoperative FEV1 of 2.0 liters indicates a patient's fitness to undergo pneumonectomy and 1.5 L a lobectomy. One must bear in mind that these rough guidelines do not factor in such things as the patient's age, body size, and predicted postoperative FEV1. If the patient's preoperative FEV1 is borderline, quantitative perfusion lung scanning or SPECT/CT can be used to obtain a predicted postoperative FEV1. Any postoperative value of less than 40% indicates a higher risk for postoperative mortality and morbidity. Additionally, preoperative DLCO less than 50% of what is predicted is associated with increased complications and mortality with pneumonectomy or lobectomy. (E) Total arterial blood gas, lung capacity, and resting minute ventilation are not included in these predictors (A, C, D).

25. C. If pulmonary function testing is within normal limits, no further testing is required, and the patient can be scheduled for surgery (B). If it is below the accepted limits, further testing is recommended, including quantitative VQ scan or SPECT/CT; this permits calculation of postoperative pulmonary reserve. The minimum acceptable predicted postoperative FEV1 is 800 mL. If the desired lobe has minimal contribution to FEV1, then the patient can still tolerate a resection (A). If the predicted FEV1 is less than 800 mL, the patient should then be referred to an oncology physician to discuss nonsurgical management. Respiratory muscle training with an incentive spirometer has not been demonstrated to improve pulmonary function test results (D). Breathing treatments may have a slight improvement in pulmonary function testing but will not correct the underlying disease (E).

26. C. The cricoid cartilage is the first cartilaginous ring of the airway and consists of an anterior arch and a posterior broad-based plate (E). The tracheal blood supply is segmental via the inferior thyroid and bronchial arteries (A). Each arterial branch supplies a 1- to 2-cm length of the trachea. Circumferential mobilization will disrupt the blood supply (B). The trachea has approximately 18 to 22 rings and is approximately 10 to 13 cm long. As much as 6 cm of length can be resected primarily using laryngeal release procedures. A tracheostomy is ideally placed between the second and third or third and fourth tracheal rings; higher placement increases the risk of tracheal stenosis and lower placement increases the risk of tracheoinnominate fistula (D).

27. C. Stage 4 nonsmall cell lung cancer is treated primarily with definitive chemotherapy and radiation therapy. There may be a role for surgical intervention for palliation of symptoms (e.g., thoracentesis or pleural window for recurrent pleural effusions), but, in general, stage 4 disease is not managed surgically. Of the aforementioned findings, malignant pleural effusion is a marker for stage 4 disease (an effusion with malignant cells is considered M1a disease) (A, B, D, E). Other clinical findings that are diagnostic of stage 4 disease include distant metastases, a positive contralateral mediastinal lymph node, and bilateral endobronchial tumors. Attempts at surgical resection are generally reserved for stages 1 to 3A. Relative contraindications to surgical intervention include recurrent laryngeal nerve involvement;

Horner syndrome; pericardial involvement; and SVC syndrome. Surgery may be indicated for selected patients with stage 3A disease in combination with neoadjuvant chemotherapy and radiotherapy. A positive ipsilateral mediastinal lymph node is N2 disease (at minimum stage 3A), a potentially resectable lesion. A contralateral mediastinal lymph node or supraclavicular node is at least stage 3B (N3 disease). Patients with stage 1 have only a 50% 5-year survival rate with resection. Stage 2 patients have a 5-year survival rate after surgery of only 30%, whereas those with stage 3A have a 17% 5-year survival rate. The stage 3B survival rate is 5%, and the stage 4 survival rate approaches zero.

Reference: National Comprehensive Cancer Network. NCCN Clinical Practice Guidelines in Oncology: Non-Small Cell Lung Cancer. National Comprehensive Cancer Network, Inc. 2015; Version 7.2015. https://www2.tri-kobe.org/nccn/guideline/archive/lung2015-2017/english/non_small.pdf

28. B. Adenocarcinoma is the most common lung cancer in nonsmokers (and overall). It is also more common in women and is most commonly a peripheral lesion. Though this could be many different types of malignancy, given the patient's age, lifelong nonsmoking status, and the findings on chest radiograph, adenocarcinoma is the most likely diagnosis (A, C–E). Additionally, the pleural effusion is concerning for stage 4 disease.

Reference: Nason KS, Maddaus MA, Luketich JD. Chest wall, lung, mediastinum, and pleura. In: Brunicardi FC, Andersen DK, Schwartz SI, eds. *Schwartz's principles of surgery.* 9th ed. McGraw-Hill; 2010.

29. D. Active tuberculosis can lead to massive hemoptysis. Most hemoptysis is due to bronchial artery bleeding and is managed via bronchial artery embolization. Rarely, hemoptysis is due to a Rasmussen aneurysm, which is a pulmonary artery aneurysm adjacent to or within a tuberculous cavity (A–C, E). Such an aneurysm would be managed by pulmonary arteriography and selective distal embolization. CT scanning is useful in hemoptysis to help localize the source and guide interventional management.

Reference: Picard C, Parrot A, Boussaud V, et al. Massive hemoptysis due to Rasmussen aneurysm: detection with helicoidal CT angiography and successful steel coil embolization. *Intensive Care Med.* 2003;29(10):1837–1839.

30. D. Thymoma is the most common neoplasm of the anterior mediastinum. Malignancy is determined based on evidence of local invasion of adjacent structures or capsular invasion, not on cellular or histologic characteristics (B). Treatment is by surgical resection (A). Thymomas are radiosensitive, so radiation therapy is used as an adjunct in locally advanced cases. As many as 50% of patients with thymomas have symptoms of myasthenia gravis. Conversely, less than 10% of patients with myasthenia gravis are found to have a thymoma on imaging (C). Nevertheless, thymectomy improves or resolves symptoms of myasthenia gravis in as many as 90% of patients without a thymoma, compared with only approximately 25% of patients with thymomas. Due to their location, large thymomas can present with SVC syndrome (E).

31. A. An increase in overall survival has been achieved with the resection of isolated lung metastases (B–E). This is especially true of osteogenic sarcoma, but it has been reported for other malignancies as well. Prior to metastasectomy, however, several conditions must be met. Ideally, lung metastases present metachronously, and the primary tumor has already been controlled; the metastatic lesion should be completely resectable, and there should be no evidence of diffuse carcinomatosis. Pulmonary metastasis occurs in as many as 40% to 60% of all primary sarcomas of the limbs within 3 years, and a 30% to 50% 5-year survival rate can be achieved with metastasectomy. In general, solitary metastases have a better prognosis. However, multiple pulmonary metastases due to osteogenic sarcoma treated with metastasectomy have achieved similar positive results as solitary metastatic lesions. Factors associated with survival following metastasectomy include a disease-free interval from primary tumor to initial evidence of metastasis, surgical resectability, tumor doubling time, and the number of metastases.

Reference: Marulli G, Mammana M, Comacchio G, Rea F. Survival and prognostic factors following pulmonary metastasectomy for sarcoma. *J Thorac Dis.* 2017;9(Suppl 12):S1305–S1315. doi:10.21037/jtd.2017.03.177

Pediatric Surgery

ALEXANDRA MOORE, VERONICA SULLINS, AND STEVEN L. LEE

22

ABSITE 99th Percentile High-Yields

I. Hernias
   A. Inguinal:
      1. Etiology is patent processus vaginalis (indirect hernia) in 99%; tx is high ligation, no mesh
      2. Risk of incarceration is inversely proportional to age (younger patients have higher risk of incarceration); 5% of patients have contralateral hernia not detected clinically
   B. Umbilical:
      1. Repair if symptomatic or at 4 years of age or older
      2. If defect is <2 cm, there is >95% chance of spontaneous resolution
   C. Congenital Diaphragmatic Hernia:
      1. Most common is Bochdalek (posterolateral), on left side; usually diagnosed on prenatal US
      2. Pulmonary hypertension causes hypoxia and significant morbidity; pulmonary arteries are anatomically different and less responsive to pulmonary vasodilators (such as nitric oxide)
      3. Pulmonary hypoplasia occurs in both lungs, with ipsilateral lungs, more affected; pulmonary hypoplasia will result in hypercapnia
      4. Management:
         a) Start with NG tube decompression and respiratory support; intubation with gentle mechanical ventilation strategy with permissive hypercapnia to minimize barotrauma; may need ECMO
         b) Surgical repair delayed, allowing pulmonary hypertension to improve or stabilize

II. Pyloric Stenosis
   A. Nonbilious, projectile vomiting in a 3- to 6-week-old; may have palpable "olive-like" abdominal mass
   B. Hypochloremic, hypokalemic metabolic alkalosis; alkalosis due to vomiting HCl; hypokalemia from renal loss of potassium (dehydration leads to activation of the renin, angiotensin, aldosterone system, aldosterone causes renal loss of potassium)
   C. Paradoxical aciduria: Urine is transiently acidic due to Na conservation with excretion of H (prevents worsening of hypokalemia)
   D. Diagnose with ultrasound, will show hypertrophied pylorus (>3 mm thick, >15 mm long)
   E. Management:
      1. Start with resuscitation! Normal saline bolus, maintenance IV fluids at 1.5× maintenance rate, add KCl to maintenance fluids once patient urinates
      2. Goal is for patient to be resuscitated with correction of electrolyte abnormalities prior to surgery; preop lab goals: pH <7.45, base excess <3.5, bicarb <26, Na >132, K >3.5, Cl >100, glucose >72; increased risk of postoperative apnea if uncorrected alkalosis prior to surgery
      3. Surgery is Fredet-Ramstedt pyloromyotomy: partial-thickness longitudinal incision in the pylorus 1 to 2 mm proximal to the duodenum, extend proximally to normal antrum; recurrence most commonly a result of not extending myotomy far enough proximally to antrum

III. Malrotation and Midgut Volvulus
   A. Presentation is typically bilious emesis ± abdominal distention
   B. Diagnosis is via UGI series (duodenum does not cross midline)
   C. If peritonitis is present, then avoid UGI and immediately go to OR
   D. Ladd procedure to minimize chance of future volvulus (create complete nonrotation anatomy)
      1. De-torse the bowel in a counterclockwise fashion ("turn back the clock")
      2. Divide Ladd bands (peritoneal attachments of right colon to paracolic gutter)
      3. Straighten the duodenum and fix the duodenum in the right upper quadrant
      4. Mobilize colon to patient's left and fix the cecum in the left lower quadrant
      5. Widen the base of the mesentery (key component)
      6. ± Appendectomy

IV. Esophageal Atresia and Tracheoesophageal Fistula
   A. Echocardiogram to rule out associated cardiac anomalies (right arch in 1%–2%)
   B. Types:

Type	Esophageal atresia	Tracheoesophageal fistula
Type A	Present	Absent
Type B	Present	Present; fistula with proximal esophagus
Type C	Present	Present; fistula with distal esophagus
Type D	Present	Present; fistula with both proximal and distal esophagus
Type E	Absent	Present, also called H-type

   C. Type C most common; treat with Immediate repair
   D. Staged repair for Type A
      1. Initial g-tube placement and allow patient to grow until two ends are close enough for repair

V. Abdominal Wall Defects

Factor	Omphalocele	Gastroschisis
Sac	Present	Absent
Location of defect	Central (through umbilicus)	To the right of the umbilicus
Umbilical cord	Inserts into sac	Normal
Defect Size	Large	Small
Contents	Bowel, liver	Bowel, gonads
Bowel	Normal	Matted
Malrotation	Present	Present
Small abdomen	Present	Present
GI function	Normal	Prolonged ileus
Associated anomalies	Common (30%–70%)	Unusual (atresia 15%)
Associated syndromes	Beckwith Wiedemann, Trisomy, Cantrell	Not observed

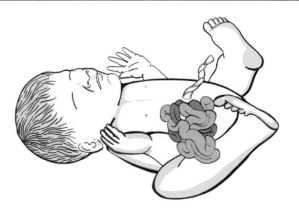

Gastroschisis

Gastroschisis is a defect in the abdominal wall defect (usually <4 cm) that is believed to arise from isolated vascular insult (rupture of intrauterine vein). It typically occurs to right of normal umbilical cord with abdominal organs herniating through the defect, there is no membranous covering sac, and the incidence of associated anomalies is low. 10% have intestinal atresia.

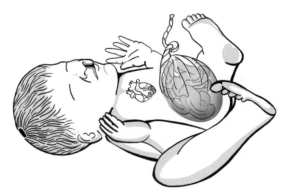

Omphalocele

Omphaloceles occur as a result of the failure of the umbilical ring to close. Intestines protrude through base of umbilical cord and herniate into a membranous sac. There is a high incidence of associated anomalies: craniofacial abnormalities, cardiac malformations, and cutis aplasia among others.

Fig. 22.1 Gastroschisis vs. Omphalocele.

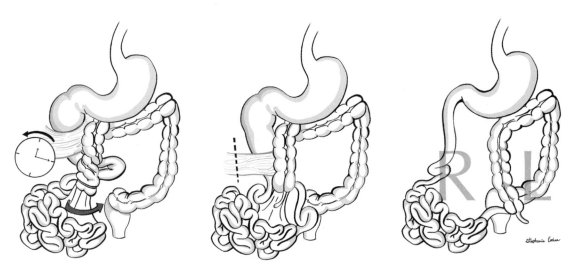

During normal development, the midgut undergoes a 270° counterclockwise rotation about the superior mesenteric artery. In malrotation, this rotation arrests or fails to occur, and the cecum and duodenum become tethered by fibrous bands called Ladd band. The Ladd procedure is aimed at preventing or alleviating midgut volvulus and vascular compromise. The first step is to rotate the bowel counterclockwise as if "turning back the hands of time". The second step is to divide the Ladd band. Ultimately, to minimize the chance of another midgut volvulus, the base of the mesentery is widened and the small bowel will be placed in the right abdomen and the colon will be placed in the left. Classically, an appendectomy is performed to avoid diagnostic confusion in the future. However, this has become controversial in modern times.

Fig. 22.2 The Ladd Procedure.

Questions

1. A 9-year-old boy is seen in the emergency room with a 1-day history of right lower quadrant abdominal pain and low-grade fever. On exam, he is focally tender in the right lower quadrant. WBC count is 15,000/mcL and US shows a 9-mm noncompressible appendix and an appendicolith. Which of the following is true about this condition?
   A. If nonoperative management with antibiotics is to be considered, a CT scan should be first obtained
   B. Success of nonoperative management in this patient is anticipated to be very high
   C. Nonoperative management tends to result in shorter hospital stay as compared to appendectomy
   D. Appendectomy is preferred in this patient
   E. Failure of nonoperative management is likely to manifest as peritonitis

2. A 10-year-old boy is a restrained passenger in a high-speed motor vehicle collision. On arrival to the emergency department, his heart rate is 140 beats per minute and his systolic blood pressure is 80 mmHg. There is an obvious deformity of his left thigh. GCS is 13. Pupils are equal and reactive. Abdomen is mildly tender to palpation. Focused assessment with sonography in trauma (FAST) is positive for peritoneal fluid. He is administered 20 mL/kg of crystalloid, and BP remains 80 mmHg. Which of the following is the most appropriate next step?
   A. CT scan of head/abdomen/pelvis
   B. Start blood product transfusion and transport to the OR for exploratory laparotomy
   C. Infuse additional bolus of isotonic crystalloid
   D. Infuse lactated ringers
   E. Infuse 3% hypertonic saline

3. A 6-month-old girl is brought to the trauma center for evaluation of a head injury. Parents report that the patient rolled off a bed. Which of the following injuries suggest abusive head trauma?
   A. Isolated skull fracture
   B. Head and neck bruising
   C. Subdural hematoma
   D. Epidural hematoma
   E. Cortical contusion

4. A 12-day-old ex-27-week premature boy was previously advancing well on enteral feeds. He becomes acutely distended. Initial abdominal radiographs reveal moderate pneumatosis intestinalis and enteral feedings were held. Three hours later, a repeat abdominal radiograph reveals pneumoperitoneum. The patient is brought emergently to the operating room for laparotomy where three areas of necrotic bowel are encountered along with numerous other areas of patchy ischemia. What is the next best step in management?
   A. Resection of necrotic bowel only, with primary anastomoses
   B. Resection of both necrotic and patchy ischemic bowel with primary anastomosis
   C. Place drains without bowel resection
   D. Resection of all necrotic and ischemic bowel with primary anastomosis and proximal diverting stoma
   E. Resection of necrotic bowel only, leave in discontinuity, second look in about 48 hours

5. A previously healthy 2-month-old girl is brought to the emergency department due to a 2-hour history of intermittent inconsolable crying, vomiting, and apparent pain. She is not eating. Her parents brought her to the hospital after she passed a loose, maroon-colored stool. There are no signs of peritonitis on exam. WBC count is normal. Which of the following is recommended?
   A. CT scan of the abdomen
   B. Laparoscopy
   C. Colonoscopy
   D. Nuclear scan
   E. Abdominal ultrasound

6. A 13-year-old female presents with severe right lower quadrant pain and emesis. At laparoscopy an ovarian torsion is found. The ovary appears swollen with a blueish-black discoloration. It remains unchanged after detorsion. The next step in management is:
   A. Biopsy
   B. Oophoropexy
   C. Oophorectomy
   D. Salpingo-oophorectomy
   E. Close and obtain serial ultrasound

7. A full-term baby girl has a diagnosis of a right-sided congenital lung malformation identified on prenatal imaging. Chest radiograph in the newborn nursery shows a cystic lesion in the right lower lobe with no mediastinal shift. She is asymptomatic and on room air. What is the next step in management?
   A. CT scan of the chest prior to discharge
   B. Discharge with CT angiogram of the chest within 6 months
   C. Right lower lobectomy
   D. Right tube thoracostomy
   E. Inpatient MRI of the chest

8. During laparoscopy for early acute appendicitis in a 5-year-old boy, you find a large, right-sided renal mass. You perform an appendectomy and:
   A. Close, then obtain further workup
   B. Biopsy the mass
   C. Right nephroureterectomy
   D. Right nephroureterectomy with ipsilateral lymph node sampling
   E. Right nephroureterectomy with ipsilateral lymph node sampling and contralateral renal biopsy

9. A 2-week-old boy presents with constipation and abdominal bloating. He failed to pass meconium on the first 2 days of life. Contrast enema demonstrates a slightly dilated sigmoid colon with a constricted rectum. What is the next most appropriate step in management?
   A. Rectal irrigations and IV antibiotics
   B. Creation of a leveling ostomy
   C. Suction rectal biopsy
   D. Change to an elemental formula
   E. Obtain a UGI contrast series with small bowel follow-through

10. A newborn is in severe respiratory distress and has a markedly scaphoid abdomen. Which of the following is true regarding this condition?
    A. A chest tube should be promptly placed
    B. The patient should be ventilated with bag-mask ventilation
    C. Severe cases may benefit from extracorporeal membrane oxygenation
    D. Ventilation with high-frequency oscillation is contraindicated
    E. Urgent thoracotomy is required

11. A full-term, healthy newborn boy is noted to have imperforate anus. After 24 hours, no meconium is visualized in the perineal area. The most appropriate management should be:
    A. Observation for another 24 hours
    B. Diverting ileostomy
    C. Sigmoid colostomy
    D. Primary repair through the perineum
    E. Laparoscopic primary repair

12. A 2-month-old infant has persistent jaundice. Ultrasonography fails to demonstrate a gallbladder. Technetium-99m hepatobiliary iminodiacetic acid (HIDA) scanning with phenobarbital pretreatment reveals uptake in the liver but not in the intestine. α1-Antitrypsin and cystic fibrosis determination is normal. The most appropriate surgical management would be:
    A. Kasai operation (hepatoportoenterostomy)
    B. Liver transplantation
    C. Percutaneous transhepatic liver drainage
    D. Endoscopic biliary stent placement
    E. Choledochojejunostomy

13. A 1-day-old full-term infant presents with bilious emesis. Abdominal x-rays show multiple loops of dilated bowel. A contrast enema shows a microcolon. What is the pathophysiology behind this obstruction?
    A. A fetal mesenteric vascular accident
    B. Failure of recanalization of the bowel
    C. Lack of proper rotation of the bowel
    D. Lack of ganglion cells in the bowel
    E. A duplication of a segment of bowel

14. A newborn baby is born with an abdominal wall defect. The defect involves the umbilicus and has a membrane associated with it. Which of the following is true regarding this type of defect?
    A. This patient requires immediate surgical closure
    B. Mortality is most often the result of persistent sepsis
    C. The etiology is due to an umbilical vein vascular accident
    D. The defect is usually associated with intestinal atresia
    E. These patients commonly have associated cardiac and genetic abnormalities

15. The most common indication for extracorporeal membranous oxygenation (ECMO) in neonates is:
    A. Congenital diaphragmatic hernia
    B. Respiratory distress syndrome
    C. Meconium aspiration
    D. Persistent pulmonary hypertension
    E. Congenital cardiac abnormalities

16. Which of the following is true regarding Bochdalek type of congenital diaphragmatic hernia (CDH)?
    A. Urgent surgical repair is indicated upon diagnosis
    B. Associated pulmonary hypoplasia leads to hypocarbia
    C. Most defects are on the right
    D. Pulmonary hypertension is a prominent feature
    E. The diaphragmatic defect is anteromedial

17. A full-term baby is born with drooling, coughing, and cyanosis after the first feeding, but these resolve quickly and spontaneously. The next step in management should be:
    A. Immediate intubation
    B. Placement of orogastric tube
    C. Two-view abdominal x-ray
    D. Two-view chest x-ray
    E. Upper gastrointestinal (UGI) contrast series

18. A patient is diagnosed with pyloric stenosis after 3 days of nonbilious emesis. This patient's electrolyte and acid/base balance will result in:
    A. Respiratory alkalosis
    B. Hyperkalemia
    C. Aciduria
    D. Hyperchloremia
    E. Hyponatremia

19. A 900-g premature infant develops formula intolerance with vomiting, abdominal distention, and bloody stools. Labs show an elevated white blood cell (WBC) count and platelets of 100,000/mcL. Abdominal x-rays show dilated loops of bowel with pneumatosis intestinalis. The most appropriate treatment would be:
    A. Blood and platelet transfusions
    B. Antibiotics and bowel rest/decompression
    C. Ultrasound and paracentesis
    D. Placement of a bedside peritoneal drain
    E. Exploratory laparotomy

20. A healthy 2-week-old girl develops bilious emesis. On exam, her abdomen is nontender and nondistended. What is the most appropriate study to make the diagnosis?
    A. 2-view abdominal x-ray
    B. Ultrasound
    C. UGI series
    D. Contrast enema
    E. Computed tomography (CT) scan of abdomen/pelvis

21. Operative management for a patient with malrotation and midgut volvulus typically includes reduction of the volvulus, division of Ladd bands, and which of the following?
    A. Placement of the small intestine in the left lower quadrant
    B. Cecopexy and gastropexy
    C. Broaden base of the small bowel mesentery
    D. Placement of the cecum in the right upper quadrant
    E. Reconstruction of the ligament of Treitz

22. A full-term baby boy is noted to have facial features of trisomy 21 and bilious emesis. The rest of his exam is normal. Abdominal x-rays show a double-bubble sign with no distal gas. Which of the following is the best next step in management?
    A. Serial abdominal x-rays
    B. UGI contrast study
    C. Contrast enema
    D. Operative exploration
    E. Echocardiogram

23. A 2-year-old child presents with an abdominal mass, "raccoon eyes," and "blueberry muffin" skin lesions. These most likely represent:
    A. Rhabdomyosarcoma
    B. Neuroblastoma
    C. Wilms tumor
    D. Hepatoblastoma
    E. Teratoma

24. The most common anomaly associated with gastroschisis is:
    A. Cardiac
    B. Renal
    C. Limb
    D. Malrotation
    E. Down syndrome

25. A newborn baby is born with a distended abdomen and bilious emesis. Both parents are carriers for cystic fibrosis. On examination, the patient has a distended but soft abdomen. Abdominal x-rays show dilated loops of bowel with a ground-glass appearance. The most appropriate initial management is:
    A. Water-soluble contrast enemas
    B. Resection of terminal ileum with stoma
    C. Resection of terminal ileum with primary anastomosis
    D. UGI with small bowel follow-through
    E. Small bowel enterotomy with evacuation of meconium

26. A 6-month-old boy presents to the ED crying in pain and has bilious emesis. On exam, he has a distended abdomen, and there is a tender mass in the right groin. Appropriate management would be:
    A. Ultrasound of right groin
    B. Bedside incision and drainage (I&D) of right groin
    C. IV antibiotics
    D. Attempt reduction
    E. Operative exploration

27. A 4-year-old girl presents with recurrent jaundice. Ultrasound shows a 5-cm fusiform dilation of the common bile duct. During surgery, the posterior aspect of the cystic mass is firmly adherent to the portal vein. The most appropriate management is:
    A. Abort surgery, IV antibiotics, and reoperate in 3 months
    B. Place a drain into the cyst, IV antibiotics, and reoperate in 3 months
    C. Resect the anterior cyst, mucosectomy of the posterior cyst with reconstruction
    D. Internal drainage of the cyst with a Roux-en-Y cystojejunostomy
    E. Resect the cyst and portal vein with reconstruction of the portal vein and common bile duct (CBD)

28. A 2-week-old, ex-25-week premature boy is in the neonatal ICU (NICU) and is diagnosed with a left inguinal hernia. His current weight is 1 kg and he requires supplemental oxygen. The hernia is easily reducible. The next appropriate step in management is:
    A. Ultrasound evaluation
    B. Immediate open operative repair
    C. Immediate laparoscopic repair
    D. Repair just prior to discharge
    E. Delay repair until 1 year of age

29. The pathogenesis of necrotizing enterocolitis (NEC) is thought to be related to:
    A. A genetic predisposition
    B. An enzyme deficiency
    C. A period of intestinal hypoperfusion
    D. Preexisting intestinal atresia
    E. An antibiotic reaction

30. A newborn baby with a prenatal diagnosis of gastroschisis is born with the entire small intestine outside of the abdomen. The bowel appears ischemic and the abdominal wall defect is small and tight. The most appropriate next step in management is:
    A. Place a bedside silo
    B. Primary reduction and closure
    C. Open the abdominal wall defect
    D. Resect the ischemic bowel
    E. Create a diverting ileostomy

31. A 1-week-old full-term baby with abdominal distention, fever, tachycardia, and low urine output is transferred to the NICU. The patient has not passed meconium. He had a suction rectal biopsy showing aganglionosis. Digital rectal examination shows explosive, foul-smelling liquid stools. Despite broad-spectrum IV antibiotics and rectal irrigation, he is clinically deteriorating. The next step in management is to:
    A. Perform contrast enema
    B. Perform loop colostomy
    C. Perform subtotal colectomy and ileostomy
    D. Perform abdominal decompression for abdominal compartment syndrome
    E. Add additional antifungal coverage

32. A 4-week-old infant presents with bilious vomiting, irritability, abdominal wall edema, and erythema. Plain films reveal proximal dilated bowel, with a paucity of distal bowel gas. Which is true regarding this patient?
    A. An urgent UGI series is indicated
    B. A trial of nasogastric tube decompression is often helpful
    C. Endoscopic decompression is often beneficial
    D. A CT scan of the abdomen and pelvis should be obtained
    E. Delay in management may lead to a need for intestinal transplantation

33. A neonate is found to have bilateral undescended testes that are not palpable in the inguinal canal. Which of the following is true regarding this condition?
    A. A bilateral orchiopexy should be performed by 1 year of age
    B. Orchiopexy does not improve fertility potential
    C. It is not associated with prune belly syndrome
    D. Chorionic gonadotropin does not aid in testicular descent
    E. The testicular arteries must be preserved during operation

Answers

1. D. Appendectomy is the preferred treatment strategy for this patient because of the presence of a fecolith. While appendectomy has been the gold standard for the treatment of uncomplicated appendicitis, multiple studies have demonstrated that nonoperative management of uncomplicated appendicitis is safe and effective. Nonoperative management consists of initial broad-spectrum IV antibiotics and IV fluids. Patients can be transitioned to oral antibiotics and discharged when their pain improves, fever resolves, and they are able to tolerate a diet. The total antibiotic course should be 7 days. Nonoperative management is initially successful in 85% to 92% of patients. Patients managed nonoperatively have a higher readmission rate within 1 year, primarily due to recurrent appendicitis. Due to recurrence of appendicitis, the 1-year success rate of avoiding appendectomy is 67%. Most would recommend only offering nonoperative management in children aged 5 to 17 years meeting the following criteria: uncomplicated appendicitis confirmed on imaging (US, CT, or MRI) (A), WBC between 5000 and 18,000, pain for <48 hours, localized tenderness, and no appendicolith. Appendicolith has been associated with failure of nonoperative management of appendicitis (B). Failure of nonoperative management can manifest as worsening or persistent symptoms or as systemic sepsis despite antibiotic treatment; and usually does not manifest as diffuse peritonitis (E). While some studies have demonstrated that children treated nonoperatively for appendicitis may return to school sooner, the hospital length of stay is longer with nonoperative management than with appendectomy (C).

References: Minneci PC, Sulkowski JP, Nacion KM, et al. Feasibility of a nonoperative management strategy for uncomplicated acute appendicitis in children. *J Am Coll Surg.* 2014;219(2):272–279.

Patkova B, Svenningsson A, Almström M, Eaton S, Wester T, Svensson JF. Nonoperative treatment versus appendectomy for acute nonperforated appendicitis in children: five-year follow up of a randomized controlled pilot trial. *Ann Surg.* 2020;271(6):1030–1035.

Shindoh J, Niwa H, Kawai K, et al. Predictive factors for negative outcomes in initial non-operative management of suspected appendicitis. *J Gastrointest Surg.* 2010;14(2):309–314.

2. B. Trauma is the most common cause of childhood mortality. Compared to adults, children remain hemodynamically compensated until 30% to 45% of their blood volume is lost. Crystalloid resuscitation should be initiated due to its immediate availability, although infused volumes should be limited to 20 mL/kg in the child who is a hemodynamic nonresponder. In patients who do not respond to a single 20 mL/kg isotonic fluid bolus, pRBC transfusion is the next most appropriate step in resuscitation (D). Trauma patients with a positive FAST who are hemodynamically unresponsive to fluid or blood resuscitation require operative exploration (A). Hypertonic saline may be useful in trauma patients with closed-head injuries that are suspected to have elevated intracranial pressure (e.g., blown pupil on exam suggesting uncal herniation) (E). Excessive crystalloid resuscitation leads to the hemodilution of clotting factors, worsening coagulopathy, and metabolic acidosis should be avoided in patients who have clearly experienced significant hemorrhage (C). Hypervolemia should also be avoided in patients with traumatic brain injury as it can result in secondary insults to the brain. Although massive transfusion has been variably defined, the most widely accepted pediatric definition is the transfusion of blood products in excess of 40 mL/kg over the first 24 hours following injury. This pragmatic threshold reliably identified critically injured children at risk for 24-hour and in-hospital mortality in a combat-injury trauma cohort of patients less than 18 years of age. While there is good evidence in adults that the implementation of massive transfusion protocols is associated with improved mortality and morbidity and decreased total blood use, the evidence in children is less clear, with no studies to date showing reduced mortality or morbidity associated with the implementation of an MTP in a pediatric trauma center.

References: Acker SN, Ross JT, Partrick DA, DeWitt P, Bensard DD. Injured children are resistant to the adverse effects of early high volume crystalloid resuscitation. *J Pediatr Surg.* 2014;49(12):852–1855.

Duchesne JC, Heaney J, Guidry C, et al. Diluting the benefits of hemostatic resuscitation: a multi-institutional analysis. *J Trauma Acute Care Surg.* 2013;75(1):76–82.

Leeper CM, McKenna C, Gaines BA. Too little too late: hypotension and blood transfusion in the trauma bay are independent predictors of death in injured children. *J Trauma Acute Care Surg.* 2018;85(4):674–678.

Magoteaux SR, Notrica DM, Langlais CS, et al. Hypotension and the need for transfusion in pediatric blunt spleen and liver injury: an ATOMAC+ prospective study. *J Pediatr Surg.* 2017;52(6):979–83.

Notrica DM, Eubanks JW, 3rd, Tuggle DW, et al. Nonoperative management of blunt liver and spleen injury in children: evaluation of the ATOMAC guideline using GRADE. *J Trauma Acute Care Surg.* 2015;79(4):683–693.

3. B. The American Academy of Pediatrics prefers the term *abusive head trauma* (AHT) to "shaken baby syndrome." In children less than 2 years of age, nonaccidental trauma accounts for 10% of head injuries. However, AHT accounts for over half of serious head injury morbidity and mortality. Improved diagnosis is important because up to one-third of AHT cases are missed on initial presentation leading to additional repeated injury. AHT is typically the result of vigorous shaking leading to an acceleration-deceleration force. This type of force causes disruption of cortical veins resulting in interhemispheric subdural or subarachnoid hemorrhage. Additional associated injuries include diffuse axonal injury, shear injury, white matter tears, and retinal hemorrhage, (C). In contrast, the most frequent accidental head injuries result from impact, producing linear skull fractures, epidural hematomas, localized homogenous subdural hemorrhages, and cortical contusion (A, D, E). A metaanalysis identified retinal hemorrhage, lack of adequate history, subdural hemorrhage, and metaphyseal and rib fractures as the most indicative findings of abusive head trauma.

Reference: Piteau SJ, Ward MG, Barrowman NJ, Plint AC. Clinical and radiographic characteristics associated with abusive and nonabusive head trauma: a systematic review. *Pediatrics.* 2012;130(2):315–323.

4. E. This infant is presenting with surgical necrotizing enterocolitis (NEC). Very low birthweight infants are at the highest risk for NEC. The etiology of NEC is mucosal compromise in the presence of pathogenic bacteria. NEC is frequently associated with the introduction of enteral feedings. This leads to bowel injury and an inflammatory cascade. Pneumoperitoneum is an absolute indication for surgical intervention. Areas of frank necrosis should be resected. In cases with patchy ischemia where the viability of the bowel is unclear, potentially salvageable bowel should not be resected to reduce the risk of short gut syndrome. (B, D) In these cases, the necrotic segments should be resected, left in discontinuity, and dropped back into the abdomen ("clip and drop") with plans for reexploration in 24 to 48 hours. When areas of ischemia are present, primary anastomoses should not be attempted until the viability of all bowel segments has been established (A). In some cases, patients will develop total intestinal necrosis with no apparent viable bowel. These patients should be closed without resection so that a thorough discussion can occur with the family about the implications of potential operative intervention (C). A common teaching is that NEC classically presents with bloody stools after the first feeding. However, the earliest signs are nonspecific, including apnea, bradycardia, lethargy, and temperature instability. The most common GI symptoms are feeding intolerance and high gastric residuals, while the most common sign is abdominal distention. Grossly bloody stools are infrequently seen. Management is initially conservative with NPO, fluid resuscitation, broad-spectrum IV antibiotics, TPN, and decompression with an orogastric tube. Surgical intervention is indicated for failure of conservative management, free air on plain films or CT, and peritonitis.

References: Dominguez KM, Moss RL. Necrotizing enterocolitis. In: Holcomb GW III, Murphy JP, Ostlie DJ, St. Peter SD, eds. *Ashcraft's pediatric surgery.* 6th ed. Saunders; 2014:454–473.

Ron O, Davenport M, Patel S, et al. Outcomes of the "clip and drop" technique for multifocal necrotizing enterocolitis. *J Pediatr Surg.* 2009;44(4):749–754.

5. E. This patient is presenting with classic signs of intussusception. These symptoms include colicky abdominal pain and "currant jelly" maroon stools. The first-line imaging modality is abdominal ultrasound, which will demonstrate a target-sign (A). A patient in this age group and with no other prior history is most likely to have ileocolic intussusception, with a target-sign visualized in the right lower quadrant. The most common etiology is hypertrophy of Peyer patches, which are circumferentially located and more closely spaced in the distal ileum, accounting for the ileocolic intussusception being the most common location. Pathologic lead points account for roughly 5% of intussusceptions in children under 3 to 4 years of age. Pathologic lead points may cause intussusception in locations other than the ileocolic. Examples of pathologic lead points include Meckel diverticulum, staple line from prior bowel resection, thick stool in cystic fibrosis, intestinal atresias (seen in the neonatal setting), polyps, appendicitis, intestinal lymphoma, submucosal hemorrhage, foreign bodies, and intestinal duplication. The most common pathologic lead point for intussusception in children is a Meckel diverticulum. A nuclear scan can be used to diagnose a Meckel diverticulum; however, this presentation is more concerning for intussusception, so ultrasound should

be done to confirm the diagnosis (D). Once diagnosed, about 80% of patients with intussusception are successfully treated with pneumatic or hydrostatic reduction, so laparoscopy at this point would not be appropriate (B). Repeat cases should again undergo pneumatic or hydrostatic reduction as long as the patient is stable and without peritonitis. Colonoscopy is not indicated in the initial workup for intussusception (C).

References: Columbani PM, Scholz S. Intussusception. In: Coran AG, ed. *Pediatric surgery.* 7th ed. Mosby; 2012:1093–1110.

Jiang J, Jiang B, Parashar U, Nguyen T, Bines J, Patel MM. Childhood intussusception: a literature review. *PLoS One.* 2013;8(7):e68482.

6. E. While the description of a swollen, bluish-black ovary even after detorsion may seem indicative of ovarian necrosis, this appearance is most often due to vascular and lymphatic congestion and *not* necrosis. Frank ovarian necrosis at the time of surgery is rare and would appear as a gelatinous or poorly defined structure that falls apart when manipulated. The color of the ovary after detorsion is not predictive of follicular development or future pregnancy, and studies of patients undergoing detorsion alone show follicular recovery on follow-up ultrasound. Furthermore, the pathology of ovarian torsion in adolescents is predominantly benign. It is for these reasons that every effort should be made to spare the ovary. A follow-up ultrasound in 3 months should be performed to evaluate the ovary for follicles or a mass that could not be seen at the time of surgery. Unfortunately, a study of a large inpatient nationwide database demonstrated that oophorectomy is performed in nearly 80% of females less than 18 years old with ovarian torsion (C). Biopsy or salpingo-oophorectomy are not indicated (A, D). There is no clear evidence to support oophoropexy with a first episode of unilateral ovarian torsion. However, it may be performed in recurrent or bilateral ovarian torsion or in a patient who has previously lost an ovary (B).

References: Geimanaite L, Trainavicius K. Ovarian torsion in children: management and outcomes. *J Pediatr Surg.* 2013;48(9):1946–1953.

Sola R, Wormer BA, Walters AL, Heniford BT, Schulman AM. National trends in the surgical treatment of ovarian torsion in children: an analysis of 2041 Pediatric Patients Utilizing the Nationwide Inpatient Sample. *Am Surg.* 2015;81(9):844–848.

Fuchs N, Smorgick N, Tovbin Y, et al. Oophoropexy to prevent adnexal torsion: how, when, and for whom? *J Minim Invasive Gynecol.* 2010;17(2):205–208.

7. B. Management of asymptomatic congenital cystic lung malformations is somewhat controversial, and if surgical resection is performed, it is typically within the first 6 months of age. The data regarding asymptomatic lesions becoming symptomatic is variable. However, in radiographically identifiable lesions, up to 85% of patients may become symptomatic, and there is a 4% risk of malignancy. Regardless of management strategy, it is important to obtain cross-sectional imaging to further characterize the lesion and inform decisions. Computerized tomography (CT) angiogram of the chest (B) can distinguish a congenital pulmonary airway malformation (CPAM) from a pulmonary sequestration or hybrid lesion. Compared to a CPAM, a bronchopulmonary sequestration does not communicate with the native airway and has a systemic feeding artery that often arises from the intraabdominal aorta. CT can also differentiate between subtypes of CPAMs based on the size of the cystic components (microcystic versus macrocystic). Immediate postnatal CT scans (A) are often suboptimal, so it is recommended to defer CT scan of asymptomatic patients until closer to potential intervention. Similarly, MRI (E) is not necessary in an asymptomatic patient and may require unnecessary sedation. Immediate surgical intervention (C–D) is not typically performed in asymptomatic patients.

References: Downard CD, Calkins CM, Williams RF, et al. Treatment of congenital pulmonary airway malformations: a systematic review from the APSA outcomes and evidence based practice committee. *Pediatr Surg Int.* 2017;33(9):939–953.

Durell J, Thakkar H, Gould S, Fowler D, Lakhoo K. Pathology of asymptomatic, prenatally diagnosed cystic lung malformations. *J Pediatr Surg.* 2016;51(2):231–235.

8. A. This child most likely has a Wilms tumor, the most common primary renal tumor in children less than 15 years of age. In this case, only the appendectomy should be performed, and the patient should have a proper staging workup (A). This includes an ultrasound of the abdomen to confirm that the mass is originating from the kidney, evaluating the contralateral kidney, and assessing for extension into the renal collecting system and inferior vena cava. The patient should also have a CT scan or MRI of the abdomen and CT of the chest to evaluate for extrarenal or metastatic disease. Surgical management includes nephroureterectomy with ipsilateral lymph node sampling (D–E). Lymph node sampling is a critical part of the evaluation and staging operation for pediatric renal tumors. Nodal status determines the overall stage and risk stratification group and therefore the chemotherapeutic regimen. Unfortunately, in a study evaluating surgical protocol violations over 10 years, lack of lymph node sampling (C) accounted for 67% of all violations. Absence of adequate lymph node sampling mandates treatment as Stage III disease and exposes the patient to potentially unnecessary abdominal radiation and additional chemotherapeutic agents. Similarly, performing a biopsy at the time of surgery (B) may upstage the disease to stage 3. There is no role for biopsy of the contralateral kidney in a nonsyndromic patient with a unilateral Wilms tumor, and in this particular scenario, a proper staging workup should be completed prior to any surgical management.

References: Ehrlich PF, Gow K, Hamilton TE, et al. Surgical protocol violations in children with renal tumors provides an opportunity to improve pediatric cancer care: a report from the Children's Oncology Group. *Pediatr Blood Cancer.* 2016;63(11):1905–1910.

Kieran K, Ehrlich PF. Current surgical standards of care in Wilms tumor. *Urol Oncol.* 2016;34(1):13–23.

9. C. Hirschsprung disease is characterized by an absence of ganglion cells in the Auerbach plexus and hypertrophy of associated nerve trunks. The cause is thought to be a defect in the migration of neural crest cells. The rectosigmoid junction is affected in 75% of cases, the splenic flexure or transverse colon in 17%, and the entire colon with variable extension into the small bowel in 8%. The presentation of the disease is characterized as a functional distal intestinal obstruction. Similar to ulcerative colitis, the disease is always present distally and extends a variable distance proximally and continuously. In the neonatal period, the most common symptoms are abdominal distention, failure to pass meconium, and bilious emesis. Infants can also present with enterocolitis, which is characterized by abdominal

distention and tenderness and is associated with manifestations of systemic toxicity. Enterocolitis is the most common cause of death in uncorrected Hirschsprung disease. The initial management of a patient with Hirschsprung-associated enterocolitis is rectal irrigation and IV antibiotics (A). The definitive diagnosis of Hirschsprung disease is made by rectal biopsy at least 2 cm above the dentate line to avoid sampling error. A contrast enema is useful because it will often help localize the transition zone between the dilated proximal ganglion containing the colon and the narrowed aganglionic distal segment, but it is not as helpful in the immediate neonatal period because the proximal segment may not be as markedly dilated yet. A small bowel follow-through is not helpful because the obstruction is in the colon (E). Multiple surgical operations exist for the management of Hirschsprung disease. Recently, primary repair with a pull-through procedure without a temporary colostomy has been performed. A leveling colostomy may be performed as part of a staged procedure. However, this is only done after the diagnosis is made (B). Most patients with Hirschsprung disease will tolerate breast milk or normal formulas after surgery and will not require an elemental formula (D).

References: Carcassonne M, Guys JM, Morrison-Lacombe G, Kreitmann B. Management of Hirschsprung's disease: curative surgery before 3 months of age. *J Pediatr Surg.* 1989;24(10):1032–1034.

Langer JC. Chapter 101 - Hirschsprung Disease. In: Coran AG, ed. *Pediatric Surgery.* 7th ed. Mosby; 2012:1265–1278. ISBN 9780323072557, https://doi.org/10.1016/B978-0-323-07255-7.00101-X.

10. C. Neonates normally have a protuberant abdomen, so the presence of a scaphoid abdomen, combined with respiratory distress at birth, should raise the suspicion of congenital diaphragmatic hernia (CDH). Overall survival is about 60% to 80%. The abdomen is scaphoid because the majority of the abdominal contents are herniated into the chest. In infants with CDH, both lungs are hypoplastic (the ipsilateral lung is worse than the contralateral lung) and there is decreased bronchial and pulmonary artery branching. Infants are prone to the development of pulmonary hypertension. Pulmonary vasculature is distinctly abnormal in that the medial muscular thickness of the arterioles is excessive and extremely sensitive to the multiple local and systemic factors known to trigger vasospasm. Between 80% and 90% occur on the left side, and the defect is posterolateral (Bochdalek hernia), as opposed to the Morgagni hernia, which is an anteromedial defect. Initial management should be focused on respiratory support. Ventilation with high-frequency oscillation is effective, as is the use of inhaled nitric oxide (D). Refractory cases should be placed on extracorporeal membrane oxygenation (ECMO). Placement of a nasogastric tube is also important to prevent gastric distention, which may slightly worsen the lung compression, mediastinal shift, and ability to ventilate. Because of the lung hypoplasia, prompt reduction of the bowel contents does not immediately improve ventilatory function (E). Once the patient is stabilized, they should be taken to the operating room to reduce the bowel, repair the defect with or without mesh, and run the entire bowel to look for associated anomalies such as malrotation. Chest tubes are not indicated because these may injure the underlying lung and worsen the prognosis (A). Bag-mask ventilation will distend the stomach and GI tract leading to further lung compression and worsen the patient's condition (B).

Reference: Stolar CJH, Dillon PW. Chapter 63 - Congenital Diaphragmatic Hernia and Eventration. In: Coran AG, ed. *Pediatric Surgery*. 7th ed. Mosby; 2012:809–824. ISBN 9780323072557, https://doi.org/10.1016/ B978-0-323-07255-7.00063-5.

11. C. In patients with an imperforate anus, the rectum fails to descend through the external sphincter complex. The pathophysiology is thought to be due to the failure of the urorectal septum to descend. The rectal pouch ends blindly in the pelvis, above (high lesion) or below (low lesion) the levator complex. Sixty percent of males have high lesions compared with only 30% of females. In most cases, the blind rectal pouch communicates more distally with the genitourinary system or with the perineum through a fistulous tract. In male patients with a high imperforate anus, the rectum usually ends up as a fistula somewhere along the urethra. In females, a high imperforate anus often occurs in the context of a persistent cloaca. Approximately 60% of patients have an associated malformation; the most common is a urinary tract defect. Skeletal defects are also seen, and the sacrum is most commonly involved. Spinal cord anomalies are common, especially with high lesions. Imperforate anus is also associated with VACTERL (vertebral defects, anal atresia, cardiac defects, tracheoesophageal fistula, renal anomalies, and limb abnormalities) syndrome. Evaluation should include plain radiographs of the spine as well as an ultrasound scan of the spinal cord. A plain chest radiograph and a careful clinical evaluation of the heart should be conducted. The most common defect is an imperforate anus with a fistula between the distal colon and the urethra in boys or to the vestibule of the vagina in girls. When there is no visible meconium in the perineal area after 24 hours, the patient is considered to have a high imperforate anus malformation. Patients with a high lesion should undergo primary sigmoid colostomy followed by a definitive pull-through at 3 to 6 months of life (B). Waiting an additional 24 hours may lead to worsening abdominal distention and respiratory compromise (A). Low lesions can be repaired by a perineal procedure at birth (D). High lesions may be repaired through a posterior sagittal approach (PSARP) or a laparoscopic-assisted approach (E). Low lesions have a better prognosis with respect to continence as the anatomy more closely resembles complete descent and development.

References: Georgeson KE, Inge TH, Albanese CT. Laparoscopically assisted anorectal pull-through for high imperforate anus–a new technique. *J Pediatr Surg*. 2000;35(6):927–931.

Levitt MA, Peña A. Chapter 103 - Anorectal Malformations. In: Coran AG, ed. *Pediatric Surgery*. 7th ed. Mosby; 2012:1289–1309. ISBN 9780323072557, https://doi.org/10.1016/ B978-0-323-07255-7.00103-3.

12. A. Jaundice within the first 24 hours of life or jaundice that persists beyond 2 weeks after birth is generally considered pathologic. Pathologic jaundice may be caused by biliary obstruction, increased hemoglobin load, or liver dysfunction. One must rule out obstructive disorders, including biliary atresia, choledochal cyst, and inspissated bile syndrome; ABO incompatibility; Rh incompatibility; spherocytosis; metabolic disorders; α1-antitrypsin deficiency; galactosemia; and congenital infection including syphilis and rubella. The most common cause of neonatal jaundice requiring surgery

is biliary atresia, which is an obliterative process of the extrahepatic bile ducts and is associated with hepatic fibrosis. The infant produces acholic stools and demonstrates a failure to thrive. Left untreated, it will progress to liver failure and portal hypertension. Nuclear scanning after pretreatment with phenobarbital is a useful study. One is specifically looking to see whether the radionuclide appears in the intestine, which would confirm that the extrahepatic bile ducts are patent. This finding excludes biliary atresia. If the radionuclide is normally concentrated in the liver but not excreted and the metabolic screen results are normal, this is highly suggestive of biliary atresia. The presence of a gallbladder does not exclude the diagnosis of biliary atresia. The diagnosis can be confirmed with a biopsy demonstrating bile plugging and periportal fibrosis. The most effective initial treatment of biliary atresia is portoenterostomy, as described by Kasai. The procedure involves anastomosing an isolated limb of the jejunum to the transected ducts at the portal plate of the liver. The likelihood of surgical success is increased if the procedure is performed before the infant reaches the age of 2 months. If the patient remains symptomatic after the Kasai operation, he or she will require liver transplantation (B). Independent risk factors that predict failure of the procedure include bridging liver fibrosis at the time of surgery and postoperative cholangitis episodes. Percutaneous drainage does not offer long-term decompression and does not address the lack of enteric bile (C). Options D and E are not possible because of a lack of extrahepatic biliary tree in this disease.

References: Cowles RA. Chapter 105 - The Jaundiced Infant: Biliary Atresia. In: Coran AG, ed. *Pediatric Surgery*. 7th ed. Mosby; 2012:1321–1330. ISBN 9780323072557, https://doi.org/10.1016/ B978-0-323-07255-7.00105-7.

Ohhama Y, Shinkai M, Fujita S, Nishi T, Yamamoto H. Early prediction of long-term survival and the timing of liver transplantation after the Kasai operation. *J Pediatr Surg*. 2000;35(7):1031–1034.

13. A. This patient has jejunal or ileal atresia. Intestinal atresias are caused by in utero mesenteric vascular accidents leading to segmental loss of the intestinal lumen. Due to small bowel atresia, the colon has been unused in utero and is therefore of small diameter. They are classified into four types based on their severity. Infants with jejunal or ileal atresia present soon after birth with bilious vomiting and progressive abdominal distention. More distal obstructions produce more distension on physical exam and radiographs. In cases in which the diagnosis of complete intestinal obstruction is ascertained by the clinical picture and the presence of staggered air–fluid levels on plain abdominal films, the child can be brought to the operating room after appropriate resuscitation. In these circumstances, there is little extra information that can be gained by a barium enema. When the diagnosis is uncertain, a contrast enema may be used. The initial treatment of jejunal atresia is nasogastric tube decompression and fluid resuscitation. Definitive treatment involves surgical resection of the atretic loop and primary reanastomosis. Failure of recanalization of the bowel is associated with esophageal and duodenal atresias (B). Lack of proper 270-degree counterclockwise rotation of the bowel is a feature of malrotation (C). Lack of ganglion cells in the bowel is seen with Hirschsprung disease, whereas a duplication would lead to duplication cysts (D, E).

Reference: Frischer JS, Azizkhan RG. Chapter 82 - Jejunoileal Atresia and Stenosis. In: Coran AG, ed. *Pediatric Surgery.* 7th ed. Mosby; 2012:1059–1071. ISBN 9780323072557, https://doi.org/10.1016/B978-0-323-07255-7.00082-9.

14. E. Omphalocele refers to a congenital defect of the abdominal wall at the midline in which the bowel and solid viscera are covered by peritoneum and the amniotic membrane. The abdominal wall defect can measure 4 cm or more in diameter and is caused by a lack of complete development of the abdominal wall muscles (C). An omphalocele is less of a surgical emergency than a gastroschisis because the bowel is protected by the covering (A). Conversely, omphalocele is associated with many other congenital abnormalities that are not seen with gastroschisis. The most common anomalies associated with omphalocele are cardiac and musculoskeletal. The size of the defect may be small or so large that it contains most of the abdominal viscera. There is an increased occurrence of cardiac and chromosomal abnormalities. Omphalocele is associated with premature and intrauterine growth retardation, while gastroschisis is associated with intrauterine rupture of the umbilical vein. Immediate treatment of an infant with omphalocele consists of maintaining normal vital signs and body temperature. The omphalocele should be covered with saline-soaked gauze, and the trunk should be wrapped circumferentially. No attempt should be made to manually reduce the abdominal contents because this maneuver may increase the risk of sac rupture or interfere with abdominal venous return. Gastroschisis, on the other hand, may be associated with intestinal atresia (10%–15%) (D). Mortality for omphalocele is largely based on the underlying comorbidities and is usually not due to sepsis (B). Additionally, omphalocele has a higher mortality rate than gastroschisis due to associated congenital anomalies.

References: Wagner JP, Lee SL. Infant born with abdominal wall defect. In: de Virgilio C, Frank PN, Grigorian A, eds. *Surgery: a case based clinical review.* 1st ed. Springer; 2015:349–357.

Benjamin B, Wilson GN. Anomalies associated with gastroschisis and omphalocele: analysis of 2825 cases from the Texas Birth Defects Registry. *J Pediatr Surg.* 2014;49(4):514–519.

15. C. In neonates with respiratory distress syndrome, management includes high-frequency ventilation, surfactant, and inhaled nitric oxide. When those interventions fail, ECMO is used. ECMO can be performed by either venovenous or venoarterial cannulation. The major indications for ECMO include meconium aspiration, respiratory distress syndrome (B), persistent pulmonary hypertension (D), sepsis, and CDH (A). Meconium aspiration is the most common indication for neonatal ECMO. ECMO has also been used to temporize infants with decompensation due to a congenital cardiac abnormality (E). The most dreaded complication of ECMO is intracranial hemorrhage secondary to the heparin required to prevent circuit clotting. Additionally, premature neonates have an underdeveloped cerebral microvasculature and an intolerance of physiologic insults, further increasing the risk of intracranial bleeding.

References: Hall J, Hardiman K, Lee S, et al. The American society of colon and rectal surgeons clinical practice guidelines for the treatment of left-sided colonic diverticulitis. *Dis Colon Rectum.* 2020;63(6):728–747.

Hines MH. ECMO and congenital heart disease. *Semin Perinatol.* 2005;29(1):34–39.

Hirschl RB, Bartlett RH. Chapter 8 - Extracorporeal Life Support for Cardiopulmonary Failure. In: Coran AG, ed. *Pediatric Surgery.* 7th ed. Mosby; 2012:123–132. ISBN 9780323072557, https://doi.org/10.1016/B978-0-323-07255-7.00008-8.

16. D. Approximately 90% of CDHs occur on the left side (C). Rarely, they may be bilateral. The cause of CDH is unknown, but it is believed that they result from the failure of normal closure of the pleuroperitoneal canal in the developing embryo. As a result, the abdominal contents herniate through the defect in the diaphragm and compress both lungs, with the ipsilateral lung being more severely affected. Compression of the developing lungs leads to pulmonary hypoplasia, which is clinically manifested with hypercarbia (B). There is a higher incidence of malrotation in patients with CDH. A Bochdalek hernia is in the posterolateral location and most commonly on the left side (E). The most significant physiologic abnormality in patients with CDH is pulmonary hypertension, which can lead to significant hypoxia. Extracorporeal membrane oxygenation (ECMO) may be required in some patients with significant pulmonary hypertension. For this reason, urgent surgical intervention is not indicated because reducing the hernia will not correct the pulmonary hypertension. In fact, surgical repair may temporarily worsen pulmonary compliance and hypertension. Thus, the infant's condition should be medically optimized before performing the repair (A). Although there is no ideal time to repair a CDH, most surgeons will wait until the infant's pulmonary vascular resistance drops, which occurs several days to weeks after birth. Bochdalek hernias are distinguished from Morgagni hernias, which are another type of congenital hernia and typically of the anteromedial diaphragm. The Morgagni hernia defect is small and asymptomatic and typically presents as a density on a chest radiograph in adulthood.

Reference: Lally KP, Paranka MS, Roden J, et al. Congenital diaphragmatic hernia. Stabilization and repair on ECMO. *Ann Surg.* 1992;216(5):569–573.

17. B. Esophageal atresia (EA) and tracheoesophageal fistula (TEF) are congenital interruptions or discontinuities of the esophagus, resulting in esophageal obstruction. Most present at birth with excessive drooling and choking or coughing after an attempted feed. There are five types (A–E). The most common type is type C, in which there is proximal EA with a distal TEF. The most appropriate next step is to attempt to place an orogastric tube. In patients with proximal EA and distal TEF, the tube will not be able to be passed into the stomach but will curl in the upper esophageal pouch. A two-view chest x-ray should follow to confirm the diagnosis (D). An esophagram or UGI series is not needed to make the diagnosis and increases the risk of aspiration (E). An abdominal x-ray is obtained after attempted placement of the orogastric tube (C). The abdominal x-ray will help determine the presence of a TEF by showing gas in the intestines. A gasless abdomen suggests an isolated EA. Intubation and positive pressure ventilation should be avoided because they increase the risk of ventilating through the TEF, resulting in respiratory failure (A).

Reference: Rothenberg S. Esophageal atresia and tracheoesophageal fistula malformations. In: Holcomb GW III, Murphy JP, Ostlie DJ, St. Peter SD, eds. *Ashcraft's pediatric surgery.* 6th ed. Saunders; 2014:365–384.

18. C. Pyloric stenosis occurs in 1 in 300 live births. Most often, it occurs in males between 3 and 6 weeks of age. Infants with pyloric stenosis present with projectile, nonbilious vomiting. As the disease progresses, an almost complete gastric outlet obstruction develops, and the infant is no longer able to tolerate even clear liquids. The classic electrolyte disorder that results from protracted vomiting is a hypochloremic, hypokalemic metabolic alkalosis (A, B, D). The urine pH level is high initially because of the alkalosis but eventually becomes acidic and is known as paradoxic aciduria. The explanation for this is that the renal tubule initially reabsorbs sodium in exchange for potassium. However, gastric juice has a high potassium concentration, and as vomiting continues, serum potassium levels drop. To conserve potassium as well, the renal tubule switches to reabsorbing sodium in exchange for hydrogen ions in the urine (E).

References: Fujimoto T, Lane GJ, Segawa O, Esaki S, Miyano T. Laparoscopic extramucosal pyloromyotomy versus open pyloromyotomy for infantile hypertrophic pyloric stenosis: which is better? *J Pediatr Surg.* 1999;34(2):370–372.

Jabaji Z, Sullins VF, Lee SL. Infant with nonbilious emesis. In: de Virgilio C, Frank PN, Grigorian A, eds. *Surgery: a case based clinical review.* 1st ed. Springer; 2015:343–349.

19. B. In all infants suspected of having necrotizing enterocolitis (NEC), feedings are discontinued, an orogastric tube is placed for decompression, and broad-spectrum parenteral antibiotics are given. Staging of NEC can be done with the Bell criteria. Patients with Bell stage 1 (suspicious for NEC) are ruled out for NEC and kept NPO and on IV antibiotics for 3 to 7 days before enteral nutrition is reinitiated. Patients with Bell stage 2 (definite NEC) require close observation for 7 to 14 days. Infants with Bell stage 3 (advanced NEC) either have definite intestinal perforation or have not responded to nonoperative therapy and thus require surgery. These patients have signs of peritonitis, acidosis, sepsis, and disseminated intravascular coagulation, all of which are associated with a high mortality rate. This patient is Bell stage 2 and should continue treatment with antibiotics and bowel rest/decompression. Blood transfusions should be based on the patient's clinical status and hemoglobin/hematocrit. A platelet count of 100,000/mcL does not require transfusion (A). Options C, D, and E are reserved for patients with Bell stage 3. Ultrasound and paracentesis may guide the decision to proceed with operative intervention. Surgical intervention may be with a peritoneal drain or exploratory laparotomy.

References: Bell MJ, Ternberg JL, Feigin RD, et al. Neonatal necrotizing enterocolitis. Therapeutic decisions based upon clinical staging. *Ann Surg.* 1978;187(1):1–7.

Dominguez KM, Moss RL. Necrotizing enterocolitis. In: Holcomb GW III, Murphy JP, Ostlie DJ, St. Peter SD, eds. *Ashcraft's pediatric surgery.* 6th ed. Saunders; 2014:454–473.

20. C. The diagnosis of malrotation with midgut volvulus should be suspected in an infant presenting with bilious vomiting and evidence of a bowel obstruction. Plain radiographs are likely to be normal or nondiagnostic (A). Some authors have recommended ultrasonography to look for a sonographic clockwise whirlpool pattern of the superior mesenteric vein and mesentery around the superior mesenteric artery; however, the gold standard for diagnosis is a UGI series (B). Historically, contrast enemas were used to make the diagnosis but are less accurate than a UGI series (D). CT scan of the abdomen/pelvis may suggest malrotation in older children or adults with vague symptoms (E).

Reference: Sullins VF, Lee SL. Infant with bilious emesis. In: de Virgilio C, Frank PN, Grigorian A, eds. *Surgery: a case based clinical review.* 1st ed. Springer; 2015:335–343.

21. C. After malrotation and midgut volvulus is diagnosed, the infant should be urgently taken to the operating room because a delay risks the development of gangrene of the entire small bowel. The first step is to reduce the volvulus. The goal of the Ladd procedure is to broaden the narrow base of the mesentery to prevent the volvulus from recurring. The bands between the cecum and abdominal wall and between the duodenum and terminal ileum are sharply divided to splay out the superior mesenteric artery and its branches. This brings the duodenum into the right abdomen and the cecum into the left lower quadrant and anatomically creates a complete nonrotation (A, D, E). The appendix is typically removed to avoid diagnostic errors later in life, but this is not absolutely required because imaging techniques and diagnostic capabilities have improved. The cecum and stomach are not fixed to the abdominal wall because this will increase the risk of a twist at these sites (B).

References: Pracros JP, Sann L, Genin G, et al. Ultrasound diagnosis of midgut volvulus: the "whirlpool" sign. *Pediatr Radiol.* 1992;22(1):18–20.

Sullins VF, Lee SL. Infant with bilious emesis. In: de Virgilio C, Frank PN, Grigorian A, eds. *Surgery: a case based clinical review.* 1st ed. Springer; 2015:335–343.

22. E. The history and radiograph findings are consistent with duodenal atresia. Duodenal atresia occurs because of failure of recanalization of the duodenum from its solid core state. It is associated with prematurity, Down syndrome, maternal polyhydramnios, malrotation, annular pancreas, and biliary atresia. In most cases, the duodenal obstruction is distal to the ampulla of Vater, and infants present with bilious emesis in the neonatal period. The classic radiographic finding is the "double-bubble sign" (an air-filled stomach, a functioning pylorus, and a distended proximal duodenal bulb). If there is no distal bowel gas, complete atresia is confirmed and no further studies are necessary (A–C). Conversely, if distal air is present, a UGI contrast study should be done to rule out malrotation and midgut volvulus. The finding of distal air in association with a double bubble could also indicate a duodenal stenosis or web or an annular pancreas that does not cause a complete obstruction. Patients may also have associated cardiac malformations for which an echocardiogram is needed before surgical intervention (D). The treatment of duodenal atresia is surgical bypass of the obstruction as either a side-to-side or proximal transverse-to-distal longitudinal duodenoduodenostomy or a duodenojejunostomy. When the proximal duodenum is markedly dilated, a tapering duodenoplasty may be performed.

Reference: Sullins VF, Lee SL. Infant with bilious emesis. In: de Virgilio C, Frank PN, Grigorian A, eds. *Surgery: a case based clinical review.* 1st ed. Springer; 2015:335–343.

23. B. Neuroblastoma is the most common solid abdominal malignancy in children <2 years of age. Wilms tumor is the most common after 2 years of age. The presenting symptoms of neuroblastoma depend on the site of the primary tumor, the presence of metastatic disease, the age of the patient, and the metabolic activity of the tumor. The most common presentation is a fixed lobular mass extending from the flank toward the midline. The tumor can also extend into the neural foramina and cause symptoms of spinal cord compression. It tends to metastasize to cortical bones, bone marrow, and the liver, and patients may present with localized swelling and tenderness, limp, or refusal to walk. Periorbital metastases account for proptosis and ecchymosis, resulting in "raccoon eyes." In infants, liver metastases may expand, causing hepatomegaly. Metastatic lesions to the skin produce the blueberry muffin appearance. Wilms tumor (C) also presents as an abdominal mass, in association with Beckwith-Wiedemann syndrome (macroglossia, hypoglycemia, gigantism, and visceromegaly), and as part of the WAGR complex (Wilms tumor, aniridia, genitourinary abnormalities, and mental retardation). Rhabdomyosarcoma is a soft-tissue tumor (A). The most common primary sites are the head and neck. Sacrococcygeal teratoma is the most common type of teratoma (E). It presents as a large mass extending off the sacrum in the newborn period. Hepatoblastoma, although the most common liver malignancy in children, is a rare solid organ malignancy (D).

Reference: Davidoff AM. Neuroblastoma. In: Holcomb GW III, Murphy JP, Ostlie DJ, St. Peter SD, eds. *Ashcraft's pediatric surgery.* 6th ed. Saunders; 2014:883–905.

24. D. Gastroschisis, unlike omphalocele, is not typically associated with systemic or chromosomal abnormalities (A–C, E). There is an abdominal wall defect to the right of the umbilicus and the bowel herniates through without a peritoneal covering. Because the bowel is eviscerated and exposed, this condition is a surgical emergency. The bowel can be thickened and covered with an exudate. All patients with gastroschisis will have intestinal malrotation. However, midgut volvulus is unlikely due to the adhesions created from the gastroschisis. Intestinal atresia is also seen in 10% to 15% of patients with gastroschisis. If the defect cannot be primarily closed, a staged-closure utilizing a silo may be required.

Reference: Wagner JP, Lee SL. Infant born with abdominal wall defect. In: de Virgilio C, Frank PN, Grigorian A, eds. *Surgery: a case based clinical review.* 1st ed. Springer; 2015:349–357.

25. A. Meconium ileus is a result of cystic fibrosis, in which the meconium becomes thick and viscous due to deficits in pancreatic enzymes. It creates a small bowel obstruction, and as such, the infant may present with bilious vomiting. In the most severe forms, it can lead to intestinal perforation. The radiograph typically demonstrates a "ground-glass" appearance, which represents small pockets of gas trapped inside the thickened meconium. The treatment strategy depends on whether the patient has complicated or uncomplicated meconium ileus. Patients with uncomplicated meconium ileus can be treated nonoperatively. Administering a water-soluble enema such as dilute gastrografin per rectum allows the meconium to soften as it takes on more water. Optimally, the contrast should reach the dilated portion of the ileum under fluoroscopic visualization. The enema may be repeated every 12 hours over several days as needed. A UGI with SBFT is not indicated or used in the initial management of meconium ileus (D). Surgery is required if nonoperative management fails or if the patient already has evidence of perforation. Complicated cases are usually amenable to bowel resection

and primary anastomosis (B, C, E), provided there is no evidence of giant cystic meconium peritonitis.

References: Rescorla FJ, Grosfeld JL. Contemporary management of meconium ileus. *World J Surg.* 1993;17(3):318–325.

Ziegler MM. Chapter 83 - Meconium Ileus. In: Coran AG, ed. *Pediatric Surgery.* 7th ed. Mosby; 2012:1073–1083. ISBN 9780323072557, https://doi.org/10.1016/ B978-0-323-07255-7.00083-0.

26. D. This patient presents with an incarcerated right inguinal hernia (RIH). The bilious emesis and abdominal distention are highly suggestive of a small bowel obstruction. Thus, the most appropriate management is to attempt a reduction of the incarcerated RIH. If reduction of the hernia is successful, the patient should be admitted for observation and repair within 24 to 48 hours. The edema from the incarcerated RIH makes immediate surgical repair more difficult. Repairing the hernia after 24 to 48 hours will allow the edema to resolve. Incarcerated hernias should be diagnosed based on history and physical exam without the need for ultrasound (A). Ultrasound may be useful if testicular torsion is suspected. Erythematous masses may be misdiagnosed as abscesses. However, in this case, the history and physical exam are consistent with an incarcerated inguinal hernia. IV antibiotics and possible incision and drainage is the treatment for abscesses (B, C). Operative exploration is performed if the incarcerated hernia cannot be reduced (E). When an incarcerated hernia cannot be reduced, there should be a heightened suspicion for the presence of ischemic bowel.

Reference: Fraser JD, Snyder CL. Inguinal hernias and hydroceles. In: Holcomb GW III, Murphy JP, Ostlie DJ, St. Peter SD, eds. *Ashcraft's pediatric surgery.* 6th ed. Saunders; 2014:689–701.

27. C. Choledochal cysts have been classified into five types. The most common is type I, which is a fusiform dilatation of the bile duct. Type II is a diverticulum of the CBD. Type III is a choledochocele. Type IV is multiple cysts. Type V is known as Caroli disease, which involves cysts limited to the intrahepatic bile ducts. The cysts lead to recurrent bouts of cholangitis and have a risk of malignancy. The treatment of a type I choledochal cyst is resection of the cyst and reconstruction with a Roux-en-Y choledochojejunostomy or a simple choledochoduodenostomy. If the cyst is adherent to the portal vein, the anterior portion of the cyst should be excised along with mucosectomy of the posterior cyst to prevent future malignant degeneration. Antibiotics and/or drainage will not result in a more favorable operation (A, B). Cholangitis should be treated with antibiotics before definitive surgery. Internal drainage alone will still predispose the patient to a future risk of malignant degeneration (D). The portal vein should not be resected during this operation (E).

Reference: Liem NT, Holcomb GW III. Choledochal cyst and gallbladder disease. In: Holcomb GW III, Murphy JP, Ostlie DJ, St. Peter SD, eds. *Ashcraft's pediatric surgery.* 6th ed. Saunders; 2014:593–606.

28. D. Inguinal hernias result from the processus vaginalis failing to close. Inguinal hernias occur more commonly in males and premature infants and are more common on the right side. The diagnosis of an inguinal hernia should be based on history and physical examination without the need for ultrasound (A). The timing of herniorrhaphy in premature infants is debatable and based on the clinical scenario. If the hernia is easily reducible, many surgeons will repair the hernia at the time of discharge (rather than immediately). By repairing the hernia before discharge, the risk of re-presenting to the ED with an incarcerated inguinal hernia is eliminated. Some surgeons would discharge patients and repair the hernia when the postconceptional age (the gestational age + age of patient) is around 55 weeks (in this infant that would be 30 weeks after birth). However, waiting until the infant reaches 1 year of age would increase the risk of incarceration (E). By waiting, there is a lower anesthetic risk, and the operation is not as challenging. Thus, the decision to repair should be considered at the time of discharge. Immediate repair in premature infants is technically more difficult and associated with a higher rate of recurrence and postoperative apnea (B, C). Inguinal hernias in children only require high ligation of the sac. Mesh is rarely ever required in pediatric patients with inguinal hernias.

Reference: Fraser JD, Snyder CL. Inguinal hernias and hydroceles. In: Holcomb GW III, Murphy JP, Ostlie DJ, St. Peter SD, eds. *Ashcraft's pediatric surgery*. 6th ed. Saunders; 2014:689–701.

29. C. The pathogenesis of NEC is thought to be intestinal hypoperfusion (A, B, D, E). This occurs most frequently in the setting of perinatal stress. The period of hypoperfusion is followed by a period of reperfusion, and the combination of ischemia and reperfusion leads to mucosal injury. The damaged intestinal mucosa barrier becomes susceptible to bacterial translocation, which initiates an inflammatory cascade. Various proinflammatory mediators are released, which in turn lead to further epithelial injury and the systemic manifestations of NEC. It is postulated that maintenance of the gut barrier is essential for the protection of the host against NEC. It has always been taught that NEC classically presents with bloody stools after the first feeding. However, the earliest signs are nonspecific, including apnea, bradycardia, lethargy, and temperature instability. The most common GI symptoms are feeding intolerance and high gastric residuals, while the most common sign is abdominal distention. Grossly bloody stools are infrequently seen. Management is initially conservative with NPO, fluid resuscitation, broad-spectrum IV antibiotics, TPN, and decompression with an orogastric tube. Surgical intervention is indicated for failure of conservative management, free air on plain films or CT, and peritonitis.

Reference: Dominguez KM, Moss RL. Necrotizing enterocolitis. In: Holcomb GW III, Murphy JP, Ostlie DJ, St. Peter SD, eds. *Ashcraft's pediatric surgery*. 6th ed. Saunders; 2014:454–473.

30. C. Management of a newborn with gastroschisis involves stabilizing the airway, preventing hypothermia, orogastric decompression, establishing IV access, and administering IV fluids and antibiotics. The bowel should also be placed in a sterile, clear plastic wrap to prevent further volume and heat loss. The bowel must also be carefully inspected for signs of ischemia. If the bowel appears ischemic, the bowel must be inspected to rule out a simple twist or kink in the mesentery. The defect is also examined to be sure that it is not tight and the cause of the ischemia, as in this case. If the defect is too tight, it must be opened immediately. The best direction to open the defect would be to the patient's right (away from the umbilicus) in order to avoid

the umbilical structures/vessels. After the defect is opened up, a silo is typically indicated (A). Primary reduction and closure should only be attempted when there is no risk to the bowel (B). Resection of ischemic bowel should be reserved for grossly necrotic bowel because patients with gastroschisis are at risk of developing short gut syndrome (D). Any questionable bowel should be observed with serial exams. A diverting ileostomy is not indicated in this patient (E).

Reference: Wagner JP, Lee SL. Infant born with abdominal wall defect. In: de Virgilio C, Frank PN, Grigorian A, eds. *Surgery: a case based clinical review*. 1st ed. Springer; 2015:349–357.

31. B. This patient has a diagnosis of Hirschsprung disease (HD). The patient then developed Hirschsprung-associated enterocolitis (HAEC). The initial management for HAEC is IV antibiotics, bowel rest, and rectal irrigations. However, if the patient deteriorates, then urgent colostomy is needed to decompress the colon and may be lifesaving. A contrast enema is contraindicated in patients with active HAEC (A). Because the level of HD is not known, a colectomy should not be performed. In addition, patients are often too sick to withstand a prolonged operation (C). This patient does not have abdominal compartment syndrome or fungal sepsis (D, E).

Reference: Langer JC. Meckel diverticulum. In: Holcomb GW III, Murphy JP, Ostlie DJ, St. Peter SD, eds. *Ashcraft's pediatric surgery*. 6th ed. Saunders; 2014:474–491.

32. E. The infant is exhibiting signs of malrotation with midgut volvulus. By the time abdominal wall edema is evident, there is a high likelihood of intestinal gangrene. As such, no further studies are indicated, and the infant requires urgent laparotomy (A, B). Confirmation with an upper GI series is only indicated when the patient is stable and the diagnosis is unclear. Endoscopy has no role in diagnosis or treatment (C). Resection of extensive dead bowel may result in short-gut syndrome and necessitate intestinal transplantation to avoid long-term parenteral nutrition. Ladd bands extend from the cecum to the lateral abdominal wall (D), crossing the duodenum, which increases the potential for obstruction. Additional clues to the presence of advanced ischemia include erythema of the abdominal wall. Sometimes, gangrenous loops of bowel may be seen transabdominally as a discolored mass. If left untreated, the infant will progress to shock and death. It must be reemphasized that the index of suspicion for this condition must be high because abdominal signs are minimal in the early states. Abdominal films show a paucity of gas through the intestine with a few scattered air–fluid levels. In early cases, the patient does not appear ill initially, and the plain films may suggest partial duodenal obstruction. Under these conditions, the patient may have malrotation without volvulus. This is best diagnosed by an upper GI series that shows incomplete rotation with the duodenojejunal junction displaced to the right. When volvulus is suspected, early surgical intervention is mandatory if the ischemic process is to be avoided or reversed. Volvulus occurs clockwise and should be untwisted counterclockwise.

Reference: Sullins VF, Lee SL. Infant with bilious emesis. In: de Virgilio C, Frank PN, Grigorian A, eds. *Surgery: a case based clinical review*. 1st ed. Springer; 2015:335–343.

33. A. Children born with bilateral undescended testes have a much higher rate of subsequent infertility. It is associated with prune belly syndrome (a lack of abdominal wall muscles) (C). When the testicle is not in the scrotum, it is subjected to higher temperatures, resulting in decreased spermatogenesis. When the testicles are placed in the scrotum, fertility is improved but still lower than in those without cryptorchidism (B). It is recommended that undescended testicles be repositioned by 1 year of age to maximize the chances of improving fertility. The use of chorionic gonadotropin sometimes is effective in achieving descent in patients with bilateral undescended testes, suggesting that they may have a hormonal deficiency (D). If the intraabdominal testes cannot be effectively mobilized to reach down into the scrotum, a 2-stage Fowler-Stephens procedure is used. In the first stage, the testicular vessels are clipped laparoscopically. In addition to the testicular arteries, the testicles receive collateral blood from the cremasteric artery, a branch of the inferior epigastric artery, and the artery to the vas (a branch of the superior vesical artery). Thus, division of the testicular artery is usually well tolerated and usually does not result in testicular necrosis (E). The orchiopexy is then performed through the groin approximately 6 months later, after which time collateral flow has increased.

References: Lee JJ, Shortliffe LMD. Undescended testes and testicular tumors. In: Holcomb GW III, Murphy JP, Ostlie DJ, St. Peter SD, eds. *Ashcraft's pediatric surgery*. 6th ed. Saunders; 2014:689–701.

Chan E, Wayne C, Nasr A, FRCSC for Canadian Association of Pediatric Surgeon Evidence-Based Resource. Ideal timing of orchiopexy: a systematic review. *Pediatr Surg Int*. 2014;30(1):87–97.

Plastic Surgery 23

AMANDA C. PURDY AND MYTIEN GOLDBERG

ABSITE 99th Percentile High-Yields

I. Skin–Grafts

A. Split-thickness versus full-thickness skin grafts:

		Split-thickness skin graft (STSG)	Full-thickness skin graft (FTSG)
Contains…		All of epidermis & *part of* dermis	All of epidermis & all of dermis
Donor site	Common sites	Thigh, buttocks, back, abdomen	Behind ear, groin, neck
	Harvesting	Dermatome (0.013–0.018 in thick) + /– meshing	Freehand with a scalpel
	Healing Mechanism	Epithelialization from dermal hair follicles & wound border	Needs to be primarily closed
Used for…		Larger wounds in noncosmetically sensitive areas	Small wounds on face or hands, joints, cosmetically sensitive areas
Primary contraction *Immediate shrinking after harvesting but before grafting*		Less; fewer elastic fibers and dermal extracellular matrix components	MORE; more dermal elastin
Secondary contraction *The degree of shrinking during healing*		MORE	Less
Chance of graft survival		Better Contain less dermis & therefore have a lower metabolic requirement; meshed STSG have the best survival/ engraftment rate; they become vascularized more rapidly	Worse requires a healthier wound bed to heal; cannot be meshed

B. Steps of graft take (engraftment):
1. Adherence (first day)—fibrin strands link collagen and elastin to bring the graft closer to the wound bed
2. Plasmatic Imbibition (in the first 3 days)—the graft absorbs transudative fluid from the recipient site, serves to nourish the graft until it becomes vascularized
3. Inosculation (in 3–4 days)—cut ends of graft vessels join with the ends of similar-sized recipient blood vessels from the wound bed
4. Neovascularization (in 5 days)—the growth of new vessels from the wound bed into the graft

Questions

1. Which of the following is true regarding component separation for abdominal wall reconstruction?
   A. A patient with a prior colostomy is not an appropriate candidate
   B. Transverse abdominis release (TAR) should be routinely performed with component separation
   C. Prior deep inferior perforator flap is a relative contraindication
   D. An intraoperative enterotomy requires aborting the procedure
   E. The semilunaris line is reconstructed

2. A 21-year-old female has a flash burn to her face, sustaining a 3-cm full-thickness wound to her right cheek. Which of the following would be the best skin graft?
   A. Full thickness from behind the ear
   B. Full thickness from the waist at the inguinal fold
   C. Full thickness from the wrist fold
   D. Split thickness from the anterior thigh
   E. Split thickness from the posterior thigh

3. The most important reason to avoid split-thickness skin grafts (STSGs) over an extremity joint is:
   A. There is an increased risk of infection over joints
   B. The rate of contracture over a joint can be debilitating
   C. There is a higher risk of graft necrosis
   D. There is a high rate of seroma formation compared with other areas on the body
   E. There is reduced imbibition

4. Which of the following is true regarding skin grafts?
   A. Full-thickness skin grafts (FTSGs) are more amenable to imbibition compared with split-thickness skin grafts (STSGs)
   B. Allografts will eventually get vascularized
   C. The most common reason for skin graft loss is a nonviable wound bed
   D. The degree of primary contraction is inversely proportional to the amount of dermis in the skin graft
   E. Secondary contraction is greater with FTSG

5. A 64-year-old male with chronic obstructive pulmonary disease (COPD) presents to the ED with full-thickness burns to the majority of the right arm after his robe caught on fire while he was cooking. Several days later, he undergoes a planned split-thickness skin graft (STSG) using his left anterior thigh as a donor site. Halfway through the anticipated harvest of donor skin using the dermatome, the surgeon notes visible fat. Which of the following is the best next step?
   A. Terminate the procedure and reschedule
   B. Continue harvesting with the dermatome at the same site while attempting to aim more superficially to obtain the planned STSG
   C. Continue harvesting with the dermatome at the same site with no change to the angle of the dermatome in an attempt to now harvest full-thickness skin graft
   D. Stop the dermatome at the current site, and attempt harvesting at another site
   E. Stop the dermatome at the current site, suture the skin, and attempt harvesting at another site

6. Which of the following is an important reason to use meshed split-thickness skin-graft (STSG) as opposed to non meshed STSG?
   A. Meshed STSG allows for use in a wound bed with poor granulation tissue
   B. Meshed STSG allows for use in an ischemic wound bed
   C. Meshed STSG allows drainage of fluid and blood
   D. Widely meshed skin is associated with less scarring
   E. Meshed STSG allows for increased amounts of adnexal structures

7. Which of the following is the recommended surveillance regimen to detect silent rupture for a 45-year-old woman with silicone gel–filled bilateral breast implants?
   A. Annual ultrasound
   B. Ultrasound as needed for pain/discomfort
   C. Magnetic resonance imaging (MRI) 3 years after implant surgery and then every 2 years for life of the implant
   D. Annual plain films
   E. Computed tomography (CT) every 5 years for the life of the implant

8. A 40-year-old female who has a desire for reconstructive breast surgery after a mastectomy is offered a deep inferior epigastric perforator (DIEP) flap. What is the disadvantage to performing a DIEP flap compared to a standard pedicle flap in this patient?

   A. It has a higher rate of flap necrosis
   B. It has an elevated rate of donor site morbidity
   C. Patients have permanent nerve dysfunction
   D. Patients have increased pain
   E. It is a longer operation

9. What is the most common early postoperative complication in gynecomastia surgery?

   A. Wound infection
   B. Hematoma
   C. Under-resection of tissue
   D. Asymmetry of breast tissue
   E. Nipple/areola depression

10. Which of the following is the most important principle in repair of a lip laceration?

    A. Closure of the mucosal layer
    B. Primary closure of the muscularis
    C. Reapproximation of the vermilion-cutaneous junction
    D. Minimal stitching
    E. Alignment of the underlying teeth

11. Which of the following is a contraindication for negative-pressure wound therapy (NPWT)?

    A. Newly grafted skin
    B. Wounds with a fistula
    C. Diabetic wounds
    D. Ischemic wounds
    E. Venous stasis wounds

12. Which of the following is required along with vitamin C to complete cross-linking of proline residues in collagen?

    A. Oxygen
    B. Oxygen and vitamin A
    C. Iron and alpha-ketoglutarate
    D. Oxygen, iron, and alpha-ketoglutarate
    E. Oxygen, iron, and penicillamine

13. Pair the dominant vascular supply of the rectus abdominis muscle with the correct feeding vessel:

    A. Superficial epigastric artery from the internal thoracic artery
    B. Inferior epigastric artery from the external iliac artery
    C. Superficial epigastric artery from the intercostal arteries
    D. Inferior epigastric artery from the internal iliac artery
    E. Deep circumflex iliac artery from the internal iliac artery

14. Which of the following bones is the most common isolated orbital bone fracture?

    A. Ethmoid
    B. Frontal
    C. Maxillary
    D. Lacrimal
    E. Zygomatic

15. What is the mainstay of postoperative flap monitoring?

    A. Doppler ultrasound
    B. Pulse oximetry
    C. Clinical observation
    D. Quantitative fluorometry
    E. Surface temperature probing

16. Which of the following is an appropriate candidate for repair of a cleft lip?

    A. 1-year-old female with hemoglobin of 9 g/dL
    B. 6-month-old male with a body weight of 9 pounds
    C. 12-week-old male with hemoglobin of 11 g/dL
    D. 1-year-old male with prealbumin less than 3 mg/dL
    E. 6-month-old female with concurrent pulmonic stenosis

Answers

1. C. Complex hernia is a term used to describe abdominal wall defects that are characterized by loss of abdominal domain and/or those associated with parastomal hernias, enterocutaneous fistulas, nonmidline hernias, hernias that abut bony landmarks, and recurrent hernias. A component separation is a technique utilized for complex hernias with the goal of primarily closing the fascial defect without tension. Previous violation of the rectus, including a prior colostomy, is not considered a contraindication (A). Component separation may also be a useful technique to consider in the setting of a contaminated field when prosthetic mesh cannot be used (D). However, this procedure is best reserved for patients fully optimized to prevent hernia recurrence after abdominal wall reconstruction. This includes optimizing nutrition, complete cessation of smoking and diet/exercise with weight loss. Component separation was first described by Ramirez et al. as a technique to repair large ventral abdominal wall defects. It begins with:

1. Rectus muscle separated from the posterior rectus sheath
2. External oblique muscle separated from the internal oblique at the linea semilunaris
3. Once the external oblique muscle is released from its fascia, the compound flap of rectus muscle and the attached internal oblique/transversus abdominis is advanced toward the midline for primary closure of the fascia. The compound flap can be advanced at the epigastrium: 5 cm, waist: 10 cm, and suprapubic: 3 cm per side.

The main supply of the rectus muscle is the superior and deep inferior epigastric arteries. Therefore, prior deep inferior epigastric perforator flap is a relative contraindication to component separation because in the DIEP flap procedure, the deep inferior epigastric artery is harvested, and thus the health of the rectus muscle may be compromised. In cases where additional length is required, TAR is performed (B). Posterior component separation with TAR allows for an advancement of 8 to 12 cm per side. Approximately 0.5 cm medial to the linea semilunaris, the posterior rectus sheath is incised, and the transversus abdominis muscle fibers are divided with electrocautery, affording additional length to the posterior rectus sheath. The posterior rectus sheath can then be reapproximated with sutures. Mesh should be placed in the retrorectus space (on top of the reapproximated posterior rectus sheath) in a sublay fashion to reinforce the repair. The anterior rectus sheath is then reapproximated on top of the mesh to reconstruct the linea alba (E).

References: Heller L, McNichols CH, Ramirez OM. Component separations. *Semin Plast Surg.* 2012;26(1):25–28.

Garvey PB, Bailey CM, Baumann DP, Liu J, Butler CE. Violation of the rectus complex is not a contraindication to component separation for abdominal wall reconstruction. *J Am Coll Surg.* 2012;214(2):131–139.

2. A. FTSG harvested from the upper eyelids, posterior auricular region, or supraclavicular fossa are the ideal donor sites for defects on the face versus split-thickness skin graft (D,E). FTSG harvested behind the ear as opposed to the wrist and inguinal fold gives the best color match, texture, and thickness (B). Additionally, FTSGs undergo less secondary wound contracture and thus less distortion of the face once it is healed. The wrist crease can also be used, but many do not like the future appearance of the scar on the wrist (C).

3. B. STSG has the highest secondary contracture (the degree of shrinkage during wound healing). STSG will yield a higher rate of contracture over a joint resulting in debilitating hand function. Therefore, FTSG is the preferred graft over any joints in the extremity. Contraction resulting from centrifugal forces in the center of the wound constitutes an important wound closure mechanism. Myofibroblasts, specialized fibroblasts characterized by intracellular smooth muscle actin filaments, contribute to this. There is no increased risk of joint infection with STSG (A). Skin grafts over a joint have a higher rate of failure due to sheer force and not because of seroma formation (D). Thus, it is important to immobilize the joint during the healing phase to allow for graft take (C, E). Rehabilitation with stretching, exercise, and splinting can minimize contracture development. Surgical release of tight bands may also be necessary to restore normal function.

4. B. Full-thickness and most deep-partial-thickness wounds will require skin grafting. This should take place after the wound has been debrided and a healthy, viable wound bed is available. If the wound bed is not ready for skin grafting, biologic coverage can be achieved with either allograft/homograft (cadaver skin) or xenograft (bovine skin). Unlike xenograft, allograft will eventually vascularize. However, both will be rejected and are thus only used as a temporary measure. The only permanent solution is autograft (using the patient's own skin). The surface area and location of the wound will determine if STSG (which contains all epidermis and some dermis) or FTSG (which contains all epidermis and dermis) will be needed. The FTSG donor site will need to be primarily closed, and thus FTSG is appropriate only for small wounds in the face and hands to ensure a cosmetically and functionally sound repair. In the case of STSG, meshing the harvested skin in a 1:1 to 4:1 ratio will allow for coverage of a larger area. The grafts are subjected to immediate shrinkage, or primary contraction, as well as secondary contraction. Primary contraction is dependent on the recoil of elastic fibers in the dermis; thus, this occurs more frequently with FTSG. The degree of secondary contraction is inversely proportional to the amount of dermis in the skin graft and thus occurs more commonly with STSGs (D, E). The newly grafted skin survives by three main mechanisms. For the first 3 days, the graft passively absorbs nutrients from the wound bed by simple diffusion (imbibition). On days 3 and 4, inosculation allows for a direct connection of the skin graft to vessels in the wound bed. By day 5, neovascularization and angiogenesis have occurred, allowing the graft to survive with its own blood supply. STSGs have a higher chance of survival because the thinner skin makes it easier for imbibition and inosculation to occur early in the healing process (A). Skin grafts fail by four main mechanisms, with the most common being hematoma or seroma formation, preventing the necessary contact of the skin graft to the wound bed (C). Other mechanisms of failure include infection, poor wound bed, and sheer forces.

Reference: Mathes SJ. *Reconstructive surgery: principles, anatomy and techniques.* Elsevier Science; 1997.

5. E. Patients with home oxygen are at a higher risk for burn injuries. This includes patients with COPD. This patient suffered a full-thickness burn to the majority of the upper extremity and thus will require split-thickness skin grafting. Full-thickness skin grafting is not appropriate for a large wound bed. STSGs are around 0.015 inches deep and take about 7 to 14 days to reepithelialize. The harvesting of skin is highly dependent on both the user and the dermatome. If the angle, set depth, and pressure are not correct, one risks harvesting skin that is too thin or cutting too deep. Seeing visible fat indicates that the graft was harvested as a full-thickness graft. The technical error is either due to the user using too much force or the dermatome being set at an inappropriate depth. In this case, the best next step is to stop the dermatome, suture the skin, and attempt harvesting at an alternative site (A–D).

References: Kim S, Chung SW, Cha IH. Full thickness skin grafts from the groin: donor site morbidity and graft survival rate from 50 cases. *J Korean Assoc Oral Maxillofac Surg.* 2013;39(1):21–26.

Weber RS, Hankins P, Limitone E, et al. Split-thickness skin graft donor site management. A randomized prospective trial comparing a hydrophilic polyurethane absorbent foam dressing with a petrolatum gauze dressing. *Arch Otolaryngol Head Neck Surg.* 1995;121(10):1145–1149.

6. C. STSG contains epidermis and various amounts of dermis. Meshing of the graft increases the surface area, allowing for increased tissue coverage as well as drainage of fluid and blood. However, a widely meshed skin graft is subject to increased scarring and longer healing times (D). Poor granulation tissue and an ischemic or infected wound bed are relative and absolute contraindications for skin grafting, respectively (A, B). Adnexal structures are contained in the dermis and thus are more abundantly available with FTSG (E).

7. C. Breast implants are not lifetime devices and will often need reoperation for implant removal with or without replacement. Common indications for reoperation include capsular contracture, rupture, poor cosmesis, infection, and pain. MRI is the most sensitive and specific modality available to detect silent rupture of breast implants. The Food and Drug Administration issued guidelines in 2011 recommending that all recipients of silicone gel-filled breast implants receive MRI screening 3 years after implant surgery and then every 2 years for the life of the implant. CT is less sensitive for the detection of silent rupture and exposes patients to unnecessary radiation (E). Ultrasound can also be used but is not as accurate as MRI (A, B). Plain films are not used in the detection of ruptured breast implants (D).

Reference: Centers for Devices and Radiological Health. *FDA Update on the Safety of Silicone Gel-Filled Breast Implants.* US Food and Drug Administration; June 2011.

8. E. A DIEP flap is a fasciocutaneous flap, also known as a perforator flap, whereby the skin and subcutaneous fat are removed from a distant or adjacent part of the body to be used to reconstruct another site. The major advantage of a perforator flap is that it reduces the morbidity at the patient's donor site, mainly because it does not require the sacrifice of the fascia or muscle (B). Because the fascia stays intact, so too do the nerves innervating the muscle, and thus nerve dysfunction is kept to a minimum, and without nerve or muscle damage, the pain is reduced (C, D). Finally, keeping the fascia intact reduces the risk of hernias from the donor site. The major disadvantage is that it must be done by a microsurgery specialist and takes a longer time compared to a standard pedicle flap. When comparing a DIEP to a pedicle transverse rectus abdominis musculocutaneous (TRAM) flap, the DIEP is associated with a shorter hospital stay, a decreased rate of donor site hernias, and a statistically significantly lower rate of fat necrosis (17.7% versus 58.5%) (A).

Reference: Garvey PB, Buchel EW, Pockaj BA, et al. DIEP and pedicled TRAM flaps: a comparison of outcomes. *Plast Reconstr Surg.* 2006;117(6):1711–1719.

9. B. Gynecomastia is a condition resulting from the abnormal benign proliferation of glandular breast tissue in men. Most patients seek surgical treatments for symptoms such as pain, hypersensitivity of the nipple, and psychologic well-being. This can be done with surgical excision, suction-assisted lipectomy, or ultrasound-assisted liposuction. If surgical excision is chosen, a periareolar incision is made at the junction of the areola and the skin. Next, a cuff of tissue 1 to 1.5 cm in thickness is preserved directly deep in the nipple/areola complex. This maneuver prevents postoperative nipple/areola depression or adherence of the nipple/areola to the pectoralis major muscle (E). The most common early complication after gynecomastia surgery is hematoma. The hematoma should be evacuated, if possible. Under-resection of tissue is the most common long-term complication of gynecomastia surgery (C). Postoperative wound infection is uncommon because it is a clean operation (A). The use of prophylactic antibiotics, particularly in liposuction cases, may account for the low incidence of this complication. Newer techniques allow for superior cosmesis, and as such, asymmetry is uncommon (D).

Reference: Thorne C. Techniques and principles in plastic surgery. In: Thorne CH, Gurtner GC, Chung KC, et al., eds. *Grabb and Smith's plastic surgery.* 7th ed. Lippincott Williams and Wilkins; 2013:1–12.

10. C. The reapproximation of the vermilion-cutaneous junction is the main goal of lip laceration repair. A vermillion border mismatch of 1 mm is visible to the naked eye. Thus, repair of the vermillion border under loop magnification is paramount to recreating the lip borders. This will optimize both cosmesis and function following repair. The vermilion border is initially closed with interrupted sutures. This is followed by closure of the muscularis and then interrupted absorbable sutures in the mucosa (A, B). Because each layer will need to be closed, multiple stitches will be used (D). The teeth are not a priority in this situation and can be fixed at a later time (E).

11. D. NPWT works by multiple mechanisms, including reduction of edema and removal of wound fluid rich in destructive enzymes that are produced by both the patient and local bacterial contamination. In addition, employing the cyclic compression mode allows stimulation of the mechanotransduction pathways in the wound, resulting in increased growth factor release, matrix production, and cellular proliferation. Common clinical scenarios amenable to NPWT include lymphatic leaks, venous stasis wounds, diabetic wounds, wounds with fistula, sternal wounds, orthopedic wounds, and abdominal wounds (B, C, E). Likewise, NPWT is frequently used as an alternative to bolster dressings for split skin grafts, reducing the risk of a seroma or hematoma under the graft (A). There are several contraindications to the use of NPWT, and these include the presence of malignancy, use on wounds characterized by ischemia, as well as inadequately debrided or badly infected wounds. There have been reports of extension of the zone of necrosis when used on ischemic wounds. Patients with ischemic wounds should be considered for revascularization before application of NPWT.

Reference: Thorne C. Techniques and principles in plastic surgery. In: Thorne CH, Gurtner GC, Chung KC, et al., eds. *Grabb and Smith's plastic surgery*. 7th ed. Lippincott Williams and Wilkins; 2013:1–12.

12. D. Oxygen, iron, vitamin C, and alpha-ketoglutarate all participate in the hydroxylation and subsequent cross-linking in collagen (A, C). Vitamin A is essential because it promotes epithelialization in collagen synthesis for wound healing, but it does not participate in cross-linking of proline residues in collagen (B). Penicillamine is associated with a reduction in numbers of T-lymphocytes, inhibition of macrophage function, decreased numbers of IL-1, and rheumatoid factor. In addition, it prevents collagen from cross-linking (E).

Reference: Thorne C. Techniques and principles in plastic surgery. In: Thorne CH, Gurtner GC, Chung KC, et al., eds. *Grabb and Smith's plastic surgery*. 7th ed. Lippincott Williams and Wilkins; 2013:1–12.

13. B. The rectus abdominis muscle has a dual-dominant blood supply. The upper vessel is the superior epigastric artery, which is one of the terminal branches of the internal thoracic artery (previously known as the internal mammary artery). The lower vessel is the inferior epigastric artery, arising from the external iliac artery above the level of the inguinal ligament (D). The *superficial* (not superior) epigastric artery arises from the femoral artery (A, C) and does not supply the rectus abdominis. The deep circumflex iliac artery arises from the external iliac artery and supplies the iliac crest (E).

14. C. Most isolated orbital fractures involve the orbital floor, which is made up mainly of the maxillary bone (A, B, D, E). Most pure blowout fractures involve the orbital floor. The most common complication after an orbital floor fracture is entrapment. There are two uncommon complications after orbital bone fracture. *Superior orbital fissure syndrome* results from compression of structures contained in the superior orbit. These include cranial nerves III, IV, and VI. Compression of these structures leads to symptoms of eyelid ptosis, globe proptosis, and paralysis of extraocular muscles. If the optic nerve is also involved, symptoms include blindness, and the syndrome is dubbed *orbital apex syndrome*. Both of these syndromes are medical emergencies, and steroid therapy or surgical compression should be considered.

15. C. Flap color, capillary refill, tissue bleeding, and flap temperature are all assessed to ensure adequate flap perfusion. The gold standard for assessing the viability of transferred tissue is clinical examination (A, B, D, E). Identification of a failing or insufficiently perfused flap can occasionally be challenging for even the most experienced microsurgeon. A Doppler probe can be a useful adjunct to assess vascular flow within the pedicle and/or specific areas of the flap. Experienced personnel are essential for monitoring a flap postoperatively. Doppler monitoring is, however, subject to error (both false-positive and false-negative) and thus should never replace clinical assessments. A number of clinical signs (present either singly or in combination) may suggest malperfusion. Pale flap color, reduction in flap temperature, loss of capillary refill, and loss of flap turgor may indicate arterial insufficiency. Venous insufficiency, on the other hand, can result in a purple or blue hue in the flap, congestion, swelling, and rapid capillary refill in the early stages, followed by eventual loss of capillary refill. Venous congestion may be addressed by surgical measures as well as the application of medical *Hirudo medicinalis* leeches or by chemical "leeching," which is topical heparin combined with dermal punctures.

References: Losee J. E., Gimbel M. L., Rubin J, et al. Plastic and reconstructive surgery. In: Brunicardi F, Andersen DK, Billiar TR, Dunn DL, Hunter JG, Matthews JB, Pollock RE. eds. *Schwartz's principles of surgery*. 10th ed. McGraw Hill Education; 2015.

Thorne C. Techniques and principles in plastic surgery. In: Thorne CH, Gurtner GC, Chung KC, et al., eds. *Grabb and Smith's plastic Surgery*. 7th ed. Lippincott Williams and Wilkins; 2013:1–12.

16. C. Cleft lip is one of the most common congenital deformities. Intervention is aimed at restoring facial appearance and oral function. There is still debate as to the ideal timing for repair, but the "rule of 10s" is a general guideline to help select appropriate candidates for repair. This includes a hemoglobin greater than 10 g/dL, age above 10 weeks, and a body weight more than 10 pounds (A, B). Contraindications to repair include severe malnutrition and concurrent cardiac anomalies requiring repair (D, E). Cleft palate involves the hard palate anterior to the incisive foramen and repair should be delayed until 1 year of age to prevent interference with maxillofacial growth. Too-early repair risks an increased incidence of middle ear infections and resultant hearing loss.

Genitourinary 24

AMANDA C. PURDY AND JEREMY M. BLUMBERG

ABSITE 99th Percentile High-Yields

I. Anatomy
   A. Renal hilum from anterior to posterior: renal Vein, renal Artery, renal Pelvis (VAP)
   B. Right renal artery courses posterior to the IVC; left renal vein courses anterior to the aorta; right adrenal vein drains into IVC; left adrenal, gonadal, lumbar veins drain into left renal vein

II. Testicular Torsion
   A. Usually in infants or during puberty; presents with acute testicular pain; testicle can be high-riding, lying horizontally, swollen, tender, and hyperemic; absent cremasteric reflex; Prehn sign: elevation of testicle does not relieve pain in torsion but does relieve pain in epididymitis
   B. Workup: ultrasound with doppler shows decreased testicular perfusion; imaging is not necessary for diagnosis and if high clinical suspicion, should go to OR
   C. Must treat urgently to salvage testicle—if detorsion done within 6 hours, salvage rate is near 100%, salvage rate decreases to 50% by 12 hours and 10% if more than 24 hours
   D. Management: surgical detorsion and bilateral orchiopexy with midline scrotal incision; if torsed testicle not viable, perform orchiectomy and contralateral orchiopexy

III. Epididymitis (Inflammation of the Epididymis, Usually Due to Infection)
   A. In men <35, most due to chlamydia and/or gonorrhea; in men >35, most due to E. coli
   B. Presentation: acute scrotal pain, point tenderness to posterior testicle, improvement of pain with elevation of the testicle
   C. Diagnosis is clinical; urinalysis and culture (however, urinalysis often negative and negative test does not rule out epididymitis), nucleic acid amplification test (NAAT) for chlamydia and gonorrhea
   D. Management: NSAIDs, scrotal elevation, antibiotics; if suspect chlamydia/gonorrhea, treat with IM ceftriaxone ×1 dose, and oral doxycycline or azithromycin for 10 days; if do not suspect STI, treat with levofloxacin for 10 days

IV. Hydrocele (Asymptomatic Fluid Collection Around Testicle That Transilluminates)
   A. Communicating hydroceles are due to a patent processus vaginalis with free flow of fluid between the scrotum and peritoneal cavity; more common in infants
   B. Size of hydrocele will fluctuate, shrink when supine and enlarge when upright (helps differentiate from varicocele which does not fluctuate in size)
   C. Noncommunicating hydroceles due to accumulation of secretions within the tunica vaginalis; this is more common in adults
   D. Presents with a cystic scrotal mass that transilluminates
   E. In babies, most will resolve spontaneously by 1 year of age

F. Communicating hydroceles come with a risk for indirect inguinal hernia and should be repaired if they persist after a child is 1 to 2 years old; repair is high ligation of the patent processus vaginalis

G. Noncommunicating hydroceles that are symptomatic can be treated with hydrocelectomy; most common complication of this procedure is postoperative hematoma

V. Cryptorchidism (a Testicle Not Within the Scrotum by 4 Months of Age)

A. Testis should descend by 4 months of age; undescended testicle most commonly in the superficial inguinal ring, followed by the inguinal canal

B. Associated with increased risk of decreased fertility, testicular cancer (especially seminoma), inguinal hernia, and torsion

C. Treat with unilateral orchiopexy if contralateral testicle has normally descended (should be done after 6 months old, before 1-year-old); bilateral orchiopexy considered if clinical scenario indicates potential for testicular torsion including bell-clapper deformity (long mesenteric attachment of testicle allowing it to rotate)

VI. Testicular Cancer

A. A solid testicular mass is cancer until proven otherwise

B. Initial workup is with ultrasound, tumor markers (AFP, beta-hCG, LDH); then get tissue diagnosis with transinguinal radical orchiectomy; don't approach via scrotum because scrotal lymphatics will be violated, which increases local recurrence and alters patterns of metastasis

C. 90% are germ cell tumors, which can be seminomas or nonseminomas; seminomas most common, radiosensitive, and always have normal AFP; nonseminomas (including embryonal carcinoma, yolk sac tumor, teratoma, and choriocarcinoma) are not radiosensitive and may have elevated AFP

D. First site of metastasis for testicular cancer usually the retroperitoneal lymph nodes; choriocarcinoma is the exception—spreads hematogenously

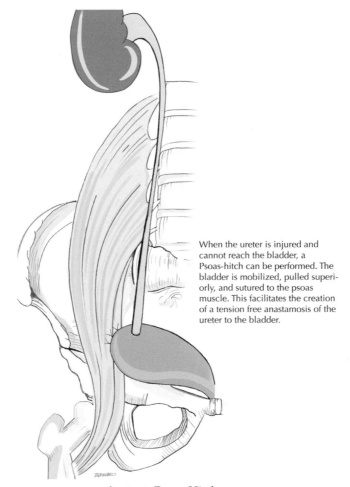

When the ureter is injured and cannot reach the bladder, a Psoas-hitch can be performed. The bladder is mobilized, pulled superiorly, and sutured to the psoas muscle. This facilitates the creation of a tension free anastamosis of the ureter to the bladder.

Fig. 24.1 Psoas-Hitch

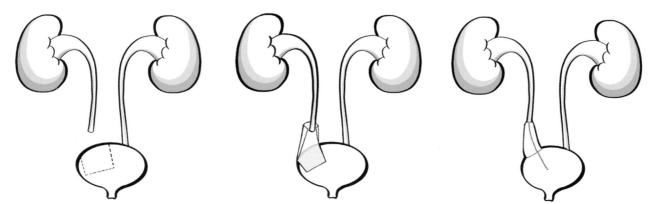

Fig. 24.2 If a psoas hitch cannot adequately bridge the gap between the injured ureter and the bladder, a Boari flap may be used. A wide flap of the anterior bladder wall is created and then tubularized to meet the distal end of the diseases or injured ureter.

Questions

1. A 25-year-old man presents for a palpable mass in his right testicle that has been present for a few months. On ultrasound, there is a solid 2-cm mass in his right testicle that appears well defined, homogenous and hypoechoic. AFP, beta-hCG, and LDH are normal. What is the most appropriate next step?
   A. MRI of the abdomen and pelvis
   B. Core needle biopsy
   C. Transscrotal orchiectomy
   D. Transinguinal orchiectomy
   E. Transinguinal orchiectomy with retroperitoneal lymph node dissection

2. On routine examination of a 12-month-old boy, it is noted that only one testicle is present in the scrotum, on the right. A mass is palpated in the left inguinal region. What is the most appropriate next step?
   A. Reexamination in 6 months
   B. Ultrasound of the groin and scrotum
   C. Laparoscopic division of the testicular vessels
   D. Left orchiopexy
   E. Bilateral orchiopexy

3. A 22-year-old male presents to the ED with an erection that has lasted for 9 hours and is becoming exceedingly painful. He denies genitourinary trauma, drug use, or recreational use of phosphodiesterase-5 inhibitors. He also denies any personal or family history of hematologic diseases. He had a similar episode 8 months ago that resolved spontaneously after 4 hours, but now he is having severe worsening penile pain. Management of his condition involves:
   A. Oxygen, IV hydration, and close monitoring
   B. Oral phenylephrine
   C. Penile Doppler ultrasound
   D. Corporal aspiration and irrigation with saline
   E. Urgent cavernoglandular shunt

4. A 35-year-old woman is in the hospital after undergoing elective sigmoidectomy for recurrent diverticulitis. On postoperative day 3, she complains of abdominal discomfort and her abdominal drain puts out 300 mL of clear fluid. Her heart rate is 123 beats per minute. Analysis of the fluid shows significantly elevated creatinine compared to serum creatinine. Which of the following is true about the most likely complication?
   A. Ureteral stents placed prior to surgery decrease the risk of ureteral injury
   B. Optimal management is to continue abdominal drainage and nephrostomy tube placement
   C. If ureteral injury is confirmed, the patient should return to the operating room for repair
   D. The rate of ureteral injury is higher in laparoscopic surgery than in open surgery
   E. Optimal management is ureteral stent placement with delayed operative repair

5. A 24-year-old female is about to undergo elective surgery for an umbilical hernia. A preoperative urinalysis is positive for nitrite and leukocyte esterase with some bacteria identified but no squamous cells present. She denies urinary frequency, urgency, or dysuria. Which of the following is the best next step in management?
   A. Proceed to surgery
   B. Proceed to surgery after administering a single dose of IV antibiotics to cover gram-negatives
   C. Delay surgery and administer a 3-day course of oral antibiotics
   D. Delay surgery, administer a 3-day course of oral antibiotics, then repeat urinalysis
   E. Repeat urinalysis and proceed to surgery only if repeat urinalysis is negative

6. Which of the following is true regarding renal anatomy?
   A. The renal vein is posterior to the renal artery in the hilum
   B. If the left renal vein needs ligation, it is best to do so near the renal hilum
   C. Glisson capsule surrounds the kidney
   D. The left renal vein crosses posterior to the aorta
   E. The right renal artery crosses posterior to the IVC

7. A 14-year-old boy presents to the ED with nausea, vomiting, and severe left scrotal pain that woke him from sleep 3 hours ago. He denies scrotal trauma or recent infections. He had a similar episode 6 months ago that resolved within minutes. Physical exam reveals an enlarged, firm, and tender left testicle that appears to be high in scrotum with abnormal lie. Stroking the left inner thigh does not elicit elevation of the hemiscrotum. Manual elevation of the scrotum does not relieve the pain. Which of the following is the best next step in management?
   A. Testicular Duplex ultrasound
   B. Attempt left testicular detorsion in the ED and, if successful, admit for close observation
   C. Attempt left testicular detorsion in the ED followed by left testicular orchiopexy in the OR
   D. Take to the OR to perform left testicular detorsion and bilateral orchiopexy
   E. Attempt left testicular detorsion in the ED and if successful perform testicular Duplex scan

8. A 45-year-old male presents to clinic with his wife to discuss having a vasectomy. Which of the following is true regarding this procedure?
   A. It is typically performed by a urologist in the operating room (OR) under general anesthesia
   B. It involves ligating the vas deferens
   C. The patient can safely have intercourse 1 month after the procedure with little risk of pregnancy
   D. Reversal of vasectomy is associated with a pregnancy rate of less than 10%
   E. There is an increased risk for testicular cancer

9. A 67-year-old male undergoes an uneventful radical prostatectomy for prostate cancer. Eight days later, he has a fever and feculent material is noted in his urine. Pelvic CT reveals a 9- × 8-cm heterogeneous perirectal fluid collection. The best course of management is administering parenteral antibiotics, percutaneous drainage of the fluid collection, and:
   A. Repeat CT in 2 weeks
   B. Initiation of total parenteral nutrition
   C. Initiation of enteric feeding via a Dobhoff tube
   D. Insertion of a suprapubic cystostomy tube
   E. Diverting colostomy creation

10. A 57-year-old male presents to the ED with a severe headache that started suddenly. His systolic blood pressure is 220 mm Hg which improves with labetalol. He does not have any medical problems but has recently reported some scrotal discomfort. On exam, his left testicle has a painless soft mass, external to the testicle, that feels like a "bag of worms." When he lies supine, the mass does not disappear. Urinalysis demonstrates 18 red blood cells per high power field. Which of the following is the best next step in management?
   A. Computed tomography (CT) of the head
   B. Testicular ultrasound
   C. CT of the abdomen/pelvis
   D. Renal ultrasound
   E. Reassurance and referral to primary care physician to begin antihypertensives

11. An otherwise healthy 62-year-old male presents with pneumaturia, urinary frequency, and dysuria for several weeks. He is afebrile and hemodynamically stable. Urinalysis is negative for blood. Urine culture grows multiple organisms. CT scan shows air in the bladder with colonic diverticulosis. Cystoscopy is negative and colonoscopy is negative other than diverticula. Optimal management consists of:
   A. Total parenteral nutrition, bowel rest, and antibiotics
   B. Colon resection with primary closure of bladder
   C. Colon resection and excision of cuff of bladder
   D. Eight-week course of oral antibiotics
   E. Fulguration via cystoscopy

12. A 45-year-old male presents to the ED with nausea, vomiting, and a sharp right groin pain that started 6 hours ago. He is unable to find a comfortable position and moves around frequently in the hospital bed. He is afebrile and hemodynamically stable. CT abdomen/pelvis without contrast reveals a 4-mm right-sided stone at the ureterovesical junction (UVJ) with mild hydronephrosis and some periureteral stranding. He has no dysuria and his urinalysis is negative for infection. His pain and nausea improve with medical therapy. Which of the following is the most appropriate course of management?
   A. Medical expulsive therapy (tamsulosin, nonsteroidal antiinflammatory drugs [NSAIDs]) and outpatient follow-up
   B. Ureteral stent placement
   C. Extracorporeal shock wave lithotripsy (ESWL)
   D. Ureteroscopy and laser lithotripsy
   E. Percutaneous nephrostomy tube placement

13. An 18-year-old woman presents to the ED following a motorcycle collision. She is hemodynamically stable but has an obvious pelvic fracture. On exam, blood is found at the vaginal introitus. CT abdomen/pelvis demonstrates a severe pelvic fracture with normal-appearing kidneys. The best next step is:
  A. Urethral catheter
  B. Cystogram
  C. Retrograde urethrogram and cystogram
  D. Urethroscopy, vaginoscopy, and cystogram
  E. Suprapubic bladder catheter

14. A 36-year-old female is admitted to the hospital after being struck by an automobile while riding her motorcycle. Plain films demonstrate a fracture at her inferior pubic ramus. Upon urethral catheter placement, she was found to have gross hematuria. CT cystogram revealed contrast extravasation into the extraperitoneal space with no bony structures within the bladder wall. The patient is hemodynamically stable. Laboratory studies are unremarkable. The next step is:
  A. Prolonged indwelling urethral catheter
  B. Replace urethral catheter with suprapubic cystostomy
  C. Open operative repair of bladder injury
  D. Cystoscopy to visualize bladder perforation site
  E. Bilateral nephrostomy tubes for temporary urinary diversion

15. A 19-year-old male presents to the ED with a stab wound to his left lower back. He is hemodynamically stable and has no evidence of peritonitis. A CT scan of the abdomen and pelvis with oral and intravenous (IV) contrast demonstrates a subcapsular hematoma of the left kidney and a small posterior left kidney laceration with no extravasation of contrast or injury to the collecting system. There is no fluid or free air in the peritoneum. Distal ureters are intact bilaterally. The next best step is:
  A. Observation
  B. Retrograde ureteropyelogram
  C. IV methylene blue and local exploration of wound
  D. Retroperitoneal exploration and renal reconstruction
  E. Exploratory laparotomy, retroperitoneal exploration, and renal reconstruction

16. A 32-year-old male is brought to the ED by ambulance after a motorcycle accident at 45 mph. Abdominal CT scan with contrast demonstrates a deep renal laceration with urinary extravasation into the retroperitoneum. After observation for 10 days, a repeat CT urogram shows persistent urinary extravasation with development of a small urinoma. There is no hydronephrosis. He is hemodynamically stable and afebrile. The most appropriate next step is:
  A. Continued observation
  B. Surgical exploration and repair
  C. Insertion of a ureteral stent
  D. Percutaneous nephrostomy drainage
  E. Percutaneous perinephric drainage

17. A 49-year-old male undergoes a low anterior resection for rectal cancer. During mobilization and dissection of the sigmoid colon, the left ureter is injured. The injured segment measures 1 cm in length and is located above the pelvic brim. The patient is hemodynamically stable. Which of the following is the appropriate management for this ureteral injury?
  A. Resect injured segment and perform a primary end-to-end ureteral anastomosis over a stent
  B. Ligate ureter and place a percutaneous nephrostomy tube
  C. Mobilize ureter and reimplant into the bladder after performing a psoas hitch
  D. Perform a nephropexy and ureteroureterostomy
  E. Perform an ileum interposition

18. A 27-year-old male presents to the ED after sustaining a gunshot wound to the pelvis. He undergoes exploratory laparotomy and is found to have a left sigmoid colon injury, which is repaired primarily. He is hemodynamically stable. On examination of the left distal ureter, it appears to be contused. Intravenous indigo carmine is administered, and no extravasation is seen from the ureter. Which of the following is the most appropriate next step?
  A. Observation
  B. Ureteral stent
  C. Percutaneous nephrostomy
  D. Resect damaged ureter and reimplant ureter into bladder
  E. Resect damaged ureter and repair with end-to-end ureteral anastomosis

Answers

1. D. A solid testicular mass is cancer until proven otherwise. Initial workup includes scrotal ultrasound and tumor markers, including AFP, beta-hCG, and LDH. Seminomas are classically well defined, oval, homogenous, and hypoechoic on ultrasound, whereas nonseminomas appear nonhomogeneous, hyperechoic, with calcifications, cystic areas, and indistinct margins. In the presence of a solid mass, the next step is obtaining a tissue diagnosis, which is done via transinguinal orchiectomy. It is important not to violate the scrotum while obtaining tissue diagnosis, as this can lead to lymphatic disruption (B, C). Imaging to assess for distant metastasis is not necessary until the diagnosis of testicular cancer is confirmed (A). Tumor markers should be repeated after orchiectomy. A retroperitoneal lymph node dissection may be indicated for nonseminomas. However, this would not be done during the initial operation before a tissue diagnosis is established (E). The patient should be counseled on testicular prosthesis, which may be placed during the orchiectomy. In addition, the patient should be counseled on sperm banking prior to orchiectomy if they have risk factors for infertility (atrophic contralateral testis, history of infertility).

Reference: Gilligan T, Lin DW, Aggarwal R, et al. Testicular Cancer, version 2.2020, NCCN clinical practice guidelines in oncology. *J Natl Compr Canc Netw.* 2019;17(12):1529–1554.

2. D. This patient has cryptorchidism. In the majority of infants, the testicles reach the scrotum by 3 to 4 months old, and spontaneous descent into the scrotum after 4 months is unlikely. In patients with cryptorchidism, the undescended testicle(s) are exposed to increased temperatures, which leads to stunted growth, decreased spermatogenesis, and an increased risk for subsequent infertility. These patients also have a higher risk of developing testicular cancer and torsion. The treatment for this is orchiopexy of the affected testicle. Orchiopexy, especially when done early, improves fertility, improves testicular growth, minimizes torsion risk, and *may* decrease testicular cancer risk. While there is no clear consensus about whether orchiopexy decreases testicular cancer risk, it at least allows for easier detection of testicular masses. Orchiopexy should be done between 6 and 12 months of age and only needs to be done on the affected side (E). Reexamination would be inappropriate as the child would be older than 12 months (A). Imaging is not needed prior to surgery in this patient with a palpable undescended testicle (B). The majority of undescended testicles are located in the superficial inguinal ring (most common), or the inguinal canal. Less than 10% of patients will have an intraabdominal testicle or an absent testicle. Even in the event the patient has a unilateral nonpalpable testicle, imaging does not need to be performed prior to exam under anesthesia with possible exploratory surgery as it does not decrease the need for eventual surgery. In the event the patient is found to have an intraabdominal testicle that cannot reach the scrotum, division of the testicular vessels may be necessary to mobilize the testicle to the scrotum. However, that is unnecessary in this case (C).

References: Chan E, Wayne C, Nasr A, FRCSC for Canadian Association of Pediatric Surgeon Evidence-Based Resource. Ideal timing of orchiopexy: a systematic review. *Pediatr Surg Int.* 2014;30(1):87–97.

Tasian GE, Copp HL. Diagnostic performance of ultrasound in nonpalpable cryptorchidism: a systematic review and meta-analysis. *Pediatrics.* 2011;127(1):119–128.

3. D. This patient is suffering from ischemic priapism, a urologic emergency requiring urgent intervention to prevent permanent erectile dysfunction. This is due to decreased venous outflow from the cavernosa and subsequent increased intracavernosal pressure. This also results in decreased arterial inflow, causing stasis of blood and resultant local hypoxia and acidosis. On exam, the patient has a fully erect, rigid, and tender penis, but the glans and corpus spongiosum are soft (corpora cavernosa are the involved compartments in priapism). Early intervention is very important. In the ED, the patient should undergo a corporal aspiration and irrigation with normal saline to drain static blood from the corpora and to flush out old clots; this achieves detumescence. Phenylephrine may be injected intracorporally as well, but the patient must be on a cardiac monitor before doing so because of the risk of hypertension, tachycardia, reflex bradycardia, and arrhythmia if the phenylephrine is systemically absorbed. If detumescence is not successfully achieved by corporal aspiration/irrigation, the patient should undergo a cavernoglandular shunt procedure, though this is more invasive and has a higher risk of permanent erectile dysfunction (E). Oral phenylephrine has not been shown to be beneficial for priapism (B). In sickle cell patients with priapism, first-line management is medical therapy with oxygen, IV hydration, and pain control (A). Blood exchange transfusions to reduce the concentration of HbS are indicated in sickle cell patients if initial medical therapy fails. Penile Doppler ultrasound is not routinely done for priapism, though it may be useful to differentiate ischemic from nonischemic priapism (nonischemic priapism is managed conservatively and often resolves with observation) (C). Nonischemic priapism is nontender and partially rigid. It is usually due to penile trauma causing a fistula between the corporal tissue and the cavernous artery and is not an emergent condition.

References: Broderick, G., et al. (2010). Priapism recommendations. Sexual Medicine: Sexual Dysfunction in Men and Women. Third International Consultation on Erectile Dysfunction (3rd ICUD). In F. Montorsi, et al., (Eds.), *Plymouth.* United Kingdom: Health Publication Ltd. https://www.auanet.org/guidelines/guidelines/priapism-guideline

Tay YK, Spernat D, Rzetelski-West K, Appu S, Love C. Acute management of priapism in men. *BJU Int.* 2012;109 Suppl 3:15–21.

4. C. Iatrogenic ureteral injuries are a rare but well-known complication during gynecologic, urologic, colorectal, and vascular surgeries. The risk of ureteral injury in colorectal surgery has been shown to be slightly higher in open surgery, and lower in laparoscopic surgery (D). Ideally, these injuries are discovered intraoperatively, so they can be repaired without subjecting the patient to a subsequent operation. While ureteral stents have not been shown to decrease the risk of ureteral injury, they may help surgeons identify injuries intraoperatively (A). In this case, the injury was not discovered until the postoperative period. Patients may present with abdominal pain or distension, ileus, oliguria, fever, tachycardia, leakage of clear fluid from their incisions, and/or increased clear drain output. If a drain is present, fluid analysis can be done. High fluid creatinine (higher than serum creatinine, similar to urine creatinine) supports the diagnosis of a urine leak. The diagnosis should be confirmed with imaging, such as a CT urogram. The management of a postoperative ureteral injury depends on the timing of diagnosis. Those diagnosed within the first 5 to 7 postoperative days, and with systemic signs (tachycardia) should return to the operating room for repair. If the diagnosis is delayed more than 7 days after surgery, the injury should be temporized and treated with delayed surgical repair. Methods to temporize the ureteral injury include stent placement for incomplete injuries or a nephrostomy tube for complete transections. Neither of which are appropriate in this case because it is only postoperative day 3 (B, E).

References: Bothwell WN, Bleicher RJ, Dent TL. Prophylactic ureteral catheterization in colon surgery. A five-year review. *Dis Colon Rectum.* 1994;37(4):330–334.

Halabi WJ, Jafari MD, Nguyen VQ, et al. Ureteral injuries in colorectal surgery: an analysis of trends, outcomes, and risk factors over a 10-year period in the United States. *Dis Colon Rectum.* 2014;57(2):179–186.

5. A. The above patient has asymptomatic bacteriuria, which is defined by the presence of bacteria or markers thereof (positive for leukocyte esterase, nitrites) in an appropriately collected urinalysis (absence or low number of squamous cells) and without any signs or symptoms of a UTI (e.g., urinary frequency, urgency, dysuria). With the exception of pregnancy and those undergoing urologic intervention (e.g., prostatectomy, prostate biopsy), adult patients with asymptomatic bacteriuria do not require any treatment (B–E). In contrast, all symptomatic patients require treatment. Women are at a higher risk for *symptomatic* UTIs owing to their shorter and straighter urethra. Additionally, its close proximity to the vaginal orifice colonized by bacteria makes them vulnerable to infection. Most uncomplicated cases can be managed with a 3-day course of nitrofurantoin or trimethoprim-sulfamethoxazole (TMP-SMX). Due to increasing microbial resistance to ciprofloxacin, it should be reserved for demographics with TMP-SMX resistance or in cases where nitrofurantoin or TMP-SMX cannot be used due to availability, allergy, or intolerance. Complicated cases require a 7-day course of oral antibiotics and include those with previous urinary manipulation, abnormal anatomy, and all male patients. Given the rarity of symptomatic UTI in young men, one should suspect abnormal anatomy predisposing him to bacteriuria and subsequent infection. Young males and most women with recurrent infections should be referred to a urologist to undergo renal ultrasound and measurement of postvoid residual bladder volume.

Reference: Gallegos Salazar J, O'Brien W, Strymish JM, Itani K, Branch-Elliman W, Gupta K. Association of screening and treatment for preoperative asymptomatic bacteriuria with postoperative outcomes among US veterans. *JAMA Surg.* 2019;154(3):241–248.

6. E. There are two kidneys, but humans can survive with just one without a clinically significant decrease in renal function or rise in creatinine. The Gerota capsule surrounds the kidney while the Glisson capsule surrounds the liver (C). The renal vein is the most anterior structure in the renal hilum, the renal pelvis is the most posterior structure, and the renal artery is between the two (A). The right renal vein is short and drains immediately into the inferior vena cava (IVC), while the longer left renal vein is joined by collateral vessels before entering the IVC. Since the left kidney has a longer renal vein, it is the preferred side for a donor kidney. The left renal vein is joined by the left adrenal vein superiorly, the left gonadal vein inferiorly, and the left lumbar vein posteriorly. The left renal vein can be ligated but should be performed close to the IVC (B); this still permits venous drainage via collaterals without irreversible renal damage or hydronephrosis. The right renal artery passes posterior to the IVC while the left renal vein passes anterior to the aorta (D). Rarely, a retroaortic left renal vein is present. This variant can present problems during infrarenal aortic surgery because the vein is prone to injury and is difficult to repair.

7. D. This patient presents with the classic clinical picture of testicular torsion. Incidence of torsion occurs in a bimodal pattern; infant boys (due to the tunica vaginalis not yet secured to the gubernaculum in the scrotum) and adolescent boys (rapidly growing testicles during puberty) are at the highest risk of torsion, though it can occur at any age. Torsion presents with acute onset of severe testicular pain, with or without swelling. Many have associated nausea and vomiting that may initially confuse the diagnosis. This patient's history also suggests possible intermittent torsion that resolved spontaneously, though this is difficult to diagnose definitively. Physical exam findings include a tender firm testicle, horizontal lie of the testicle, high-riding testicle, and an absent cremasteric reflex (stroking the inner thigh elicits elevation of the hemiscrotum). In contrast to epididymitis, patients with testicular torsion have a negative Prehn sign (manual elevation of the scrotum relieves pain). Torsion is diagnosed clinically, and surgical exploration should not be delayed to perform other imaging studies if suspicion is high, as in this case (A). If the diagnosis is questionable, a scrotal Doppler ultrasound is a reasonable option. This would demonstrate an absence of flow and a more heterogeneous texture of the testicular parenchyma compared with the contralateral testis. A torsed testicle is usually viable if detorsed within 6 hours. When the suspicion for torsion is high, the patient should be taken directly to the operating room. Attempting detorsion in the ED is an option prior to surgery, particularly if there will be an anticipated delay in getting to the OR, or if a urologist is unavailable. This can be attempted in the ED with proper pain medication but still necessitates an urgent bilateral orchiopexy in the OR (B, C, E). After surgical detorsion, both testes are sutured to the scrotal dartos muscle (orchiopexy) to prevent future torsion episodes (contralateral testis has a higher risk of torsion as well, necessitating concurrent contralateral orchiopexy). A common imitator of testicular torsion is epididymo orchitis, differentiated by pain relief with testicular elevation, normal or increased flow in the testicle or epididymis on Doppler ultrasound (increased flow indicating inflammation), and a urinalysis suggesting bacteriuria. Sexually transmitted infections must also be ruled out if epididymo orchitis is suspected. If the testicle is found to be ischemic and does not recover color and appearance after detorsion, testicular infarction has resulted and an orchiectomy is necessary.

References: DaJusta DG, Granberg CF, Villanueva C, Baker LA. Contemporary review of testicular torsion: new concepts, emerging technologies and potential therapeutics. *J Pediatr Urol.* 2013;9(6 Pt A):723–730.

Johnston BI, Wiener JS. Intermittent testicular torsion. *BJU Int.* 2005;95:933–934. Sharp VJ, Kieran K, Arlen AM. Testicular torsion: diagnosis, evaluation, and management. *Am Fam Physician.* 2013;88(12):835–840.

8. B. Vasectomy is a very effective method for male contraception. It is less costly, safer, and associated with a shorter recovery time compared with tubal ligation. However, vasectomy is performed less frequently, which is likely related to patient misinformation and public stigma. There are a variety of methods to perform a vasectomy, and it can be done by urologists as well as general surgeons, typically in the office with local anesthesia (A). The guiding principle involves ligation of the vas deferens, which can be achieved with two small scrotal incisions. Although the success rate exceeds 95%, patients should not have unprotected intercourse for 3 months after the procedure and only after confirming sterility with a semen analysis to look for azoospermia (C). The probability of obtaining a natural pregnancy following vasectomy reversal is 50% (D). There is no evidence to suggest that patients who have undergone vasectomy have an increased risk for testicular cancer (E).

References: Aradhya KW, Best K, Sokal DC. Recent developments in vasectomy. *BMJ.* 2005;330(7486):296–299.

van Dongen J, Tekle FB, van Roijen JH. Pregnancy rate after vasectomy reversal in a contemporary series: influence of smoking, semen quality and post-surgical use of assisted reproductive techniques. *BJU Int.* 2012;110(4):562–567.

9. E. A rare but feared complication of radical prostatectomy is rectal injury, with an incidence of 1.5%. If identified intraoperatively, it may be repaired primarily. If the bowel injury is recognized postoperatively as a vesicorectal fistula (as in this case), conservative management is not appropriate (A–D). Since the patient has systemic signs of infection, he needs to be started on parenteral antibiotics and the fluid collection needs to be drained. Additionally, a large fluid collection suggests a sizeable rectal injury and perforation; this will need to be treated with a colostomy to temporarily divert his stool with the intent to perform a delayed repair.

References: Harpster LE, Rommel FM, Sieber PR, et al. The incidence and management of rectal injury associated with radical prostatectomy in a community based urology practice. *J Urol.* 1995;154(4):1435–1438.

Rovner ES. Urinary tract fistula. In: Campbell MF, Wein AJ, Kavoussi LR, eds. *Campbell-Walsh urology.* 9th ed. Saunders Elsevier; 2007.

10. C. Scrotal discomfort accompanied by a mass that feels like a "bag of worms" is characteristic of a varicocele, but if it right sided, acute onset, or fails to decompress while lying supine, it is concerning for proximal venous obstruction. A left-sided varicocele that fails to decompress is concerning for obstruction at the left renal vein, whereas a right-sided one for IVC compression/obstruction. Renal cell carcinoma (RCC) is one concerning etiology in this setting. The classic triad for RCC includes a flank mass, flank pain,

and hematuria, but less than 10% have all three findings. In addition, RCC can initially present with a paraneoplastic syndrome that includes hypertension from renin secretion (likely in the above patient), hypercalcemia from parathyroid hormone (PTH)-related peptide secretion, polycythemia from erythropoietin secretion, hypoglycemia from insulin secretion, and hepatic dysfunction (Stauffer syndrome), all of which resolve with treatment of RCC. About 40% of patients with RCC have an elevated renin level. Risk factors for RCC include smoking, alcohol, obesity, cystic disease of the kidney, and diabetes. The next best step for this patient is to order a CT scan of the abdomen/pelvis with a urogram phase to evaluate for a renal mass and visualize his upper urinary tracts (A, B, D, E). Although metastasis accounts for the majority of renal tumors (typically from breast cancer), the most common primary renal tumor is RCC. The lung is the most frequent site of distant spread. Tissue diagnosis is required before surgical intervention. Patients with resectable disease and without distant spread can undergo partial nephrectomy for smaller tumors, or radical nephrectomy for larger tumors or those with local invasion (such as this patient).

Reference: Palapattu GS, Kristo B, Rajfer J. Paraneoplastic syndromes in urologic malignancy: the many faces of renal cell carcinoma. *Rev Urol.* 2002;4(4):163–170.

11. B. Definitive treatment of a colovesical fistula due to diverticulitis involves colon resection with primary closure of the bladder (C). Though there are some case reports of nonoperative management, particularly in high-risk patients, this is not the standard recommendation (A, D). An exception is in patients with Crohn disease. Due to the chronic relapsing nature of the disease, medical management with antibiotics, azathioprine, steroids, and/or infliximab may resolve the fistula, obviating the need for resection of part of the bladder. If the colovesical fistula were due to malignancy, then an en bloc resection would be recommended. With operative management of a colovesical fistula, an omental flap is placed between the repaired bladder and bowel to prevent overlapping suture lines and provide a well-vascularized surface for healing. Cystoscopy with fulguration and endoscopic stenting are not used in the management of colovesical fistulas (E).

Reference: Zhang W, Zhu W, Li Y, et al. The respective role of medical and surgical therapy for enterovesical fistula in Crohn's disease. *J Clin Gastroenterol.* 2014;48(8):708–711.

12. A. This patient presents with an obstructing 4-mm right UVJ stone causing acute pain. The majority are calcium-oxalate stones, which are radiopaque. Uric acid stones account for 10% of all nephroliths and are radiolucent, which is why the initial workup should include a noncontrast stone protocol CT. In the setting of an obstructing distal ureteral stone without evidence of urinary tract infection, it is reasonable to observe and medically treat the patient with tamsulosin 0.4 mg daily (relaxes ureteral smooth muscle and facilitates stone passage) and NSAIDs, assuming the patient's pain is well controlled and oral intake is adequate. Given the stone's location, there is greater than a 75% chance of spontaneously passing this stone within 3 weeks. Medical expulsive therapy is less successful for stone passage if it is larger than 7 mm or if it is in the proximal ureter. ESWL and ureteroscopy/laser lithotripsy are not initially indicated because this stone has a high chance of passing with medical management alone, but may be indicated later if his symptoms persist (C, D). If the patient meets criteria for prompt intervention, ureteral stent placement and percutaneous nephrostomy tube placement would be indicated to decompress the urinary system (B, E). This includes the following: (1) high-grade unilateral urinary obstruction, (2) bilateral urinary obstruction, (3) urinary obstruction to solitary kidney, (4) urinary obstruction with urinary infection or sepsis, (5) inability to tolerate oral intake from nausea/vomiting, and (6) severe pain not controlled by oral analgesics.

References: Coll DM, Varanelli MJ, Smith RC. Relationship of spontaneous passage of ureteral calculi to stone size and location as revealed by unenhanced helical CT. *AJR Am J Roentgenol.* 2002;178(1):101–103.

Miller OF, Kane CJ. Time to stone passage for observed ureteral calculi: a guide for patient education. *J Urol.* 1999;162(3 Part 1):688–691.

Parsons JK, Hergan LA, Sakamoto K, Lakin C. Efficacy of alpha-blockers for the treatment of ureteral stones. *J Urol.* 2007;177(3):983–987.

Preminger GM, Tiselius HG, Assimos DG, et al. 2007 guideline for the management of ureteral calculi. *J Urol.* 2007;178(6):2418–2434.

13. D. Open pelvic fractures are associated with very high impact injuries. It occurs most commonly following high-speed motorcycle accidents. They have a high rate of significant bleeding and associated injuries and can lead to life-threatening pelvic sepsis, particularly if a rectal injury goes unrecognized. Thus, in the setting of a pelvic fracture, it is essential to examine the perineum for evidence of external wounds, as well as for blood in the rectum or vagina (and never assume that vaginal bleeding is due to menses). Any external perineal wounds or rectal/vaginal blood should be presumed to be due to an open pelvic fracture until proven otherwise. Given the blood found at the vaginal introitus, this patient is at risk of having sustained injury to the urethra, vagina, bladder, or rectum. She will require an exam under anesthesia, a urethroscopy, a vaginoscopy, and a cystogram to evaluate for vaginal, urethral, or bladder trauma (B). A retrograde urethrogram is technically difficult to perform in a younger female because of a short urethra (around 4 cm); therefore, it is not used in the diagnosis of female urethral trauma (C). A suprapubic bladder catheter is not necessary without evaluation of the urethra (E). A urethral catheter should be delayed until a urethral injury is ruled out given the gross blood (A).

References: Kong JPL, Bultitude MF, Royce P, Gruen RL, Cato A, Corcoran NM. Lower urinary tract injuries following blunt trauma: a review of contemporary management. *Rev Urol.* 2011;13(3):119–130.

Morey AF, Dugi DD. Genital and lower urinary tract trauma. In: Campbell MF, Kavoussi LR, Wein AJ, eds. *Campbell-Walsh urology.* 10th ed. Elsevier Saunders;2012.

14. A. Bladder injury is usually caused by a pelvic fracture or by blunt trauma to the lower abdomen when the bladder is distended. Bladder injuries include bladder contusions (hematuria without extravasation), extraperitoneal bladder rupture, and intraperitoneal bladder rupture. Gross hematuria is the most common presenting sign of rupture and can be accompanied by concurrent pelvic fracture and suprapubic discomfort/tenderness. Bladder rupture is diagnosed with a cystogram; the bladder is filled with 300 to 400 cc of contrast

through a Foley catheter and observed for contrast extravasation. Intraoperative bladder ruptures can be similarly diagnosed by filling the bladder with colored dye (methylene blue, indigo carmine) to assess for leakage. Management of an extraperitoneal bladder rupture is managed by a 2-week course of an indwelling Foley catheter and a repeat cystogram to ensure bladder healing. Replacing the Foley catheter with a suprapubic cystostomy is invasive and unnecessary (B). However, in the setting of persistent hematuria, concomitant pelvic organ injury, bladder foreign bodies (bullets, bone fragments), persistent urine leak, or penetrating trauma, operative repair of an extraperitoneal bladder rupture is indicated. Open surgical repair is also necessary for intraperitoneal ruptures as soon as feasible to prevent peritonitis. Intraperitoneal ruptures typically occur at the bladder dome, which is lined by peritoneum. The bladder is closed in 2 to 3 layers with absorbable suture (using nonabsorbable suture for bladder wall closures results in calcification of the suture line and bladder stones) (C). Occasionally, bladder injuries are not immediately detected, and a urinoma may develop. If there is concern for infected urinoma, the patient may benefit from interventional radiology (IR) drainage, though adequate bladder drainage is usually sufficient. Cystoscopy is a diagnostic option for intraoperative bladder perforations. However, in the setting of a traumatic bladder rupture, a cystogram is the best diagnostic approach because it is quicker, less invasive, and can differentiate between intraperitoneal and extraperitoneal perforations (D). In poor operative candidates who have persistent urine leakage from the bladder despite urethral drainage, bilateral nephrostomy tubes may help divert the urine temporarily and allow a better opportunity for the bladder to heal (E).

References: Morey AF, Dugi DD. Genital and lower urinary tract trauma. In: Campbell MF, Kavoussi LR, Wein AJ, eds. *Campbell-Walsh urology.* 10th ed. Elsevier Saunders;2012.

Mundy AR, Andrich DE. Pelvic fracture-related injuries of the bladder neck and prostate: their nature, cause and management. *BJU Int.* 2010;105(9):1302–1308.

15. A. Historically, the general recommendation has been that penetrating trauma to the kidney mandates surgical exploration. However, that algorithm has recently been challenged. In select cases in which the patient is hemodynamically stable, the penetrating injury is due to a stab wound or a low-velocity gunshot wound, there are no intraabdominal injuries, and the renal injury is low grade, a nonoperative approach can be implemented (B–E). The main concern with a penetrating flank or back wound would be a missed colon injury. Renal trauma is graded according to the severity of renal parenchymal injury and disruption of the renal pelvis and renal vascularity. Grade I is a subcapsular renal hematoma or renal contusion with no renal laceration. Grade II is a parenchymal laceration less than 1 cm in depth with the hematoma contained within the Gerota fascia. Grade III is a laceration larger than 1 cm in depth into the medulla with the hematoma contained in the Gerota fascia. Grade IV is a laceration into the collecting system or the renal pelvis or a disruption of the ureteropelvic junction (seen oftentimes in children). Injury to a segmental renal artery or vein also qualifies as Grade IV. A Grade V injury is a disruption of the main renal artery or vein or a shattered kidney. If the patient is already undergoing a laparotomy for a penetrating abdominal injury and a renal injury is noted, the question arises as to whether the renal injury should be explored. Similarly, if there is no large or expanding hematoma and no active bleeding, such an injury is now increasingly being observed without exploration. Exploring such wounds requires opening the Gerota fascia and releasing its tamponade effect, which in turn may lead to bleeding and a nephrectomy (in other words, destabilizing a stable condition). As a general rule, Grades I and II rarely need operative management. Grades III and IV can be observed if no intraperitoneal injuries are noted. Delayed bleeding occurs in 20% of Grade III to IV renal injuries and can be managed with arteriographic embolization. Grade V injuries should be explored in the OR.

References: Buckley JC, McAninch JW. Revision of current American Association for the Surgery of Trauma Renal Injury grading system. *J Trauma*. 2011;70(1):35–37.

Heyns CF. Renal trauma: indications for imaging and surgical exploration. *BJU Int*. 2004;93(8):1165–1170.

Santucci R, Wessells H, Bartsch G. Evaluation and management of renal injuries: consensus statement of the renal trauma committee. *BJU Int*. 2004;93(7):937–954.

16. C. Blunt injuries to the kidney are often managed conservatively with observation alone, even in the presence of urinary extravasation on early imaging studies. Extravasation resolves spontaneously in 85% of renal injuries without further intervention. However, patients with persistent extravasation should be managed by drainage of urine with an internal ureteral stent. A Foley catheter may also be needed to maximally decompress the bladder and prevent urine from refluxing up the stented ureter to allow closure of the collecting system injury. Percutaneous nephrostomy tubes are difficult to place without hydronephrosis and provide no advantage over internal stents in the above case (D). Perinephric drainage is unnecessary without evidence of infection or large urinoma formation (E). Surgical exploration is excessively invasive and may result in more damage to the kidney (B).

Reference: Alsikafi NF, McAninch JW, Elliott SP, Garcia M. Nonoperative management outcomes of isolated urinary extravasation following renal lacerations due to external trauma. *J Urol*. 2006;176(6 Pt 1):2494–2497.

17. A. Ureteral injury and repair is an important part of general surgery training because it is a well-known complication during pelvic dissection and mobilization of the iliac arteries (ureters cross anterior to the common iliac vessel bifurcation). Ureteral repair is divided into thirds and depends on whether a large (>2 cm) or small (<2 cm) segment is missing. The upper and middle thirds of the ureter are defined as being above the pelvic brim. If a small segment is injured above the

pelvic brim, the recommended management is resection of the injured segment followed by a primary end-to-end ureteral anastomosis over a stent. For small injuries to the distal third, the recommended management is reimplantation into the bladder. For larger injuries to the upper and middle third, nephropexy (anchoring the kidney caudad) to bring the ureteral ends closer together to create a tension-free end-to-end ureteral anastomosis (ureteroureterostomy) is an option (D). For large injuries to the distal third of the ureter, reimplantation into the bladder is recommended. However, with larger distal ureteral injuries, the ureter may not reach, so the bladder will need to be mobilized. This can be performed with a psoas hitch maneuver in which the bladder is pulled up and anchored to the psoas muscle to reach the injured ureter (C). Additionally, a Boari bladder flap can be performed in which the bladder is tubularized to create additional length. In cases where the patient is unstable, the surgeon can ligate the ureter and place a percutaneous nephrostomy tube (B). The patient can be brought back at a later date for repair, which may include ileal interposition (E). Absorbable sutures should always be used to avoid stricturing and calculi formation and to prevent a nidus for infection. Most surgeons prefer to leave drains for ureteral injuries.

18. B. Blast injury can cause extensive direct and indirect soft tissue damage. The initial blast can cause immediate tissue damage, but there is oftentimes tissue injury that appears later. Victims suffer burns from the heat discharged from the explosive device or the blast. Gunshot wounds resemble such blast injuries. The degree of injury corresponds to the type of weapon, caliber of bullet, and distance from the projectile to the victim. Bullet velocity has the greatest effect on soft tissue damage. The faster the bullet, the larger the temporary cavity created, indicating a greater extent of soft tissue injury. These blast injuries tend to evolve with time and become more widespread after several days. A minor ureteral contusion is managed with ureteral stent placement to prevent ureteral narrowing from resultant scar tissue. If the ureteral damage was greater, the microvascular supply to the ureter would be compromised, leading to ureteral breakdown or stricture that would manifest days to weeks after the initial injury. This would necessitate excision of the damaged ureteral segment and either end-to-end anastomosis of the remaining ureter (ureteroureterostomy) or reimplantation of the remaining ureter into the bladder (ureteroneocystostomy) (A, D–E). Percutaneous nephrostomy is not indicated in this case because ureteral stenting is possible (C).

Reference: McAninch W, Santucci RA. Renal and ureteral trauma. In: Campbell MF, Wein AJ, Kavoussi LR, eds. *Campbell-Walsh urology*. 9th ed. Saunders Elsevier; 2007.

Gynecology 25

AMANDA C. PURDY AND TAJNOOS YAZDANY

ABSITE 99th Percentile High-Yields

1. Ectopic Pregnancy (Associated With Pelvic Inflammatory Disease)
   A. Presents with lower abdominal pain, vaginal bleeding, period of amenorrhea; only 50% have all three
   B. Vast majority located in the fallopian tube (other locations: ovary, cervix, intraabdominal)
   C. Diagnose with beta-human chorionic gonadotropin (hCG) and transvaginal ultrasound
      1. Consider if no IUP on ultrasound with beta-hCG >2000
   D. Management options:
      1. Methotrexate
         a) Indicators that methotrexate therapy will be successful: Mild symptoms, beta-hCG <5,000, absent embryonic cardiac activity, gestational sac <4cm
         b) Absolute contraindications for methotrexate use: Hemodynamic instability, ruptured ectopic (may see peritoneal free fluid), immunocompromised, breastfeeding, renal or hepatic dysfunction, pulmonary disease, peptic ulcer disease, hematologic abnormalities
         c) After methotrexate, need to follow with serial beta-hCG days 4 and 7; if it fails to decline more than 15%, then 2nd dose is given, follow hCG until normal
      2. Surgery
         a) Laparoscopic surgery usually sufficient; can perform salpingotomy in antimesosalpinx portion of tube (preferred) or salpingectomy

2. Ovarian Torsion (Most Associated With Benign Ovarian Cysts)
   A. Presents with acute lower abdominal pain (radiating to groin), nausea, vomiting; fever if ovarian ischemia develops, increase risk during pregnancy
   B. Doppler ultrasound for diagnosis: check ovarian blood flow and evaluate for ovarian cyst/mass (most are >5 cm); (normal ovarian blood flow does not rule out torsion)
   C. Management: emergent laparoscopy, most can be successfully detorsed; even if the ovary is "bluish-black" and enlarged, it is most likely due to venous congestion and not necrosis; in these cases, still perform detorsion and not oophorectomy; if large cyst, perform cystectomy; if ovary is grossly necrotic on exploration (rare) or malignancy is suspected, then perform salpingo-oophorectomy

3. Pelvic Inflammatory Disease (PID)
   A. Inflammation of the upper genital tract; usually an ascending polymicrobial infection from the vagina/cervix; chlamydia and gonorrhea are common inciting pathogens
   B. Minimum diagnostic criteria: pelvic or lower abdominal pain AND tenderness with cervical motion or over uterus or adnexa; other supporting criteria: fever >38.3°C, abnormal discharge, leukocytes on microscopy of vaginal secretions, elevated CRP and/or ESR, confirmed chlamydia and/or gonorrhea
   C. Complications of PID = infertility, tubo-ovarian abscess (TOA), ectopics, Fitz-Hugh-Curtis syndrome (RUQ pain, perihepatic inflammation with "violin string adhesions" and mild transaminitis)

D. Management of PID: if mild-moderate disease, can treat as outpatient with antibiotics (IM ceftriaxone ×1 and oral doxycycline +/− metronidazole ×14 days); if severe disease, pregnancy, or TOA, treat as inpatient with IV antibiotics

E. Management of TOA: in stable premenopausal patients, start with antibiotics (most respond to antibiotics alone); if *no improvement* on antibiotics in 48 hours, next step is image-guided drainage; if *worsening* on antibiotics, next step is surgical drainage

4. Endometrial Cancer (Most Common Gynecologic Malignancy)

   A. Risk factors: unopposed estrogen (hormone replacement, tamoxifen, obesity, polycystic ovarian syndrome), Lynch syndrome

   B. Can present with postmenopausal uterine bleeding or abnormal perimenopausal bleeding

   C. Diagnose with endometrial biopsy

   D. Staging is surgical—hysterectomy, bilateral salpingo-oophorectomy, pelvic and paraaortic lymph node dissection, and peritoneal washings; if metastasis is found, consider cytoreduction

5. Ovarian Cancer (Second Most Common Gynecologic Malignancy; Deadliest Gynecologic Malignancy)

   A. Risk factors: increased number of ovulations (early menarche, late menopause, nulliparity), diabetes, *BRCA tumor suppressor* mutation; *BRCA1* has a higher risk for ovarian cancer than *BRCA2*; smoking is NOT a risk factor

   B. Oral contraceptives are protective (may increase risk of breast cancer)

   C. Nonspecific presentation of bloating, abdominal discomfort; usually diagnosed late when disease is advanced; may have elevated CA-125; stage 1: cancer limited to one or both ovaries only (no peritoneal or diaphragmatic metastasis)

   D. Initial treatment is usually surgical; consider neoadjuvant chemotherapy in patients medically unable to undergo surgery or for very bulky disease where cytoreduction isn't possible

   E. Most common subtype is papillary serous cystadenocarcinoma, second is mucinous

   F. Staging is surgical: hysterectomy, bilateral salpingo-oophorectomy, pelvic and paraaortic lymph node dissection, peritoneal washings, omentectomy

   G. If metastasis found during staging, and it is possible to remove most of the disease (goal is <1cm of residual disease): primary cytoreductive surgery

   H. Most patients get adjuvant chemotherapy

6. Cervical Cancer

   A. Screening: Pap smears starting at age 21, screen every 3 years

   B. Risk factors: HPV (especially types 16 and 18), immunocompromised (HIV), and smoking

   C. May present with abnormal uterine bleeding or postcoital bleeding

   D. Staged CLINICALLY with physical exam (can include colposcopy, hysteroscopy, cystoscopy, proctoscopy) and plain films (chest x-ray, IV pyelogram, skeletal x-rays)

   E. Most common subtype is squamous

   F. For cervical dysplasia only or early-stage microscopic disease (patient desires fertility): consider local excision only with cold knife cone

   G. For less advanced disease (lesions <4 cm within cervix or into upper two-thirds of the vagina): radical hysterectomy (total hysterectomy + removal of parametrium and the top portion of the vagina) and pelvic lymph node dissection OR radiation

   H. For more advanced disease: cisplatin-based chemoradiation + brachytherapy

Questions

1. A 35-year-old G2P2 woman presents with significant pelvic pain and dyspareunia that has been occurring for the past few years. The pain is cyclical, mostly occurs a few days before menses, and lasts until a few days after menses. On bimanual exam, there are palpable nodules on the uterosacral ligament. Which of the following is true about her condition?
   A. Transvaginal ultrasound is the gold standard for diagnosis
   B. Diagnosis requires image-guided biopsy
   C. This condition can present with pneumothorax
   D. CA-125 is most commonly normal
   E. Medical management improves infertility

2. A 45-year-old woman with both a personal and family history of breast cancer decides to undergo *BRCA* mutation testing. Which of the following is true?
   A. Patients with either a *BRCA1* or *BRCA2* mutation should be offered prophylactic bilateral salpingo-oophorectomy (BSO)
   B. Only those with a *BRCA1* should be offered prophylactic BSO
   C. The risk of ovarian cancer is higher with *BRCA2* than *BRCA1*.
   D. *BRCA* mutations are autosomal recessive
   E. *BRCA2* is an oncogene

3. A 38-year-old G1P1 female presents with abnormal vaginal bleeding. She reports having intermittent spotting throughout the month with some pelvic discomfort. This has persisted for the past several months. She denies any recent sexual activity. Serum beta-hCG is negative. Which of the following is the most important study or procedure for this patient?
   A. CT scan of the abdomen/pelvis
   B. Magnetic resonance imaging (MRI) abdomen/pelvis
   C. Endometrial biopsy
   D. Transvaginal ultrasound
   E. Pelvic examination

4. A 42-year-old female presents to her obstetrician complaining of heavy menstrual bleeding that appears to be worsening. She is having significant abdominal cramping with her menses and is having trouble with urinary frequency and urgency. Which of the following is true regarding the most likely condition?
   A. The condition tends to improve during pregnancy
   B. MRI is most often required to confirm the diagnosis
   C. Most cases are associated with vaginal bleeding
   D. This is most likely a benign condition
   E. Uterine artery embolization is preferred in younger women

5. Which of the following is true regarding adnexal torsion?
   A. Adnexal torsion is most commonly due to an ovarian malignancy
   B. Doppler ultrasound may demonstrate vascular compromise caused by torsion
   C. CT imaging is the preferred method to confirm diagnosis
   D. If the ovary is frankly necrotic, oophorectomy with pexy of the contralateral ovary is the recommended treatment
   E. The majority will detorse on their own

6. Which of the following is true in regard to ovarian cancer?
   A. It is the most common malignant tumor in the female genital tract
   B. It is staged similarly to cervical cancer
   C. Bilateral ovary involvement is considered stage 4 disease
   D. Krukenberg tumor classically demonstrates signet ring cells
   E. Oral contraceptive pills increase the risk of ovarian cancer

7. A 23-year-old female has had two Pap smears over the last 24 months, showing atypical squamous cells of undetermined significance (ASC-US). On subsequent cervical biopsy, she is found to have mild dysplasia. Which of the following is the most appropriate treatment?
   A. Pap smear in 1 year
   B. Pap smear in 6 months
   C. Cryoablation
   D. Loop electrosurgical excision procedure (LEEP)
   E. Cold knife conization

8. A 28-year-old female would like to know if she is currently pregnant. Which of the following combinations of imaging and lab threshold is most likely to accurately demonstrate an intrauterine gestational sac the earliest?
   A. Transabdominal ultrasound with a serum beta-hCG of 3500 mIU/mL
   B. Transvaginal ultrasound with a urine beta-hCG of 1500 mIU/mL
   C. Transvaginal ultrasound with a serum beta-hCG of 2000 mIU/mL
   D. Transvaginal ultrasound with a urine beta-hCG of 2500 mIU/mL
   E. Transabdominal ultrasound with a serum beta-hCG of 5500 mIU/mL

9. A 35-year-old woman presents to the emergency department (ED) complaining of abdominal pain and irregular vaginal spotting. Her last menstruation was 8 weeks ago. On physical exam, she has tenderness in her right adnexa. Laboratory data demonstrates leukocytosis of 18,000 cells/mL and beta-hCG of 3,000 mIU/mL. She is hemodynamically stable. Which of the following is true regarding the most likely condition?
   A. This is most commonly seen in women after HPV infection
   B. Intrauterine devices (IUDs) increase one's risk of this condition
   C. Immediate laparotomy is warranted
   D. Immediate laparoscopy is warranted
   E. Methotrexate can successfully treat this condition

10. A 32-year-old female presents to the ED 1 week after vaginal delivery of her first child. She has persistent right lower quadrant abdominal pain, nausea, and leukocytosis. Pelvic examination is unremarkable. A Duplex ultrasound demonstrates a tubular hypoechoic structure that extends superiorly from the adnexa, with absence of flow on Doppler. Which of the following is true about this condition?
    A. MRI is generally not helpful in establishing the diagnosis
    B. Therapeutic anticoagulation and IV antibiotics should be started
    C. Exploratory laparotomy should be performed
    D. Diagnostic laparoscopy should be performed
    E. She likely has retained products of contraception

11. A 33-year-old female who is 18 weeks pregnant presents to the ED with hypotension, altered mental status, and tachycardia. The paramedics report that she was in a car accident earlier in the day and that they were called when she became altered. She has obvious vaginal bleeding, and the bedside nurse states that she is persistently bleeding from her peripheral IV site. Which of the following is true about this condition?
    A. Low fibrinogen levels are rare
    B. Transfusion of blood products is the cornerstone of management
    C. This condition can be excluded in cases with no vaginal bleeding
    D. Ultrasound is the best initial screening test
    E. Delivery of the fetus should be performed

Answers

1. C. This patient has endometriosis characterized by endometrial glands and stroma found outside of the uterine cavity. Patients often present with chronic cyclical pelvic pain and may report dyspareunia, dysuria, and dyschezia, depending on where the implants are located. Catamenial pneumothorax (usually on the right) occurs in temporal relation to menstruation and is caused by endometrial implants found in the visceral lung pleura or abnormal diaphragm fenestrations. A physical exam is usually normal, but sometimes there can be palpable nodules on the uterosacral ligament or rectovaginal septum. The diagnosis of endometriosis can be empirically made if symptoms are ameliorated after a short 3-month trial of Gonadotropin-releasing hormone agonist therapy; however, laparoscopy is the gold standard for

diagnosis (A, B). Endometriosis is associated with infertility due to pelvic adhesions, distorted pelvic anatomy, and bilateral tubal blockage. Medical management does not improve infertility, but surgery may improve the spontaneous pregnancy rate (E). Although not sensitive or specific, CA-125 is often elevated in patients with endometriosis (D). First-line therapy is medical management with NSAIDs and combined oral contraceptives (C). The goal of medical management is to improve symptoms. If patients fail medical management, surgery can be considered. The options for surgery include laparoscopic excision or ablation of the endometrial lesions with or without hysterectomy. The addition of a hysterectomy significantly decreases the recurrence of symptoms and the need for reoperation. However, laparoscopic excision/

ablation is still effective and should be offered to women undergoing surgery for endometriosis who want to preserve their fertility.

Reference: Shakiba K, Bena JF, McGill KM, Minger J, Falcone T. Surgical treatment of endometriosis: a 7-year follow-up on the requirement for further surgery. *Obstet Gynecol.* 2008;111(6):1285–1292. Erratum in: *Obstet Gynecol.* 2008 Sep;112(3):710.

2. A. *BRCA1* and *BRCA2* are autosomal dominant mutations in tumor suppressor genes that increase the carrier's risk of cancer, especially breast and ovarian cancers (D, E). The risk of ovarian cancer is greater in patients with a *BRCA1* mutation than in those with a *BRCA2* mutation (C). In one study, 44% of women with *BRCA1* and 17% of women with *BRCA2* developed ovarian cancer by the age of 80. Although ovarian cancer is more common in patients with *BRCA1* mutations, risk-reducing BSO should be offered to patients with both *BRCA1* and *BRCA2* mutations (B). It is recommended that patients consider prophylactic BSO when childbearing is finished, by the age of 35 to 40.

Reference: Kuchenbaecker KB, Hopper JL, Barnes DR, et al. Risks of breast, ovarian, and contralateral breast cancer for *BRCA1* and *BRCA2* mutation carriers. *JAMA.* 2017;317(23):2402–2416.

3. C. There is a large differential diagnosis in a patient with abnormal vaginal bleeding including intrauterine pregnancy, ectopic pregnancy, endometriosis, adenomyosis, fibroids, and malignancy. The American Congress of Obstetricians and Gynecologists (ACOG) recommends that all women with abnormal vaginal bleeding receive a full history and physical examination, including pelvic exam, and blood work including a pregnancy test with serum beta-hCG (initial laboratory study in the workup) (A, E). This should be followed by diagnostic imaging such as a transvaginal ultrasound (D). Additionally, all patients younger than 45 years of age with persistent abnormal uterine bleeding, or those with unopposed estrogen exposure, should undergo endometrial biopsy to rule out endometrial cancer. Additionally, all women over 45 years of age with abnormal uterine bleeding should undergo endometrial biopsy. MRI, while potentially useful to identify a mass, would not be needed during the initial examination in a patient with abnormal bleeding (B).

Reference: Sweet MG, Schmidt-Dalton TA, Weiss PM, Madsen KP. Evaluation and management of abnormal uterine bleeding in premenopausal women. *Am Fam Physician.* 2012;85(1):35–43.

4. D. Uterine fibroids, also known as uterine leiomyomas, are benign smooth muscle tumors of the uterus. These most commonly become symptomatic in patients between 40 and 50 years old, with prevalence ranging from 20% to 80%. However, most are asymptomatic; bleeding caused by leiomyomas is the most common indication for hysterectomy in the United States (C). Malignant degeneration occurs in less than 1% of cases and is usually encountered in the postmenopausal years. High levels of pregnancy hormones (estrogen and progesterone) frequently cause significant enlargement of preexisting myomas, which may lead to distortion of the uterine cavity resulting in recurrent miscarriages, intrauterine growth restriction, abruption, preterm labor, and pain from degeneration (A). Diagnosis is usually made by transvaginal ultrasound, but MRI, CT, and hysterosalpingography can also be performed and help to distinguish submucosal and intrauterine myomas (B). Conservative management includes oral contraceptive pills, medroxyprogesterone acetate, gonadotropin-releasing hormone (GnRH) agonists, uterine artery embolization, and myomectomy. Uterine artery embolization is contraindicated in patients desiring fertility (E). GnRH should be given for 3 months before surgery to reduce blood loss and assist in normalizing the hematocrit.

5. B. Adnexal torsion occurs when the ovary and/or fallopian tubes become twisted and the vascular supply becomes compromised. Adnexal torsion is generally a disease of reproductive-aged women. Torsion is commonly related to ovarian or tubal enlargement, including benign neoplasms (benign cystic teratoma, paraovarian cyst, cystadenoma, fibroma) and pregnancy-related changes (corpus luteum cyst, ovarian enlargement from ovulation induction). It is rarely related to an ovarian malignancy (A). While CT imaging can be used to assist with the diagnosis of adnexal torsion (C), ultrasound is the preferred method of imaging. In patients with signs of ovarian necrosis intraoperatively, adnexectomy is the treatment of choice (D), without intervention for the contralateral ovary. Once a diagnosis has been confirmed, the patient needs to be taken to the operating room immediately to determine viability of the adnexa (E). Laparoscopic detorsion can usually be performed in the majority of patients.

References: Chang KH, Hwang KJ, Kwon HC, et al. Conservative therapy of adnexal torsion employing color Doppler sonography. *J Am Assoc Gynecol Laparosc.* 1998;5(1):13–17.

Jung SI, Park HS, Jeon HJ, et al. CT predictors for selecting conservative surgery or adnexectomy to treat adnexal torsion. *Clin Imaging.* 2016;40(4):816–820.

Sommerville M, Grimes DA, Koonings PP, Campbell K. Ovarian neoplasms and the risk of adnexal torsion. *Am J Obstet Gynecol.* 1991;164(2):577–578.

6. D. Although ovarian cancer is considered the leading gynecologic cause of death, the most common malignant tumor in the female genital tract is endometrial cancer (A). A woman's lifetime risk of being diagnosed with ovarian cancer is 1.5%. Since most women with early-stage ovarian cancer have very few symptoms, nearly two-thirds of cases are diagnosed in the later stages. Risk factors include early menarche, nulliparity, and late menopause; all of these increase the total number of ovulations in a woman's lifetime. Oral contraceptive pills prevent ovulation and decrease the risk of ovarian cancer (E). They can increase the risk of breast cancer, which can persist for about 10 years after the cessation of oral contraceptive pills. After this time, the risk returns to baseline. Krukenberg tumor refers to an ovarian tumor that has metastasized from another site, classically the stomach. The classic pathology associated with this is a signet ring cell. Women with ovarian cancer may complain of vague abdominal pain or pressure, nausea, early satiety, constipation, abdominal swelling, loss of weight, urinary frequency, and abnormal vaginal bleeding. Transvaginal ultrasound and CA-125 should be performed during the initial workup. However, staging is completed with surgery (unlike cervical cancer) (B). This allows for the best evaluation of the extent of disease and thus determines the need for adjuvant therapy. Interestingly, bilateral ovarian involvement is still considered stage 1 disease (C). In patients with localized ovarian cancer (stage 1 and some cases of stage 2) who wish to retain fertility, a unilateral oophorectomy, peritoneal biopsies, and unilateral lymphadenectomy may be performed, with hysterectomy and contralateral oophorectomy delayed until after completion of childbearing. In all other situations, a total abdominal hysterectomy with BSO is recommended. Although few randomized clinical trials have evaluated the concept of "debulking surgery" to reduce the volume of ovarian cancer to a microscopic residual, it is generally accepted that patients with smaller volumes of tumor following staging laparotomy have an improved survival when cytoreduction is performed compared with patients in whom cytoreduction is unable to be performed. The goal of cytoreduction is to minimize the diameter of the remaining disease because survival is directly proportional to the tumor volume following cytoreduction.

References: NIH Consensus Development Panel on Ovarian Cancer. Ovarian cancer: screening, treatment, and follow-up. *JAMA.* 1995;273(6):491–497.

Ries LAG, Eisner MP, Kosary CL, et al., eds. *SEER cancer statistics review, 1975–2001.* National Cancer Institute; 2004.

7. A. The goal of screening for cervical cancer is to circumvent progression of cancer while avoiding the overtreatment of lesions that are likely to regress. This patient had a concerning pap smear result that required follow-up with colposcopy and biopsy. Prior to colposcopy, biopsy was done with a large excisional procedure, such as LEEP or cold knife conization. However, directed biopsies are now possible with colposcopy. Cervical intraepithelial neoplasia (CIN) is a premalignant condition ranging from low to high grade that can be identified on cervical biopsy and is grouped into three broad categories: CIN 1 is mild dysplasia, CIN 2 is moderate to marked dysplasia, and CIN 3 is severe dysplasia. Because cervical biopsies with colposcopy don't sample the entire cervix, invasive cancer can't be confirmed (or excluded). Thus, CIN is most useful to help identify women who would most benefit from excisional cervical biopsies to rule out cancer or can simply proceed with less invasive screening. CIN 2-3 has a much simpler algorithm for management compared to CIN 1. Since the risk of concurrent cancer and/or progression to cancer is high, treatment is recommended for all women (C–E). With the advent of colposcopy, this can be performed with ablative (cryoablation or laser ablation) or excisional methods. Ablative options are popular among reproductive-aged women as the risk of adverse outcomes such as preterm delivery and prenatal mortality is lower than with excisional techniques. The decreased risk of adverse events is possible because the depth of tissue destruction is lower when compared to excisional techniques. This explains why excision offers a more accurate sample and is preferred in older women or younger women who are not concerned with future fertility. The management of CIN 1, or mild dysplasia, depends on the age of the patient. Women aged 21 to 24 are at a very low risk for cervical cancer, so these women can be managed conservatively with a repeat pap smear in 1 year (not 6 months) (B). If the Pap smear is concerning at that time, repeat colposcopy and biopsy should be performed. For women older than 25 with CIN 1, the management is tailored based on current HPV status, results of any previous Pap smears, and patient preference, but most would agree

that repeat pap smear in 1 year along with HPV testing is appropriate.

References: Khan MJ, Smith-McCune KK. Treatment of cervical precancers: back to basics. *Obstet Gynecol.* 2014;123(6):1339–1343.

Massad LS, Einstein MH, Huh WK, et al. 2012 updated consensus guidelines for the management of abnormal cervical cancer screening tests and cancer precursors. *Obstet Gynecol.* 2013;121(4):829–846.

8. B. Either transvaginal or transabdominal ultrasound can be used concurrently with serum or urine beta-hCG level to identify and estimate the gestational age of an intrauterine pregnancy. Transvaginal ultrasound is a more accurate way of determining gestational age at a significantly earlier point in the pregnancy. With the advent of quantitative urine tests, the accuracy and sensitivity of detecting pregnancy is comparable to serum beta-hCG. The earliest an intrauterine gestational sac can be visualized is with a transvaginal ultrasound in a patient with a urine or serum beta-hCG greater than 1500 mIU/mL (A, C–E). In fact, nonvisualization of an intrauterine sac on transvaginal ultrasound in a patient with a urine or serum beta-hCG of more than 1500 mIU/mL is concerning for an ectopic pregnancy. The intrauterine sac is visible on trans-abdominal ultrasound when the urine or serum beta-hCG is greater than 6000 mIU/ml.

Reference: Grossman D, Berdichevsky K, Larrea F, Beltran J. Accuracy of a semi-quantitative urine pregnancy test compared to serum beta-hCG measurement: a possible screening tool for ongoing pregnancy after medication abortion. *Contraception.* 2007;76(2):101–104.

9. E. A common and potentially life-threatening cause of abdominal pain in women is ectopic pregnancy. An ectopic pregnancy is defined as gestation in which implantation has taken place in a site other than the endometrium; 97% of cases occur in the fallopian tubes. In a patient who is hemodynamically stable and is interested in reproduction later in life, methotrexate can be given in a single dose with a median success rate of 84%. Methotrexate has a higher rate of failure if the beta-hCG level is greater than 5000 mIU/mL, if the intrauterine gestational sac is greater than 4 cm with no fetal cardiac activity, or if the intrauterine gestational sac is greater than 3.5 cm with fetal cardiac activity. Ectopic pregnancies are often seen in patients with pelvic inflammatory disease (PID). Women with HPV are not at risk for PID (A). Even though patients with IUDs have a 5% risk of ectopic pregnancy, the overall risk is still lower than those who do not use contraception (B). Based on multiple studies, the data have consistently shown laparoscopic surgery to be safer than open laparotomy (D). However, laparotomy should be performed in patients with an acute abdomen that are hemodynamically unstable (C). These patients have shorter hospital stays, less blood loss, and less use of postoperative narcotics. Finally, patients that are Rh-negative will need to receive an anti-D globulin injection within 72 hours of medical or surgical intervention.

References: Hajenius PJ, Engelsbel S, Mol BW, et al. Randomised trial of systemic methotrexate versus laparoscopic salpingostomy in tubal pregnancy. *Lancet.* 1997;350(9080):774–779.

Murphy AA, Nager CW, Wujek JJ, Kettel LM, Torp VA, Chin HG. Operative laparoscopy versus laparotomy for the management of ectopic pregnancy: a prospective trial. *Fertil Steril.* 1992;57(6):1180–1185.

10. B. This patient has ovarian vein thrombophlebitis (OVT). Patients with OVT usually present with fever and abdominal pain within 1 week after delivery or surgery. The majority (80%) occur on the right side. Some patients may also have nausea and/or ileus. Postpartum pelvic thrombophlebitis is often preceded by Virchow triad involving (1) endothelial damage with delivery, (2) venous stasis as a result of pregnancy-induced ovarian venous dilatation and low postpartum ovarian venous pressures, and (3) the hypercoagulable state of pregnancy. The diagnosis is often challenging and a diagnosis of exclusion, but one clinical clue is often persistent fever despite broad-spectrum IV antibiotics. There is no single imaging modality that has proven to be most effective in assisting with a diagnosis. Ultrasound can be useful but may be limited by bowel gas. Both CT and MRI are useful (A). The current recommended management is antibiotic therapy in conjunction with systemic anticoagulation (C–E).

Reference: Nezhat C, Farhady P, Lemyre M. Septic pelvic thrombophlebitis following laparoscopic hysterectomy. *JSLS.* 2009;13(1):84–86.

11. E. Disseminated intravascular coagulation (DIC) is a pathologic disruption of hemostasis. Massive activation of the clotting cascade results in widespread thrombosis, which leads to the depletion of platelets and coagulation factors and excessive thrombolysis. In DIC, excessive production of thrombin leads to widespread intravascular fibrin deposition and fibrinolysis (A). This results in the depletion of coagulation factors and platelets, along with the production of fibrin degradation products, causing a profound bleeding diathesis. This can result in massive hemorrhage, thrombosis, and multiorgan failure. Since DIC is considered a consumptive process, blood transfusions are not considered the definitive management. In fact, they may worsen symptoms. The best management is to treat the underlying cause (B). DIC in pregnancy occurs in 0.03% to 0.035% of cases but does not occur in isolation; most cases are initiated by a trigger. In pregnancy, these triggers include postpartum hemorrhage, preeclampsia, HELLP syndrome (hemolysis, elevated liver enzymes, low platelet count), acute fatty liver disease, amniotic fluid embolism, sepsis, and traumatic placental abruption (as in the above patient). Although placental abruption is often accompanied by vaginal bleeding, patients with a concealed placental abruption can present with an absence of vaginal bleeding (C). Since the above patient is unstable with DIC secondary to traumatic placental abruption, the best management is delivery of the fetus. This will often resolve obstetric conditions initiating DIC. Ultrasound can be a useful adjunct in equivocal cases of placental abruption (D).

Head and Neck 26

ZACHARY N. WEITZNER AND JAMES WU

ABSITE 99th Percentile High-Yields

I. High Yield Anatomy
   A. Branches of external carotid artery: superior thyroid artery, ascending pharyngeal artery, lingual artery, facial artery, occipital artery, posterior auricular artery, maxillary artery, superficial temporal artery
   B. The external branch of the superior laryngeal nerve runs with the superior thyroid artery; supplies motor innervation to the cricothyroid muscle; if injured, pitch of voice is altered
   C. The recurrent laryngeal nerve runs with the inferior thyroid artery; supplies motor innervation to all intrinsic laryngeal muscles besides the cricothyroid and moves vocal cords into an adducted position; if unilateral injury, will have hoarseness; if bilateral injury, will have stridor and compromised airway
   D. Phrenic nerve runs on anterior surface of anterior scalene
   E. Long thoracic nerve runs along middle scalene
   F. Lymph node levels of the neck:
      1. Levels I–V: these lymph nodes are removed during a lateral neck dissection
      2. Level VI: these lymph nodes are removed during a central neck dissection
   G. Landmarks for surgical airway:
      1. Cricothyroidotomy: made in the cricothyroid membrane (inferior to the thyroid cartilage, superior to the cricoid cartilage)
      2. Tracheostomy: usually between the 2nd and 3rd tracheal rings; if lower than the 4th tracheal ring—increased risk for tracheoinnominate fistula

II. Eyes, Ears, Nose
   A. Temporal bone fractures: facial nerve can be injured proximally (leads to ipsilateral facial droop); evaluate for cerebrospinal fluid (CSF) leak and sensorineural hearing loss
   B. Rhinorrhea: evaluate for CSF leak (test for tau protein and beta-2-transferrin)
   C. Epistaxis: anterior can be packed, posterior is more likely to require intervention—embolization of internal maxillary or ethmoid artery
   D. Lacerations:
      1. Eyelid: orbicularis oculi closed in separate layer
      2. Lip: vermillion border must be approximated
      3. Auricle: hematomas drained to prevent cauliflower ear; cartilage must be covered
      4. Facial nerve: if anterior to vertical line from lateral canthus, nerve does not need to be repaired; if posterior, nerve should be repaired

III. Oropharynx
   A. Squamous cell carcinoma (SCC)
      1. Risk factors: HPV 16 and 18, Plummer-Vinson syndrome (glossitis, iron deficiency anemia, esophageal web); HPV-related head and neck masses are most commonly found in the oropharynx
   B. Benign disease (always start with airway, breathing, circulation)

1. Ludwig angina: parapharyngeal abscess or infection of floor of mouth which can lead to mediastinitis and airway compromise; treat with drainage of lateral neck
2. Peritonsillar abscess: untreated pharyngitis causing dysphagia, trismus, dysphagia, uvular deviation; treat with drainage
3. Retropharyngeal abscess: fever, odynophagia, pooling secretions; secure airway emergently then drain

IV. Nasopharynx
  A. Malignancies linked to Epstein-Barr virus (EBV), Asian ethnicities
  B. Benign disease
    1. Nasopharyngeal angiofibroma: vascular tumor causing epistaxis in young patients, treat with embolization and resection

V. Salivary Glands
  A. Major salivary glands: parotid, submandibular, sublingual
  B. Benign tumors in order of frequency: pleomorphic adenoma, monomorphic adenoma, Warthin tumor, oncocytoma
    1. Treat with excision, superficial parotidectomy with facial nerve preservation
    2. Warthin can present bilaterally; it is also known as papillary cystadenoma lymphomatosum
  C. Malignant tumors: mucoepidermoid carcinoma (most common), adenoid cystic carcinoma
    1. Treat by local excision, may need total parotidectomy if invades deep lobe
  D. Sialadenitis and parotitis: seen in elderly and dehydrated patients; due to obstruction of salivary gland; most common bacteria *Staphylococcus aureus*; treat with IVF, lozenges, massage, and antibiotics; should rule out cancer; may need to incise duct and remove stone

VI. Neck
  A. Thyroglossal duct cyst
    1. Extends from residual foramen cecum at tongue base to lower anterior neck: midline mass that rises with swallow
    2. Treatment is Sistrunk procedure (excision of the cyst, tract, and central hyoid bone) to reduce risk of infection and malignancy
  B. Branchial cleft cysts
    1. First: associated with external auditory canal and parotid
    2. Second: superior anterior border of sternocleidomastoid muscle between internal carotid artery and external carotid artery to tonsils
    3. Third: middle anterior border of sternocleidomastoid muscle posterior to common carotid artery to pyriform sinus
  C. Radical neck dissection: removal of nodes in levels I to V, sternocleidomastoid muscle, internal jugular vein, CN XI
  D. Modified radical neck dissection: removal of nodes with preservation of one or more of the sternocleidomastoid muscle, internal jugular vein, CN XI
  E. When performing a neck dissection, raise platysmal flaps more than 1.5 cm below the inferior border of the mandible to avoid injury to the marginal mandibular nerve

VII. Workup of New Neck Mass
  A. Differential: SCC, melanoma, thyroid cancer, lymphoma, brachial cleft cyst
  B. Evaluation:
    1. History, exam of skin and scalp, oral cavity, flexible laryngoscopy
    2. Neck ultrasound
    3. Fine-needle aspiration
    4. If SCC: Direct laryngoscopy under anesthesia, esophagoscopy, bronchoscopy (panendoscopy)
    5. Possible to have SCC in neck node with unknown primary, manage with modified radical neck dissection

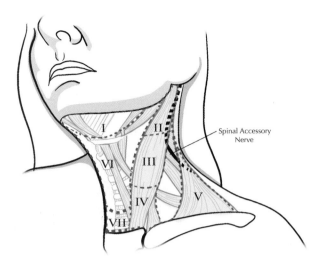

Compartment 6 is dissected for medullary thyroid caner. During a compartment V dissetion, much care must be taken to avoid injuring the spinal accessory nerve which innervates the sternocleidomastoid and trapezius muscles.

Fig. 26.1 Neck Dissection.

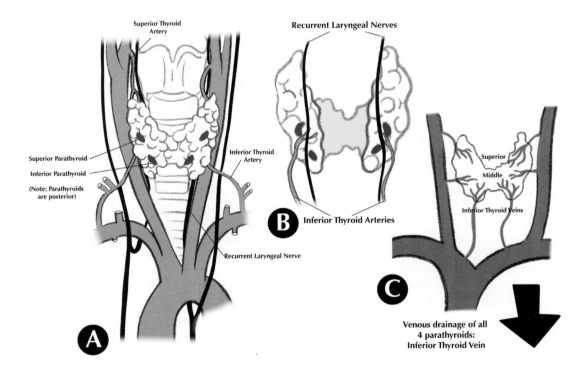

The relationships between the parathyroid glands, recurrent laryngeal nerve, and the inferior thyroid artery are illustrated in Figures A and B: The inferior thyroid artery is superior to the inferior parathyroids but inferior to the superior parathyroid glands. The recurrent laryngeal nerve is lateral and posterior to the inferior parathyroids and medial and anterior to the superior parathyroids. Figure C illustrates that all four parathyroid glands drain into the inferior thyroid vein.

Fig. 26.2 Relationship Between Neck Nerves are Vasculature.

Questions

1. A 4-year-old boy presents to clinic with progressive neck swelling over the past few weeks. He has felt otherwise well without fevers, weight loss, or decreased playfulness. A 2-cm mass is palpable beneath the angle of the mandible without fluctuance. The overlying skin is violaceous but without drainage. He has no cranial neuropathy. Fine needle aspirate demonstrates acid-fast bacteria. What is the best treatment for this condition?
   A. A 10-day course of amoxicillin
   B. Incision and drainage
   C. Lymphadenectomy
   D. Azithromycin and rifampin until symptom resolution
   E. Chemotherapy

2. Which of the following is true regarding cleft lip and cleft palate?
   A. The majority of cases of cleft lip and cleft palate are due to congenital syndromes
   B. Repair of cleft palate should be delayed until approximately 12 months of age
   C. For cleft palate, echocardiography for cardiac abnormalities is unnecessary
   D. Repair of cleft lip should be performed within a week of birth in full-term infants
   E. Tube feeding is usually necessary for cleft palate to ensure preoperative growth and development

3. A 6-year-old male with recurrent otitis media presents to the ED with fever and right-sided earache. Methylene blue confirms a sinus tract from the right submandibular area to the external auditory canal. Which of the following branchial cleft cysts does this patient most likely have?
   A. First
   B. Second
   C. Third
   D. Fourth
   E. Fifth

4. The brachial plexus is located:
   A. Posterior to the middle scalene muscle
   B. Anterior to the middle scalene muscle
   C. Anterior to the anterior scalene muscle
   D. Posterior to the posterior scalene muscle
   E. Anterior to the posterior scalene muscle

5. A 44-year-old male with recurrent melanoma of the posterior scalp and cervical adenopathy arrives at clinic to discuss the risks of cervical lymph node dissection. The nerve most likely to be injured during this procedure is the:
   A. Spinal accessory nerve
   B. Long thoracic nerve
   C. Lesser occipital nerve
   D. Transverse cervical nerve
   E. Phrenic nerve

6. Which of the following is true regarding nasopharyngeal carcinoma?
   A. It is not associated with alcohol
   B. Most patients present with cervical lymph node metastasis
   C. The standard of care involves surgical excision followed by chemoradiation
   D. Plummer-Vinson syndrome increases the risk for its development
   E. It is commonly confused with otitis externa

7. Which of the following is true regarding epistaxis?
   A. The vast majority of bleeds are from the posterior part of the nose
   B. Posterior bleeds most commonly arise from the sphenopalatine artery
   C. Anterior bleeds have a significant mortality risk
   D. Posterior bleeds are best managed by applying digital pressure to the nose
   E. Anterior bleeds often require packing combined with a Foley catheter

8. Which of the following statements is true regarding parotid gland tumors?
   A. The majority are malignant
   B. Pleomorphic adenoma (benign mixed tumor) is the most common type
   C. Pleomorphic adenomas are managed by total parotidectomy
   D. For malignant tumors resection of the facial nerve is usually required
   E. For benign tumors, the most commonly injured nerve during resection is the facial nerve

9. A 65-year-old male presents with a persistent firm lateral neck mass that measures approximately 2.5 cm. Careful history and physical examination of the head and neck are negative. The next step in the management is:
   A. Positron emission tomography
   B. Computed tomography scan of the head and neck
   C. Fine-needle aspiration of the neck mass
   D. Chest radiograph
   E. Panendoscopy (esophagoduodenoscopy, bronchoscopy, laryngoscopy)

10. A 12-week-old male infant with trisomy 21 presents with a large posterolateral neck mass extending into the axilla that transilluminates. The mass has been growing continuously for the past several weeks. Optimal management would consist of:
    A. Radiation therapy
    B. Repeat needle aspirations
    C. Radical wide excision
    D. Observation
    E. Conservative excision

11. A 54-year-old man presents with a tender left neck mass with a draining sinus. Microscopic examination reveals sulfur granules. Optimal management would be:
    A. Penicillin
    B. Radical excision
    C. Penicillin and surgical drainage
    D. Trimethoprim-sulfamethoxazole
    E. Trimethoprim-sulfamethoxazole and surgical drainage

12. A 50-year-old male presents with a right-sided slow-growing rounded neck mass located anterior to the sternocleidomastoid. The mass appears to move side to side only. CT of the neck is performed and demonstrates widening of the carotid bifurcation by a well-defined tumor blush. The mass is 3 cm. Optimal management consists of:
    A. Radiographic embolization
    B. Radiation therapy
    C. Chemotherapy
    D. Surgical excision
    E. Radiographic embolization followed by surgical excision

13. A 2-year-old male presents with a well-defined anterior neck mass, located midline and above the cricoid cartilage. The mother reports no other medical history. It elevates when he swallows and is nontender. He has no cervical adenopathy. Which of the following is recommended before considering surgical excision?
    A. Computed tomography (CT) scan of the neck
    B. Thyroid scintigraphy
    C. Fine-needle biopsy
    D. Magnetic resonance imaging (MRI) of the neck
    E. Ultrasound

14. A 45-year-old male with squamous cell carcinoma at the floor of the mouth is recovering from a resection, a mandibular flap reconstruction, and a tracheostomy performed at the third tracheal ring. Several hours later, the surgical resident gets called to the postoperative recovery suite because the patient develops some bleeding at the tracheostomy site. Which of the following is true?
    A. Making the tracheostomy at the second tracheal ring could have prevented this complication
    B. He should be taken to the operating room (OR) to undergo a median sternotomy
    C. He likely has a traumatic injury of the anterior jugular vein
    D. Immediate bronchoscopy should be performed
    E. Overinflating the tracheostomy cuff should be avoided

15. A 15-year-old male arrives at the emergency department (ED) with recurrent right-sided epistaxis and nasal obstruction. Vital signs are normal. Nasal endoscopy reveals a flesh-appearing mass in the right nares. His hemoglobin is 12 g/dL. MRI demonstrates a mass in the pterygopalatine fossa with anterior bowing of the posterior maxillary wall. Treatment consists of:
    A. Placing nasal packing and discharging home
    B. Intraoperative biopsy of mass
    C. Administering flutamide
    D. Radiation therapy
    E. Endoscopic surgical excision of the mass

16. The most common cause of hearing loss in an adult is:
    A. Acute otitis media
    B. Chronic otitis media
    C. Otosclerosis
    D. Cerumen
    E. Presbycusis

17. An elderly patient being treated with chemotherapy for metastatic colon cancer presents with swelling of the cheek and pain. WBC is normal and patient is afebrile. Initial treatment for this condition consists of:
    A. Bedside incision and drainage
    B. Parotid massage, lozenges, and hydration
    C. Superficial parotidectomy
    D. IV antibiotics
    E. Endoscopic duct exploration

18. The most likely site of origin for a metachronous cancer in a patient with a history of laryngeal cancer is the:
    A. Esophagus
    B. Lung
    C. Floor of mouth
    D. Tongue
    E. Hypopharynx

19. Which of the following is true regarding carcinoma of the lip?
    A. Upper lip carcinoma is more common
    B. The majority present with nodal metastasis
    C. Squamous cell carcinoma is the most common type of cancer in the lower lip
    D. Radiation therapy is the treatment of choice for most lip cancers
    E. Prophylactic neck dissection is usually indicated

20. Which of the following is true regarding salivary gland tumors?
    A. Parotid tumors are more likely to be malignant than submandibular gland tumors
    B. Submandibular gland tumors are more likely to be malignant than minor salivary gland tumors
    C. Pleomorphic adenomas may undergo malignant degeneration
    D. Warthin tumors are malignant
    E. Facial nerve palsy is common in benign tumors

Answers

1. C. This boy presents with likely nontuberculous mycobacterial lymphadenitis (scrofula), and diagnosis can be confirmed with FNA stained for acid-fast bacteria. This condition typically affects healthy children under the age of 5 years old and is most frequently due to Mycobacterium avium. Scrofula typically presents as a nonpainful mass with significant overlying skin discoloration that progresses to fistulization and sinus tracts. The treatment for uncomplicated isolated mycobacterial lymphadenitis is lymphadenectomy without antimicrobials. In the event the patient is not a candidate for lymphadenectomy, which can be due to parent preference or neurovascular involvement, a course of macrolide plus rifampin or ethambutol can be chosen (D). Unfortunately, antimicrobial therapy alone frequently leads to prolonged course of illness with increased likelihood of disfiguring complications compared to lymphadenectomy. Incision and drainage is the treatment of choice for simple abscesses, and incising mycobacterial lymphadenitis leads to fistulization (B). Antimicrobials combined with lymphadenectomy may be required in the setting of bacterial superinfection (A). Chemotherapy is reserved for the treatment of lymphoma, which typically presents as a neck mass without overlying skin changes associated with B cell symptoms such as fevers, weight loss, and fatigue (E).

2. B. Cleft lip and cleft palate are common congenital abnormalities seen in newborns. Variants include isolated cleft lip, cleft lip with cleft palate, and isolated cleft palate. Developmentally, cleft lip is the result of the failure of fusion of the lateral, median, and maxillary mesodermal processes. As such, cleft lip may present either unilaterally or bilaterally, and rarely in the midline. Cleft palate results from failure of fusion of bilateral palatal shelves and thus always occurs in the midline. The majority of cases of cleft lip and cleft palate are nonsyndromic, but many congenital syndromes may be associated with cleft lip and cleft palate, such as Treacher-Collins syndrome, DiGeorge syndrome, and Pierre Robin sequence (A). Because of this, evaluation of newborns with cleft lip and cleft palate should include assessment for concomitant cardiovascular, skeletal, and neurologic abnormalities (C). Postnatally, the management of cleft lip and cleft palate revolves around airway management and feeding optimization to ensure optimal growth and development. This can usually be accomplished with frequent oral feedings (E). Surgical repair of cleft lip may occur earlier than cleft palate, as early repair of cleft palate may result in midface hypoplasia. Cleft lip repair optimally occurs between 2 and 6 months of age, while cleft palate repair occurs between 9 and 18 months of age (D).

References: Lewis CW, Jacob LS, Lehmann CU, SECTION ON ORAL HEALTH. The primary care pediatrician and the care of children with cleft lip and/or cleft palate. *Pediatrics.* 2017;139(5):e20170628.

Cockell A, Lees M. Prenatal diagnosis and management of orofacial clefts. *Prenat Diagn.* 2000;20(2):149–51.

3. A. There are only four branchial cleft cysts (E). The above patient has a first branchial cleft cyst presenting with recurrent infection. The accompanying sinus tract typically traverses from the submandibular area to the external auditory canal, and it is a result of incomplete closure of the ectoderm during development. Definitive intervention involves a superficial parotidectomy. The most common branchial cleft cyst is a second branchial cleft cyst, which appears anterior to the sternocleidomastoid muscle and can also present with recurrent infections (B). Third branchial cleft cysts are rare but most commonly appear on the left side near the lateral neck (C). Fourth branchial cleft cysts also appear on the lateral neck and can lead to neck swelling and airway compromise (D).

References: Pincus RL. Congenital neck masses and cysts. In: Bailey BJ, ed. *Head and neck surgery—otolaryngology.* 3rd ed. Lippincott Williams and Wilkins; 2001.

Zhong Z, Zhao E, Liu Y, Liu P, Wang Q, Xiao S. Management and classification of first branchial cleft anomalies. *Lin Chuang Er Bi Yan Hou Tou Jing Wai Ke Za Zhi.* 2013;27(13):691–694.

4. B. The subclavian vein, artery, and brachial plexus are all part of the posterior neck triangle, and their relative relation to the scalene muscles is important to appreciate during neck and upper extremity dissection. Additionally, the pathway that each of these structures takes in the neck, upper thorax, and upper extremity helps in understanding the pathophysiology of thoracic outlet syndrome (TOS). The most common type of TOS is neurogenic, presenting with sensory and motor loss in the ulnar nerve distribution. The brachial plexus and subclavian artery pass posterior to the anterior scalene muscle but anterior to the middle scalene muscle (A, C–E). The subclavian vein passes anterior to the anterior scalene muscle and can develop an area of narrowing between the first rib and clavicle.

5. A. Although all the nerves listed are at risk during a cervical lymph node dissection, the most commonly injured nerve during cervical dissection is the spinal accessory nerve also known as cranial nerve eleven (CN XI) (B–E). The superficial course of this nerve at the posterior neck triangle makes it particularly susceptible to injury. It travels through the sternocleidomastoid muscle. It can lead to trapezius palsy presenting with shoulder weakness and pain. The phrenic nerve travels anterior to the anterior scalene muscle and passes posterior to the subclavian vein before entering the chest.

References: Lima LP de, Amar A, Lehn CN. Spinal accessory nerve neuropathy following neck dissection. *Braz J Otorhinolaryngol.* 2011;77(2):259–262.

Wiater JM, Bigliani LU. Spinal accessory nerve injury. *Clin Orthop Relat Res.* 1999;368(368):5–16.

6. B. Nasopharyngeal carcinoma is associated with Epstein-Barr virus. In fact, Epstein-Barr virus titers can be used to follow the response to treatment. Nasopharyngeal carcinoma is endemic in certain areas of southern China. Previously, alcohol was not thought to increase the risk for nasopharyngeal carcinoma, but a recent systemic review suggests heavy alcohol use may have a contributing role (A). Plummer-Vinson syndrome has not been shown to be associated with nasopharyngeal carcinoma (D). Nasopharyngeal carcinoma often presents with a middle ear effusion and can initially be confused with otitis media (E). The majority of patients (up to 90%) have cervical lymph node metastasis on presentation. Whites born in the United States have a lower risk of developing nasopharyngeal carcinoma, whereas whites born in China have an increased risk. Several studies have demonstrated that a combination of chemotherapy and radiation yields a higher survival rate than either modality alone.

In a randomized study, the 3-year survival rate was 46% for patients randomized to radiation therapy and 76% for the chemotherapy and radiation therapy group. Surgery is generally not indicated (C).

References: Al-Sarraf M, LeBlanc M, Giri PG, et al. Chemoradiotherapy versus radiotherapy in patients with advanced nasopharyngeal cancer: phase III randomized Intergroup study 0099. *J Clin Oncol.* 1998;16(4):1310–1317.

Chen L, Gallicchio L, Boyd-Lindsley K, et al. Alcohol consumption and the risk of nasopharyngeal carcinoma: a systematic review. *Nutr Cancer.* 2009;61(1):1–15.

Tomita N, Fuwa N, Ariji Y, Kodaira T, Mizoguchi N. Factors associated with nodal metastasis in nasopharyngeal cancer: an approach to reduce the radiation field in selected patients. *Br J Radiol.* 2011;84(999):265–270.

7. B. It is important to recognize that epistaxis has the potential to be life threatening. Epistaxis has anterior and posterior sources. Anterior epistaxis is most common (A) and is caused by trauma in most cases, which causes rupture of superficial mucosal vessels (Kiesselbach plexus). Most anterior bleeds stop with simple direct pressure (E) and are not considered to be dangerous (C). If this fails, then anterior packing is performed. Posterior bleeds are more dangerous and potentially life threatening. Bleeding is most commonly from a branch of the sphenopalatine artery, the terminal branch of the internal maxillary artery. It is associated with hypertension and atherosclerosis. Direct pressure cannot tamponade posterior bleeds. Treatment involves posterior packing (D). Posterior packing has the potential to compromise the airway and cause hypoventilation; therefore, patients need to be admitted to a monitored setting. Part of the mortality risk associated with posterior bleeds can be attributed to the patient population that is frequently affected—the elderly with significant underlying disease.

8. B. Most salivary gland tumors are in the parotid gland, and approximately 80% of parotid gland tumors are benign (A). Submandibular and sublingual gland tumors are approximately 50% malignant, and minor salivary gland tumors are predominantly malignant. The largest salivary gland is the parotid gland. The most common type of parotid gland tumor is a pleomorphic adenoma (also called a benign mixed tumor). Bilateral lesions are extremely rare (0.2% of all parotid gland tumors). The most commonly injured nerve in parotid surgery is the greater auricular nerve (E). The treatment of choice for benign parotid tumors is a superficial parotidectomy (C). For malignant tumors, every effort should be made to preserve the facial nerve if it is not invaded by the tumor (D).

Reference: Huang JT, Li W, Chen XQ, Shi RH, Zhao YF. Synchronous bilateral pleomorphic adenomas of the parotid gland: Bilateral pleomorphic adenomas. *J Investig Clin Dent.* 2012;3(3):225–227.

9. C. In adults, the most likely etiology of a persistent neck mass larger than 2 cm is cancer. Most often the cancer is from the head and neck and is squamous cell carcinoma. Careful physical examination is essential. If the physical examination is unremarkable, the next step is to establish whether the mass is malignant. This is best achieved by fine-needle aspiration. Once metastatic cancer is confirmed, panendoscopy with guided biopsies is performed in the OR under general anesthesia to locate the primary mass (E). CT scan of the head and neck and chest radiograph are also performed to assist in locating the mass (B, D). If the primary mass is still not localized, the role of positron emission tomography is debatable (A). Several studies have shown that it has a low sensitivity and does not alter outcome. If the mass is not localized after panendoscopy, an excisional biopsy should be performed. Adenocarcinoma would suggest a primary lung, breast or gastrointestinal tumor.

References: Grau C, Johansen LV, Jakobsen J, Geertsen P, Andersen E, Jensen BB. Cervical lymph node metastases from unknown primary tumours. Results from a national survey by the Danish Society for Head and Neck Oncology. *Radiother Oncol.* 2000;55(2):121–129.

Kole AC, Nieweg OE, Pruim J, et al. Detection of unknown occult primary tumors using positron emission tomography. *Cancer.* 1998;82(6):1160–1166. McGuirt WF. The neck mass. *Med Clin North Am.* 1999;83(1):219–234.

10. E. The presentation is consistent with a cystic hygroma (CH) given the age of the patient, the location of the mass, and the fact that it transilluminates. CH occurs more commonly in patients with trisomy 21 and Turner syndrome. CH is a lymphatic malformation. Most present in the posterior neck, and the next most common site is the axilla. More than half present at birth, and the remainder become apparent within the first 2 years of life as baby fat recedes. On occasion, intralesional bleeding can cause the mass to grow significantly in a short amount of time. Complete surgical excision is preferred; however, if the mass is adjacent to nerves, it is best managed with a conservative excision (C). Radiation has no role in the management of CH (A). Although repeated needle aspirations (B) may shrink the mass, it will only be a temporary intervention. Observing the mass is an appropriate consideration for patients that are asymptomatic (e.g., the mass is not growing) (D).

11. C. Actinomyces israelii and other Actinomyces species occur in the normal flora of the mouth and tonsillar crypts. They are anaerobic, gram-positive, branching filamentous bacteria. They do not stain acid-fast positive (unlike M. tuberculosis or Actinomycetes). The face and neck are the most common sites of infection and usually develop after minor trauma or tooth extraction. Actinomyces infections generally occur in association with other bacteria. The infection tends to form abscesses that later drain. Microscopic examination may reveal the classic appearance of sulfur granules, which are masses of filamentous organisms. Optimal treatment is with penicillin and surgical drainage, not antibiotics alone (A). Surgical excision can be considered for complicated cases (e.g., fibrotic lesions, extensive abscesses) (B). However, it is rarely successful without concurrent antibiotic therapy. Although Nocardia is also an anaerobic, gram-positive, branching filamentous bacteria, it is considered a weakly acid-fast organism. It is treated with trimethoprim-sulfamethoxazole (D, E).

12. D. Widening of the carotid bifurcation by a well-defined tumor blush (lyre sign) on CT is considered a pathognomonic finding for a carotid body tumor. Patients typically present in the fourth or fifth decade with a slow-growing rounded neck mass. It is usually located anterior to the sternocleidomastoid near the angle of the mandible. Carotid body tumors can only be moved from side to side, not up or down, because of their location within the carotid sheath (Fontaine sign). Treatment of carotid body tumors is surgical. One dangerous pitfall in excising these tumors is that,

in an effort to excise completely, the dissection is carried too close to the artery. Because of their vascular nature, biopsy is contraindicated. Routine preoperative embolization is not necessary but should be considered in large tumors (>4 cm) (A, E). Radiation therapy may be considered for long-term tumor control in patients that are not candidates for surgery (e.g., inaccessible site) (B). Chemotherapy has no role in the management of these tumors (C). Excising the carotid bifurcation should be avoided (E).

References: Davidovic LB, Djukic VB, Vasic DM, Sindjelic RP, Duvnjak SN. Diagnosis and treatment of carotid body paraganglioma: 21 years of experience at a clinical center of Serbia. *World J Surg Oncol.* 2005;3(1):10.

Hinerman RW, Amdur RJ, Morris CG, Kirwan J, Mendenhall WM. Definitive radiotherapy in the management of paragangliomas arising in the head and neck: a 35-year experience. *Head Neck.* 2008;30(11):1431–1438.

13. E. This patient has a thyroglossal duct cyst, a remnant of thyroid gland descent and the most common midline congenital malformation of the neck. Though present at birth, these do not often appear until age 2 as baby fat recedes. It presents as an anterior midline cystic mass that moves with swallowing or sticking out the tongue. Definitive management involves surgical intervention. The operation, known as the Sistrunk procedure, removes the cyst, tract, and central portion of the hyoid bone, as well as a portion of the tongue base up to the foramen cecum. However, given the increased association of an ectopic thyroid gland in patients with a thyroglossal duct cyst, preoperative imaging needs to be performed to confirm the correct anatomic location of the thyroid gland. This will help avoid excising an ectopic thyroid gland inadvertently during the Sistrunk procedure. Ultrasonography is the preferred option since it is noninvasive, widely available, and cost effective. Thyroid scintigraphy is equally as effective but is used less often (B). Additionally, ultrasound has several advantages over scintigraphy, including the absence of ionizing radiation, and it has the ability to characterize the thyroglossal duct cyst with high fidelity. MRI or CT scan is not required for the diagnosis and should not be performed in young patients (A, D). Fine-needle aspiration (FNA) biopsy is appropriate for a suspected thyroid nodule (C). Serial exams/observation would not be appropriate because these cysts have an increased risk of recurrent infections and malignant transformation.

14. C. Bleeding from around the tracheostomy site could have dire consequences and should be evaluated quickly. The lag time between tracheostomy creation and hemorrhage helps narrow down the possible etiology. Hemorrhage within the first 48 hours is more likely to be secondary to local trauma such as injury to the inferior thyroid artery or anterior jugular veins. Additionally, this patient has likely received heparin since he had a flap reconstruction performed. Systemic coagulopathy could also contribute to continued bleeding in the immediate postoperative period. The first line of management involves applying direct pressure, which can be performed by overinflating the tracheostomy cuff (E). If this does not control bleeding and the patient continues to have stable vital signs, a bronchoscopy can be considered (D). However, if there is any concern for massive hemorrhage or airway compromise, the patient should be immediately returned to the OR for neck exploration.

Tracheoinnominate fistula (TIF) is a rare and fatal complication that requires, at a minimum, 48 hours to develop. It often presents with a herald bleed that will progress to massive exsanguination. Performing a tracheostomy above the third tracheal ring will help decrease the risk of developing this complication (A). If TIF is suspected, placing one's finger through the tracheostomy with digital pressure applied between the TIF and the posterior surface of the sternum can control bleeding until the patient is taken to the OR to have a median sternotomy and fistula ligation performed (B).

References: Grant CA, Dempsey G, Harrison J, Jones T. Tracheo-innominate artery fistula after percutaneous tracheostomy: three case reports and a clinical review. *Br J Anaesth.* 2006;96(1):127–131.

Muhammad JK, Major E, Wood A, Patton DW. Percutaneous dilatational tracheostomy: haemorrhagic complications and the vascular anatomy of the anterior neck. A review based on 497 cases. *Int J Oral Maxillofac Surg.* 2000;29(3):217–222.

15. E. A young adolescent male presenting with severe unilateral epistaxis and a flesh-appearing nasal mass has juvenile nasal angiofibroma until proven otherwise. This is a highly vascular benign neoplasm arising from around the pterygopalatine fossa. Patients may report history of recurrent epistaxis, nasal obstruction, and/or discharge. If there is any concern about airway compromise due to massive bleeding, the patient should be intubated. If the patient has symptomatic blood loss, he should be transfused with blood products. The next step is to confirm the diagnosis with MRI or CT scan and look for extension of the fibroma into the sinuses. Biopsy of the mass is avoided because it can lead to life-threatening hemorrhage (B). Nasal packing should be used initially to help stop bleeding. However, the patient should be admitted and observed (A). Additionally, nasal packing for a prolonged period of time can lead to toxic shock syndrome secondary to Staphylococcus aureus, and as such, a patient discharged with nasal packing that is to remain in place for a prolonged period of time should also be given oral antibiotics. The testosterone receptor blocker flutamide has been reported to shrink small tumors but is not the standard recommendation (C). If bleeding continues, the patient will need to be taken to the angiography suite for embolization of the internal maxillary artery. The definitive intervention is surgical excision, which can now be performed with a transnasal endoscopic approach (E). Coagulation studies would be indicated. Radiation therapy used to be a treatment option, but it is no longer performed, particularly in adolescents (D).

References: English GM, Hemenway WG, Cundy RL. Surgical treatment of invasive angiofibroma. *Arch Otolaryngol Head Neck Surg.* 1972;96(4):312–318.

Gullane PJ, Davidson J, O'Dwyer T, Forte V. Juvenile angiofibroma: a review of the literature and a case series report. *Laryngoscope.* 1992;102(8):928–933.

Nicolai P, Schreiber A, Bolzoni Villaret A. Juvenile angiofibroma: evolution of management. *Int J Pediatr.* 2012;2012:412545.

16. D. Hearing loss can be divided into two categories including conductive and sensorineural loss. Conductive hearing loss occurs more commonly with cerumen (earwax) being the major contributor. Otosclerosis can also lead to conductive hearing loss (C). The majority of patients are asymptomatic, and contrary to popular belief, cerumen should not always be removed because it serves as a protective layer for the skin of the ear canal and helps protect against infection. Patients that present with hearing loss, earache, or fullness should have cerumen removed. Otitis media is more likely to result in hearing loss in children (A, B). Presbycusis is a sensorineural hearing loss and affects older patients (E).

References: Isaacson JE, Vora NM. Differential diagnosis and treatment of hearing loss. *Am Fam Physician.* 2003;68(6):1125–1132.

Roland PS, Smith TL, Schwartz SR, et al. Clinical practice guideline: cerumen impaction. *Otolaryngol Head Neck Surg.* 2008;139(3 Suppl 2):S1–S21.

17. B. This patient presents with uncomplicated parotitis. Initial treatment consists of parotid massage, sialagogues, and IV hydration (B). Parotitis is frequently seen in elderly patients with poor oral intake and dehydration. Occlusion of Stensen duct by a stone can lead to bacterial infection, most frequently with *S. aureus*. However, with normal vital signs and white blood cell levels, it is unlikely this patient has suppurative parotitis at this time. Initial treatment for suppurative parotitis is IV antibiotics (D), and if treatment fails or patient demonstrates signs of sepsis, incision and drainage, endoscopic duct exploration, or even parotidectomy may be required (A, C, E). The most common gland to develop sialolithiasis is the submandibular gland (produces over 90% of stones).

Reference: Pfaff J, Moore GP. Otolaryngology. In: Marx JA, Rosen P, eds. *Rosen's emergency medicine: concepts and clinical practice.* Vol. II, 5th ed. Mosby; 2002:55–88.

18. B. Patients with head and neck cancers have an approximately 14% risk of developing a second primary tumor. Most of these are metachronous (beyond 6 months). For laryngeal cancer patients, the most common metachronous malignancy is lung cancer (C–E). For patients with oral cavity and pharyngeal cancers, the most common metachronous cancer is esophageal (A).

19. C. Ninety percent to 95% of lip cancers occur in the lower lip (A). Sun exposure and tobacco use are the most important risk factors. Lip cancers occur most often in elderly white men. They are most often due to squamous cell carcinoma. Upper lip cancers are usually basal cell carcinomas. The most common presentation is an ulcerative lesion on the vermilion or skin surface (B). Early-stage lesions can be treated with surgery or radiation therapy, but surgical resection is preferred and is the treatment of choice for larger lesions (D, E).

20. C. Salivary gland neoplasms are rare. Most arise in the parotid gland. The ratio of malignant to benign tumors varies by site. Parotid gland tumors are 80% benign and 20% malignant, submandibular gland and sublingual gland tumors are 50% benign and 50% malignant, and minor salivary gland tumors are 25% benign and 75% malignant (A, B). Warthin tumor is the second most common benign salivary tumor and is strongly related to smoking (D). Facial nerve involvement is highly suggestive of a malignant tumor (E). Although benign, pleomorphic adenomas have a known risk of malignant transformation that becomes as high as 10% to 25% when present beyond 15 years. Fine-needle aspiration is useful in the diagnosis.

Nervous System

27

ERIC O. YEATES AND RICHARD EVERSON

ABSITE 99th Percentile High-Yields

I. Traumatic Brain Injury (TBI)
   A. Glasgow Coma Scale (GCS): useful for classifying injury severity and prognostication
      1. GCS ≤ 8 is severe TBI (consider intubation), GCS 9 to 12 is moderate TBI, GCS ≥ 13 is mild TBI
   B. Treatment goals (prevent secondary insults to the brain)
      1. ICP goal < 20 mmHg; CPP = MAP-ICP, CPP goal ≥ 60 mmHg (adults), CPP goal ≥ 40 mmHg (pediatrics); consider pressors after appropriate volume resuscitation to achieve CPP goal
      2. Temperature 36.0 to 37.0°C
      3. PaO_2 80 to 120 mmHg, $PaCO_2$ 35 to 40 mmHg
      4. Sodium 145 to 155, hemoglobin > 7, platelets ≥ 75, INR ≤ 1.4, glucose 80 to 180
   C. ICP monitoring
      1. Indications: GCS < 8 with structural damage on CT, GCS < 8 with normal CT and 2 of the following: age > 40-years, systolic blood pressure < 90 mmHg, abnormal motor posturing
      2. External ventricular drain (EVD) is preferred as it is diagnostic and therapeutic
   D. Approach to management of elevated ICP
      1. In order of intervention to be attempted: head of bed to 30 degrees, sedation, hypertonic saline or mannitol (contraindicated if systemic hypotension), short-term mild hyperventilation ($PaCO_2$ 30–35 mmHg), ventricular drainage, barbiturates, paralysis, and decompressive craniectomy
      2. Hypertonic saline and/or mannitol should both be given as boluses and not continuous infusions as they will equilibrate and thus become ineffective; the goal of these interventions is to create an *acute* osmotic disequilibrium, which can only be achieved with a bolus
   E. Nutrition: start enteric feeding within 24 to 48 hours, postpyloric preferred
   F. Venous thromboembolism (VTE) prophylaxis: very high risk of VTE in TBI
      1. Brain Trauma Foundation guidelines (2016) leave the timing and choice of agent to the clinician's judgment; however, most start low-molecular weight heparin (LMWH) 48 hours after the last stable CT
   G. Anticoagulation reversal agents

Drug	Reversal	Half-life (hrs)
Warfarin	Prothrombin complex concentrate (preferred), vitamin-K	20–60
Dabigatran	Idarucizumab	10–20
Edoxaban	Andexanet alpfa	10–15
Rivaroxaban	Andexanet alpfa	5–10
Apixaban	Andexanet alpfa	10–12

II. Spinal Cord Injuries

Syndrome	Epidemiology	Affected spinal tracts	Clinical presentation	Prognosis
Central cord	Most common incomplete spinal cord injury syndrome, commonly in elderly with cervical spondylosis and spinal stenosis, hyperextension injury	Bilateral central corticospinal and lateral spinothalamic tracts	Motor deficits in upper extremities more than lower extremities	Good prognosis although full functional recovery is rare
Anterior cord	Infarction of anterior spinal artery or trauma (e.g., penetrating trauma, burst fracture of vertebra, flexion injury)	Corticospinal and spinothalamic tracts	Motor loss, pain, and temperature loss (proprioception and vibratory sense preserved)	Worst prognosis of incomplete syndrome; low chance (10%–20%) of motor recovery
Posterior cord	Very rare, caused by infarction of posterior spinal artery, trauma (e.g., penetrating trauma), multiple sclerosis	Posterior columns	Loss of proprioception, light touch, vibratory sense (motor, pain, and temperature sensation preserved)	Recovery variable and related to completeness of lesion
Brown-Séquard	Most commonly due to penetrating injury	Hemisection of the cord	Ipsilateral motor and proprioception loss, contralateral pain and temperature loss	Best prognosis for functional motor activity recovery (99% ambulate)

Questions

1. Which of the following is true regarding the management of severe traumatic brain injury (TBI) in adults?
   A. A CT scan is required prior to placement of an intracranial monitoring device
   B. External ventricular drains (EVD) are preferred over intraparenchymal intracranial pressure monitors if both are available
   C. The goal cerebral perfusion pressure (CPP) is greater than 40 mmHg
   D. Decompressive craniectomy does not lower mortality in cases of refractory intracranial hypertension as compared to medical management
   E. Heparin is the preferred agent for VTE chemoprophylaxis

2. Which of the following is true regarding gunshot wounds to the head?
   A. Suicide attempts have the same mortality rate as assaults or accidents
   B. The incidence of vascular injury is low
   C. Extended antibiotic prophylaxis is recommended
   D. Bihemispheric injuries are a significant risk factor for mortality
   E. GCS on arrival is not a significant predictor of mortality

3. Which of the following is true regarding primary brain tumors?
   A. Medulloblastomas are the most common malignant tumors in adults
   B. Adults with glioblastoma have a 5-year survival rate of around 30%
   C. Corticosteroids are used for symptomatic peritumoral vasogenic edema
   D. Brain tumors in infants typically present with focal neurologic deficits
   E. In children over the age of 10, infratentorial tumors are more common than supratentorial

4. A 26-year-old intubated male is opening his eyes to voice and attempts to open his mouth. His only consistent motor movement is to occasionally withdraw from painful stimuli. What is his current GCS score?
   A. GCS 4T
   B. GCS 8T
   C. GCS 9T
   D. GCS 11T
   E. GCS 13T

5. An 88-year-old female is brought by ambulance to the ED after being struck by a vehicle while crossing the street. She is only responsive to painful stimuli and is promptly intubated for airway protection. Her secondary exam reveals only a small abrasion to the left forehead. Her systolic blood pressure suddenly increases to the 200s, and her left pupil becomes dilated and unresponsive to light. What is the next best course of action?
   A. Hypertension control with nicardipine continuous infusion
   B. Placement of intraparenchymal intracranial pressure monitor
   C. Immediate mannitol bolus
   D. Rectal lorazepam and initiation of levetiracetam
   E. Raise head of bed

6. A 17-year-old boy presents to the ED via ambulance after new-onset seizure activity that started 30 minutes ago. He is unable to provide a good history because of word finding issues but is able to convey that his head hurts. His parents state that he felt completely normal until about 4 weeks ago when he began to complain of left ear pain. Vital signs reveal a mild tachycardia and high fever. Physical exam shows absent light reflex in the left eye and papilledema. Which of the following is contraindicated in the workup and subsequent treatment of his condition?
   A. Lumbar puncture
   B. Computed tomography with intravenous contrast
   C. Stereotactic needle aspiration
   D. Surgical debridement
   E. Corticosteroids

7. Which of the following is true regarding Cushing triad?
   A. The pulse pressure narrows
   B. The heart rate increases
   C. It does not lead to changes on electrocardiogram
   D. It is associated with hypocarbia
   E. It is a late manifestation of increased intracranial pressure

8. Which of the following is true regarding ruptured intracranial aneurysms?
   A. Following repair, fluid restriction is recommended
   B. Most arise from the posterior circulation
   C. The initial study of choice is a contrast-enhanced head CT
   D. Following repair, the risk of cerebral vasospasm causing stroke persists for 3 weeks
   E. Outcomes are overall quite favorable

9. An 85-year-old female presents to the ED after falling and striking her chin on the kitchen counter. She is unable to lift her arms or hands off the bed and does not respond to painful stimuli. However, she is able to wiggle her toes and seems to feel pain at her feet. She has a history of cervical radiculopathy. A digital rectal exam reveals good sphincter tone and squeeze pressure. What is the most likely incomplete spinal cord injury that she has sustained?
   A. Posterior cord syndrome
   B. Anterior cord syndrome
   C. Cauda equina syndrome
   D. Brown-Séquard syndrome
   E. Central cord syndrome

10. Which of the following is true regarding head trauma and/or intracranial hemorrhage?
    A. The most common cause of subarachnoid hemorrhage is rupture of a berry aneurysm
    B. Epidural hematoma is typically associated with acceleration-deceleration injuries
    C. A single episode of systolic blood pressure (BP) less than 90 mmHg doubles the mortality rate in patients with head trauma
    D. Xanthochromia is virtually pathognomonic for acute subdural hemorrhage
    E. In the absence of other findings, reimaging for cerebral contusion is generally unnecessary

11. A 25-year-old male is being evaluated in the emergency department (ED) after sustaining a blow to the head with an unknown object during an assault. He has a 6 cm, stellate laceration with an underlying scalp hematoma. Computed tomography (CT) scan shows evidence of a skull fracture. In which of the following situations can this patient be managed nonoperatively?
    A. Fracture penetrates dura but not brain
    B. 0.5 cm of skull depression
    C. Involvement of the frontal sinus only
    D. Pneumocephalus
    E. Gross wound contamination

12. A 45-year-old female arrives at the ED after diving head-first into a half-empty swimming pool. She is combative and appears intoxicated. She is not able to move her lower extremities or trunk. You observe her lifting her arms and bending at the elbows but are unable to assess any movement in her hands. It has been 30 minutes since she first sustained her injury. Which of the following is true regarding this patient?
    A. The likely site of her injury is C3-C4
    B. In the absence of other injuries, methylprednisolone should be administered immediately
    C. This is a rare spinal cord injury after a diving accident
    D. Anticoagulation should be started within 2 to 3 days and continued for 2 to 3 months
    E. Mean arterial pressure should be maintained between 65 and 75 mmHg for the first 7 days

13. Neurogenic thoracic outlet syndrome most commonly affects which nerve?
    A. Radial
    B. Ulnar
    C. Median
    D. Musculocutaneous
    E. Axillary

14. A 4-day-old female infant weighing 1400 g born at 28 weeks' gestation is being monitored in the neonatal critical care unit because of multiple episodes of apnea and difficulty with feeding. Supplemental oxygen has been sufficient to maintain saturations. Over the last several hours, she has had waxing and waning alertness and decreased spontaneous eye movements. Her fontanelle appears to be full. Which of the following is the most appropriate next step?
    A. Immediate administration of furosemide and acetazolamide
    B. Bedside intracranial ultrasound
    C. Lumbar puncture
    D. Noncontrast CT of head
    E. Administer IV steroid bolus

Answers

1. B. One of the first decision points in managing a patient with severe TBI is the placement of an intracranial pressure (ICP) monitor. ICP monitors are indicated in patients with a CT scan showing intracranial hemorrhage and who have a GCS of less than 8 (or higher than 8 but with a high risk of progression). Additionally, ICP monitors are also indicated in patients with a low GCS who are having emergent extracranial surgery (A). A CT scan is not needed in this scenario. Though EVDs and intraparenchymal pressure monitors can both be used to measure ICP, EVDs are preferred as they are both diagnostic and therapeutic (B). Once an ICP monitor is placed, CPP can be calculated with CPP = mean arterial pressure (MAP)–ICP. The goal CPP is greater than 60 mmHg in adults (C). However, the goal CPP is >40 mmHg for pediatrics patients.

All efforts should be made to maintain an adequate CPP with techniques including sedation, ventricular drainage, mannitol, hypertonic saline, and paralytics. If intracranial hypertension persists despite these measures, decompressive craniectomy is often utilized, though there is still some controversy regarding its outcomes. In a randomized controlled trial in 2016, decompressive craniectomy for refractory intracranial hypertension resulted in lower mortality compared to medical treatment alone (D). Although Brain Trauma Foundation guidelines leave the choice of VTE chemoprophylaxis to the clinician's judgement, a national database study including over 10,000 patients demonstrated LMWH to be associated with reduced mortality and thromboembolic complications, regardless of timing of prophylaxis initiation in severe TBI patients (E).

References: ACS Trauma Quality Improvement Program. *Best Practices in the Management of Traumatic Brain Injury.* American College of Surgeons, Committee on Trauma; January 2015. https://www.facs.org/-/media/files/quality-programs/trauma/tqip/tbi_guidelines.ashx.

Kolias PJ, Timofeev AG, IS, et al. Trial of decompressive craniectomy for traumatic intracranial hypertension. *N Engl J Med.* 2016;375(12):1119–1130.

Benjamin E, Recinos G, Aiolfi A, Inaba K, Demetriades D. Pharmacological thromboembolic prophylaxis in traumatic brain injuries: low molecular weight heparin is superior to unfractionated heparin. *Ann Surg.* 2017;266(3):463–469.

2. D. Gunshot wounds to the head have a high morbidity and mortality. In a large meta-analysis, factors predictive of mortality included age greater than 40 years, GCS less than 9 on arrival, fixed and dilated pupils, dural penetration, bihemispheric injuries, multilobar injuries, tranventricular injuries, and suicide attempts (A, D, E). In fact, suicides had a six times higher rate of mortality compared to assaults or accidents. Another interesting finding in this study was that vascular injuries were very common (38%–50%) with intracranial aneurysm, arterial dissection, arterial occlusion, and arteriovenous fistulas being the most common types in descending order of incidence (B). There is a lack of high-quality evidence regarding the management of this type of injury. Though surgery is associated with lower mortality, it is unclear whether this is a result of surgery itself or due to patient selection. The rate of CNS infection after penetrating TBI is less than 10% and there is no reduction in the risk of infection with prophylactic antibiotics (C). However, surgical intervention and ICP monitoring appear to be risk factors for infection, regardless of prophylactic use.

References: Maragkos GA, Papavassiliou E, Stippler M, Filippidis AS. Civilian gunshot wounds to the head: prognostic factors affecting mortality: meta-analysis of 1774 patients. *J Neurotrauma.* 2018;35(22):2605–2614.

Harmon LA, Haase DJ, Kufera JA, et al. Infection after penetrating brain injury-An Eastern Association for the Surgery of Trauma multicenter study oral presentation at the 32nd annual meeting of the Eastern Association for the Surgery of Trauma, January 15–19, 2019, in Austin, Texas. *J Trauma Acute Care Surg.* 2019;87(1):61–67.

3. C. The types and presentations of brain tumors are significantly different in children and adults. In adults, the majority of tumors are benign, with meningiomas being the most common. The most common malignant tumor is glioblastoma, which carries a 5-year survival rate of 5% (A, B). The management is typically focused on maximal resection and is sometimes followed by radiation. Other considerations are seizure management and corticosteroid use for symptomatic peritumoral vasogenic edema (C). In children, brain tumors are relatively more common and are the most common cause of death among childhood cancers. In children up to 14 years old the most common brain tumor is a glioma, but pituitary tumors are the most common in children 15 years and older. The most common malignant brain tumor in children is a medulloblastoma. The location of brain tumors in children also varies by age, with children aged 4 to 10 years old being more likely to have infratentorial tumors. All other ages are more likely to have supratentorial tumors (E). Supratentorial tumors tend to present with focal neurologic deficits depending on the exact location, and infratentorial tumors tend to

have cranial nerve palsies or cerebellar dysfunction. The caveat to this rule is in infants (who will not noticeably display these deficits) who more commonly present with macrocephaly, irritability, failure to thrive, loss of developmental milestones, and vomiting (D).

References: Lapointe S, Perry A, Butowski NA. Primary brain tumours in adults. *Lancet.* 2018;392(10145):432–446.

Udaka YT, Packer RJ. Pediatric brain tumors. *Neurol Clin.* 2018;36(3):533–556.

4. B. The Glasgow Coma Scale uses the combined scores from the motor, verbal, and speech sections to give an estimate of a patient's level of functional status. The scoring is as follows. For eye opening: 4: Spontaneously, 3: To verbal command, 2: To pain, 1: No response. Best motor response scores: 6: Obeys command, 5: Localizes pain, 4: Flexion withdrawal, 3: Flexion abnormal (decorticate), 2: Extension (decerebrate), 1: No response, and for Best verbal response: 5: Oriented and converses, 4: Disoriented and converses, 3: Inappropriate words; cries, 2: Incomprehensible sounds, 1: No response. If the patient is intubated, the maximum score that he or she can get in the verbal category is 1T (the letter T indicating intubated) and maximum overall score of 11T. This patient opens his eyes to voice commands but not spontaneously, which correlates with an eye score of 3. The best calculated motor score is a 4 for withdrawing from pain. This places his total GCS at 1T (verbal) + 3 (eye opening) + 4 (motor) = 8T.

5. C. Without a CT scan, one cannot be sure of the exact etiology of these neurologic findings, but, based on the history and physical exam findings, this likely represents a closed head injury with an elevated intracranial pressure (ICP). A "blown" pupil in the setting of head trauma is consistent with uncal herniation, which is often fatal and will cause permanent neurologic deficits if not treated promptly. Systolic blood pressure greater than 180 mmHg can aggravate vasogenic brain edema and intracranial hypertension. However, systemic hypertension may be a physiologic response to reduced cerebral perfusion. Thus, early and aggressive treatment of hypertension should be avoided until ICP monitoring has been established (A). While this patient likely needs an ICP monitor, a diagnosis still needs to be made before surgical treatment or invasive monitoring (B). Additionally, an external ventricular drain is a better choice in this patient because it allows therapeutic drainage of cerebrospinal fluid. Current indications for a mannitol bolus are for situations just like the above—a quick bailout maneuver to be used as a bridge to more definitive therapies. Mannitol immediately improves cerebral perfusion due to the fact that it decreases blood viscosity and therefore increases cerebral blood flow and cerebral oxygen delivery. Its osmotic properties take 15 to 30 minutes to work. There is some evidence that prolonged or scheduled use will render it ineffective at best and potentially harmful. Immediately following mannitol, the patient needs a CT scan and should be evaluated for possible surgical drainage of an intracranial hematoma. Lorazepam and levetiracetam (Keppra) are both medications used for the treatment of seizures, which is not consistent with her exam at this time (D). Raising the head of the bed can lower ICP, but with a blown pupil, the patient needs more aggressive treatment (E).

Reference: Brain Trauma Foundation, American Association of Neurological Surgeons, Congress of Neurological Surgeons. Guidelines for the management of severe traumatic brain injury. *J Neurotrauma*. 2007;24 Suppl 1:S91–S95.

6. A. The triad of headache, focal neurologic deficits, and fevers should raise concern for brain abscess; however, this classic presentation is present in less than half of all patients. The most common presenting symptom is a headache, which is present in approximately 70% of patients. They arise primarily by two forms of spread: hematogenously from distant sites and direct spread from contiguous sites of infection (otitis media being most common). This leads to a wide array of potential pathogens, though the most common are Streptococcus spp. and Staphylococcus spp. Initial diagnosis should be obtained by CT scan with contrast, which will show a rim-enhancing collection (B). Lumbar puncture is generally not diagnostic and contraindicated in the setting of elevated ICP. Changes in cerebrospinal fluid volume in this setting can precipitate herniation. All patients should be started on broad-spectrum antibiotics, which can be tailored once cultures are obtained. Total duration of treatment is typically 4 to 6 weeks. Traditional management included surgical drainage and excision of the abscess cavity (D). However, serial needle aspiration has now become the treatment of choice unless the abscess is traumatic in origin (potentially has foreign debris), fungal, multiloculated, or does not improve with needle aspiration (C). Corticosteroids are controversial in this setting but may be considered when there is substantial mass effect from the abscess (E).

References: Brouwer MC, Coutinho JM, van de Beek D. Clinical characteristics and outcome of brain abscess: systematic review and meta-analysis. *Neurology*. 2014;82(9):806–813.

Muzumdar D, Jhawar S, Goel A. Brain abscess: an overview. *Int J Surg*. 2011;9(2):136–144.

7. E. Cushing triad is a vasomotor and respiratory response to an elevated ICP that includes bradycardia, irregular breathing, and elevation in systolic blood pressure with a widened pulse pressure (A). The increased ICP leads to impaired respiration, which worsens hypercarbia (D). Typically, Cushing triad is a late sign of elevated ICP and suggests imminent herniation. In addition to bradycardia on ECG, Mayer waves can be seen with elevated ICP (B). The waves are cyclic changes in arterial blood pressure brought about by oscillations in baroreceptor and chemoreceptor reflex control systems and are noted on ECG (C).

8. D. Intracranial aneurysms affect 4% of the population but are asymptomatic in the majority of cases, and most patients are unaware of the diagnosis. Risk factors include female gender, polycystic kidney disease, and Marfan syndrome. The majority of the aneurysms occur in the circle of Willis with the anterior communicating artery being the most frequent site (B). When the aneurysm ruptures, it can result in intraparenchymal and subarachnoid hemorrhage, which is a catastrophic event with a mortality rate up to 50% (E). Noncontrast CT head is the study of choice to confirm the diagnosis (C). Bleeding on brain parenchyma elicits a vasospasm response, which can result in stroke and patients are at increased risk for 21 days; thus, most neurosurgeons will start calcium channel blockers. Because

cerebral autoregulation is compromised, these patients should be given volume to maintain adequate cerebral perfusion pressure (A).

Reference: Keedy A. An overview of intracranial aneurysms. *McGill J Med*. 2006;9(2):141–146.

9. E. Central cord syndrome is the most common type of incomplete spinal cord injury and is primarily found in patients that suffered a hyperextension injury in the setting of previous cervical spine abnormalities. Symptoms include muscle weakness of the upper extremities with relative sparing of the lower extremities. Sensory function is variable. Posterior cord syndrome is a relatively rare entity typically caused by infarction of the posterior spinal artery. Classic presentation includes sparing of muscles with the loss of proprioception and vibration sensation below the level of the lesion with preservation of most motor function (A). Anterior cord syndrome can be caused by either infarction of the anterior spinal artery or, less frequently, by fracture or dislocation of vertebrae. It is characterized by loss of motor function, pain sensation, and temperature sensation but preservation of touch and proprioception (B). Cauda equina syndrome can be caused by trauma, mass lesions, or lumbar spinal stenosis and occurs at the level that the spinal cord has split into nerve roots. Symptoms can be variable but generally include paresthesia of the perineum, anus, and external genitalia ("saddle anesthesia"), bilateral or unilateral paralysis, and incontinence of bowel and bladder (C). Brown-Séquard syndrome is hemisection of the spinal cord from a mass lesion or more commonly trauma. It causes an ipsilateral loss of motor, proprioception, and vibration sensation with contralateral loss of pain and temperature sensation (D).

10. C. Traumatic brain injuries are among the most common presenting symptoms in emergency departments in the United States, with over 1.7 million admissions each year. The early recognition and management of brain injury is critical in this patient population because it is considered the most common cause of trauma-related death in patients reaching the hospital alive. Preventing secondary injury is an important part of management, and this involves maintaining cerebral perfusion pressure greater than 60 mmHg. One prospective trial found that a single episode of hypotension with a systolic blood pressure of less than 90 mmHg doubled mortality in patients with brain injury. Trauma is considered the most common etiology of subarachnoid hemorrhage, followed by rupture of berry aneurysms (A). In nontraumatic cases, patients may report mild "sentinel" headaches in the prior weeks leading up to a severe, unrelenting, "thunderclap" headache. Noncontrast computed tomography (CT) scan is the diagnostic tool of choice to look for hyperdensities suggestive of acute bleeding. Additionally, xanthochromia of cerebrospinal fluid is considered pathognomonic for subarachnoid hemorrhage (D). Epidural hematoma is generally the result of direct trauma to the skull causing disruption of arterial vessels, particularly the middle meningeal artery. It initially presents with unconsciousness from the concussive effects of the injury, followed by a "lucid" interval that progresses to somnolence, lethargy, and eventually a coma as the hematoma grows. Noncontrast CT scan will demonstrate a lentiform (biconvex), hyperdense clot that does not cross suture lines. Acute subdural hematoma is generally the result of acceleration-deceleration injuries that tear the bridging veins as the brain shifts in relation to the dura (B). Patients are often unconscious from the moment of impact. Noncontrast CT scan will demonstrate a hyperdense, lunar (crescent-shaped) lesion that does not cross the midline. Cerebral contusion is due to the brain directly striking the skull in either a coup or countercoup mechanism after a closed head injury. Lesions on noncontrast CT scans are typically scattered, hyperdense, and intraparenchymal, though they can also present as hypodense lesions. There is a significant propensity for these lesions to worsen, and repeat imaging is typically recommended in the first 24 hours (E).

References: Chesnut RM, Marshall LF, Klauber MR, et al. The role of secondary brain injury in determining outcome from severe head injury. *J Trauma.* 1993;34(2):216–222.

Faul M, Xu L, Wald MM, Coronado VG. *Traumatic brain injury in the United States: emergency department visits, hospitalizations and deaths 2002–2006.* Centers for Disease Control and Prevention, National Center for Injury Prevention and Control; 2010. https://www.cdc.gov/traumaticbraininjury/pdf/blue_book.pdf

11. B. Any skull fracture with an overlying laceration is considered an open fracture. Traditional teaching is that all of these patients should be taken to the operating room to prevent infection. However, there seems to be a subset of patients that can be treated expectantly without significant increases in morbidity. Nonoperative management of open skull fracture can be considered in patients without evidence of dural penetration, significant intracranial hematoma, frontal sinus involvement, wound infection, pneumocephalus, or gross wound contamination (A, C–E). Additionally, patients with less than 1 cm of skull depression can be managed nonoperatively.

Reference: Bullock MR, Chesnut R, Ghajar J, et al. Surgical management of depressed cranial fractures. *Neurosurgery.* 2006;58 (3 Suppl):S56–60.

12. D. Although it is difficult to ascertain the exact level of spine injury in a noncooperative patient, complete paralysis of the lower extremities and the trunk with preservation of her shoulders and elbows most likely indicates an injury at C5 or below (A). The most common spinal injury after a diving accident is C5 followed by C6 (C). The use of steroids in spinal cord injury has been controversial. However, recent level 1 evidence recommends against the use of steroids in the management of acute spinal cord injury (B). Among trauma victims, patients with spinal cord injury and head injury have the highest risk of venous thromboembolic events (VTEs). Without prophylaxis, the risk of VTE is about 40% after complete spinal cord injury. Mechanical prophylaxis with compression devices should be started immediately. Anticoagulation should be started within 72 hours and continued for 2 to 3 months. Low-molecular-weight heparin is preferred over heparin. Mean arterial pressure should be maintained between 85 and 90 mmHg for the first 7 days (E).

References: Bailes JE, Herman JM, Quigley MR, et al. Diving injuries of the cervical spine. *Surg Neurol.* 1990;34(3):155–158.

Theodore N, et al. Guidelines for the management of acute cervical spine and spinal cord injuries: 2013 update. *Neurosurgery.* 2013;72(2):1–259.

13. B. Neurologic symptoms occur in 95% of cases of thoracic outlet syndrome. The lower 2 nerve roots of the brachial plexus, C8 and T1, are most commonly (90%) involved, producing pain and paresthesias in the ulnar nerve distribution (A, C–E). The second most common anatomic pattern involves the upper three nerve roots of the brachial plexus, C5, C6, and C7, with symptoms referred to the neck, ear, upper chest, upper back, and outer arm in the radial nerve distribution.

14. B. Intraventricular hemorrhage (IVH) occurs in approximately 15% to 20% of infants born with a birth weight of less than 1500 g. Because of the frequency of this condition, serial ultrasound screening is recommended for all premature infants and any infants that show signs of IVH. In premature infants, the relative fragility of the germinal matrix makes them sensitive to changes in cerebral blood flow with subsequent hemorrhage into the ventricles. Predisposing factors in addition to prematurity include maternal chorioamnionitis or preeclampsia, and neonatal respiratory distress, hypotension, or anemia. While 25% to 50% of infants can have clinically silent IVH, symptoms range from nonspecific changes in alertness to stupor or coma. Once it has been diagnosed, management is largely supportive to prevent long-term complications such as posthemorrhagic hydrocephalus (PHH). Prior to the advent of intracranial ultrasound, CT scan was utilized to make the diagnosis, but has now been largely abandoned (D). Once the diagnosis is established, treatment is supportive, including correction of anemia (patients can suffer major bleeding), hypotension, acidosis, and ventilatory support. Treatments to try to prevent hydrocephalus have been largely ineffective. Though furosemide and acetazolamide have been used in older children with PHH, they do not seem to alter the course in premature infants and could potentially be deleterious (A). Serial lumbar puncture has been tried with no significant change in deterioration or progression to permanent ventricular drainage procedures (C, E). Temporary ventricular drainage with transition to permanent drainage procedures if necessary is currently the treatment of choice for PHH with elevated intracranial pressures. Ultimately, if significant hydrocephalus persists, the infant may need a ventriculoperitoneal shunt.

References: Mazzola CA, Choudhri AF, Auguste KI, et al. Pediatric hydrocephalus: systematic literature review and evidence-based guidelines. Part 2: management of posthemorrhagic hydrocephalus in premature infants. *J Neurosurg Pediatr.* 2014;14 Suppl 1:8–23.

Robinson S. Neonatal posthemorrhagic hydrocephalus from prematurity: pathophysiology and current treatment concepts: a review. *J Neurosurg Pediatr.* 2012;9(3):242–258.

Anesthesia

28

ERIC O. YEATES AND CATHERINE M. KUZA

ABSITE 99th Percentile High-Yields

I. American Society of Anesthesiologists Physical Status (ASA PS)

ASA PS	Definition	Examples
I	Normal healthy patient	Young with no comorbidities
II	Mild systemic disease	Well-controlled hypertension, current smoker
III	Severe systemic disease	Poorly controlled hypertension, morbid obesity, stable angina, prior myocardial infarction, controlled congestive heart failure with no symptoms, end-stage renal disease on scheduled dialysis
IV	Severe systemic disease that is a constant threat to life	Unstable angina, congestive heart failure with symptoms, sepsis, end-stage renal disease not on scheduled dialysis
V	Moribund patient not expected to survive without the operation	Ischemic bowel, intracranial hemorrhage with midline shift, ruptured abdominal aortic aneurysm
VI	Brain-dead patient undergoing organ donation	Traumatic brain-injured patient with no brain stem reflexes

II. Opioid Equivalents

Opioid	Oral	Parenteral
Morphine	30 mg	10 mg
Hydromorphone	7.5 mg	1.5 mg
Hydrocodone	30 mg	N/A
Fentanyl	N/A	0.1 mg
Codeine	200 mg	N/A
Oxycodone	20 mg	N/A
Tramadol	120 mg	N/A

III. Local Anesthetic Maximum Dose

Medication	Without epinephrine	With epinephrine
Lidocaine	5 mg/kg	7 mg/kg
Bupivacaine/Ropivacaine	2.5 mg/kg	3 mg/kg

0.5% = 5 mg/ml, 1% = 10 mg/ml, 2% = 20 mg/mg

IV. Common Intravenous Induction Agents

Medication	Mechanism of action	Side effects
Propofol	GABA agonist	Hypotension, propofol infusion syndrome
Etomidate	Mechanism unclear, modulates or activates GABA	Adrenal suppression, myoclonus
Ketamine	NMDA receptor antagonist	Emergence delirium, hypertension, arrhythmias, increased intracranial pressure
Midazolam	GABA agonist	Nausea, vomiting, delirium

V. Neuromuscular Blocking Drugs for Rapid Sequence Intubation

Medication	Mechanism of action	Onset (min)	Histamine release	Metabolism	Side effects	Reversal agent
Succinylcholine	Depolarizing	1–1.5	Yes	Plasma cholinesterase	Hyperkalemia, malignant hyperthermia, bradycardia	N/A
Rocuronium	Nondepolarizing	1.5–3	Yes	Hepatic, metabolites excreted renally	Allergy	Sugammadex
Vecuronium	Nondepolarizing	3–4	No	Hepatic	Allergy	Sugammadex
Cisatracurium/ atracurium	Nondepolarizing	5–7	No	Hofmann elimination	Bronchospasm	Neostigmine

VI. Steroid Potency: hydrocortisone < prednisone < methylprednisolone < dexamethasone

VII. Malignant Hyperthermia: rare, severe reaction to medications used during general anesthesia
   A. Genetics: rare, autosomal dominant disorder caused by a mutation in the ryanodine receptor, located on the sarcoplasmic reticulum (in skeletal muscle)
   B. Triggering medications: volatile anesthetics (halothane, sevoflurane, desflurane, isoflurane, enflurane) or depolarizing muscle relaxants (succinylcholine, decamethonium)
   C. Signs/symptoms: can occur immediately and as late as 24 hours postoperatively
      1. Hyperthermia, tachycardia, increased end-tidal CO_2, muscle rigidity, rhabdomyolysis, lactic acidosis
   D. Diagnosis: acutely, the diagnosis is clinical
      1. Confirmatory testing or testing of close relatives who have suffered from malignant hyperthermia; this includes a skeletal muscle biopsy followed by a caffeine-halothane contracture test (CHCT); the muscle is exposed to halothane and caffeine with a positive test causing significant muscle contraction; testing must take place in centers specialized in diagnosing malignant hyperthermia
   E. Treatment: stop all anesthetics, administer 2.5 mg/kg of IV dantrolene which inhibits calcium ion release from the sarcoplasmic reticulum (can administer additional 1–2.5 mg/kg boluses, max cumulative dose of 10 mg/kg), cooling, correction of hyperkalemia, and fluid resuscitation.
   F. Outcomes: mortality approximately 5%

VIII. Propofol Infusion Syndrome: rare syndrome triggered by high dose (>4 mg/kg/hr) infusion >48 hours
  A. Mechanism: unknown, but possibly due to the impairment of fatty acid metabolism
  B. Risk factors: children, concomitant catecholamine or steroid infusion, severe critical illness
  C. Signs/symptoms: metabolic acidosis, arrhythmias (most often bradycardia), rhabdomyolysis, hyperlipidemia, hepatomegaly (not splenomegaly), renal failure, cardiovascular collapse
  D. Treatment: immediate cessation of propofol, early hemodialysis, supportive care
  E. Screening tool: daily CPK and lactate levels

IX. Differential Diagnosis of Intraoperative Changes in End-Tidal CO_2

Rising end-tidal CO_2	Dropping end-tidal CO_2
Hypoventilation	Hyperventilation
Rebreathing	Circuit disconnected
Malignant hyperthermia	Inadvertent extubation
Sepsis	Endotracheal tube obstruction
Hyperthyroidism (thyroid storm)	Hypothermia
Pheochromocytoma	Pulmonary embolism
Rhabdomyolysis	Cardiac arrest
	Reduced cardiac output
	Tension pneumothorax

QUESTIONS

1. A 35-year-old man involved in a motorcycle cycle collision sustains a large laceration to his right thigh. The decision is made to washout and close the wound at bedside with the assistance of procedural sedation. The patient has an oral airway in place, is breathing spontaneously, and is maintaining adequate oxygen saturation with a simple face mask. With painful stimulation, he awakens briefly and is able to follow simple commands. What level of sedation is this patient currently under?
   A. Minimal sedation
   B. Moderate sedation
   C. Conscious sedation
   D. Deep sedation
   E. General anesthesia

2. Which of the following is associated with opioid tolerance?
   A. Characterized by pronounced cravings and compulsive drug taking
   B. Decreased analgesic effect of opioids develops before decreased effects on respiratory depression
   C. Increased sleeping and eating, depression, and pupillary constriction
   D. Constipation resolves over time with long-term opioid use
   E. Genetic components associated with opioid use have not been identified

3. A 68-year-old woman is undergoing a laparoscopic liver resection. An arterial line and central line are placed prior to surgical incision. As the hepatic parenchyma is being divided, the anesthesiologist reports sudden hypotension and a drop in end-tidal CO_2. There is no break in the ventilatory circuit. There is only minimal bleeding at this time. There are ST changes noted on the EKG. Which if the following is the next best step in management of this condition?
   A. Transthoracic echocardiography (TTE) examination of the heart
   B. Administer epinephrine
   C. Administer fluid bolus
   D. Emergently place a pulmonary artery catheter line
   E. Release (desufflate) pneumoperitoneum

4. Which of the following is most likely associated with opioid abuse and postsurgical prescribing patterns?
   A. The majority of opioids abused in the US originate from international drug cartels
   B. Heroin users rarely report previously abusing prescription opioids
   C. 30 pills of 5 mg oxycodone are the recommended amount to be prescribed after laparoscopic cholecystectomy
   D. New persistent opioid use after surgery is more common after major procedures compared to minor procedures
   E. Preoperative tobacco use is a significant risk factor for new persistent opioid use after surgery

5. A 75-year-old woman is brought to the operating room for laparoscopic cholecystectomy. She has a history of progressive dementia and is unable to provide a medical history. Fifteen minutes into the operation performed under general anesthesia, the anesthesiologist reports difficulty ventilating the patient, and she develops a diffuse maculopapular rash with urticaria. Which of the following is the most likely offending agent?
   A. Rocuronium
   B. Latex
   C. Cefazolin
   D. Sevoflurane
   E. Propofol

6. A 29-year-old man undergoes a laparoscopic cholecystectomy for symptomatic cholelithiasis. Shortly after induction, the anesthesiologist notes an increase in core body temperature and end-tidal CO2. After administration of dantrolene and aborting the operation, his status improves. Which of the following is most likely associated with this diagnosis?
   A. It is an autosomal recessive disorder
   B. Genetic analysis is required for diagnostic confirmation
   C. It is more common in elderly patients
   D. It may present as late as 24 hours after anesthesia
   E. Mortality rate is less than 1%

7. After excision of multiple subcutaneous lipomas under local anesthesia, a 42-year-old woman seizes violently. What is the maximum safe dose of a local anesthetic agent in a 70-kg woman?
   A. 10 to 20 mL 1% lidocaine
   B. 40 to 50 mL 2% lidocaine with epinephrine
   C. 40 to 50 mL 1% lidocaine with epinephrine
   D. 40 to 50 mL 0.5% lidocaine
   E. 40 to 50 mL 1% lidocaine without epinephrine

8. A 20-year-old man is about to undergo arthroscopic surgery on his left shoulder. During anesthetic induction with succinylcholine, the anesthesiologist noted trismus that persisted for >2 minutes, and the mouth could not be opened to perform direct laryngoscopy or place an endotracheal tube. The anesthesiologist was able to bag mask ventilate the patient. The end-tidal CO_2, heart rate, and temperature remained normal. Which of the following is the next best step in management?
   A. Administer an additional dose of succinylcholine
   B. Proceed with surgery if the patient can be intubated
   C. Cancel surgery and send the patient home
   D. Cancel surgery, administer dantrolene, and admit for 24-hour observation
   E. Cancel surgery, admit for 24-hour observation, and refer for muscle biopsy

9. Which of the following is the best immediate way to confirm placement of an endotracheal tube in the airway after intubation?
   A. Direct visualization of tube passing through the vocal cords
   B. Auscultation of lungs
   C. Observation of condensation within tube
   D. Pulse oximetry
   E. Capnography

10. A 65-year-old man is undergoing urgent surgery for gangrenous cholecystitis. The patient has a history of moderate aortic valve stenosis that was recently diagnosed on echocardiography but he denies any symptoms. Which of the following would be most important goal in the anesthetic management?
    A. Preload reduction
    B. Afterload reduction
    C. Avoidance of hypotension
    D. Heart rate goal of >90 beats per minute
    E. Use of ephedrine for hypotension

11. A 9-year-old boy has been in the pediatric intensive care unit for the last 7 days after presenting to the hospital with influenza infection leading to respiratory failure requiring mechanical ventilation. He is receiving continuous fentanyl and propofol infusions for pain control and sedation, respectively. This morning he developed bradycardia, and his urinary output decreased. He is noted to have hepatomegaly on physical examination. Laboratory values show an elevated creatinine, hyperlipidemia, hyperkalemia, and lactic acidosis. Which of the following is the best next step in management?
    A. Start bicarbonate infusion
    B. Perform liver biopsy
    C. Initiate hemodialysis
    D. Initiate treatment with low-dose epinephrine
    E. Discontinue propofol and start dexmedetomidine infusion

12. A 55-year-old diabetic man underwent a right-sided video-assisted thoracoscopic surgery (VATS) for an empyema yesterday. This morning he is complaining of pain along his medial left forearm and has paresthesia of his fourth and fifth digits. Which of the following risk factors are most likely associated with this complication?
    A. Male sex
    B. Emergency surgery
    C. Supine positioning during surgery
    D. Hyperthermia during surgery
    E. Diabetic neuropathy

13. Which of the following is true regarding invasive lines used for the monitoring of surgical patients?
    A. Trauma patients show improved mortality with placement of a pulmonary artery catheter (PAC)
    B. A normal Allen Test before radial artery cannulation will reduce incidence of hand ischemia
    C. PAC will provide direct measurement of systemic vascular resistance
    D. Systolic blood pressure measured on a radial artery catheter will typically be higher than the aortic pressure
    E. A right bundle branch block seen on electrocardiogram is considered a contraindication for PAC placement

14. A 47-year-old woman is recovering from pneumonia complicated by multiorgan system dysfunction. She is currently receiving hemodialysis after developing renal failure secondary to sepsis. This morning, a rapid response was called for respiratory depression and confusion, which improved after the administration of naloxone. Which of the following medications most likely contributed to her respiratory compromise?
    A. Fentanyl
    B. Hydromorphone
    C. Morphine
    D. Methadone
    E. Oxycodone

15. A 37-year-old woman underwent a percutaneous bedside tracheostomy tube placement. On postoperative day 1, she developed significant subcutaneous emphysema of the neck over the course of an hour, and her current oxygen saturation is 80%. A respiratory therapist attempted directional suctioning, but they were unable to pass the catheter. What is the most appropriate next step in management?
    A. Remove the tracheostomy tube and attempt recannulation with a smaller caliber cannula
    B. Remove the tracheostomy tube and recannulate over a suction catheter
    C. Remove the tracheostomy tube and recannulate over a fiberoptic bronchoscope
    D. Replace the tracheostomy tube using a percutaneous tracheostomy kit
    E. Bag mask ventilation and prepare for orotracheal intubation

16. Which of the following correctly pairs the invasive mechanical ventilation mode with its mechanism of action?
    A. Synchronized intermittent mechanical ventilation (SIMV): every breath has a mandated volume
    B. Airway pressure release ventilation (APRV): maintains continuous positive airway pressure (CPAP) with an intermittent release phase
    C. Assist-control (AC) ventilation: patient determines the rate and volume of breaths
    D. CPAP: two different pressure settings for inhalation and exhalation
    E. High-frequency oscillatory ventilation (HFOV): high respiratory rate with large tidal volumes

17. Which of the following parameters is most likely to predict successful discontinuation of mechanical ventilation?
    A. Rapid shallow breathing index (RSBI) (f/VT) less than 105
    B. Negative inspiratory force (NIF) −20 to −30 cm H2O
    C. Successful spontaneous breathing trial (SBT)
    D. Respiratory rate less than 30 breaths per minute
    E. Tidal volume greater than 5 mL/kg

18. A 66-year-old woman presents in septic shock due to a perforated duodenal ulcer. She is taken urgently to the operating room for an exploratory laparotomy. Due to persistent hypotension, dopamine is infused by the anesthesiologist and is eventually titrated to a rate of 15 mcg/kg per minute. At that rate, which of the following receptors is exerting the predominant effect?
    A. α1-Adrenergic
    B. α2-Adrenergic
    C. β1-Adrenergic
    D. β2-Adrenergic
    E. Dopaminergic

19. A 55-year-old man with a history of chronic obstructive pulmonary disease (COPD) undergoes an interscalene regional block with bupivacaine for surgery of a left humerus fracture. Soon after placement of the block, the patient develops significant dyspnea. Breath sounds are equal to auscultation and clear. Which of the following factors is the most likely cause of his shortness of breath?
    A. Pneumothorax
    B. COPD exacerbation
    C. Inadvertent intravascular injection of bupivacaine
    D. Air embolism
    E. An elevated left hemidiaphragm

20. At the end of a surgery, an anticholinesterase is administered to a patient to reverse the neuromuscular blockade. Which of the following muscles would be expected to recover first?
    A. Diaphragm
    B. Adductor pollicis
    C. Ocular muscles
    D. Pharyngeal
    E. Quadriceps femoris

21. A 40-year-old man with obesity, hypertension, cirrhosis, diabetes mellitus, and chronic kidney disease (CKD) stage 1 undergoes general anesthesia for repair of an incarcerated inguinal hernia. He takes insulin, echothiopate, amlodipine, and simvastatin at home. Propofol and pancuronium are used for induction. At the end of the procedure, a peripheral nerve stimulator demonstrates no recovery of muscle twitches despite 60 minutes of time elapsing. Which of the following underlying factors is most likely responsible for this condition?
    A. Diabetes mellitus
    B. Obesity
    C. Stage 1 CKD
    D. Pancuronium
    E. Simvastatin

22. Which of the following is associated with barbiturate toxicity?
    A. Myocardial depression
    B. Acute tubular necrosis
    C. Hepatotoxicity
    D. Peripheral neuropathy
    E. Seizures

23. A patient is given benzocaine spray in anticipation of a bedside flexible laryngoscopy. After several minutes, he develops a headache and shortness of breath. Pulse oximetry shows an SpO2 of 85%, while an arterial blood gas shows an SaO2 of 80% with a PaO2 of 150 mmHg. Which of the following is the most appropriate treatment?
    A. Intubation
    B. Intravenous methylene blue
    C. Discontinue benzocaine and administer prilocaine
    D. Metoclopramide
    E. Thiosulfate

ANSWERS

1. D. Level of sedation is a continuum defined by the patient's response to the medications administered. During minimal sedation, patients have a normal response to verbal stimulation (A). During moderate sedation, patients have purposeful responses to verbal or tactile stimulation (B). While under deep sedation, repeated verbal or painful stimulation is needed to achieve purposeful movements. Intervention on the airway may be required at this level of sedation. Under general anesthesia, the patient is unarousable even with painful stimulus (E). Moderate sedation and conscious sedation are terms that are often used interchangeably (C).

Reference: Practice guidelines for moderate procedural sedation and analgesia 2018: a report by the American Society of Anesthesiologists Task Force on Moderate Procedural Sedation and Analgesia, the American Association of Oral and Maxillofacial Surgeons, American College of Radiology, American Dental Association, American Society of Dentist Anesthesiologists, and Society of Interventional Radiology. *Anesthesiology.* 2018;128(3):437–479.

2. B. Long-term opioid use commonly results in tolerance and physical dependence. Tolerance describes a decrease in opioid potency with repeated administration. Tolerance to analgesic effects of opioids develops more quickly than

tolerance to respiratory depression, which partially explains the high overdose rates. Tolerance within the colon typically does not develop and results in chronic constipation (D). Dependance is characterized by the unpleasant response to stopping or reducing intake of the drug, also referred to as withdrawal symptoms. Opioid withdrawal symptoms include lacrimation, piloerection, muscle aches, nausea, vomiting, diarrhea, pupillary dilation, insomnia, tachycardia, hyperreflexia, and hypertension (C). Addiction is much less predictable and less common than both tolerance and dependance and is characterized by pronounced cravings, obsessive thinking, compulsive drug taking, and an inability to refrain from use (A). It is also now believed that opioid addiction has a fairly strong genetic component with heritability rates similar to diabetes and hypertension (E).

References: Volkow ND, McLellan AT. Opioid abuse in chronic pain–misconceptions and mitigation strategies. *N Engl J Med.* 2016;374(13):1253–1263.

Akbarali HI, Inkisar A, Dewey WL. Site and mechanism of morphine tolerance in the gastrointestinal tract. *Neurogastroenterol Mot.* 2014;26(10):1361–1367.

3. E. Given the unexplained hypotension and decrease in end-tidal CO_2, this patient most likely has a CO_2 embolism.

Clinically significant CO_2 embolism is very rare during laparoscopic surgery but has a mortality rate of approximately 28%. CO_2 embolism is thought to be caused by either intravascular injection of CO_2 into a vessel with either a Veress needle or trocar during initial insufflation, or by gas entering an injured vessel later during the operation. Signs of a CO_2 embolism are unexplained hypotension, hypoxia, or a sudden decrease in end-tidal CO_2. Transesophageal echocardiography (TEE) is the most sensitive method for detecting CO_2 embolism, though often not necessary when clinical suspicion is high (A). Precordial doppler is the most sensitive noninvasive test. If CO_2 embolism is suspected, insufflation should be stopped and the abdomen desufflated immediately. Though historically it has been recommended to place the patient in the left lateral and Trendelenburg position to move the air bubble out of the pulmonary artery, new evidence suggests that neither of the above positions results in significant hemodynamic improvements. Rather, for procedures below the level of the heart, the patient should be placed in the reverse Trendelenburg position to reduce further air entrainment. Vasopressor administration and a fluid bolus are reasonable interventions for persistent hypotension, but should be done after reducing the risk of further air entrapment (B, C). Pulmonary artery catheters have been shown to be ineffective at aspirating air with a success rate between 6% and 16% and should not be the next step in management (D). A "mill-wheel" murmur is present in less than half of patients.

References: Cottin V, Delafosse B, Viale JP. Gas embolism during laparoscopy: a report of seven cases in patients with previous abdominal surgical history. *Surg Endosc.* 1996;10(2):166–169.

Mirski M, Lele AV, Fitzsimmons L, et al. Diagnosis and treatment of vascular air embolism. *Anesthesiology.* 2007;106:164–177.

4. E. Opioid abuse has risen substantially in the US in recent years, prompting research investigating the causes of this new epidemic. Though the majority of opioids abused in the US originate from legitimate prescriptions, only 20% of opioid users were the intended recipients of the initial prescription (A). The majority of opioid abusers received pills for free from family members or friends with excessive pills or from other methods of diversion. Opioid abuse can also lead to further illicit drug use, as 50% to 85% of heroin users report having previously abused prescription opioids (B). As excessive opioid prescriptions appear to be one of the inciting factors in opioid abuse, additional attention has been placed on prescribing patterns after surgery. A large retrospective study showed that new persistent opioid use was fairly common after both major and minor surgical procedures, with an incidence of around 6%. The incidence was not significantly different between major and minor surgeries indicating that pain is not the driving factor for this postsurgical complication (D). Risk factors independently associated with new persistent opioid use include preoperative tobacco use, alcohol and substance abuse disorders, mood disorders, anxiety, and preoperative pain disorders (E). To address the overprescribing of opioids after surgery, one study identified the number of pills (equivalent to 5 mg oxycodone) that would fully supply the needs of 80% of patients undergoing a number of different operations. Examples of these needs include 5 pills after a partial mastectomy, 15 pills after a laparoscopic cholecystectomy, and 15 pills after an open inguinal hernia repair (C).

References: Brummett CM, Waljee JF, Goesling J, et al. New persistent opioid use after minor and major surgical procedures in US adults. *JAMA Sur.* 2017;152(6):e170504.

Hill MV, McMahon ML, Stucke RS, et al. Wide variation and excessive dosage of opioid prescriptions for common general surgical procedures. *Ann Surg.* 2017;265(4):709–714.

5. A. A study done in France from 1997 to 2004 looked at all patients who had immediate hypersensitivity reaction presumed to be from allergic reaction. Of the 1816 patients that met criteria for the study, the top three offending agents for immediate hypersensitivity reaction were neuromuscular blocking agents (58%), latex (20%), and antibiotics (13%) (B, C). Allergy to inhaled anesthetics and hypnotics was much less common (D, E). In children, latex was more common than neuromuscular blocking agents, but the sample size for this population was much lower.

References: Butterworth J, Mackey D, Wasnick J, et al., eds. Inhalation anesthetics. In: *Morgan & Mikhail's clinical anesthesiology.* 5th ed. McGraw-Hill; 2013;44–88.

Butterworth J, Mackey D, Wasnick J, et al., eds. Intravenous anesthetics. In: *Morgan & Mikhail's clinical anesthesiology.* 5th ed. McGraw-Hill; 2013;141–156.

Di Leo E, Delle Donne P, Calogiuri GF, Macchia L, Nettis E. Focus on the agents most frequently responsible for perioperative anaphylaxis. *Clin Mol Allergy.* 2018;16:16.

Mertes PM, Alla F, Tréchot P, Auroy Y, Jougla E, Groupe d'Etudes des Réactions Anaphylactoïdes Peranesthésiques. Anaphylaxis during anesthesia in France: an 8-year national survey. *J Allergy Clin Immunol.* 2011;128(2):366–373.

6. D. This patient likely has malignant hyperthermia, a rare autosomal dominant disorder of skeletal muscle (A). The condition is characterized by a hypermetabolic state triggered by exposure to inhalation anesthetics (sevoflurane, desflurane, isoflurane) and/or succinylcholine. The older anesthetic agents associated with this reaction include halothane and enflurane. It is not caused by nitrous oxide, intravenous anesthetic agents, or other neuromuscular blockers (except for succinylcholine). Malignant hyperthermia occurs when uncontrolled amounts of intracellular calcium accumulate in skeletal muscle. Symptoms may develop as early as 30 minutes after anesthetic administration and as late as 24 hours postoperatively. Even after treatment with dantrolene, patients need to be monitored because they can have a refractory response and go back into a malignant hyperthermic crisis. The initial clues occur in the operating room after induction. Rather than achieving complete paralysis, the anesthesiologist may notice rigidity in the masseter muscle. Other findings include an increase in end-tidal CO2, tachycardia, and an increase in temperature. It is imperative that all anesthetics are immediately stopped and dantrolene given (2.5 mg/kg every 5 minutes) until resolution of symptoms. Dantrolene stabilizes muscle channels in the sarcoplasmic reticulum. The mortality rate was previously 30%, but recent evidence suggests the mortality rate is now approximately 5% (E). A functional test on skeletal muscle biopsy (caffeine halothane contracture test) is used for diagnosis (B). More than 50% of the families show linkage of the in vitro contracture test phenotype to the gene encoding the skeletal muscle ryanodine receptor. The test requires a muscle biopsy with exposure of the muscle to halothane and caffeine. A positive test will cause significant muscle contraction. The majority of cases occur in children or young adults (C).

References: Jurkat-Rott K, McCarthy T, Lehmann-Horn F. Genetics and pathogenesis of malignant hyperthermia. *Muscle Nerve.* 2000;23(1):4–17.

Ellinas H, Albrecht MA. Malignant hyperthermia update. *Anesthesiol Clin.* 2020;38(1):165–181.

7. C. There are relatively few side effects of local anesthetic agents such as lidocaine, unless they are inadvertently injected intravenously or administered in doses higher than recommended. Toxicity begins with neurologic signs and symptoms such as light-headedness, facial paresthesias, blurred vision, and tinnitus. It can progress to lethargy, tremors, and tonic-clonic seizures. Neurologic symptoms precede the more severe cardiovascular symptoms, which include hypertension and tachycardia (early symptoms) and later hypotension, cardiovascular collapse, bradycardia or conduction abnormalities, and even cardiac arrest. The maximum doses for local injection of lidocaine are 5 mg/kg without epinephrine and 7 mg/kg with epinephrine because the vasoconstriction delays the systemic release of lidocaine. Because a 1% solution of lidocaine contains 10 mg/mL, an easy way to remember this is to multiply the patient's weight by either 5 (no epinephrine) or 7 (with epinephrine) and then divide by 10. Therefore, for this patient: 70 kg × 5 mg/kg = 350 mg and divide by 10 mg/mL = 35 mL of 1% lidocaine. For lidocaine with epinephrine, 70 kg × 7 mg/kg = 490 mg and divide by 10 = 49 mL of 1% lidocaine. For a 2% lidocaine solution, one would divide by 20 (24.5 mL and 17.5 mL, respectively, with and without epinephrine), and for a 0.5% solution, one would divide by 5 (70 mL and 98 mL, respectively, with and without epinephrine). Patients who experience local anesthetic systemic toxicity (LAST) should be treated by discontinuing the local anesthetic, administering fluids, support with 100% FiO_2, hyperventilation, and administering 20% intralipid with a bolus of 1 to 1.5 mL/kg over one minute. The bolus can be repeated every 3 minutes up to a total dose of 3 mL/kg, followed by an infusion of 0.25 mL/kg/min which is continued until the patient is hemodynamically stable for at least 10 minutes. CPR and epinephrine should be used in cardiac arrest, and bicarbonate should be used in acidosis. Benzodiazepines are preferred over propofol to manage seizures.

References: Warren JA, Thoma RB, Georgescu A, Shah SJ. Intravenous lipid infusion in the successful resuscitation of local anesthetic-induced cardiovascular collapse after supraclavicular brachial plexus block. *Anesth Analg.* 2008;106(5):1578–1580.

Neal JM, Mulroy MF, Weinberg GL, American Society of Regional Anesthesia and Pain Medicine. American Society of Regional Anesthesia and Pain Medicine checklist for managing local anesthetic systemic toxicity: 2012 version. *Reg Anesth Pain Med.* 2012;37(1):16–18.

Cao D, Heard K, Foran M, Koyfman A. Intravenous lipid emulsion in the emergency department: a systematic review of recent literature. *J Emerg Med.* 2015;48(3):387–97.

8. E. Masseter muscle rigidity, or trismus, is considered a normal reaction to the administration of neuromuscular blocking agents. However, if this condition persists for more than 20 to 30 seconds, it is considered an abnormal response, and the clinician needs to have a high level of concern for malignant hyperthermia, and nonemergent surgeries should be canceled (B). Persistent trismus is not a sign of inadequate neuromuscular blockade, and thus additional neuromuscular blocker administration is not indicated (A). Masseter spasm is an early indicator of susceptibility to malignant hyperthermia. Other markers for malignant hyperthermia include fevers, increased end-tidal CO_2, generalized muscle rigidity, autonomic instability, and rhabdomyolysis. The incidence of patients who develop masseter spasms and go on to develop malignant hyperthermia is unknown. It should be noted that isolated masseter spasm is not pathognomonic for malignant hyperthermia. The surgery should be canceled and the patient admitted for at least 24 hours of observation to watch for the development of rhabdomyolysis or malignant hyperthermia; the patient should not be sent home prior to 24 hours of observation and monitoring in the hospital (C). In the absence of hemodynamic instability, elevated CO2, or fever, it is unnecessary to administer dantrolene (D). However, these patients should be referred to a center that can perform the necessary testing, including genetic testing and a caffeine halothane contracture test (muscle biopsy test). After muscle biopsy, the tissue is only viable for several hours, so testing must take place in centers specialized in diagnosing malignant hyperthermia (E).

References: Schneiderbanger D, Johannsen S, Roewer N, Schuster F. Management of malignant hyperthermia: diagnosis and treatment. *Ther Clin Risk Manag.* 2014;10:355–362.

Bauer SJ, Orio K, Adams BD. Succinylcholine induced masseter spasm during rapid sequence intubation may require a surgical airway: case report. *Emerg Med J.* 2005;22:456–458.

Sheikh MM, Riaz A, Umair HM, Waqar M, Muneeb A. Succinylcholine-induced masseter muscle rigidity successfully managed with propofol and laryngeal mask airway: a case report and brief review. *Cureus.* 2020;12(7):e9376.

9. E. Although direct visualization of the tube passing through the vocal cords, auscultation of the lungs, visualization of condensation within the tube, and pulse oximetry are good adjuncts to confirm initial placement of the endotracheal tube, interpretation is subjective and not as accurate as more objective methods for confirming the position of the endotracheal tube within the trachea (A–C). Both the American College of Emergency Physicians and the American Society of Anesthesiologists recommend capnography or end-tidal CO_2 detection devices as the preferred confirmatory test for tracheal intubation (E). Patients should have a continuous uniform waveform of end-tidal CO_2 with similar amplitudes to confirm tracheal intubation; however, this does not differentiate a tracheal from a bronchial intubation. A capnographic waveform that shows end-tidal CO_2 detection but does not have a continuous waveform or the amplitudes get smaller and smaller until no additional end-tidal CO_2 can be detected is indicative of an esophageal intubation. Direct visualization of the tube passing through the cords is not always reliable, as the cords can be misidentified or the tube can be dislodged from the trachea before it is secured (A). Auscultation of the lungs is not always reliable because it is possible to get referred sounds from the stomach (B). Condensation within the tube can occur even with esophageal intubation (C). Pulse oximetry is also not reliable, as hypoxia with esophageal intubation can be very delayed if the patient is preoxygenated well (D).

References: American Society of Anesthesiologists Task Force on Management of the Difficult Airway. Practice guidelines for management of the difficult airway: an updated report by the American Society of Anesthesiologists Task Force on Management of the Difficult Airway. *Anesthesiology.* 2003;98(5):1269–277.

Grmec S. Comparison of three different methods to confirm tracheal tube placement in emergency intubation. *Intensive Care Med.* 2002;28(6):701–704.

10. C. While asymptomatic aortic stenosis is not a contra-indication to surgery, it requires careful intraoperative monitoring. The increased pressures required to overcome the stenosis cause concentric hypertrophy of the left ventricle, which in turn reduces the compliance of the ventricle. This makes these patients heavily preload dependent for ventricular filling, and careful attention should be paid to maintaining adequate intravascular volume (A). In addition, up to 40% of the left ventricular end-diastolic volume (LVEDV) is provided by the atrial kick. Atrial arrhythmias can quickly lead to heart failure and should be aggressively treated, preferably with defibrillation. Bradycardia (<50 bpm) should also be avoided because patients have a fixed stroke volume and cardiac output is dependent on the heart rate. Hypotension and reductions in afterload will reduce coronary artery filling and increase the likelihood of cardiac ischemia (B). Hypotension should be preferentially treated with selective α-adrenergic agents such as phenylephrine, which increase SVR and prevent tachycardia (C, E). Sinus tachycardia and hypertension can precipitate ischemia and should be treated by increasing the depth of anesthesia (D). Because of the potential for bradycardia and hypotension with beta-blockers, these agents should be used with caution, and short-acting agents, such as esmolol, are preferred. To summarize, the goals of anesthesia in patients with aortic stenosis are to avoid hypotension, ensure adequate LVEDV, and maintain coronary perfusion pressure, normal sinus rhythm, and preload.

References: Christ M, Sharkova Y, Geldner G, Maisch B. Preoperative and perioperative care for patients with suspected or established aortic stenosis facing noncardiac surgery. *Chest.* 2005;128(4):2944–2953.

Anesthesia for patients with cardiovascular disease. In: Butterworth IV JF, Mackey DC, Wasnick JD, eds. *Morgan & Mikhail's clinical anesthesiology.* 6th ed. McGraw-Hill; 2018.

11. E. Propofol infusion syndrome is a clinical condition that is associated with higher doses of propofol infusion (>4 mg/kg/hr) that is continued for more than 48 hours. It is associated with metabolic acidosis, arrhythmias (most often bradycardia), rhabdomyolysis, hyperlipidemia, hepatomegaly (not splenomegaly), renal failure, and eventual cardiovascular collapse. A liver biopsy is not needed for diagnosis (B). The first case report was in the pediatric population, and though the correlation with age is unclear, children may be at a higher risk. Once it has been diagnosed, the first step in management is immediate cessation of propofol, and another sedating medication should be started (E). However, treatment is largely ineffective, especially in the setting of arrhythmias. Renal replacement may be utilized in patients who develop hyperkalemia and rhabdomyolysis but is not the most important next step (C). Sodium bicarbonate administration to treat lactic acidosis is not recommended (A). The combination of high-dose propofol with exogenous catecholamines (i.e., phenylephrine, norepinephrine, epinephrine) or steroid administration appears to trigger the syndrome. Catecholamines and steroids aggravate propofol inhibition of fatty acid metabolism, promoting rapid and irreversible peripheral and cardiac muscle injury (D). A screening tool for this condition has been proposed that includes daily CPK and lactate levels because these may be the first indications that propofol infusion syndrome has developed.

References: Fodale V, La Monaca E. Propofol infusion syndrome: an overview of a perplexing disease. *Drug Saf.* 2008;31(4):293–303.

Hemphill S, McMenamin L, Bellamy MC, et al. Propofol infusion syndrome: a structured literature review and analysis of published case reports. *Br J Anaesth.* 2019;122(4):448–459.

Ichikawa T, Okuyama K, Kamata K, et al. Suspected propofol infusion syndrome during normal targeted propofol concentration. *J Anesth.* 2020;34(4):619–623.

Mirrakhimov AE, Voore P, Halytskyy O, et al. Propofol infusion syndrome in adults: a clinical update. *Crit Care Res Pract.* 2015;2015:260385.

Schroeppel TJ, Fabian TC, Clement LP, et al. Propofol infusion syndrome: a lethal condition in critically injured patients eliminated by a simple screening protocol. *Injury.* 2014;45(1):245–249.

12. E. The American Society of Anesthesiologists has identified perioperative peripheral nerve injuries as among the top three medical malpractice claims directed at anesthesiologists and operating room staff. Despite the fact that over 60% included documentation of appropriate padding and position, almost half of the cases involved payment. Of these injuries, ulnar and brachial plexus injuries appear to be the most common. These injuries appear to happen by one of several mechanisms: direct nerve damage, stretch/compression, and ischemia or toxicity of locally injected medications. Risk factors related to the patient include hypertension, diabetes, smoking, extremes in body mass index, and malnutrition (A, E). Chronically dysfunctional nerves (such as in a patient with diabetic neuropathy) may be particularly susceptible to an acute insult. Intraoperative risk factors include hypothermia, hypovolemia, hypotension, hypoxemia, and electrolyte abnormalities (B–D). Because it can take several days for denervation of the affected muscles to take place, EMG is often normal in the immediate postoperative period. However, EMG should still be done early because any abnormalities likely represent a preexisting neuropathy that was simply exacerbated by the operation. Most of these injuries will heal with time. However, operative intervention can be performed depending on the severity of injury and failure to improve with conservative measures.

References: Chui J, Murkin JM, Posner KL, Domino KB. Perioperative peripheral nerve injury after general anesthesia: a qualitative systematic review. *Anesth Analg.* 2018;127(1):134–143.

Lalkhen AG, Bhatia K. Perioperative peripheral nerve injuries. *Contin Educ Anaesth Crit Care Pain.* 2012;12(1):38–42.

Welch MB, Brummett CM, Welch TD, et al. Perioperative peripheral nerve injuries: a retrospective study of 380,680 cases during a 10-year period at a single institution. *Anesthesiology.* 2009;111(3):490–497.

Winfree C, Kline DG. Intraoperative positioning nerve injuries. *Surg Neurol.* 2005;63(1):5–18.

13. D. Though invasive hemodynamic monitoring of the critically ill patient provides valuable information, complications of placement must always be measured against the potential advantages. PAC was considered the standard of care for many critically ill patients but is being used less frequently now because of multiple studies showing no improvement in mortality (A). Based on these findings, invasive hemodynamic monitoring is no longer recommended for routine use. However, there may still be a role in patients with unknown volume status, severe cardiogenic shock, pulmonary artery hypertension, or severe underlying cardiopulmonary disease. Before placement, an electrocardiogram must be obtained to rule out left bundle branch block (LBBB). There is a high incidence of a temporary right bundle branch block with placement, and in the setting of an LBBB, a complete heart block could be incited. However, there is no contraindication to placement in most other arrhythmias (E). The PAC directly measures cardiac output, central venous pressure, mixed venous oxyhemoglobin saturation, right-sided cardiac pressures, and pulmonary artery pressures. From this information, systemic vascular resistance, cardiac index, and oxygen delivery/uptake can be calculated (C). Invasive arterial blood pressure monitoring provides continuous measurement of blood pressure as well as easy access to arterial blood gas samples. However, it too comes with potential complications, the most significant being arterial thrombosis. The radial artery is generally preferred because of adequate collaterals through the ulnar, relative ease of cannulation, and lower incidence of infection. Though the Allen test is currently considered mandatory before radial arterial line placement, it does not seem to accurately predict risk of hand ischemia. Several trials looking at the Allen test have shown disagreement on what constitutes a positive test, high variability among observers, and inconsistent prediction of collateral flow when compared with less subjective tests such as ultrasound (B). It is also important to remember that systolic blood pressure in the radial artery will be higher than in the aorta but mean arterial pressure should be preserved. A higher systolic pressure occurs with distal progression, smaller arterial caliber, and older age.

References: Barone JE, Madlinger RV. Should an Allen test be performed before radial artery cannulation? *J Trauma.* 2006;61(2):468–470.

Fischer J, ed. Cardiovascular monitoring and support. In: *Fischer's mastery of surgery.* 6th ed. Wolters Kluwer Health/Lippincott Williams & Wilkins;2012.

Vincent JL. The pulmonary artery catheter. *J Clin Monit Comput.* 2012;26(5): 341–345.

14. C. Opioid pain medications undergo metabolism predominantly in the liver into a variety of metabolites that are generally excreted in the urine. Morphine is metabolized via glucuronidation by the liver, brain, and kidney into the active metabolites morphine-3-glucuronide and morphine-6-glucuronide. The glucuronide metabolites are then eliminated via bile and predominantly urine. Morphine-6-glucuronide is more selective for mu-receptors and is a more potent analgesic than morphine. In the setting of renal injury, the metabolites can persist for long periods of time and cause respiratory depression. Thus, morphine and codeine (which is a prodrug that is metabolized into morphine) should be avoided in renal failure and in patients on dialysis. Hydromorphone does have an active metabolite, but it does not have increased potency as is seen with morphine's metabolites (B). Fentanyl and methadone are likely the safest medications to use in dialysis patients because all of the metabolites are inactive (A, D). Oxycodone is metabolized into noroxycodone (which is five times less potent than oxycodone) and oxymorphone (which is 8 times as potent as oxycodone). However, both these metabolites are metabolized to noroxymorphone, which is weakly active, and oxycodone and all its metabolites also undergo glucuronidation, resulting in metabolites which are inactive at the mu-receptor, and thus do not have significant opioidergic effects. Since the metabolites do not appear to have significant active effects on opioid receptors, it is deemed safe to use in renal patients, although it is considered a second-line agent. Furthermore, hemodialysis increases the clearance of oxycodone

and all its metabolites, so it may be used in dialysis-dependent patients (E).

References: Dean M. Opioids in renal failure and dialysis patients. *J Pain Symptom Manag.* 2004;28(5):497–504.

Leuppi-Taegtmeyer A, Duthaler U, Hammann F, et al. Pharmacokinetics of oxycodone/naloxone and its metabolites in patients with end-stage renal disease during and between haemodialysis sessions. *Nephrol Dial Transplant.* 2019;34(4):692–702.

Schumacher, M et al. Opioid agonists & antagonists. In: Katzung BG, Trevor AJ, eds. *Basic & clinical pharmacology.* 13th ed. McGraw-Hill; 2014.

15. E. Early dislodgement of the tracheostomy tube is an infrequent but potentially devastating complication associated with placement. In general, the first tube exchange happens between postoperative days 3 and 7. Accidental removal before a planned exchange can potentially cause loss of the airway. Additionally, manipulation of the endotracheal tube by ancillary staff may promote a false passage. Despite positioning of the tracheostomy in a false passage, patients may be able to maintain some oxygenation despite its location. This can manifest as respiratory distress (in a nonventilated patient) and with subcutaneous emphysema. Replacement of the tracheostomy tube can be attempted via multiple methods including trying to use a small caliber cannula, using a suction catheter or fiberoptic bronchoscope as a guide, or using the equipment in a percutaneous tracheostomy kit (A–D). However, if the patient is unstable and rapidly desaturating, securing the airway is the main priority and oral endotracheal is warranted.

References: Halum SL, Ting JY, Plowman EK, et al. A multi-institutional analysis of tracheotomy complications. *Laryngoscope.* 2012;122(1):38–45.

Subroto, P, Colson, Y. (2014). Tracheostomy. In: Sugarbaker DJ, Bueno R, Colson YL, Jaklitsch MT, Krasna MJ, Mentzer S, eds. *Adult chest surgery.* 2nd ed. McGraw-Hill Professional; 2014.

16. B. Data showing improved survival of one mode of ventilation over another in specific disease states is inconsistent at best. However, theoretically, each mode of ventilation offers certain advantages and disadvantages. The conventional modes of mechanical ventilation can be considered on a spectrum based on the amount of support that is provided to the patient and how the machine supports patient-initiated breaths. At the lowest end of the spectrum is CPAP, in which all breaths are triggered by the patient and no additional support is provided. The mechanical ventilator simply provides a constant pressure and allows patients to breath at a rate and volume that they determine (D). Pressure support ventilation (PSV) allows the patient to determine the rate and volume of breaths but provides additional pressure to support a patient-triggered breath. SIMV allows the clinician to mandate a certain number of breaths per minute at a set volume or pressure but allows the patient to breath spontaneously in between the machine-triggered breaths. It is frequently combined with PSV to provide additional pressure to support the patient-triggered breaths. Proponents advocate that it allows patients to exercise their respiratory muscles, but this comes at the expense of an increased effort of breathing, which can potentially fatigue the diaphragm (A). AC allows patients to trigger breaths, but every breath has a mandated volume or pressure (C). This allows patients to change their work of breathing simply by increasing the respiratory rate (RR), and, because every breath is machine delivered, it has the lowest associated work of breathing. APRV is a mode designed to maximize alveolar recruitment by maintaining relatively constant higher pressures with an intermittent release phase. In this mode, there is a high pressure (P high) which is set for a prolonged time (T high) to recruit alveoli and maintain adequate lung volume, with a time-cycled release phase to a lower pressure (P low) for a shorter amount of time (T low), where CO2 removal occurs. This mode of ventilation uses an extreme inverse I:E (inspiratory:expiratory) ratio (which distinguishes it from BiPAP (biphasic positive airway pressure)) to allow for more time at a higher pressure to promote alveolar opening and recruitment. APRV is not routinely used and it is reserved as a rescue mode for treating acute respiratory distress syndrome (ARDS) or acute lung injury (ALI). Its advantages include: increased comfort for the patient, allowing spontaneous ventilation and decreased sedation requirements, alveolar recruitment, improved oxygenation, and hemodynamic stability. HFOV is a mode of ventilation that works off of the assumption that high airway pressures can be tolerated by patients as long as they are not sustained for prolonged periods of time. The goal is to maintain the lungs at a relatively constant mean airway pressure with sinusoidal flow oscillation, which can recruit alveoli but does not result in overdistention. Therefore, patients receive small tidal volumes, which are below the volume of dead space (E) with a high RR. Current approved ventilators in the United States do not support spontaneous breathing with HFOV; heavy sedation or paralysis is generally required with HFOV. Additionally, it can result in hemodynamic instability, pulmonary barotrauma (e.g., pneumothorax), and increased infections. This is also a rescue mode of ventilation that may be used in patients with ALI/ARDS or burn patients with inhalation injury. Current recommendations are to limit its use to high-volume centers because of the increased training required of the staff and the time-intensive nature of treatment.

References: Brochard L, Lellouche F. Pressure-support ventilation. In: Tobin MJ, ed. *Principles and practice of mechanical ventilation.* 3rd ed. McGraw-Hill Medical; 2013.

Froese A, Ferguson N. High-frequency ventilation. In: Tobin MJ, ed. *Principles and practice of mechanical ventilation.* 3rd ed. McGraw-Hill Medical; 2013.

Higgins J, Estetter B, Holland D, Smith B, Derdak S. High-frequency oscillatory ventilation in adults: respiratory therapy issues. *Crit Care Med.* 2005;33(3 Suppl):S196–S203.

Mancebo J. Assist-control ventilation. In: Tobin MJ, ed. *Principles and practice of mechanical ventilation.* 3rd ed. McGraw-Hill Medical; 2013.

Putensen C. Airway pressure release ventilation. In: Tobin MJ, ed. *Principles and practice of mechanical ventilation.* 3rd ed. McGraw-Hill Medical; 2013.

Sassoon C. Intermittent mandatory ventilation. In: Tobin MJ, ed. *Principles and practice of mechanical ventilation.* 3rd ed. McGraw-Hill Medical; 2013.

17. C. The term *weaning* when describing discontinuation of mechanical ventilation refers to an old concept of slowly reducing ventilator support until a patient is ready to take over the work of breathing on his or her own. Because this practice is no longer encouraged, there has been a push to change the term to *liberation* from the mechanical ventilator. In 2001, "Evidence-Based Guidelines for Weaning and Discontinuing Ventilatory Support" was published in *Chest* by a task force specifically assembled to assess current weaning strategies. The basis of these recommendations was that daily evaluation of readiness for extubation should be done, underlying conditions corrected, and that the ventilator should be discontinued as early as possible. Delaying extubation in patients ready for spontaneous breathing was associated with an increase in mortality, increased nosocomial pneumonia, and a prolonged hospital stay. The most predictive factor for successful extubation was successful SBT (A, B, D, E). Current recommendations include a daily screening for SBT readiness; which includes an improvement in the underlying disease state, adequate gas exchange (high PaO_2, low FiO_2, low $PEEP:FiO_2$ ratio), hemodynamic stability, and either the discontinuation of vasopressors or decreasing vasopressor requirements, and the patient's ability to generate a spontaneous breath. Patients should also ideally be able to follow simple commands, be neurologically intact (in order to protect their airway once extubated), and not require frequent suctioning of secretions (i.e., suctioning every 1 hour would not make the patient a good candidate for extubation trial). Once these parameters are met, the patient should undergo an SBT. The modality of the SBT (CPAP versus pressure support versus T-piece) is not significant, as one has not been demonstrated to be superior to the others. Clinicians should use the modality their institution uses, and the one with which they have the most experience. A patient is considered to have "failed" an SBT if any of the following criteria are met: worsening gas exchange, hemodynamic instability, significant increase in respiratory rate (RR), change in mental status, diaphoresis, or signs of increased work of breathing. Patients that pass an SBT should be considered for immediate extubation. Though several specific values help guide clinicians in determining a patient's readiness to extubate (e.g., RSBI <105, tidal volume 4–6 mL/kg, NIF −20 to −30 cm H_2O, minute ventilation 10–15 L/min, RR <30 bpm), studies have demonstrated that they are not individual predictors of extubation success. RSBI is considered an excellent predictor of failed extubation but should not be used solely to determine readiness for extubation, nor is it a predictor of successful extubation. Although the goal is early extubation, patients really need to be optimized and demonstrate that they have a high likelihood of extubation, as premature extubation may result in reintubation, which is associated with an 8-fold increased risk of nosocomial pneumonia and a 6- to 12-fold increased risk of mortality.

References: Celli B. Mechanical ventilatory support. In: Kasper DL, Fauci AS, Hauser SL, Longo DL, Jameson JL, Loscalzo J, eds. *Harrison's principles of internal medicine.* 19th ed. McGraw-Hill; 2015.

MacIntyre NR, Cook DJ, Ely EW Jr, et al. Evidence-based guidelines for weaning and discontinuing ventilatory support: a collective task force facilitated by the American College of Chest Physicians; the American Association for Respiratory Care; and the American College of Critical Care Medicine. *Chest.* 2001;120(6 Suppl):375S–95S.

McConville JF, Kress JP. Weaning patients from the ventilator. *N Engl J Med.* 2012;367(23):2233–2239.

18. A. Dopamine is an α- and β-adrenergic agonist that exerts a variable effect dependent on the dose. However, regardless of dose, its effect on α- and β-adrenergic receptors is generally weaker than epinephrine and norepinephrine (B, D). At lower doses (1–2 mcg/kg per minute), its predominant effect is on the dopaminergic receptors, causing renal and visceral vasodilation (E). As you increase the dose to 3 to 10 mcg/kg per minute, the β1-adrenergic receptors predominate; this is most similar to the effects of dobutamine or low-dose epinephrine. This causes an increase in cardiac output, primarily by increasing stroke volume (C). As you increase the dose further to greater than 10 mcg/kg per minute, the α1-adrenergic receptors predominate, leading to peripheral vasoconstriction; this is most similar to the effects of phenylephrine. Dopamine infusions do not significantly affect α2- and β2-adrenergic receptors.

Reference: Han J, Cribbs SK, Martin GS. Sepsis, severe sepsis, and septic shock. In: Hall JB, Schmidt GA, Kress JP, eds. Principles of critical care. 4th ed. McGraw-Hill; 2014.

19. E. An interscalene nerve block is a frequently performed and generally well-tolerated anesthesia adjunct for upper extremity surgery. Local anesthetic is injected into the interscalene groove, which then disperses to block the brachial plexus (C5-T1). However, the origin of the phrenic nerve (C3-C5 nerve roots) is in close proximity to the targeted area of the block, especially high in the neck, and ipsilateral diaphragmatic paralysis is possible. One small study showed a 100% incidence of diaphragm dysfunction when evaluated with ultrasound. This complication is generally well tolerated by patients with an adequate pulmonary reserve, but it can be very problematic for patients with lung disease. Ultrasound guidance, targeting the brachial plexus at a lower level in the neck, and lower volumes of anesthetic agent are used to help prevent this complication, but cranial spread of the agent is still possible. Pneumothorax is a known complication, but with bilateral breath sounds it would be unlikely (A). COPD exacerbation is also unlikely with such an acute onset and clear breathing sounds (B). Air embolism is also unlikely with a percutaneous block (D). The toxic doses of intravenous bupivacaine are associated with cardiac and neurotoxicity, not isolated dyspnea (C).

Reference: Urmey WF, Talts KH, Sharrock NE. One hundred percent incidence of hemidiaphragmatic paresis associated with interscalene brachial plexus anesthesia as diagnosed by ultrasonography. *Anesth Analg.* 1991;72(4):498–503.

20. A. Not all muscles respond in the same fashion to neuromuscular blockade. In general, central muscles (e.g., diaphragm) have a greater blood supply and will have a quicker onset and quicker recovery from paralysis compared with peripheral muscles (e.g., quadriceps femoris), which will have slower onset and slower recovery (E). Because of the variability in muscle relaxant duration and the potentially devastating complications of incomplete recovery before extubation, many argue that quantitative train of four testing should be routine for all cases. One important exception to this rule involves the muscles of the upper airway and pharynx, which have quick onset but slow offset (D). The ocular muscles tend to behave like central muscles and, for this reason, are an ideal muscle group to monitor at induction and during the operation because they will serve as a surrogate for measuring adequate blockade of the central muscles (C). Conversely, adductor pollicis is a good muscle group to monitor at the end of anesthesia because return of function will ensure that the central muscles and pharynx have recovered from blockade (B).

Reference: McGrath CD, Hunter JM. Monitoring of neuromuscular block. *Contin Educ Anaesth Crit Care Pain.* 2006;6(1):7–12.

21. D. Failure to regain muscle twitches after neuromuscular blockade should raise concern for a pseudocholinesterase deficiency. This patient was given succinylcholine for induction and because pseudocholinesterase is necessary for the degradation of succinylcholine, neuromuscular blockade was not reversed. Pseudocholinesterase deficiency can be either acquired or due to genetic abnormality, inherited in an autosomal recessive fashion. Conditions that lower plasma pseudocholinesterase are chronic infections (i.e., tuberculosis), extensive burns, liver disease, malnutrition, malignancy, and uremia (A–C). Medications that lower plasma pseudocholinesterase are anticholinesterase inhibitors, chlorpromazine, contraceptives, cyclophosphamide, echothiophate eye drops, esmolol, glucocorticoids, metoclopramide, and pancuronium, among others (E). Unfortunately, treatment is mainly supportive and patients must be maintained on mechanical ventilation until spontaneous recovery takes place. Pseudocholinesterase also affects the metabolism of ester local anesthetics and up to 50% of the metabolism of cocaine, which increases their risk of life-threatening cocaine toxicity. The diagnosis is confirmed by a laboratory assay demonstrating decreased plasma cholinesterase enzyme activity.

Reference: Soliday FK, Conley YP, Henker R. Pseudocholinesterase deficiency: a comprehensive review of genetic, acquired, and drug influences. *AANA J.* 2010;78(4):313–320.

22. A. Barbiturates are a class of medications that were previously used for anesthetic induction and seizures. However, they have largely been replaced by other agents for these two indications. As such, barbiturate toxicity is relatively rare. They are central nervous system depressants and can cause effects ranging from drowsiness to general anesthesia. They inhibit neuron firing and are protective against seizures, as they decrease the seizure threshold (E). Higher doses of barbiturates inhibit the respiratory drive and normal rhythmic respiration. Hepatotoxicity is not seen in barbiturate toxicity; however, it does inhibit CYP enzymes, which can increase concentrations of other drugs that undergo hepatic degradation (C). At the level of the peripheral nervous system, barbiturates decrease transmission through the autonomic nervous system and suppress nicotinic receptors, which contribute to hypotension but not peripheral neuropathy (D). At anesthetic doses, barbiturates do minimally suppress cardiac reflexes because of suppression of the autonomic ganglia, which is only problematic in patients with underlying cardiac disease. However, at toxic doses, there is direct suppression of cardiac contractility. Renal injury is likely secondary to hypotension rather than having any direct effect on the kidneys (B).

Reference: Mihic S, Harris R. Hypnotics and sedatives. In: Brunton LL, Chabner BA, Knollmann BC, eds. *Goodman & Gilman's: the pharmacological basis of therapeutics.* 12th ed. McGraw-Hill; 2015.

23. B. Benzocaine toxicity can manifest as methemoglobinemia. In this condition, the ferrous component of hemoglobin is oxidized to form ferric hemoglobin, which does not effectively carry oxygen. Mild to moderate methemoglobinemia can cause marked cyanosis but is generally well tolerated and does not typically require mechanical intubation (A). Pulse oximetry will not reliably assess the degree of hypoxemia. It will be falsely elevated initially and can be falsely low after treatment with methylene blue. Methemoglobinemia will result in a falsely low saturation when SaO_2 is greater than 85%, and a falsely high saturation when SaO_2 is <85%. The partial pressure of oxygen in the blood (PaO_2) will remain normal, so standard arterial blood gas analyzers, which calculate the oxygen saturation based off of the PaO_2, will show a falsely elevated oxygen saturation. Treatment is with supplemental oxygen and intravenous methylene blue, which will reduce hemoglobin back to the ferrous state (B). Prilocaine has similar toxicity to bupivacaine and will not treat the underlying issue (C). Metoclopramide is used for delayed gastric emptying (D). Thiosulfate is used in the treatment of cyanide toxicity (E).

Reference: Blanc P. Methemoglobinemia. In: Olson KR, ed. *Poisoning & drug overdose.* 6th ed. McGraw-Hill; 2012.

Fluids, Electrolytes, and Acid-Base Balance

29

JORDAN M. ROOK, AREG GRIGORIAN, AND CHRISTIAN DE VIRGILIO

ABSITE 99th Percentile High-Yields

I. Physiology/Pathology
   A. Total body water in liters = 0.6 × weight in kg (in males); 0.5 × weight in kg (in females)
      1. Intracellular water is 40% of total body weight and extracellular water is 20% of total body weight; plasma accounts for about 5% of total body weight

II. Resuscitative Fluids: replaces water and electrolyte losses secondary to pathologic processes
   A. Crystalloids: contains water-soluble molecules
      1. Sepsis: adults, initial bolus: 30 mL/kg (20 mL/kg in children)
      2. Common crystalloid/colloid:
         a) Lactated Ringer's: 5 electrolytes—Na (130 mEq/L), K (4 mEq/L), Ca (2.7 mEq/L), Cl (109 mEq/L), lactate (28 mEq/L)
         b) Normal saline (0.9%): 2 electrolytes—Na, Cl (both 154 mEq/L)

III. Pathology
   A. Vomiting/high nasogastric tube output
      1. Metabolic disturbance: hypochloremia, hypokalemia, metabolic alkalosis
      2. Mechanism: loss of HCl and volume -> kidneys retain bicarb and Na^+ and excrete K^+, H^+, Cl^-
      3. Treatment: normal saline
   B. High output ostomy, fistula, diarrhea
      1. Metabolic disturbance: non–anion gap metabolic acidosis
      2. Mechanism: pancreatic fluid, enteric fluid (small intestine), and diarrhea rich in bicarb
      3. Treatment: lactated Ringer's
   C. Syndrome of inappropriate antidiuretic hormone secretion (SIADH)
      1. Metabolic disturbance: euvolemic hyponatremia
      2. Diagnosis: urine osmolality abnormally high
      3. Treatment: fluid restriction, hypertonic saline, vasopressin antagonist in severely symptomatic refractory cases (tolvaptan or demeclocycline)
   D. Diabetes Insipidus (DI) (most commonly occurs after brain injury)
      1. Nephrogenic DI: kidneys unresponsive to vasopressin/DDAVP; Central DI: posterior pituitary does not release vasopressin/DDAVP; both types of DI result in lack of aquaporin channels in distal convoluted tubules and subsequent inability to reabsorb free water
      2. Metabolic disturbance: hypovolemic hypernatremia
      3. Diagnosis: urine osmolality abnormally low (<300 mmol/L) with high serum osmolarity (>280 mmol/L) and serum sodium (>142 mEq/L)
      4. Treatment: central DI responds to exogenous ADH (desmopressin); nephrogenic DI managed with supportive care and free water

E. Refeeding syndrome (shift from fat to carbohydrate metabolism)
  1. Metabolic disturbance: hypophosphatemia (carbohydrate leads to insulin spike and subsequent extracellular phosphate driven intracellular to produce ATP), hypokalemia, hypocalcemia, hypomagnesemia
  2. Diagnosis: electrolyte abnormalities in malnourished patient being fed; hypophosphatemia can lead to respiratory distress (diaphragm needs lots of ATP)
  3. Most common cause of mortality is cardiac complication
  4. Treatment: aggressive electrolyte repletion; slowly increase calorie intake

IV. Important formulas:
  A. Anion gap: $AG = (Na^+ + K^+) - (Cl^- + HCO_3^-)$
    1. Abnormal is >10–15
    2. Aniongap: MUDPILES—methanol, uremia, diabetic ketoacidosis, paraaldehyde, isoniazid, lactic acidosis, ethylene glycol, salicylates
    3. Non–anion gap: diarrhea, nasogastric tube losses, high ileostomy output, small bowel fistula
  B. Osmolarity: $Osm = (2 \times Na^+) + (BUN/2.8) + (Glucose/18)$

V. Hyponatremia (Na^+ <135 mEq/L)
  A. Symptoms: lethargy, headaches, nausea, vomiting, confusion, seizures
  B. Diagnosis
    1. Hypertonic (osmolality >290 mOsm/kg): dilutional drop in serum sodium due to osmotically active molecules
      a) Most often caused by hyperglycemia (can also occur with mannitol and contrast)
      b) Sodium correction: add 2 mEq/L of Na^+ for each 100 mg/dL the blood glucose is above 100 mg/dL
    2. Isotonic (osmolality 275–290 mOsm/kg): pseudohyponatremia
      a) Laboratory error due to over-dilution in the presence of abnormally high amounts of solute
      b) Most common causes are hypertriglyceridemia, familial hypercholesterolemia, multiple myeloma
    3. Hypotonic (osmolality <275 mOsm/kg): excess free water
      a) Low urine osmolality (<285 mOsm/kg): antidiuretic hormone (ADH) independent
        (1) Tea and toast/Beer potomania: due to low solute intake
          (a) Treatment: high solute diet
        (2) Psychogenic polydipsia: excessive water intake
          (a) Treatment: water restriction
      b) High urine osmolality (>285 mOsm/kg): ADH dependent
        (1) Hypovolemic: gastrointestinal losses, renal losses (diuretics, mineralocorticoid deficiency), third-spacing
          (a) Treatment: normal saline
        (2) Euvolemic: SIADH, adrenal insufficiency, hypothyroidism
          (a) Treatment: free water restriction, hypertonic saline, vaptans (SIADH)
        (3) Hypervolemic: heart failure, cirrhosis, nephrotic syndrome
          (a) Treatment: water and Na+ restriction, diuresis
  C. Treatment: Na^+ should be corrected at a rate <8 to 12 mEq/L over 24 hours in order to avoid osmotic demyelination syndrome (ODS) characterized by encephalopathy, seizures, dysphagia, neuromuscular weakness, lethargy, tremors, and paralysis; severe case of ODS is "locked-in syndrome"
    1. Chronic hyponatremia, hypokalemia, liver disease, malnutrition, alcoholism are higher risk for ODS and should be corrected <8 mEq/L over 24 hours; initial level of serum sodium does not necessarily correlate with the development of ODS

VI. Hypernatremia (Na^+ > 145 mEq/L): water deficit and/or excess solute
  A. Symptoms: restlessness, confusion, seizures
  B. Diagnosis
    1. Hypovolemic
      a) High urine sodium (>20 mEq/L): renal losses (diuretics, postobstructive, intrinsic renal disease)
      b) Low urine sodium (<20 mEq/L): extrarenal losses (burns, diarrhea, fistulas)

2. Euvolemic
    a) Low urine osmolality (<300 mOsm/kg) diabetes insipidus (nephrogenic or central)
    b) High urine osmolality (>300 mOsm/kg) insensible losses, hypodipsia
3. Hypervolemic
    a) High urine sodium (>20 mEq/L): hyperaldosteronism, Cushing syndrome, exogenous sodium
C. Treatment: Na⁺ should be corrected at a rate of <8 to 10 mEq/L over 24 hours to avoid cerebral edema

1. Free water deficit $= 0.6 \times kg \times (\frac{Na}{140} - 1)$

VII. Other common electrolyte abnormalities

Electrolyte abnormality	Common causes	Symptoms	EKG findings	Treatment
Hyperkalemia	Renal failure, tissue trauma, acidosis	Weakness with hyporeflexia	Peaked T waves, P wave flattening, PR prolongation, wide QRS	Calcium gluconate (stabilize cardiac membrane), insulin + glucose and albuterol (shift intracellular), Kayexalate, furosemide, dialysis
Hypokalemia	Hydrochlorothiazide, furosemide, gastrointestinal losses	Weakness, ileus	Flattened/ inverted T wave, ST depression, U wave, QTc prolonged	Potassium supplementation
Hypercalcemia	Cancer with bony metastases, multiple myeloma, hyperparathyroidism	Lethargy, nausea, vomiting, hypotension	Short ST, wide T wave	Normal saline, Lasix, calcitonin, bisphosphonates
Hypocalcemia	After parathyroidectomy or thyroidectomy, furosemide, pancreatitis, low vitamin D	Perioral numbness/ tingling, hyperreflexia, Chvostek sign, Trousseau sign	Prolonged ST, Long QTc	Calcium supplementation
Hypermagnesemia	Renal failure, laxatives, antacids	Lethargy, areflexia, paralysis, com	Prolonged PR, QRS widening	Calcium, normal saline, furosemide, dialysis
Hypomagnesemia	Diuresis, chronic TPN, EtOH abuse	Irritability, confusion, hyperreflexia, tetany, seizures	Tall T wave, ST depression	Magnesium supplementation
Hyperphosphatemia	Renal failure	Muscle cramps, perioral tingling	Prolonged QTc	Sevelamer, low phosphate in diet, dialysis
Hypophosphatemia	Refeeding syndrome	Muscle weakness, difficulty weaning off ventilator	Various	Phosphate supplementation

QUESTIONS

1. A 34-year-old G1P0 21-week pregnant female with a history of severe asthma requiring multiple prior hospitalizations is postoperative day 1 from an uncomplicated laparoscopic cholecystectomy. On morning rounds she is found to be in moderate respiratory distress with accessory muscle use, diaphoresis, and tachypnea to 30 breaths per minute despite nebulized ipratropium and albuterol and IV hydrocortisone. She is saturating 99% on 2L nasal canula. Her heart rate is 90 beats per minute. An arterial blood gas demonstrates a pH of 7.40, PaO$_2$ of 97, PaCO$_2$ of 42, and HCO$_3^-$ of 24. What is the next best step in management?

   A. CTA of the chest
   B. Intravenous (IV) magnesium sulfate
   C. Transfer to intensive care unit (ICU) for observation
   D. Continue breathing treatments
   E. Intubation

2. A 16-year-old girl arrives via ambulance after the family became concerned that she was behaving strangely. She appears disoriented and will answer simple questions but is evasive in answering questions about events leading up to her arrival. Vital signs are normal except for a respiratory rate of 7 and a body mass index (BMI) of 16. Arterial blood gas and basic metabolic panel are consistent with a metabolic alkalosis. Which of the following tests will be most helpful in establishing a diagnosis?

   A. Urine drug screen
   B. Computed tomography of the brain
   C. Spot urine chloride concentration
   D. Electrocardiogram (ECG)
   E. Abdominal ultrasound

3. A 64-year-old female with a past medical history of breast cancer with diffuse osseous metastases is admitted to the general surgery service for nonoperative management of small bowel obstruction thought to be due to adhesive disease. Her admission labs demonstrate a calcium of 12.6 mg/dL with an albumin of 2.0 g/dL. She is given a normal saline bolus followed by a drip at 200 mL/hr. IV calcitonin is also administered. What is the best next step in management?

   A. Administer IV furosemide
   B. Administer IV sevelamer
   C. Convert to maintenance fluids with lactated Ringer's
   D. Administer IV zoledronic acid
   E. Administer IV hydrocortisone

4. A 44-year-old male with poorly controlled type 2 diabetes mellitus presents with acute cholecystitis and a blood glucose of 800 mg/dL, Na$^+$ of 120 mEq/L, an anion gap of 22, and positive urine ketones. He is initiated on IV fluids, an insulin drip, and antibiotics. What is true regarding his sodium?

   A. The corrected sodium is 127 mEq/L
   B. The sodium should not be corrected faster than 5 mEq/L in 24 hours
   C. The corrected sodium is 134 mEq/L
   D. It is impossible to correct for sodium in the setting of ketones
   E. His hyponatremia is due to glucose-induced diuresis

5. A 76-year-old female is postoperative day 4 from sigmoid colon resection. Her postoperative course has been uneventful, but she has not yet started passing flatus. Overnight, the urinary output has decreased to 20 cc/hour, and the patient has had several episodes of emesis. Lab work includes a blood urea nitrogen (BUN) of 40 mg/dL and serum creatinine of 1.5 mg/dL. Urinary sodium is 10 mEq/L. What is the most likely etiology of oliguria in this patient?

   A. Postoperative ileus
   B. Intraabdominal hemorrhage
   C. Intraoperative hypotension
   D. Inadvertent ligation of the left ureter
   E. Drug-induced nephrotoxicity

6. Which of the following is true regarding sodium and water maintenance in the geriatric patient?

   A. There is an increase in the ratio of intracellular to extracellular water
   B. A hyperactive thirst response predisposes geriatric patients to hyponatremia
   C. Elevated antidiuretic hormone levels predispose patients to sodium retention
   D. Atrial natriuretic peptide level increases with aging
   E. There is a relative increase in the activity of the renin-angiotensin-aldosterone system

7. A 50-year-old type I diabetic male is admitted to the hospital for the workup of vague abdominal pain and malaise. Past medical history includes total proctocolectomy with ileostomy for ulcerative colitis. Routine laboratory values include: pH 7.26, pCO₂ 24 mm Hg, pO₂ 100 mm Hg, sodium 129 mEq/L, potassium 2.9 mEq/L, chloride 110 mEq/L, and bicarbonate 12 mEq/L. Which of the following is the most likely diagnosis?

   A. Excessive ileostomy output
   B. Kidney failure
   C. Diabetic ketoacidosis
   D. Lactic acidosis
   E. Methanol intoxication

8. A 62-year-old female was recently diagnosed on upper endoscopy with a near obstructing distal gastric tumor but was subsequently lost to follow-up. She now returns to the ED with 24 hours of nonbilious vomiting and abdominal pain. What is the most significant contributing factor to hypokalemia in this patient?

   A. Intracellular shift
   B. Increased excretion in the urine
   C. Loss of potassium with emesis
   D. Metabolic acidosis
   E. Hypokalemic fluid replacement

9. Which of the following is considered a normal physiologic change in pregnancy?

   A. Decrease in blood pH
   B. Decrease in minute ventilation
   C. Increased vital capacity
   D. Right-shift of oxyhemoglobin dissociation curve
   E. Relative leukopenia

10. Which of the following is true regarding dehydration and/or hypovolemia in children?

    A. Children only need to lose 5% of total body water to produce significant symptoms of hypovolemia
    B. Hypovolemia refers to a reduction in free water
    C. Dehydration will primarily result in extracellular fluid losses
    D. Profound hypernatremic hypovolemia should be corrected initially with hypotonic fluids
    E. Oral fluid replacement is adequate in most children with insensible fluid losses

11. A 45-year-old male with congestive heart failure is being treated in the ICU for sepsis secondary to pneumonia. Over the last 24 hours, he has received 11 L of crystalloid and was started on vasopressors for hypotension. His urine output has dropped to 20 mL/hr. Delivered tidal volumes on the mechanical ventilator have also significantly decreased. Physical exam reveals a tense abdomen, abdominal fluid wave, and anasarca. Current bladder pressure is 25 mm Hg. The most appropriate initial management is:

    A. Neuromuscular blockade
    B. Immediate decompressive laparotomy
    C. Percutaneous drainage of intraabdominal fluid
    D. Continuous renal replacement therapy
    E. Change resuscitative fluid to albumin

12. Which of the following is true regarding serum osmolarity and serum osmolality?

    A. Large proteins are the most important contributors to serum osmolality
    B. The presence of an osmolar gap indicates the presence of a foreign molecule that readily distributes across cell membranes
    C. The difference between serum osmolarity and serum osmolality is highly variable depending on the physiologic state
    D. Sodium is multiplied by two in the calculation for serum osmolarity because of its increased osmotic activity
    E. The number of molecules, and not the size, is the most important contributor to serum osmolarity

13. An elderly patient presents to the emergency department (ED) with increased thirst and urinary output. Which of the following findings would be most helpful to suggest diabetes insipidus (DI) as the likely etiology in this patient?

    A. Hypernatremia
    B. Hyperglycemia
    C. Hyponatremia
    D. Low urine osmolality
    E. High serum-to-urine osmolality ratio

14. A 58-year-old male alcoholic presents to the ED complaining of increased abdominal girth over the last several weeks. He underwent a diagnostic ultrasound 1 year ago, which showed evidence of cirrhosis. Physical exam reveals pitting edema of the lower extremities and positive abdominal fluid wave. In addition to alcohol cessation, what is the next step in management?

    A. Free water restriction
    B. Transjugular intrahepatic portosystemic shunt
    C. Intravenous furosemide with transition to PO once ascites resolves
    D. Strict sodium restriction (<1 g/day)
    E. Combination of oral furosemide and spironolactone

15. A 25-year-old female is postoperative day 1 from a laparoscopic, converted to open cholecystectomy for acute cholecystitis. Since surgery, she has had one episode of emesis, urinary output has decreased to 0.3 cc/kg per hour, and serum sodium is found to be 131 mEq/L. Serum creatinine is normal, but antidiuretic hormone (ADH) level is elevated. What is the most likely cause of these findings?

    A. Syndrome of inappropriate antidiuretic hormone secretion (SIADH)
    B. Normal physiologic response to surgery
    C. Acute kidney injury
    D. Emesis
    E. Congestive heart failure

16. A 65-year-old male with massive intracranial hemorrhage after a ruptured intracranial aneurysm is currently in the neurosurgical intensive care unit (ICU). Two days ago, he underwent intravascular coiling of the lesion. Because of increased urinary output over the last 24 hours, a urine sodium was measured and found to be 35 mEq/L. Current labs include a serum sodium of 128 mEq/L and a hemoglobin of 18 g/dL. Central venous pressure is 2 mm Hg. Which of the following is the most appropriate initial treatment?

    A. Normal saline
    B. Free water restriction
    C. Desmopressin
    D. Demeclocycline
    E. Tolvaptan

17. A 75-year-old male is in the ICU due to sepsis 5 days after a colectomy for a perforated diverticulitis. While the nurse is checking his blood pressure, his hand went into a spasm. Which of the following is the most likely etiology?

    A. Hypercalcemia
    B. Hypermagnesemia
    C. Hypomagnesemia
    D. Hyponatremia
    E. Hyperkalemia

18. A 48-year-old male with past medical history of alcoholic cirrhosis and refractory ascites is admitted to the ICU recovering from spontaneous bacterial peritonitis (SBP). He is now off the antibiotics, and there is no evidence of continued infection. Over the course of his hospitalization, his creatinine level increased from 1.0 to 1.6 mg/dL. Urinalysis reveals no evidence of proteinuria or microhematuria. Which of the following is the initial step in management?

    A. Fluid resuscitation with normal saline
    B. Cessation of diuretics
    C. Terlipressin and albumin
    D. Initiation of continuous renal replacement therapy
    E. Transjugular intrahepatic portosystemic shunt (TIPS)

19. A 24-year-old female underwent a jejunal resection complicated by abdominal compartment syndrome and an open abdomen after a motor vehicle collision. She is eventually discharged home but returns 1 week later with copious output of yellowish fluid from her midline wound. She has noted diminished urinary output, is tachycardic, and has decreased skin turgor. What combination of electrolyte abnormalities is most likely present in this patient?

    A. Hyponatremia, hypokalemia, and metabolic acidosis
    B. Hypokalemia, hypochloremia, and metabolic alkalosis
    C. Hyponatremia, hyperkalemia, and metabolic acidosis
    D. Hypernatremia and metabolic acidosis
    E. Hyperkalemia and metabolic alkalosis

20. A 55-year-old male is admitted to the hospital with altered mental status. Paramedics report that they found multiple empty beer cans in his home. He is found to have a serum alcohol concentration of 255 mg/dL and a serum sodium concentration of 118 mEq/L. Fluid resuscitation is initiated with normal saline and sodium levels return to normal by the next morning. On hospital day 5, he develops spastic quadriplegia and is unresponsive to external stimuli. Which of the following is true regarding this condition?

    A. It could have been prevented with the use of hypertonic saline
    B. Desmopressin can be used as an adjunct to fluid replacement to prevent this complication
    C. Cerebral adaptions to hyponatremia take up to a week to develop
    D. Recovery is impossible after the onset of neurologic symptoms
    E. Injury is restricted to the pons

ANSWERS

1. E. This pregnant patient is experiencing an acute asthma exacerbation with acute respiratory failure in the postoperative setting. While the patient is oxygenating well as indicated by her PaO_2 and pulse oximetry, her blood gas is concerning for impending hypercarbic respiratory failure. As a result of a progesterone-induced increase in alveolar ventilation during pregnancy, arterial PCO_2 typically falls to a plateau of 27 to 32 mm Hg. Furthermore, during acute asthma exacerbations, respiratory drive increases resulting in hyperventilation and decreased $PaCO_2$. As such, a $PaCO_2$ of 42 in this patient indicates airway narrowing and dynamic hyperinflation so severe that alveolar ventilation has already decreased despite increased respiratory drive. Given this clinical picture, the patient should be intubated for management of her hypercarbic respiratory failure and exhaustion as indicated by her use of accessory muscles of respiration, diaphoresis, and tachypnea on physical exam. The first priority in this patient should be to establish a safe airway and begin mechanical ventilation to reduce the patient's work of breathing. Furthermore, this can provide a valuable bridge while waiting for bronchodilators and glucocorticoid medications to reduce airway swelling. It would be unsafe to only continue breathing treatments or administer IV magnesium which may not reverse airway edema in a timely enough manner to account for this patient's decompensating respiratory status (B, D). Pulmonary embolism is unlikely given no evidence of hypoxia or tachycardia (A). This patient should be transferred to the ICU, but only after addressing her respiratory failure with intubation (C).

Reference: Brenner B, Corbridge T, Kazzi A. Intubation and mechanical ventilation of the asthmatic patient in respiratory failure. *Proc Am Thorac Soc.* 2009;6(4):371–379.

2. C. Severe metabolic alkalosis leads to hypoventilation due to inhibition of the respiratory center in the medulla. The etiology of metabolic alkalosis is generally clear from history (excessive emesis, diuretic use) alone. However, in scenarios where the patient is unable, or unwilling, to provide a history (such as bulimia), the measurement of urine chloride concentration can provide important diagnostic information. When metabolic alkalosis is associated with hypovolemia, the urine chloride concentration will be appropriately low (<20 mEq/L) in response to the corresponding hypochloremia and volume contraction. Examples of chloride-responsive metabolic alkalosis include excessive vomiting or laxative abuse, such as in anorexia-nervosa or bulimia-nervosa. Diuretic use is another common etiology, though recent use will increase the urine chloride concentration. Chloride unresponsive metabolic alkalosis (urine chloride concentration >20 mEq/L) can be associated with hypervolemia in the setting of excessive mineralocorticoid concentrations (primary aldosteronism) or conditions that mimic mineralocorticoid excess (licorice ingestion). Disorders that lead to increased urinary salt wasting (Bartter or Gitelman syndrome) will also be chloride unresponsive but will be associated with hypovolemia. Most drugs of abuse that would lead to altered mental status and hypoventilation

will be associated with a respiratory acidosis, not a metabolic alkalosis (A). Electrocardiogram may show signs of hypokalemia, but that is a common finding in metabolic alkalosis (D). Computed tomography and abdominal ultrasound may be useful in the workup of altered mental status, but laxative abuse or self-induced vomiting is a much more likely diagnosis in this scenario (B, E).

3. D. This patient presents with severe hypercalcemia secondary to malignancy. While this patient first appears to have moderate hypercalcemia, defined as calcium between 12 and 14 mg/dL, after correcting for low serum albumin, her calcium corrects to 14.4, which is considered severe, and therefore prompts aggressive treatment. Hypercalcemia of malignancy presents by three primary mechanisms: (1) tumor secretion of parathyroid hormone-related protein (PTHrP), (2) osteolytic metastases, and (3) tumor production of 1,25 dihydroxyvitamin D. In up to 80% of cases, hypercalcemia of malignancy is secondary to excretion of PTHrP. In approximately 20% of cases, osteolytic metastases are responsible for hypercalcemia. Breast cancer is known to cause hypercalcemia through both mechanisms. Hypercalcemic patients are often dehydrated, since the hypercalcemic state impairs the kidney's ability to concentrate urine. Initial treatment is via a normal saline bolus followed by a 200 cc/hr drip, which should be titrated for a urine output of 1 to 2 mL/kg/hr. Lactated Ringer's should be avoided due to their calcium content (C). Once the patient is rendered euvolemic, adjunct agents can be added. Calcitonin reduces osteoclast activity and, in turn, decreases serum calcium. Often volume expansion and calcitonin are all that is needed and can reduce serum calcium in 12 to 24 hours. However, in this case, the hypercalcemia is likely a long-term problem. As such, the concurrent administration of bisphosphonates is encouraged, particularly for severe cases of hypercalcemia of malignancy. Multiple randomized, controlled trials support the fact that bisphosphonates (zoledronate or pamidronate) are potent and relatively safe medications for the treatment of moderate to severe hypercalcemia of malignancy. It should be noted that this drug takes days to render its effect. Glucocorticoids are not demonstrated to have benefit in the treatment of hypercalcemia of malignancy (E). Sevelamer, a phosphate binder, is not indicated for use in hypercalcemia of malignancy (B). Furosemide has not been demonstrated as an effective medication for management of hypercalcemia of malignancy. However, loop diuretics do cause calciuresis, but they induce fluid loss, and their utility is therefore more limited (A).

References: LeGrand S, Leskuski D, Zama I. Narrative review: furosemide for hypercalcemia: an unproven yet common practice. *Ann Intern Med.* 2008;149(4):259–263.

Major P, Lortholary A, Hon J, et al. Zoledronic acid is superior to pamidronate in the treatment of hypercalcemia of malignancy: a pooled analysis of two randomized, controlled clinical trials. *J Clin Oncol.* 2001;19(2):558–567.

4. C. This patient presents with diabetic ketoacidosis as demonstrated by his elevated blood glucose, increased anion gap, and positive urine ketones. Additionally, he presents with hypertonic hyponatremia with a measured serum sodium of 120 mEq/L in the setting of hyperglycemia. The presence of elevated extracellular glucose results in increased serum tonicity and the shift of water from the intracellular to the extracellular space, thereby lowering serum sodium concentration. The calculation to correct for this is to add 2 mEq/L of Na^+ for each 100 mg/dL the blood glucose is above 100 mg/dL. As such, this patient's serum sodium corrects to 134 mEq/L (A). Clinician must be extremely diligent in correcting serum sodium in a controlled manner (less than 8–12 mEq/L per 24 hrs) so as to not cause osmotic demyelination syndrome (B). Ketones do not affect the correction of serum sodium in the setting of hyperglycemia (D). Glucosuria can contribute to significant total body depletion of sodium and potassium; however, in this case the sodium corrects to a normal value and thus is more likely to represent hypertonic hyponatremia (E).

Reference: Emmett M, Sterns RH. Fluid, electrolyte, and acid-base disturbances. *J Am Soc Nephrol.* 2013;12:191.

5. A. The first step in identifying the etiology of oliguria is an adequate history and analysis of the BUN:creatinine ratio. A BUN:creatinine ratio of greater than 20 with a history of hypoperfusion or hypotension is virtually diagnostic of prerenal azotemia. However, no such history is provided in this vignette. At this point, urinalysis is necessary. A low urinary sodium concentration (<20 mEq/L) or a low fractional excretion of sodium (<1%) is indicative of a prerenal cause of acute kidney injury. In the presence of emesis and failure to pass flatus, ileus is the most likely diagnosis (A). Ileus or small bowel obstruction can lead to significant intraabdominal fluid sequestration that, without adequate fluid resuscitation, decreases renal blood flow and subsequently urinary output. The low urinary sodium is the result of physiologically elevated ADH secondary to the hypovolemia. Though intraabdominal hemorrhage would lead to a similar clinical picture, bleeding is more common earlier in the postoperative period (POD 0-1) (B). You would also expect the consequences of intraoperative hypotension to present earlier (C). Drug-induced nephrotoxicity is an intrinsic acute kidney injury, and urinary sodium would not be low (E). Inadvertent ligation of the ureter typically does not present with oliguria unless both sides are affected (D).

6. D. Numerous physiologic changes associated with aging diminish the geriatric population's ability to adapt to changes in the environment or health, especially regarding the maintenance of water and electrolyte balance. Loss of lean body mass decreases total body water and decreases the ratio of intracellular to extracellular water (A). This results in a diminished ability to respond to fluid losses because there is less water to mobilize from the intracellular space. In addition, the older population has a diminished thirst response to changes in serum osmolality (B). The kidney itself also undergoes structural changes that result in a diminished glomerular filtration rate, which decreases the kidneys' ability to dilute urine in response to a water load. However, the kidney also shows a diminished ability to concentrate the urine in response to dehydration. This is partly due to reduced responsiveness to ADH in the aged kidney (C). On the other hand, atrial natriuretic peptide levels increase, which further

contributes to renal salt and water wasting. The renin-angiotensin-aldosterone system is also suppressed, leading to dysregulation of sodium and potassium balance (E).

References: El-Sharkawy AM, Sahota O, Maughan RJ, Lobo DN. The pathophysiology of fluid and electrolyte balance in the older adult surgical patient. *Clin Nutr.* 2014;33(1):6–13.

Miller M. Disorders of fluid balance. In: Halter JB, Ouslander JG, Tinetti ME, Studenski S, High KP, Asthana S, eds. *Hazzard's geriatric medicine and gerontology.* 6th ed. McGraw-Hill; 2009.

7. A. A low pH with a corresponding low pCO_2 and low bicarbonate is indicative of a metabolic acidosis. Calculation of the anion gap [129 (Na)–110 (Cl) – 12 (HCO_3)] reveals a value of 7, which is consistent with a non-anion gap metabolic acidosis (normal 8–16). The patient's history of total proctocolectomy and non–anion gap metabolic acidosis is consistent with gastrointestinal (GI) losses from excessive ileostomy output. All of the other answer choices listed will contribute to an anion gap (B–E).

8. B. Gastric outlet obstruction and large volume emesis result in significant volume loss in addition to hydrogen and chloride ions. Though gastric juice has a higher concentration of potassium than serum, at 10 mEq/L, the overall potassium content is low and relatively insignificant compared with the loss of hydrogen and chloride (C). This subsequently leads to a hypochloremic metabolic alkalosis, not an acidosis (D). The volume depletion, initially, is counteracted by the mobilization of extravascular fluids so the kidney maintains a relatively constant flow. Initially, the kidney responds by excreting the excess bicarbonate in the urine in combination with sodium and potassium to balance the negative charge. However, as more sodium is lost and hypovolemia becomes more apparent, the renin-angiotensin-aldosterone system is activated. This increases the absorption of sodium and water, but potassium continues to be excreted, leading to hypokalemia. Eventually, the kidney will begin to compensate for the hypokalemia by exchanging potassium ions for hydrogen ions, which perpetuates the alkalosis and causes the paradoxical aciduria associated with excessive loss of gastric contents. Though alkalosis does cause an intracellular shift of potassium ions, the effect is variable and does not account for the significant hypokalemia seen with metabolic alkalosis (A). Before replacement of the hypokalemia, volume expansion with crystalloid is recommended, which will reduce the effects of aldosterone and potassium loss in the urine (E).

References: Aronson PS, Giebisch G. Effects of pH on potassium: new explanations for old observations. *J Am Soc Nephrol.* 2011;22(11):1981–1989.

Lee Hamm L, Hering-Smith KS, Nakhoul NL. Acid-base and potassium homeostasis. *Semin Nephrol.* 2013;33(3):257–264.

9. D. Pregnancy causes a number of physiologic changes, either to improve conditions for the developing fetus or as a side effect of the increased metabolic demands placed on the mother. From a respiratory standpoint, the changes are primarily related to the increased production of progesterone and the mass effect of the uterus on the diaphragm. Progesterone acts on the central nervous system to lower CO_2 levels. In an effort to lower pCO_2, the tidal volume and respiratory rate increase, causing an increase in minute ventilation (B). This reduction in the pCO_2 causes a respiratory alkalosis

(A). The mass effect from the uterus causes a reduction in inspiratory and expiratory reserve, as well as functional and residual capacity. However, vital capacity remains relatively unchanged (C). The increased metabolic demands require an increase in oxygen delivery. This is accomplished by an increase in cardiac output. The total blood volume increases proportionally to the cardiac output, but the increase in plasma volume is greater than the increase in red blood cell mass, which causes dilutional anemia. The increased cardiac output proportionally increases the glomerular flow rate of the kidney and reduces circulating urea. The oxyhemoglobin dissociation curve also shifts to the right to facilitate unloading of oxygen to the fetus. In addition to the increased affinity of fetal hemoglobin for oxygen, there is an increase in 2,3-DPG, which further facilitates delivery of oxygen to the fetus. There is a mild reduction in platelets, likely because of increased platelet aggregation from hypercoagulability. However, there is an increase in circulating white blood cells (E).

10. E. Though frequently used interchangeably, dehydration and hypovolemia are separate clinical entities. Dehydration refers to a reduction in free water (fluid loss in excess of solute loss), while hypovolemia is a loss of circulating extracellular volume (B). This is an important distinction because of the distribution of total body water. Two-thirds of total body water is intracellular, which means that dehydration will primarily result in intracellular fluid losses (C). In fact, almost 10% of total body water needs to be lost before significant signs of hypovolemia manifest. Hypovolemia from dehydration is relatively rare in people with access to water because the increase in plasma osmolality stimulates a strong thirst response, which is why it typically only presents when people are reliant on others (children and the elderly) (A). In hypovolemia, the serum sodium will correspond with the type of fluid lost and any prehospital replacement that has taken place. Insensible losses, such as sweating, will result in hypernatremia because the fluid lost is hypotonic to plasma and increases in ADH will result in sodium and water retention. Secretory diarrhea or bleeding, on the other hand, results in fluid losses that are isotonic to plasma and don't have a direct effect on serum sodium levels. However, replacement of these losses with hypotonic fluids will lead to hyponatremia. Profound hypernatremic hypovolemia mandates rapid intravascular volume replacement with intravenous isotonic fluids. After the severe volume depletion is treated, the replacement of the free water deficit can take place more slowly. Care should be taken to avoid rapid correction of hypernatremia because it can precipitate cerebral edema (D). Unless there are direct contraindications, such as altered mental status or vascular compromise, oral replacement therapy is likely adequate and is the preferred replacement strategy by the American Academy of Pediatrics.

Reference: Spandorfer PR, Alessandrini EA, Joffe MD, Localio R, Shaw KN. Oral versus intravenous rehydration of moderately dehydrated children: a randomized, controlled trial. *Pediatrics.* 2005;115(2):295–301.

11. C. Abdominal compartment syndrome is defined as a sustained intraabdominal pressure of greater than 20 mm Hg associated with new-onset organ failure. Early clinical signs are oliguric acute kidney injury and increased peak airway pressures or decreased tidal volumes in a pressure mode of ventilation. It is further subdivided into primary and secondary depending on the etiology. Primary abdominal compartment syndrome refers to etiologies that arise in the abdomen (such as volvulus or colonic pseudo obstruction), and current recommendations are for immediate decompressive laparotomy (B). However, in secondary abdominal compartment syndrome, such as cirrhotics or patients with congestive heart failure with tense ascites, nonsurgical treatments can first be attempted. In 2011, Cheatham and others treated abdominal compartment syndrome from ascites with percutaneous drainage, and 81% of study participants were successfully treated without a decompressive laparotomy (C). While the most recent consensus guidelines released by the World Society of the Abdominal Compartment Syndrome still advocate surgical intervention for abdominal compartment syndrome, they also maintain that the use of percutaneous catheter drainage for the treatment of obvious intraperitoneal fluid contributing to abdominal compartment syndrome should be used in place of decompressive laparotomy when it is technically feasible because it may alleviate the need for surgery. While neuromuscular blockade and diuresis may help with the treatment of intraabdominal hypertension, worsening kidney and lung function require immediate intervention (A, D). The role of albumin in abdominal compartment syndrome is still controversial (E).

References: Cheatham M, Safcsak K. Percutaneous catheter decompression in the treatment of elevated intraabdominal pressure. *Chest.* 2011;140(6):1428–1435.

Kirkpatrick AW, Roberts DJ, De Waele J, et al. Intra-abdominal hypertension and the abdominal compartment syndrome: updated consensus definitions and clinical practice guidelines from the World Society of the Abdominal Compartment Syndrome. *Intensive Care Med.* 2013;39(7):1190–1206.

12. E. Osmolarity and osmolality represent the number of osmotically active solutes (osmoles) in a given solution. Osmolarity is the number of osmoles in a liter of solution, and osmolality is the number of osmoles in a kg of water. Because the volume of a solution can vary slightly depending on temperature, osmolality is technically more precise, but under normal physiologic conditions the terms are essentially interchangeable because 1 L of water weighs 1 kg (C). Because the kinetic energy of dissolved solutes is based on the number, and not the size, large proteins like albumin have a relatively low contribution compared to more abundant molecules, like sodium (A). In order to contribute osmotic pressure across a semipermeable membrane, the dissolved solute must not be able to readily diffuse across the membrane. Thus, a foreign molecule that readily distributes intracellularly does not contribute to serum osmolality or an osmolar gap (B). The equation for the calculation of serum osmolality is 2 [Na] + [glucose]/18 + [BUN]/2.8. Sodium is multiplied by two to account for the corresponding anions (chloride and bicarbonate) that would otherwise need to be added separately (D). Serum osmolality can also be directly measured, normally by freezing point depression, and compared to the calculated value. If there is a significant difference between the calculated and measured serum osmolality, it indicates the presence of an osmotically active foreign solute, like methanol.

13. E. DI is a disease process characterized by either a low level of ADH (central DI) or diminished renal response to

ADH (nephrogenic DI). The first step in the evaluation of polyuria is the measurement of serum electrolytes, serum glucose, and urine and serum osmolality. In the absence of osmotic diuresis from hyperglycemia (i.e., diabetes mellitus), primary polydipsia, central DI, and nephrogenic DI are the most common etiologies (B). All three entities will show increased production of dilute urine, or low urine osmolality (D). However, in primary polydipsia, this is a normal response to increased water intake. Serum sodium levels will generally be low because of the increased intake of water. Increased urinary output with hyponatremia, low urine osmolality, and low or normal serum osmolality is virtually diagnostic (C). Diabetes insipidus, on the other hand, will be associated with low urine osmolality in the presence of elevated serum osmolality. Though hypernatremia is possible because of the excessive loss of water in the urine, in general, patients are able to compensate for the increased urinary output with increased oral intake of water (A). Suspicions can be confirmed with a water deprivation test. In primary polydipsia, the urinary output will decrease and the urine osmolality will increase as the test progresses because the stimulus for the polyuria has been removed. However, patients with DI lack the ability to concentrate urine, so the production of dilute urine will continue, despite rising serum osmolality. Once the patient's serum osmolality increases to a sufficient level, the administration of vasopressin will differentiate between nephrogenic and central DI. In central DI, the vasopressin will allow the kidneys to concentrate the urine. In nephrogenic DI, no response to exogenous vasopressin will be expected because the problem is the kidney's response to, not the absence of, ADH.

14. E. The mobilization of ascites in cirrhotic patients requires a negative sodium balance. This is accomplished through limiting oral intake of sodium and initiating diuresis. In the absence of significant hyponatremia (<125 mEq/L), free water restriction is generally not indicated (A). The problem lies in the inappropriate retention of sodium by the kidney, not excess free water. Diuresis should be initiated with an initial goal of negative 1 L/day, though 500 mL/day is likely adequate in the absence of peripheral edema. Oral spironolactone and furosemide should be initiated at an initial dose of 100 mg and 40 mg, respectively, per day. These can be increased to a maximum daily dose of 400 mg spironolactone and 160 mg furosemide. Simultaneous administration of these two medications potentiates the natriuretic effect of each and limits the potassium imbalance that can be seen with either agent alone. Unlike ascites secondary to heart failure, intravenous administration of diuretics in cirrhotics with new-onset ascites should generally be avoided because it can frequently result in azotemia (C). While strict sodium restriction will result in faster mobilization of ascites, the diet is more difficult to adhere to and can potentially worsen any malnutrition that is present; a sodium restriction of less than 2 g/day is generally all that is required (D). All patients should be considered for liver transplant because the onset of ascites is associated with a significantly worsened prognosis. Patients with ascites refractory to diuretics can be considered for serial paracentesis or portosystemic shunt. Transjugular intrahepatic portosystemic shunt is preferred over surgical shunts (B).

References: Runyon BA. *Management of adult patients with ascites due to cirrhosis: update 2012. AASLD Practice Guideline.* American Association for the Study of Liver Diseases; 2012. https://www.aasld.org/sites/default/files/2019-06/141020_Guideline_Ascites_4UFb_2015.pdf.

Wong P, Price JC, Herlong H. Cirrhosis and its complications. In: McKean SC, Ross JJ, Dressler DD, Brotman DJ, Ginsberg JS, eds. *Principles and practice of hospital medicine.* McGraw-Hill; 2012.

15. B. After a major operation, there is both an endocrine and a cytokine response to the stress. This can be partly inhibited by blocking painful stimuli from reaching the central nervous system, but it is also mediated by the effects of local tissue damage. Of the numerous physiologic responses, the retention of sodium and water is likely the most significant. This is dependent on multiple factors, including the effects of anesthetic drugs, renal vasoconstriction from catecholamines, increased plasma cortisol and aldosterone, and increased secretion of antidiuretic hormone (ADH). During an operation, ADH levels will increase up to 100 × normal. Though they begin to drop at the end of the operation, they remain elevated for several days. This response is largely secondary to the loss of intravascular volume by sequestration in injured tissues, or "third-spacing," dehydration from prolonged fasting, and insensible losses during the operation. This results in postoperative oliguria and hyponatremia. In this setting, the elevated level of ADH is not "inappropriate"; instead, it is a normal physiologic response to stress and decreased intravascular volume. In critically ill patients, the ADH level may get inappropriately high due to dysregulation of the hypothalamus-pituitary axis, resulting in SIADH. This subsequently leads to secretion of the natriuretic peptides to induce loss of sodium and water, resulting in a euvolemic state. Additionally, the loss of sodium is much greater than that of water, such that patients with SIADH have a significantly lower level of sodium compared with the mild hyponatremia seen postoperatively (A). By definition, this patient cannot have acute kidney injury with a normal creatinine clearance (C). Excess vomiting can present as hyponatremia, but a single episode of emesis is unlikely to produce this effect (D). Congestive heart failure is an unlikely cause of hyponatremia without other associated symptoms (E).

Reference: Rassam SS, Counsell DJ. Perioperative electrolyte and fluid balance. *Contin Educ Anaesth Crit Care Pain.* 2005;5(5):157–160.

16. A. In a neurologically injured patient with hyponatremia and elevated urinary sodium, the two most likely diagnoses are SIADH or an isolated natriuresis from elevated atrial natriuretic peptide (cerebral salt wasting syndrome). SIADH can have a natriuresis component as described in question 1. Though they have similar laboratory findings, the hyponatremia in cerebral salt wasting is caused by excessive urinary losses of sodium as opposed to excess water retention with SIADH. This means that the only measurable difference between SIADH and cerebral salt wasting is the intravascular volume status of the patient; hypovolemia for the latter, and euvolemia or hypervolemia for the former. Cerebral salt wasting is classically described as a patient with a subarachnoid hemorrhage and a sudden increase in urine output, which leads to hyponatremia and hypovolemia. The cause of cerebral salt wasting syndrome has not been completely characterized, and it is unclear whether natriuretic factors are released from the brain or are simply a downstream consequences of hormonal effects from the brain injury. The proposed theoretic mechanism is excessive release of atrial natriuretic peptide (ANP) from the cardiac myocytes in the right atrium. However, there are some authors who argue that this is simply a manifestation of SIADH because ANP levels will naturally rise to counteract the effects of ADH. Regardless, the low CVP and elevated hemoglobin in this patient indicate a reduction in intravascular volume, which should be replaced with normal saline. Fluid restriction, in an attempt to treat SIADH, could potentially cause worsening cerebral ischemia (B). Desmopressin is an ADH analogue used to treat central diabetes insipidus (inadequate production of ADH), which is characterized by excessive output of dilute urine and normal to high plasma sodium (C). Demeclocycline is a tetracycline antibiotic that blocks the responsiveness of the renal collecting tubules to ADH; it is used off-label as an adjunct to treat SIADH that is unresponsive to fluid restriction (D). "Vaptans" are a category of medications that function as vasopressin receptor antagonists and have also been used to treat SIADH (E).

References: Robinson AG. The posterior pituitary (neurohypophysis). In: Gardner DG, Shoback D, eds. *Greenspan's basic & clinical endocrinology.* 9th ed. McGraw-Hill; 2011.

Ropper AH. The hypothalamus and neuroendocrine disorders. In: Ropper AH, Samuels MA, Klein JP, eds. *Adams & Victor's principles of neurology.* 10th ed. McGraw-Hill; 2014.

17. C. Hypomagnesemia is one of the most common electrolyte abnormalities in hospitalized patients (11%–65%) and particularly in critically ill patients. Most patients are asymptomatic but can become symptomatic as the level drops below 1.2 mg/dL. Symptoms can manifest as simple neuromuscular irritability, as demonstrated above by the presence of Trousseau sign (spasm of the forearm and hand with occlusion of the brachial artery) or, in more serious cases, as tetany, nystagmus, and seizures. Depletion of magnesium also leads to both atrial and ventricular arrhythmias. However, hypomagnesemia commonly presents in the presence of other electrolyte deficiencies, and the individual contribution of magnesium is often difficult to determine. Replacement therapy for symptomatic magnesium deficiency is mandatory, but the treatment of asymptomatic hypomagnesemia is less well defined. Rubeiz et al. showed increased mortality in patients with hypomagnesemia on admission to the medical ICU or ward. Similarly, a review article published in the Journal of Clinical Medicine Research, which included 20 different studies, showed a correlation between low magnesium levels and increased adverse outcomes and mortality in patients with sepsis. Hypercalcemia, hypermagnesemia, hyponatremia, and hyperkalemia would not present with neuromuscular irritability (A, B, D, E).

References: McEvoy C, Murray PT. Electrolyte disorders in critical care. In: Hall JB, Schmidt GA, Kress JP. eds. *Principles of critical care.* 4th ed. McGraw-Hill; 2014.

Rubeiz G, Thill-Baharozian M, Hardie D. Association of hypomagnesemia and mortality in acutely ill medical patients. *Critical Care Medicine.* 1993;21(2):203–209.

Velissaris D, Karamouzos V, Pierrakos C, et al., Hypomagnesemia in critically ill sepsis patients. *J Clin Med Res.* 2015;7(12): 911–918.

18. B. More than 50% of patients with cirrhosis and renal failure will die within 1 month of the diagnosis. The most common cause of renal failure in patients with cirrhosis is prerenal azotemia, so the cessation of diuretics and volume expansion with human albumin and not normal saline (A) is the initial step when acute kidney injury is suspected. Failure to respond to these measures raises concern for the hepatorenal syndrome. The current diagnostic criteria for hepatorenal system include: cirrhosis with ascites, serum creatinine greater than 1.5 mg/dL, no improvement in serum creatinine after at least 2 days of diuretic withdrawal and volume expansion with albumin, absence of shock, no current or recent treatment with nephrotoxic drugs, and the absence of parenchymal kidney disease (no proteinuria, no microhematuria, and a normal renal ultrasound). In addition, urine sodium is very low (<10 mEq/L). The most important physiologic change in hepatorenal syndrome is splanchnic vasodilation, which causes a cascade effect resulting in increased sympathetic nerve activity, increased activity of the renin-angiotensin system, increased nonosmotic vasopressin release, renal vasoconstriction, abolished autoregulation of the kidney, activation of the hepatorenal reflex, and a decrease in renal blood flow. Treatment depends on the severity of illness and whether or not the patient is in the ICU. In the critically ill, treatment with albumin and norepinephrine can be initiated. In the non–critically ill, terlipressin (a vasopressor analogue) and albumin volume expansion have shown the greatest incidence of renal recovery (C). However, in countries where terlipressin is unavailable, like the United States, therapy can be initiated with midodrine and octreotide. The ideal treatment is liver transplantation but is limited by availability. Dialysis or renal replacement therapy should only be used as a bridge to transplant because it hasn't been shown to decrease mortality or improve renal recovery (D). TIPS can be considered in patients with refractory ascites, but its role in the treatment of hepatorenal syndrome is unclear (E).

References: Israelsen M, Gluud L, Kraq A. Acute kidney injury and hepatorenal syndrome in cirrhosis. *J Gastroenterol Hepatol.* 2015;30(2):236–243.

Lenz K, Buder R, Kapun L, Voglmayr M. Treatment and management of ascites and hepatorenal syndrome: an update. *Therap Adv Gastroenterol.* 2015;8(2):83–100.

Runyon BA. *Management of adult patients with ascites due to cirrhosis: update 2012. AASLD Practice Guideline.* American Association for the Study of Liver Diseases; 2012. https://www.aasld.org/sites/default/files/2019-06/141020_Guideline_Ascites_4UFb_2015.pdf.

19. A. The corresponding electrolyte abnormalities seen with hypovolemia are heavily dependent on the composition of the corresponding secretions that are lost. Because of the relatively higher concentration of bicarbonate and potassium in small bowel and pancreatic secretions, it is common for excessive losses to result in hypokalemia and metabolic acidosis. The sodium content is generally isotonic, or even slightly hypotonic, to plasma. However, patients with an intact thirst mechanism will typically replace fluids with free water, making hyponatremia much more common on presentation. Stomach secretions are high in hydrogen and chloride, which results in a hypochloremic metabolic alkalosis. The renal response to these losses results in hypokalemia (B). The highest concentration of potassium in any gastrointestinal secretion is saliva, followed by the large intestine. Excessive losses of these fluids frequently present with hypokalemia. Sweat is typically hypotonic to plasma and effectively results in free water loss, though the sweat gland's ability to absorb sodium does diminish as output increases. If oral intake is inadequate, this can lead to a hypernatremic metabolic acidosis (D). Hyponatremia, hyperkalemia, and mild metabolic acidosis can be seen in adrenal insufficiency (C). Hyperkalemia is not typically seen in conjunction with metabolic alkalosis because the renal response to alkalosis causes the wasting of potassium in the urine (E).

20. B. Osmotic demyelination syndrome (ODS), formally known as central pontine myelinolysis, is a condition brought on by a change in serum osmolality classically described with the rapid correction of chronic hyponatremia. Chronic hyponatremia results in the loss of osmotically active solutes and water from brain cells, which protects against cerebral edema. This process starts with the initiation of hyponatremia and is generally completely in place by 48 hours (C), which is why hyponatremia that develops over this time period is generally not associated with significant symptoms. While the exact mechanism is unknown, studies in animals have shown that the areas of the brain that are slowest at replacing the lost solutes are the most likely to undergo demyelination. This process was originally described in the pons, but it has now been described in other areas of the brain as well (E). While some recovery has been described weeks after the onset of neurologic symptoms and there has been some data to support reinstitution of hyponatremia to improve prognosis (D), prevention is the mainstay of treatment. This involves slow correction of chronic or unknown chronicity hyponatremia by no more than 9 mEq/L per day. In cases of associated hypovolemia, volume replacement can remove the stimulus for ADH release, resulting in free water diuresis and an increased rate of sodium correction. For this reason, desmopressin has been advocated for use in this scenario to allow the production of more concentrated urine and prevent rapid autocorrection of sodium. The use of hypertonic saline is generally unnecessary unless the cause of hyponatremia is clearly acute by history and there are signs of cerebral edema or elevated intracranial pressures (A). As one might expect, cerebral mechanisms deal with chronic hypernatremia by increasing the concentration of these same osmotically active solutes and rapid correction can result in cerebral edema.

Reference: Mount DB. Fluid and electrolyte disturbances. In: Kasper D, Fauci A, Hauser S, Longo D, Jameson J, Loscalzo, eds. *Harrison's principles of internal medicine.* 19th ed. McGraw Hill; 2014.

Immunology

30

KRISTOFER E. NAVA AND SAAD SHEBRAIN

ABSITE 99th Percentile High-Yields

I. Innate Immunity
   A. Cells
      1. Phagocytes—dendrites, macrophages, neutrophils
      2. Mast cells, eosinophils, basophils (*mast cell is the most important cell involved in anaphylaxis*)
      3. Complement
         a) Classic pathway—activated by antigen-antibody complex (activation of classic complement pathway: IgM > IgG); factors C1, C2, C4
         b) Alternate pathway—activated by bacteria/endotoxins: factors B, D, and P (properdin)
         c) MB-lectin pathway, triggered by mannan-binding lectin, a normal serum constituent that binds some encapsulated bacteria
         d) Anaphylatoxins: C3a, C4a, C5a
         e) Opsonins: C3b, C4b
         f) Membrane attack complex: C5b-C9b

II. Acquired Immunity
   A. Lymphoid organs
      1. Primary lymphoid organs—liver, bone, thymus
      2. Secondary lymphoid organs—spleen, lymph nodes
   B. Cell-mediated immunity: effective against intracellular pathogens, major histocompatibility complex-(MHC-) restricted, that is, only recognize antigen presented on MHC
      1. CD4 "T helper" cells—cytokine release
         a) IL-1: fever (increased production of prostaglandin, PGE2, by hypothalamus)
         b) IL-2: maturation of cytotoxic T cells
         c) IL-4: maturation of B cells into plasma cells
         d) IL-6: fever, acute phase reactant
         e) IL-8: neutrophil recruitment, chemotaxis
         f) IL-10: antiinflammatory ("octreotide of the immune system")
         g) TNF-α: cachexia
         h) IFN-γ: macrophage activation
      2. CD8 "cytotoxic T" cells—kill infected cells
         a) Suppressor cells—regulate CD4 and CD8 cells
         b) Cytotoxic cells—recognize infected cells expressing MHC-I, for example, viruses, intracellular pathogens
   C. Antibody (humoral)-mediated immunity: effective against extracellular pathogens, not MHC-restricted
      1. Antibody production occurs as a result of plasma cell maturation from B cells stimulation via IL-4 (CD4 cells)
      2. Ten percent of plasma cells become memory cells, which can be reactivated for antibody production

3. Antibodies (Abs):
   a) All Abs have two antigen bindings sites (except IgM)
   b) All Abs have two regions: (1) constant region—recognized by effector cells, (2) variable region—bound to antigen
   c) IgM—largest (5 domains, 10 binding sites) → cannot cross placenta; initial Ab produced after antigen exposure, *most common Ab in spleen*; opsonin
   d) IgG—*most abundant Ab*; Ab produced after secondary antigen exposure, can cross the placenta and is responsible for neonatal immunity; opsonin
   e) IgA—present on mucosal surfaces (Peyer patches), present in breast milk
   f) IgE—type I hypersensitivity reactions and parasitic infestations

D. Antigen presentation
   1. Extracellular pathogens, for example, bacteria: pathogen is engulfed by antigen-presenting cells and fused into phagosomes, which then undergo proteolytic degradation; these proteins are then repackaged and presented on the cell surface bound to MHC-II for presentation to CD4 cells
   2. Intracellular pathogens, for example, viruses: infected cells produce viral proteins, which are loaded onto MHC-I and then presented on the cell surface to CD8 cells

E. Hypersensitivity reactions
   1. Type I: IgE binds to basophils/mast cells leading to release of histamine, 5-HT, and bradykinin; for example, allergies, anaphylaxis
   2. Type II: antigen-Ab complex (IgM or IgG), for example, ABO incompatibility, hyperacute rejection
   3. Type III: antigen-Ab complex deposition, for example, systemic lupus erythematosus, rheumatoid arthritis
   4. Type IV: delayed (T cells)—APCs presents to CD4 → macrophage activation (IFN-γ); *only hypersensitivity not related to Ab.*, for example, chronic graft rejection

Questions

1. Which immunoglobulin is responsible for neonatal immune function, and how is it transmitted?
   A. IgM, from breast milk
   B. IgA, crossing placenta
   C. IgG, from breast milk
   D. IgA, from breast milk
   E. IgM, crossing placenta

2. A 19-year-old male with a known history of HIV is noncompliant with his retroviral medication and is found to have a CD4 count of 42 cells/mm^3. What antibiotic prophylaxis is indicated?
   A. Daptomycin
   B. Cephalexin
   C. Fluconazole
   D. Azithromycin
   E. Clindamycin

3. Which of the following is true regarding apoptosis?
   A. It does not occur during embryogenesis
   B. It is characterized by a loss of membrane integrity
   C. It induces an inflammatory response
   D. CD-8 T cells can initiate apoptosis in cells that are virally infected
   E. p53 inhibits apoptosis while BCL-2 promotes apoptosis

4. Spontaneous regression of cancer due to the immune system is best exemplified by which of the following malignancies?
   A. Melanoma
   B. Thymoma
   C. Colon
   D. Pancreas
   E. Lung

5. Which of the following is true regarding the immune response to bacterial infection?
   A. CD-4 T cells transform B cells into plasma cells
   B. Class-1 MHC molecules present bacteria-derived proteins
   C. Cells infected by bacteria are destroyed by cytotoxic T cells
   D. Activated CD-4 T cells secrete antibodies
   E. Class-2 MHC cells are present on all nucleated cells

6. Which of the following is true regarding the immediate cellular response to a paper cut injury?
   A. L-selectin is expressed on endothelial cells
   B. The majority of the cytokine response is released by circulating platelets
   C. *ICAM* expressed on endothelial cells binds to beta-2 integrin on leukocytes
   D. This is not affected by diabetes mellitus
   E. Selectins are involved in platelet adhesion

7. Which of the following is true regarding cyclosporine?
   A. It is primarily excreted by the kidneys
   B. It is associated with thrombocytosis
   C. It inhibits the release of IL-2
   D. It inhibits activation of B cells
   E. It is more potent than FK-506

8. A 28-year-old male with type A blood develops a high fever, chills, jaundice, and hematuria shortly after receiving a blood transfusion. The nurse checks the blood bag and realizes this patient received type B donor blood. Which of the following is true regarding this condition?
   A. This is an example of serum sickness
   B. He developed a T cell-mediated response
   C. Direct Coombs test will demonstrate IgG bound to red blood cells
   D. His symptoms are a result of an overexaggerated response from mast cells
   E. This response does not involve complement activation

9. Which of the following is true regarding cytokines?
   A. IL-2 is a major endogenous pyrogen
   B. IL-6 is considered a potent stimulus for the production of acute phase reactants
   C. IL-10 is responsible for enhancing macrophage function
   D. Neutrophils are considered the largest producers of tumor necrosis factor (TNF)-α
   E. During an inflammatory response, C-reactive protein production is dampened

10. A 24-year-old male patient with HIV presents with fever, dry cough, and shortness of breath. Workup demonstrates *Pneumocystis carinii pneumonia*. He is admitted to the intensive care unit and treated with trimethoprim/sulfamethoxazole (TMP-SMX). The resident performs a medication reconciliation and starts the patient on highly active antiretroviral therapy (HAART) as it was present in the patient's electronic medical record. His symptoms improve the next day. However, on hospital day three, the patient has worsening leukocytosis and hypotension, requiring initiation of vasopressors. Chest x-ray demonstrates a loculated pleural effusion concerning for an empyema and surgical consultation is requested. Tracheal aspirate culture is negative for any other organisms. The patient is unable to speak in complete sentences and is using accessory muscles. He indicates that he has been noncompliant with all his medications. What is the most likely cause of his worsening symptoms?

A. Natural history of *P. carinii* pneumonia
B. Incorrect antibiotic therapy
C. Lymphocyte hyperactivity
D. Poor penetration of antibiotics in lung parenchyma
E. Superimposed bacterial infection

Answers

1. D. During the neonatal period of development, the immature immune system relies on exogenous transplacental IgG and IgA in the breast milk (B, C). IgM, the largest immunoglobulin, is too large to cross the placenta (A, E). Outside of allergens and parasitic infections, IgE does not play a major role in early in neonatal immunology.

Reference: Pierzynowska K, Woliński J, Weström B, Pierzynowski SG. Maternal immunoglobulins in infants—Are they more than just a form of passive immunity? *Front Immunol.* 2020;11:855. doi:10.3389/fimmu.2020.00855.

2. D. Antibiotic prophylaxis in patients with HIV and low CD4 counts is essential in preventing opportunistic infections. For patients with CD4 counts <200, prophylaxis with trimethoprim-sulfamethoxazole (TMP-SMX) against *Pneumocystis jirovecii* (previously *Pneumocystis carinii*) and *Toxoplasma gondii* is indicated to prevent pneumonia and encephalitis, respectively. When the CD4 count is <50, additional prophylaxis with azithromycin or clarithromycin is needed against *Mycobacterium avium complex* (MAC) which can cause pneumonia. Fluconazole is not indicated unless the patient lives in an area endemic to coccidiomycosis and has positive serology (C). Daptomycin is not indicated as a prophylactic antibiotic but can be used to treat gram-positive infections in HIV patients (A). Similarly, clindamycin and cephalexin are not used as prophylactic medications in HIV patients but can be used to treat uncomplicated skin infections within this population (B, E).

Reference: Aberg JA, Gallant JE, Ghanem KG, Emmanuel P, Zingman BS, Horberg MA. Infectious Diseases Society of America. Primary care guidelines for the management of persons infected with HIV: 2013 update by the HIV Medicine Association of the Infectious Diseases Society of America. *Clin Infect Dis.* 2014 Jan;58(1).

3. D. Apoptosis (programmed cell death) is a critical process governing homeostasis and begins during embryogenesis with the shedding of skin between digits (A). This continues lifelong and promotes the growth of healthy cells and tissue while facilitating the disposal of infected, damaged, or transformed cells that may give rise to cancer. The two pathways of apoptosis have in common the activation of caspases, which serves as the final step for cell destruction. The intrinsic pathway is regulated by two important genes; *p53* promotes apoptosis while *BCL-2* inhibits apoptosis (**p** for *p53* and **p**romotes) (E). Li-Fraumeni syndrome is characterized by an absence of *p53* and thus apoptosis does not occur, leading to large solid tumors. The extrinsic pathway is activated by several external "death" receptors that are expressed in infected cells or cells with DNA damage. CD-8 T cells are responsible for recognizing the FAS-death receptor in virally infected cells and initiating cell destruction. Apoptosis is characterized by DNA fragmentation and compartmentalization of cytoplasmic particles into apoptotic bodies, which are then broken down further by activated caspases and ultimately undergo phagocytosis by macrophages without inducing an inflammatory response (C). In contrast, cell necrosis is characterized by a violation of the cell membrane, release of cytoplasmic products, and a subsequent inflammatory response (B).

Reference: Elmore S. Apoptosis: a review of programmed cell death. *Toxicol Pathol.* 2007;35(4):495–516. doi:10.1080/01926230701320337.

4. A. Spontaneous regression of malignant tumors refers to cases of complete or partial tumor destruction and/or involution without any particular therapy. This occurs in most cancers, but certain tumors regress more commonly. Melanoma, testicular germ cell tumors, and neuroblastoma are cancers that regress with increased frequency. This is due to a combination of cell apoptosis, immune mediators, and tumor microenvironment. Regression not only occurs in primary tumors but also can occur in metastases. The remaining answer choices regress less frequently (B–E).

Reference: Ricci SB, Cerchiari U. Spontaneous regression of malignant tumors: importance of the immune system and other factors (Review). *Oncol Lett.* 2010;1(6):941–945. doi:10.3892/ol.2010.176.

5. A. The only cells capable of initiating humoral immunity to bacterial invasion are antigen-presenting cells, which include dendrites, macrophages, and B cells. This begins with endocytosis and processing of bacterial proteins, which are coupled to class 2 MHC molecules and are expressed on the cell surface (B). Next, CD-4 T cells recognize the bacterial protein motif and bind to the receptor. The newly activated CD-4 T cell finds B cells bound to the bacterial antigen and helps transform them into plasma cells (secreting antibodies) and memory B cells conferring long-term immunity to a particular bacterial antigen (D). The immune response to a viral infection works by a different mechanism. Firstly, all nucleated cells (most notably absent are red blood cells) have class 1 MHC molecules, which are able to bind to viral proteins and translocate to the cell surface (E). This is then recognized by CD-8 or cytotoxic T cells and marked for destruction (C).

6. C. The immune response involved in healing a paper cut or similar small injury is a complex one. There are three stages including platelet rolling, tight adhesion, and emigration. The damaged endothelial cell expresses E-selectin (E for endothelium), which binds to P-selectin on platelets and L-selectin on leukocytes (A). This promotes weak binding, which allows for platelet rolling initiating a platelet plug. Circulating macrophages release cytokines and chemokines, which induce the expression of various endothelial receptors and attract other immune modulators (B). One of these newly expressed endothelial receptors includes *ICAM*, a type of integrin that promotes stable binding allowing for platelet adhesion. Next, *PECAM* and *VCAM* are expressed on the endothelial surface, which facilitates emigration of circulating leukocytes from the vasculature toward the inflammatory stimulus. Selectins are involved in platelet rolling while integrins are involved in platelet adhesion (E). This response is dampened in patients with diabetes and those with chronic steroid use, which helps explain why these patients have difficulty with wound healing (D). The most notable syndrome affecting this process is leukocyte adhesion deficiency, which is characterized by defunct integrin molecules leading to recurrent bacterial infection and the classic presenting sign of delayed umbilical cord sloughing.

7. C. Cyclosporine is an immune modulator that was commonly used in transplant patients as maintenance therapy. It has largely been replaced by tacrolimus. Cyclosporine works by inhibiting cyclophilin protein on calcineurin and thereby inhibits synthesis of IL-2 and IL-4, which are interleukins that activate T cells (D). FK-506 works by a similar mechanism but is considered more potent than cyclosporine (E). The adverse effects of cyclosporine include nephrotoxicity, gingival hyperplasia, hirsutism, and thrombocytopenia (B). The drug undergoes hepatic metabolism and is primarily excreted in bile. Less than 5% undergo renal excretion (A).

Reference: Burckart GJ, Starzl TE, Venkataramanan R, et al. Excretion of cyclosporine and its metabolites in human bile. *Transplant Proc.* 1986;18(6 Suppl. 5):46–49.

8. C. This patient has developed a type II hypersensitivity reaction from receiving an incorrect blood type transfusion. The cause of ABO incompatibility in blood transfusion is clerical error as demonstrated in the above case. There are four types of hypersensitivity reactions. The first three types occur quickly and are antibody- and complement-mediated while type IV is a delayed response and is T cell-mediated. Type I is the only IgE-mediated reaction and occurs when a stimulus activates eosinophils, which in turn activate mast cells and basophils, resulting in a systemic release of bradykinin, serotonin, and histamine (D). Type I reactions are our immune system's adaptation as a protective mechanism against parasites, which is less threatening in the modern age. Instead, type I hypersensitivity reactions occur most frequently with exposure to allergens such as bee stings, peanut exposure, or hay fever. Type II hypersensitivity is an IgG- and IgM-mediated response resulting in complement activation (opsonization), cell lysis, and phagocytosis (E). In the case of ABO incompatibility, patients will present with widespread hemolysis. A direct Coombs test will demonstrate IgG bound to RBC and an indirect Coombs test will measure free antibodies in the serum. Of note, not all type II hypersensitivity reactions are cytotoxic; myasthenia gravis is a noncytotoxic variant of type II hypersensitivity. Type III hypersensitivity is an immune complex–mediated response in which immune conglomerates deposit into healthy tissue and thus inflict damage; serum sickness, systemic lupus erythematosus (SLE), and rheumatoid arthritis are examples of this (A). Type IV hypersensitivity is a delayed reaction and is preceded by T-cell sensitization (B). Tuberculosis skin test and contact dermatitis are considered type IV hypersensitivity reactions.

9. B. Cytokines are largely responsible for cell signaling during an inflammatory response. TNF-α and IL-1 are the two main cytokines responsible for propagating the inflammatory response during the early stages of injury and/or infection. The largest producers of these cytokines are macrophages (D). Both are responsible for soliciting additional cytokine production and immune cell recruitment. IL-1, in particular, is considered the primary endogenous pyrogen (A). It regulates the thermal set point in the hypothalamus (by binding to the CD-121 family receptor), resulting in fever. Alveolar macrophages producing IL-1 have classically been taught to surgical residents as being responsible for the fever seen in patients with atelectasis. Additionally, corticosteroids can inhibit production of IL-1; this may explain why patients with acute adrenal insufficiency develop a high fever (due to the disinhibition of IL-1). Some authors do not agree that atelectasis is involved in postoperative fever and others have suggested that IL-6 more closely correlates with postoperative fever. IL-2 is primarily produced by T cells and helps recruit and activate additional T cells and enhances interaction between T and B cells. IL-6 is the most potent stimulus of hepatic acute phase reactants including C-reactive protein, amyloid A, and ceruloplasmin (E). In contrast, prealbumin and transferrin production decrease during inflammation; this explains why prealbumin as a measure of nutritional status can't be interpreted without measuring one of the acute phase reactants. IL-10 is considered the largest inhibitor of the inflammatory response including the function of macrophages (C).

References: Losa García JE, Rodriguez FM, Martín de Cabo MR, et al. Evaluation of inflammatory cytokine secretion by human alveolar macrophages. *Mediators Inflamm.* 1999;8(1):43–51. doi:10.1080/09629359990711.

Mavros MN, Velmahos GC, Falagas ME. Atelectasis as a cause of postoperative fever: where is the clinical evidence? *Chest.* 2011;140(2):418–424. doi:10.1378/chest.11-0127.

10. C. This patient with HIV presents with an AIDS-defining opportunistic infection (*P. carinii pneumonia*). As such, he likely has a low CD-4 count. In fact, HIV patients with CD-4 counts <200 cells/mL should receive prophylactic treatment with TMP-SMX. This antibiotic is the drug of choice for *P. carinii pneumonia* as it has excellent lung penetration (B, D). Most patients recover with this treatment (A). Patients that are noncompliant with HAART are at risk for immune reconstitution inflammatory syndrome (IRIS). This refers to a group of inflammatory disorders that arise after the initiation of antiretroviral therapy in AIDS patients. IRIS is more likely to occur in patients who are younger, male with a low CD-4 count, or who have an active infection and are noncompliant with HAART. It usually occurs in patients whose pretreatment CD4 count is <100 cells/mm^3 and requires evidence of a positive virologic response to therapy, temporal association with initiation of therapy, systemic signs of inflammation, and ruling out other etiologies of systemic inflammation (e.g., bacterial infection, drug-drug reaction) (E). IRIS in the context of a recently treated *P. carinii pneumonia* may present with initial improvement of symptoms followed by worsening pulmonary symptoms, high fever, hypoxia, and even acute respiratory failure.

Reference: Sharma SK, Soneja M. HIV & immune reconstitution inflammatory syndrome (IRIS). *Indian J Med Res.* 2011;134(6): 866–877.

Infection and Antimicrobial Therapy

31

ERIC O. YEATES AND JEFFRY NAHMIAS

ABSITE 99th Percentile High-Yields

I. Surgical Care Improvement Project (SCIP) Recommendations: Prevention of Postoperative Infection
   A. Prophylactic antibiotics should be given within 1 hour prior to incision.
   B. Antibiotics should cover the most likely pathogens to be encountered during the operation.
   C. Prophylactic antibiotics should be discontinued after skin closure in clean and clean-contaminated cases.
   D. Maintain euglycemia in the first 2 postoperative days.
   E. Surgical site hair can be removed with electrical clippers, but not by shaving.
   F. Urinary catheters should be removed before postoperative day 2 when possible.
   G. Maintain normothermia perioperatively.

II. Surgical Wound Classification System

Classification	Description	Examples	Surgical site infection
Clean	Uninfected wounds without entry into the gastrointestinal, genitourinary, or respiratory systems	Skin mass removal, tunneled central-venous catheter placement, cardiac surgery	1%–5%
Clean/contaminated	Wounds with operative entry into the gastrointestinal, genitourinary, or respiratory system, but no gross spillage	Cholecystectomy, routine appendectomy, pancreaticoduodenectomy	3%–11%
Contaminated	Gross spillage of gastrointestinal contents	Inflamed appendicitis, bile spillage during cholecystectomy	10%–17%
Dirty/infected	Incision through or operating in existing infection	Perforated diverticulitis, incision and drainage of abscess, traumatic wound > 4 hours old	>27%

III. Common Causes of Postoperative Fever and Timing
   A. Wind (pneumonia): POD 1-5
   B. Water (urinary tract infection): POD 3-9
   C. Walk (venous thromboembolism): POD 6-11
   D. Wound (surgical site infection): POD 5-14

IV. Surviving Sepsis Guidelines
   A. Fluid resuscitation
      1. Resuscitation should begin ASAP with 30cc/kg of crystalloid within the first 3 hours

2. Fluid challenges with crystalloid (either balanced or saline) should be continued as long as hemodynamics improve
3. Mean arterial pressure goal of 65 mmHg
4. Resuscitation should attempt to normalize lactate

B. Diagnosis
   1. Appropriate cultures should be obtained prior to starting antibiotics if it results in no substantial delay

C. Antimicrobial therapy
   1. IV antibiotics (empiric broad-spectrum coverage) should be started as soon as possible and within one hour of diagnosis of sepsis or septic shock
   2. Antibiotics should be narrowed once pathogen is identified and sensitivities are established
   3. Antibiotics should continue for 7 to 10 days for most serious infections
   4. Procalcitonin can be used to support shortening duration of antibiotics

D. Source control
   1. Interventions to achieve source control should be implemented as soon as possible
   2. Intravascular devices that are possible sources of sepsis should be removed

E. Vasoactive medications
   1. Mean arterial pressure goal of 65 mmHg
   2. First-line vasopressor is norepinephrine
   3. Either vasopressin (up to 0.03 U/min) or epinephrine as second-line
   4. Recommend invasive monitoring with arterial catheter for patients requiring vasopressors

F. Corticosteroids
   1. IV hydrocortisone at 200 mg/day in divided doses (e.g., 50 mg every 6 hours) can be used for shock refractory to fluid resuscitation and vasopressors

G. Blood products
   1. RBC transfusion at <7.0 g/dL (can have higher threshold in acute myocardial ischemia, severe hypoxia, acute hemorrhage)

H. Glucose control
   1. Blood glucose goal should be less than 180 mg/dL
   2. Point-of-care testing should be interpreted with caution in patients with shock

I. Renal replacement therapy
   1. Consider continuous or intermittent renal replacement therapy (RRT) in patients with sepsis and acute kidney injury
   2. Continuous RRT should be utilized in hemodynamically unstable patients

J. Bicarbonate therapy
   1. Recommend against sodium bicarbonate therapy in patients with hypoperfusion-induced lactic acidemia with pH >7.15

K. Stress ulcer prophylaxis
   1. Proton pump inhibitor or histamine-2 receptor antagonist is recommended in patients with sepsis/septic shock who have risk factors for gastrointestinal bleeding

L. Nutrition
   1. Early enteral feeding when feasible
   2. Recommend against omega-3 fatty acid as immune supplement in critically ill patients

V. Antibiotic Mechanisms by Site of Action

A. Cell wall synthesis
   1. Beta Lactams (penicillins, cephalosporins, carbapenems, monobactams)
   2. Vancomycin

B. Nuclei acid synthesis
   1. Folate synthesis: sulfonamides, trimethoprim
   2. DNA gyrase: quinolones
   3. RNA polymerase: rifampin

C. Protein synthesis
   1. 50S: macrolides, clindamycin, linezolid
   2. 30S: tetracyclines, aminoglycosides

Questions

1. A previously healthy 55-year-old male presents with perforated diverticulitis and peritonitis. He undergoes an emergent exploratory laparotomy and is found to have purulent peritonitis. A Hartmann's procedure is performed and his abdomen is copiously irrigated. When should antibiotics be stopped in this patient?
   A. Within 24 hours after the operation
   B. Postoperative day 4
   C. Postoperative day 7
   D. Postoperative day 14
   E. Duration should be determined by procalcitonin levels

2. A 75-year-old-male with dementia is admitted for a moderate traumatic brain injury after a ground-level fall. He weighs 50 kg. His hospital course has been complicated by urinary retention and he now has an indwelling urinary catheter. On hospital day 4, he develops worsening confusion throughout the day. On evaluation, his heart rate is 105 beats per min, blood pressure is 92/64 mmHg, and his respiratory rate is 30 breaths per min. Labs reveal a lactic acid of 5.4 mmol/L and a metabolic acidosis with a pH of 7.18. Which of the following is true regarding the management of his condition?
   A. Vasopressors should be initiated immediately
   B. A 1.5 L colloid fluid bolus should be administered as soon as possible
   C. A 2 L colloid fluid bolus should be administered as soon as possible
   D. Sodium bicarbonate should be administered to correct his acidosis
   E. A 1.5 L crystalloid fluid bolus should be administered as soon as possible

3. Which of the following is true regarding the prevention of postoperative infections?
   A. Prophylactic antibiotics should be given anytime between 1 hour prior to incision and before the end of the operation
   B. Cefazolin would be an appropriate choice of prophylactic antibiotics for an elective sigmoid colectomy
   C. Electrical clipping and manual shaving prior to an operation have similar infection rates

   D. Indwelling urinary catheter use longer than 2 days after surgery is associated with a longer length of stay, but no difference in urinary tract infections
   E. Intravenous insulin infusion reduces surgical site infections after cardiac surgery compared to sliding-scale subcutaneous insulin injections

4. A 47-year-old female with history of pulmonary sarcoidosis is discovered to have a right upper lobe mass on chest radiograph that is outlined by a crescent of air superiorly. On a left lateral decubitus film, the crescent of air shifts to remain in a nondependent position. The patient is currently asymptomatic. What is the next step in management?
   A. Diagnostic bronchoscopy with bronchoalveolar lavage
   B. CT-guided biopsy
   C. IV voriconazole
   D. Pulmonary wedge resection
   E. No further workup or treatment is required

5. Which of the following profiles for hepatitis B surface antigen (HBsAg), hepatitis B surface antibody (anti-HBs), total hepatitis B core antibody (anti-HBc), and IgM antibody against hepatitis B core antigen (IgM anti-HBc) would you expect for a patient with chronic hepatitis B infection?
   A. HbsAg–, anti-HBs–, anti-HBc–, IgM anti-HBc–
   B. HbsAg–, anti-HBs+, anti-HBc+, IgM anti-HBc–
   C. HbsAg–, anti-HBs+, anti-HBc–, IgM anti-HBc–
   D. HbsAg+, anti-HBs–, anti-HBc+, IgM anti-HBc+
   E. HbsAg+, anti-HBs–, anti-HBc+, IgM anti-HBc–

6. Which of the following is true regarding occupational risk of hepatitis in health-care workers?
   A. The risk of transmission is greater for hepatitis C than for hepatitis B
   B. If the exposed person has been vaccinated for hepatitis B, no hepatitis B treatment is needed
   C. If the patient has hepatitis C, the exposed person should be given ribavirin
   D. Most hepatitis B transmissions are the result of needlestick injuries
   E. Hepatitis B virus can survive on dried blood for at least a week

7. A 32-year-old male is recovering in the ICU 1 day after extensive debridement of the left leg for a necrotizing soft-tissue infection (NSTI). He is intubated and requiring 80% FiO_2. He has leukocytosis that has been rising and an elevated serum lactate. He is on broad-spectrum antibiotics. Which of the following is the best next step in management?
   A. Amputation of left leg
   B. Second-look operation
   C. Add antifungal coverage
   D. CT scan of the leg
   E. Start pressors

8. Which of the following is least likely to contribute to a surgical site infection?
   A. American Society of Anesthesiologists physical status
   B. Length of operation
   C. Serum glucose level
   D. Body temperature
   E. Hemoglobin level

9. The organism most commonly associated with acute mesenteric lymphadenitis is:
   A. *Campylobacter jejuni*
   B. *Escherichia coli*
   C. *Enterococcus*
   D. *Yersinia enterocolitica*
   E. *Pinworms*

10. Forty-eight hours after total mastectomy, high fever, diarrhea, vomiting, redness of the skin of the entire body, and hypotension develop in a 30-year-old patient. The mastectomy incision appears unremarkable. The following day diffuse desquamation develops. The most likely etiology is:
    A. *Clostridium perfringens*
    B. *Clostridium difficile*
    C. β-Hemolytic *Streptococcus*
    D. *Staphylococcus aureus*
    E. *Staphylococcus epidermidis*

11. A 52-year-old male smoker with chronic obstructive pulmonary disease (COPD) presents to the emergency department (ED) complaining of fevers and foul-tasting sputum for the past 4 weeks. He was recently admitted to an outside hospital for treatment of a COPD exacerbation and has a history of vancomycin-resistant *S. aureus* bacteremia. Chest radiograph shows a 4-cm air-fluid level within the right lung. He reports a 20-pound weight loss over the past 5 months. Appropriate management includes:
    A. Administration of intravenous daptomycin
    B. Thoracotomy and decortication
    C. Pulmonary lobectomy
    D. Percutaneous drain placement
    E. Diagnostic bronchoscopy

12. Which of the following is true regarding the management of parapneumonic effusions?
    A. They should be drained with tube thoracostomy as soon as detected
    B. Intrapleural fibrinolytics are highly efficacious in patients with loculated effusions
    C. Large diameter chest tubes (>28 French) are required for adequate drainage
    D. Treatment of the organizing phase requires open drainage (e.g., Eloesser flap)
    E. If it progresses to an empyema, video-assisted thoracoscopic surgery should be performed if it does not respond to chest tube drainage

13. Which of the following is true regarding antibiotic mechanisms?
    A. Penicillin-derivative antibiotics bind to the bacterial cell membrane and increase its permeability
    B. Piperacillin-tazobactam works partly by binding β-lactamases
    C. Metronidazole, though limited, has some effect against aerobic bacteria
    D. Linezolid competitively inhibits the 30S ribosome
    E. Clindamycin, like the macrolides, reversibly binds the 50S ribosome

14. Which of the following should be used as part of a screening tool to identify non-ICU patients that are at increased risk of organ failure from infection?
    A. Temperature higher than 38°C
    B. Heart rate greater than 90/min
    C. Altered mentation
    D. White blood cell (WBC) count greater than 12,000/mm^3
    E. $PaCO_2$ less than 32 mmHg

15. A 56-year-old HIV-positive (with a low CD4 count) patient presented to the ED with a spontaneous pneumothorax and underwent a tube thoracostomy procedure. While trying to re-cap the 20-gauge needle used for anesthetizing the skin, the resident who performed the procedure was inadvertently stuck resulting in visible bleeding from the skin. Which of the following is true regarding this exposure?
    A. Postexposure prophylaxis with a 2-drug regimen should be administered for 8 weeks
    B. Postexposure prophylaxis with a 3-drug regimen should be administered for 4 weeks
    C. Potential HIV infection should be disclosed to future patients
    D. At least 6 months of postexposure treatment is recommended
    E. The hollow bore needle used for this procedure lowers the risk of HIV transmission

16. A 45-year-old HIV-positive male presents to the ED with perianal pain for the past two days. Physical exam reveals a small area of tenderness in the right posterolateral position distal to the external sphincter that is extremely tender. His CD4 count is 550 cells/mL, and he is currently on highly active antiretroviral therapy (HAART). Which of the following is the most correct management of this patient?
    A. Intravenous (IV) antibiotics
    B. Incision and drainage under local anesthesia in the ED
    C. Oral antibiotics and incision and drainage under local anesthesia in the ED
    D. IV antibiotics, exam under anesthesia (EUA), and if an area of fluctuance is identified, then incision and drainage and biopsy
    E. IV antibiotics, EUA, incision and drainage, and biopsy of the area of tenderness even if no fluctuance is identified

17. A 62-year-old man is postoperative day 6 from an elective laparoscopic sigmoid colectomy for recurrent diverticulitis. He had return of bowel function 2 days ago and was getting ready to be discharged home. Throughout his hospital course, he has been having low-grade fevers. He is now complaining of tenesmus and urinary retention. Which of the following represents the most appropriate next step in management?
    A. Transition to nonnarcotic pain medications
    B. Bladder scan and in-and-out catheterization as needed
    C. Abdominal radiography
    D. Computed tomography (CT)
    E. Diagnostic laparoscopy

18. A 60-year-old man presents with gas gangrene of his left leg requiring below-knee amputation. Wound cultures were positive for *Clostridium septicum*. Additional workup should include:
    A. Head CT scan
    B. Bronchoscopy
    C. Colonoscopy
    D. HIV serology
    E. Chest CT scan

19. Which of the following is true regarding tetanus?
    A. It is highly contagious
    B. Trismus is usually the first sign
    C. It is caused by a gram-negative anaerobic rod
    D. A prior history of surviving tetanus provides immunity
    E. The diagnosis is established by demonstrating the organisms in a wound

20. Which of the following is associated with an endotoxin?
    A. *Streptococcus pyogenes*
    B. *Bacteroides fragilis*
    C. *Clostridium tetani*
    D. *S. aureus*
    E. *C. perfringens*

Answers

1. B. The Study to Optimize Peritoneal Infection Therapy (STOP-IT) trial was a randomized controlled trial designed to determine the optimal length of antibiotic treatment after source control in patients with intraabdominal infections. Patients were randomized to receive antibiotics for 4 days postoperatively versus 2 days after the resolution of fever, leukocytosis, and ileus. The median duration of antibiotics was 4 days versus 8 days postoperatively, and there was no difference in surgical-site infections, recurrent intraabdominal infections, or mortality. Therefore, antibiotics should continue only for 4 days postoperatively in most cases (A, C–E). Procalcitonin may be useful in helping determine the duration of antibiotic therapy. A single absolute value is less useful than the trend over several days. It is best used in cases where systemic inflammation is present without an obvious infectious etiology. If the procalcitonin level declines with antibiotic therapy, it is reasonable to complete a 5 to 10-day course depending on the suspected source(s). However, if the level is normal and/or does not change with antibiotics, it would be reasonable to stop antibiotic therapy.

Reference: Sawyer RG, Claridge JA, Nathens AB, et al. Trial of short-course antimicrobial therapy for intraabdominal infection. *N Engl J Med.* 2015;372(21):1996–2005.

2. E. This patient is showing multiple signs of sepsis with the most likely source being a catheter-associated urinary tract infection. The Surviving Sepsis Campaign is a joint collaboration committed to reducing morbidity and mortality related to sepsis and septic shock. Updated recommendations detailing the ideal management of sepsis and septic shock are provided periodically. Fluid resuscitation should begin as soon as possible with 30 cc/kg of crystalloid (C). Albumin (colloid) bolus has not been consistently demonstrated to be associated with improved outcomes in patients with septic shock and is significantly more costly than crystalloid. As such, crystalloids are preferred over colloids (B). Empiric broad-spectrum intravenous antibiotics should also be administered within one hour. However, appropriate cultures should be obtained prior to starting antibiotics if this incurs no substantial delay. If hypotension persists despite fluid resuscitation, vasopressors should be initiated with a MAP goal of >65 mmHg (A). Additionally, intravenous hydrocortisone at 200 mg/day should be considered if shock is refractory to both fluid resuscitation and vasopressors (C). This patient has an elevated lactate which should be measured at regular intervals and utilized as an endpoint for adequate resuscitation. Though he does have a significant acidemia, administration of sodium bicarbonate is not recommended for correction as long as his pH is greater than 7.15 and certainly should not occur prior to adequate fluid resuscitation (D).

Reference: Rhodes A, Evans LE, Alhazzani W. Surviving Sepsis Campaign: international guidelines for management of sepsis and septic shock. *Crit Care Med.* 2017;45(3):486–552.

3. E. The Surgical Care Improvement Project (SCIP) is a program designed to reduce the rates of postoperative surgical infections. Their most recent recommendations address timing of antibiotics, choice of antibiotics, hair removal techniques, normothermia, euglycemia, and indwelling urinary catheter use. Prophylactic antibiotics should be given within 1 hour prior to the incision (A). Additionally, the chosen antibiotic should cover the most likely pathogen to be encountered during the operation. Cefazolin does not have appropriate anaerobic coverage for a colectomy (B). Surgical site hair should be removed with electrical clippers, rather than shaving, on the day of or day prior to surgery. Shaving has been shown to have a higher rate of mediastinitis in patients undergoing open-heart surgery (C). Indwelling urinary catheter use longer than 2 days after an operation is associated with higher rates of urinary tract infection and it is recommended to remove catheters prior to this point when possible (D). Maintaining euglycemia for the first 48 hours postoperatively has been shown to decrease surgical site infection. Additionally, intravenous insulin infusion postoperatively was associated with decreased deep sternal wound infections in open cardiac surgery compared to sliding-scale insulin injections.

References: Furnary AP, Zerr KJ, Grunkemeier GL, Starr A. Continuous intravenous insulin infusion reduces the incidence of deep sternal wound infection in diabetic patients after cardiac surgical procedures. *Ann Thorac Surg.* 1999;67(2):352–360.

Rosenberger LH, Politano AD, Sawyer RG. The surgical care improvement project and prevention of post-operative infection, including surgical site infection. *Surg Infect (Larchmt).* 2011;12(3):163–168.

4. E. *Aspergillus* species are widely dispersed in the environment and, when implicated as a pathogen, primarily affect the lungs. It typically presents as one of four syndromes: aspergilloma, allergic bronchopulmonary aspergillosis (ABPA), chronic necrotizing *Aspergillus* pneumonia, and invasive aspergillosis. Aspergilloma typically presents as an asymptomatic radiographic finding in patients with a preexisting cavitary lung disease such as sarcoidosis. A soft-tissue mass within a cavity that is surrounded by a crescent of air (Monad sign) is diagnostic, and because the aspergilloma is not adherent to the cavity walls, the air will remain in a nondependent position. Biopsy or bronchoscopy is not indicated or necessary for diagnosis (A, B). As long as the patient is asymptomatic, no further workup or treatment is necessary. The most common symptom associated with aspergilloma is hemoptysis, which can occasionally be life threatening. In this setting, an emergency bronchial artery embolization should be performed followed by surgical resection (D). ABPA is a noninvasive hypersensitivity disease that, if left untreated, can lead to fibrotic lung disease. Therapy is aimed at the treatment of acute exacerbations either with inhaled bronchodilators/steroids (mild disease) or systemic corticosteroids (severe disease) to prevent long-term sequelae. Serial chest radiographs, pulmonary function tests, and IgE levels should be monitored because permanent pulmonary damage can take place even in asymptomatic patients. Invasive aspergillosis and chronic necrotizing *Aspergillus* pneumonia are both treated with intravenous antifungals (C). Invasive disease can be rapidly fatal and is typically only found in immunocompromised hosts. High-risk transplant patients, such as bone marrow recipients, receive prophylactic agents to prevent invasive infection.

Reference: Limper AH, Knox KS, Sarosi GA, et al. An official American Thoracic Society statement: treatment of fungal infections in adult pulmonary and critical care patients. *Am J Respir Crit Care Med.* 2011;183(1):96–128.

5. E. Hepatitis B surface antigen is found on the surface of the hepatitis B virus and is found in high quantities in the serum of individuals with acute or chronic infection. Antibodies against this antigen (anti-HBs) are considered to represent an immunity to the virus either from previous infection or vaccination. All patients with chronic hepatitis B infection will be anti-HBs negative. Antibodies against hepatitis core antigen (anti-HBc) appear at the onset of symptoms and persist for life, though they do not confer immunity to the disease. Vaccination will not produce antibodies to hepatitis B core antigen. Presence of these antibodies indicates either active or previous infection with hepatitis B but does not confer a timeline associated with that infection. However, IgM against hepatitis B core antigen is only present for the first 6 months of infection, so its presence indicates a recent exposure to the virus. The aforementioned serologic profiles represent: A, susceptible to infection; B, immunity from previous infection; C, immunity from vaccination; D, acute infection; E, chronic infection.

6. E. The risk of developing hepatitis B from a needlestick injury is far greater than that of hepatitis C, particularly when the patient is hepatitis Be surface antigen (HBeAg) positive (A). If the patient's blood is both HBeAg and HBsAg positive, the risk of developing clinical hepatitis is very high (22%–31%). If the blood is HBsAg positive but HBeAg negative, the risk drops to 1% to 6% (although seroconversion is still high at 23%–37%). Hepatitis B is highly infectious, and the virus can survive on dried blood and on environmental surfaces for at least a week. The majority of health-care workers infected with hepatitis B do not recall a needlestick exposure, though they were in contact with a hepatitis B–positive patient (D). For health-care workers who have never been vaccinated for hepatitis B, or are seronegative, treatment with both HBIG (immunoglobulin prepared from human plasma known to contain a high titer of antibody to HBsAg) and the hepatitis B vaccine is recommended (B). Data on clinical hepatitis C following exposure is lacking. However, the average incidence of anti-HCV seroconversion from an HCV-positive source is very low (only 1.8%), suggesting that the risk of transmission from a needlestick injury is very low. In fact, some studies suggest that the risk of hepatitis C transmission from a solid surgical needle is negligible. No effective prophylaxis for HCV has been identified. Immunoglobulin and antiviral agents are not recommended for HCV postexposure prophylaxis (C).

Reference: Kuhar DT, Henderson DK, Struble KA, et al. *Updated U.S. public health service guidelines for the management of occupational exposures to HIV and recommendations for postexposure prophylaxis.* Division of Healthcare Quality Promotion, National Center for Emerging and Zoonotic Infectious Diseases, Center for Disease Control and Prevention (CDC); 2013. https://stacks.cdc.gov/view/cdc/20711.

7. B. NSTI is a broad term that encompasses infections limited to skin and subcutaneous tissue (necrotizing cellulitis) and those involving the fascia (necrotizing fasciitis) and muscle (myonecrosis). They can be extremely difficult to accurately diagnose early on because fewer than half present with obvious hard signs of NSTI, such as bullae, skin necrosis, gas on radiograph, and crepitus. Other signs include tense edema, violaceous skin color, severe pain, and neurologic deficit. Several laboratory values have been shown to be useful in distinguishing NSTI from simple cellulitis. The LRINEC (Laboratory Risk Indicator for Necrotizing Fasciitis) score uses the total WBC count, hemoglobin, sodium, glucose, serum creatinine, and C-reactive protein levels. A simpler model uses an admission WBC count greater than 15.4×10^9/L and/or a serum sodium level less than 135 mEq/L. This latter model is more useful for its negative predictive value (99%). A low serum sodium level is theorized to be the result of either a sepsis-induced syndrome of inappropriate antidiuretic hormone or adrenal insufficiency, but this has not been confirmed. Risk factors for NSTI include diabetes, illicit IV drug abuse, immunosuppression, and liver disease. Seventy percent to 80% of NSTIs are due to polymicrobial infection. Of those that are caused by a single organism, *Klebsiella*, *S. pyogenes*, and *C. perfringens* are the most common. The NSTI is subdivided into two categories; type I infections are caused by polymicrobial infection with aerobic and anaerobic bacteria (e.g., *Clostridium* and *Bacteroides* spp.), which work synergistically to produce infection. Type II infections are caused by group A *Streptococcus* with or without *Staphylococcus*. Treatment includes rapid administration of broad-spectrum antimicrobial agents, aggressive fluid resuscitation, and aggressive surgical debridement. The mortality rate remains at 20% to 40% and is higher with surgical delays, particularly beyond 24 hours. A rising WBC count and lactate after debridement are highly suggestive of progression of the NSTI. A second-look operation is often required and should be performed for this patient in order to ensure that no additional tissues have become involved since the initial debridement. Amputation may be necessary, but only a second-look operation will indicate whether this is the case (A). CT scan in the postoperative setting may not be useful because interpretation can be difficult secondary to postsurgical changes (D). With septic shock, pressors may be necessary, but this would not be the definitive treatment (E). Additionally, no hemodynamic parameters (blood pressure, central venous pressure) are provided that would indicate that pressors are needed. Similarly, adding antifungal coverage can be considered, but this is not a definitive intervention (C).

References: Anaya DA, Dellinger EP. Surgical infections and choice of antibiotics. In: Townsend CM, Jr, Beauchamp RD, Evers BM, Mattox KL, eds. *Sabiston textbook of surgery: the biological basis of modern surgical practice.* 17th ed. W.B. Saunders; 2004:257–282.

Dunn DL, Beilman GJ. Surgical infections. In: Brunicardi FC, Andersen DK, Billiar TR, et al., eds. *Schwartz's principles of surgery.* 8th ed. McGraw-Hill; 2005:109–128.

Wall DB, Klein SR, Black S, de Virgilio C. A simple model to help distinguish necrotizing fasciitis from nonnecrotizing soft tissue infection. *J Am Coll Surg.* 2000;191(3):227–231.

Wong CH, Khin LW, Heng KS, Tan KC, Low CO. The LRINEC (Laboratory Risk Indicator for Necrotizing Fasciitis) score: a tool for distinguishing necrotizing fasciitis from other soft tissue infections. *Crit Care Med.* 2004;32(7):1535–1541.

Yaghoubian A, de Virgilio C, Dauphine C, Lewis RJ, Lin M. Use of admission serum lactate and sodium levels to predict mortality in necrotizing soft-tissue infections. *Arch Surg.* 2007;142(9):840–846.

8. E. Risk for surgical site infections is related to several factors, including microbial contamination during surgery, length of operation, and patient factors such as diabetes, nutritional state, obesity, and immunosuppression (cancer, renal failure, immunosuppressive drugs) (B–D). The National Nosocomial Infection Surveillance Risk Index is a useful tool to assess the risk of wound infection. This index includes (1) American Society of Anesthesiologists physical status score higher than 2, (2) class III or IV wounds, and (3) duration of an operation greater than the 75th percentile for that particular procedure (A). Wounds are classified as clean (class I) (e.g., hernia repair, breast biopsy), clean/contaminated (class II) (e.g., cholecystectomy, elective gastrointestinal surgery), contaminated (class III) (e.g., bowel injury from trauma or inadvertent enterotomy), and dirty (class IV) (e.g., perforated appendicitis, diverticulitis, necrotizing soft-tissue infections [NSTIs]). Hemoglobin levels have not been shown to increase the risk of wound infection. In a randomized study of patients undergoing colorectal surgery, surgical wound infections were found in 19% who were permitted to become hypothermic but in only 6% who were actively kept normothermic. In a randomized study of clean surgery (breast, varicose vein, hernia), those who were actively warmed 30 minutes before surgery had only a 5% wound infection rate versus 14% in nonwarmed patients. Active control of glucose via continuous infusion was shown to decrease sternal wound infection in diabetic patients undergoing cardiac surgery. The main concern with aggressive glucose control, however, is that it may incite episodes of hypoglycemia. A recent study also highlighted the risk of blood transfusion in wound infection, likely the result of its immunosuppressive effects.

References: Campbell DA Jr, Henderson WG, Englesbe MJ, et al. Surgical site infection prevention: the importance of operative duration and blood transfusion–results of the first American College of Surgeons-National Surgical Quality Improvement Program Best Practices Initiative. *J Am Coll Surg.* 2008;207(6):810–820.

Furnary AP, Zerr KJ, Grunkemeier GL, Starr A. Continuous intravenous insulin infusion reduces the incidence of deep sternal wound infection in diabetic patients after cardiac surgical procedures. *Ann Thorac Surg.* 1999;67(2):352–360.

Kurz A, Sessler DI, Lenhardt R. Perioperative normothermia to reduce the incidence of surgical-wound infection and shorten hospitalization: study of Wound Infection and Temperature Group. *N Engl J Med.* 1996;334(19):1209–1215.

Melling AC, Ali B, Scott EM, Leaper DJ. Effects of preoperative warming on the incidence of wound infection after clean surgery: a randomised controlled trial. *Lancet.* 2001;358(9285):876–880.

9. D. Acute mesenteric adenitis presents most commonly in children and young adults. It can frequently be confused with appendicitis in children. Usually, an upper respiratory infection is present or has recently resolved. The abdominal pain is usually diffuse, but involuntary guarding on exam is rare. Laboratory values are of little help in establishing the diagnosis. More than 50% have an elevated WBC count. Although infection with the other answer choices can lead to mesenteric lymphadenitis, *Y. enterocolitica* is the most commonly associated organism in children (A–C, E). If the diagnosis is clear preoperatively (which is usually not the case), treatment is supportive because it is a self-limited disease. Ultrasound has emerged as a useful tool in children to suggest this diagnosis. Findings include enlarged, hypoechoic mesenteric lymph nodes (at least one more than 8 mm in diameter) and the absence of an inflamed (dilated) appendix. The diagnosis can also be made with CT by the demonstration of enlarged, clustered mesenteric lymph nodes in the right lower quadrant in the absence of acute appendicitis, but there is increasing reluctance to expose children to the radiation associated with CT scanning. The diagnosis is sometimes made during laparoscopy.

10. D. A rare cause of infection in the first 48 hours after an operation is wound toxic shock syndrome. Toxic shock syndrome is an acute onset, multiorgan illness that resembles severe scarlet fever. It was originally described in menstruating women in association with tampon use, but it has been increasingly recognized in postsurgical wounds. In the majority of cases, the illness is caused by *S. aureus* strains that express toxic shock syndrome toxin-1, enterotoxin B, or enterotoxin C. It has rarely been described in association with *S. pyogenes* (group A streptococci) (C). The remaining answer choices are not associated with toxic shock syndrome (A, B, E). Half of the postsurgical toxic shock syndrome cases present early, within 48 hours of operation. Symptoms include fever, diarrhea, vomiting, diffuse redness of the skin, and hypotension. This is followed a day or two later by diffuse desquamation. Physical examination findings of wound infection are often unremarkable. Wound drainage and antibiotics are recommended. Administration of clindamycin may be helpful because it inhibits exotoxin production.

Reference: Reingold AL, Dan BB, Shands KN, Broome CV. Toxic-shock syndrome not associated with menstruation. A review of 54 cases. *Lancet.* 1982;1(8262):1–4.

11. E. Lung abscesses typically present with an indolent course over several weeks. Patients often complain of fevers, purulent sputum, and cough. Single lung abscesses are frequently monomicrobial and are usually associated with aspiration pneumonia. As such, they are typically found in segments of the lung that are dependent in the supine position (i.e., the posterior segment of the upper lobes or the superior segments of the lower lobes). An air-fluid level on a chest radiograph and purulent sputum are virtually diagnostic of an anaerobic lung infection. However, coinfection with antibiotic-resistant gram-positive organisms is possible in patients with frequent hospitalizations. Most lung abscesses will resolve with antibiotics alone, but daptomycin cannot be used to treat lung infections because it is inhibited by pulmonary surfactant (A). In addition to intravenous (IV) antibiotics, a patient with risk factors for lung cancer (e.g., smoking, recent weight loss) should undergo bronchoscopy to rule out an underlying neoplasm (obstruction leading to infectious process). Surgical treatment may be necessary for infections that fail to respond to medical management, abscesses greater than 6 cm in size, and abscesses secondary to an obstructed bronchus from a foreign body or neoplasm. This typically involves either lobectomy or pneumonectomy (C). Percutaneous drain placement can be considered in patients who are poor surgical candidates (D). Thoracotomy and decortication are treatment options for empyema, not lung abscess (B).

References: Mandal K. Thoracic infections. In: Yuh DD, Vricella LA, Yang SC, Doty JR. eds. *Johns Hopkins textbook of cardiothoracic surgery.* 2nd ed. McGraw-Hill; 2014.

12. E. Parapneumonic effusion refers to the accumulation of pleural fluid in response to a respiratory infection. It is generally divided into three stages: exudative, fibrinopurulent, and organizing. The first (exudative) stage is characterized by the development of sterile pleural fluid in response to increased capillary permeability. After 5 days, bacteria begin to enter the fluid and inflammatory cells follow. This marks the beginning of the fibrinopurulent phase. In general, new effusions should undergo diagnostic thoracentesis to rule out an empyema. If transudative, antibiotic treatment of the pneumonia is all that is required (A). Urgent drainage via tube thoracostomy is recommended for frankly purulent effusions or those with bacteria on Gram stain or culture. The diameter of the chest tube does not seem to be important so long as smaller caliber tubes are routinely flushed to prevent blockage of the catheter (C). As the fibrinopurulent phase progresses, loculations begin to form within the collection, making drainage with a single catheter or tube thoracostomy difficult. Several studies have been done evaluating the use of intrapleural fibrinolytics, such as alteplase, to prevent progression to surgery. However, the results are controversial at best, and a 2008 Cochrane Review of the practice found no consistent benefit (B). At this stage, video-assisted thoracoscopic debridement and adhesiolysis are viable options, though a certain number of patients will still need to be converted to thoracotomy (E). After 2 to 3 weeks of untreated infection, fibroblasts begin to form a pleural peel and the final (organization) stage is reached. Once this membrane has formed, formal decortication via thoracotomy is generally necessary. In patients that are unfit for surgery, open drainage (e.g., Eloesser flap) may be considered. However, this subjects patients to months of dressing changes and significant morbidity (D).

References: Cameron R, Davies HR. Intra-pleural fibrinolytic therapy versus conservative management in the treatment of adult parapneumonic effusions and empyema. *Cochrane Database Syst Rev.* 2008;2:CD002312.

Davies HE, Davies RJO, Davies CWH, BTS Pleural Disease Guideline Group. Management of pleural infection in adults: British Thoracic Society Pleural Disease Guideline 2010. *Thorax.* 2010;65(Suppl 2):ii41–ii53.

Light RW. Parapneumonic effusions and empyema. *Proc Am Thorac Soc.* 2006;3(1):75–80.

13. B. All penicillin-derivative antibiotics (β-lactams) inhibit the final step of bacterial cell wall synthesis by binding transpeptidases or penicillin-binding proteins (A). Cephalosporins work by the same mechanism but are more resistant to degradation by β-lactamases. Tazobactam, sulbactam, and clavulanic acid bind β-lactamases and are frequently combined with penicillin-derivative antibiotics to increase their effectiveness. Examples of this include piperacillin-tazobactam and amoxicillin-clavulanic acid. Metronidazole is an antibiotic that only has action against anaerobic bacteria by inhibiting nucleic acid synthesis. It is not effective in aerobic cells because it requires reduction to its active state, which only takes place in anaerobic cells (C). Aminoglycosides and

tetracyclines inhibit the 30S ribosome. Linezolid, on the other hand, inhibits the 50S ribosome subunit. Several other antibiotics (macrolides, linezolid, chloramphenicol) also inhibit the 50S ribosome; however, it is a slightly different process (D). Clindamycin is a lincosamide antibiotic, which interferes with the amino acyl-tRNA complex (E). Aminoglycosides and tetracycline antibiotics inhibit the 30S ribosome.

14. C. The *Third International Consensus Definitions for Sepsis and Septic Shock*, published in JAMA in 2016, redefined the current definition used for sepsis and septic shock. The panel came to the conclusion that the previously used definition of sepsis (2+ SIRS criteria and a source of infection) was too nonspecific and generally unhelpful in the identification of patients at increased risk of mortality from infection (A, B, D, E). Instead, the committee recommended a bedside screening tool called the quick Sequential Organ System Failure score (qSOFA) for identification of patients that are likely to have a poor outcome as the result of an infection. If a patient meets two of the three criteria (respiratory rate >22/min, altered mental status, and systolic blood pressure <100 mmHg), further workup and treatment for sepsis is indicated. The term *sepsis* has also been changed to represent a more serious physiologic process. Sepsis is now defined as an infection with 2 or more points on the Sequential (Sepsis-Related) Organ Failure scoring system, or SOFA score. This score takes objective criteria for multiple organ systems (respiration, cardiovascular, coagulation, liver, central nervous system, and renal) and assigns a score based on the amount of organ dysfunction. A score of 2 or more is associated with a 10% or greater increase in mortality. Finally, the term *septic shock* has been redefined as sepsis that requires vasopressors to keep the mean arterial pressure (MAP) greater than 65 mmHg and a lactate level greater than 2.0 mmol/L. The term *severe sepsis* is no longer being encouraged as a formal diagnosis.

Reference: Singer M, Deutschman CS, Seymour CW, et al. The Third International Consensus Definitions for Sepsis and Septic Shock (Sepsis-3). *JAMA.* 2016;315(8):801–810.

15. B. With a blood exposure, the first step is to determine the risk (severity) of the exposure and the risk to the patient. The risk of puncture by a hollow needle with fresh blood is greater than the risk of puncture with a solid (surgical) needle, which is greater than the risk of splashing of a few blood drops on mucous membranes or nonintact skin, which is greater than the risk of blood drops on intact skin (no risk) (E). Depending on the combination of severity of exposure and severity of HIV, the recommendation is either a basic regimen of two drugs (4 weeks of zidovudine and lamivudine) or an expanded one of three drugs (basic regimen plus either indinavir or nelfinavir for 4 weeks). Given that the health-care worker had visible skin penetration by fresh blood with a hollow, large bore needle (high-exposure severity), and the patient described has a low CD4 count (high-risk HIV status), the recommendation would be a three-drug regimen (A). The 3-drug regimen is recommended whenever a hollow needlestick pierces the skin and the patient is HIV positive, regardless of his or her viral load or CD4 count. With a solid needle (as in the OR), because the risk of transmission risk is lower, the severity of HIV is considered, and a 2-drug regimen is recommended if the patient is low-risk HIV positive (no active infection, low viral load, high CD4 count); a 3-drug regimen is recommended if the patient is high-risk HIV positive. Follow-up testing to confirm HIV negative status in health-care workers is recommended 3 to 6 months later (D). Part of the initial evaluation of the exposed health-care worker should involve counseling regarding appropriate precautions including the use of barrier protection, not to donate blood, practicing safe sex, and to avoid breastfeeding if possible. If the HIV status of the patient is unknown, it depends on the perceived risk of HIV and type of exposure. So if it is a solid needle, in a patient at a low risk for HIV, prophylaxis is generally not recommended; whereas with a large-bore hollow needle, prophylaxis is generally recommended until the patient tests negative. The average risk of HIV transmission after a percutaneous exposure to HIV-infected blood is overall very low (approximately 0.3%). For health-care workers there is no need to stop working or to inform patients of a possible exposure (C). The most recent statement from the American College of Surgeons states that "HIV-infected surgeons may continue to practice and perform invasive procedures and surgical operations unless there is clear evidence that a significant risk of transmission of infection exists through an inability to meet basic infection control procedures" and that "the HIV status of a surgeon is personal health information and does not need to be disclosed to anyone."

References: American College of Surgeons. Statement on the surgeon and HIV infection. *Bull Am Coll Surg*. 2004;89(5):27–29.

Kuhar DT, Henderson DK, Struble KA, et al. Updated US Public Health Service guidelines for the management of occupational exposures to human immunodeficiency virus and recommendations for postexposure prophylaxis. *Infect Control Hosp Epidemiol*. 2013;34(9):875–892.

16. E. Anorectal disease is the most common indication for surgery in the HIV-infected patient, and it can frequently be the first presenting symptom for an undiagnosed patient. However, diagnosis can be difficult because HIV patients with anorectal abscesses may be unable to mount an adequate response; thus, patients may present without an obvious fluctuant abscess (depending on CD4 count). Additionally, they often have significant tenderness that is out of proportion to exam findings. Previously, operative interventions were avoided because of the risk of perianal sepsis. However, HAART therapy has allowed these patients to be managed with the same practice standards as the noninfected patient with similar outcomes given that they are not neutropenic. Incision and drainage is recommended for this patient (even if no fluctuance is detected) with a concurrent seton placement in the event a fistula is discovered (A). Anoscopy with biopsy should also be performed because a perianal abscess may be the presenting symptom of an anal or rectal malignancy, particularly in an HIV-positive patient. Ordinarily, antibiotics are not recommended for perianal abscess. The exception is the immunocompromised patient. Thus for the HIV patient, antibiotics are routinely used, even in the setting of adequate drainage, and wound cultures should be sent for the identification of atypical organisms (D). The procedure is best performed in the OR under anesthesia (B, C).

References: Miles AJ, Mellor CH, Gazzard B, Allen-Mersh TG, Wastell C. Surgical management of anorectal disease in HIV-positive homosexuals. *Br J Surg*. 1990;77(8):869–871.

Steele SR, Kumar R, Feingold DL, Rafferty JL, Buie WD, Standards Practice Task Force of the American Society of Colon and Rectal Surgeons. Practice parameters for the management of perianal abscess and fistula-in-ano. *Dis Colon Rectum*. 2011;54(12):1465–1474.

Vasilevsky CA. Anorectal abscess and fistula. In: Beck DE, Wexner SD, Hull TL, et al, eds. *The ASCRS manual of colon and rectal surgery*. 2nd ed. Springer; 2013:245–272.

17. D. Over 80% of all intraabdominal abscesses are postsurgical. They typically arise from one of two mechanisms: persistent walled off infection after the resolution of peritonitis or after an anastomotic breakdown or perforation that is effectively controlled by peritoneal defense mechanisms. Presentation can be highly variable depending on their location, ranging from hiccoughing with subphrenic abscesses to a palpable mass in the paracolic gutter or even sepsis. Pelvic abscesses can also present primarily with urinary or fecal symptoms such as urinary retention or tenesmus, a recurrent inclination to evacuate bowels. These typically present on postoperative days 5 to 7, and suspicious symptoms should be evaluated with an abdominal CT with intravenous and potentially oral contrast depending on the clinical scenario. Plain abdominal radiography has been essentially replaced by CT because of increased diagnostic sensitivity and specificity for intraabdominal pathology (C). Though narcotic pain medications or underlying benign prostatic disease can cause urinary retention after surgery, a more serious etiology must be ruled out first (A, B). Almost all intraabdominal abscesses can be treated with percutaneous drainage and antibiotics. In the absence of diffuse peritonitis, operative intervention is likely unnecessary (E).

Reference: Tawadros PS, Simpson J, Fischer JE, Rotstein OD. Abdominal abscess and enteric fistulae. In: Zinner MJ, Ashley SW, eds. *Maingot's abdominal operations*. 12th ed. McGraw-Hill; 2013.

18. C. *C. septicum* has been associated with colonic and hematologic malignancies. In a review of the literature involving 162 cases of *C. septicum* infection, 81% had an associated malignancy, including 34% with colon carcinoma and 40% with a hematologic malignancy. In 37%, the malignancy was occult. The survival rate was only 35%. As such, patients discovered to have an infection with *C. septicum* should have an outpatient colonoscopy scheduled (A, B, D, E).

Reference: Kornbluth AA, Danzig JB, Bernstein LH. Clostridium septicum infection and associated malignancy. Report of 2 cases and review of the literature. *Medicine (Baltimore)*. 1989;68(1):30–37.

19. B. Tetanus is an acute, often fatal, disease caused by an exotoxin produced by the gram-positive anaerobic rod, *C. tetani*, that enters the body through a wound (C). The mean incubation period is 7 to 8 days (range 3–21). In the presence of anaerobic (low oxygen) conditions, the spores germinate. *C. tetani* produces two exotoxins: tetanolysin and tetanospasmin. Tetanospasmin is a neurotoxin and causes the clinical manifestations of tetanus. The toxins act at several sites within the central nervous system (i.e., peripheral motor end plates, spinal cord, brain, and sympathetic nervous system). The toxin interferes with the release of neurotransmitters, blocking inhibitor impulses, leading to unopposed muscle contraction and spasm. It is characterized by generalized rigidity and convulsive spasms of skeletal muscles. It typically involves the jaw muscles (hence the term *lockjaw*) and neck (trismus) and then becomes generalized. The back spasms can be so intense that they can lead to vertebral fractures. Intense facial spasms can lead to a classic appearance known as risus sardonicus (sardonic smile, a smile of contempt or of pain). Laryngospasm and/or spasm of the muscles of respiration leads to interference with breathing. There are no characteristic laboratory findings of tetanus. Culture of the wound or blood is not helpful. The diagnosis is clinical (E). Treatment includes human tetanus immunoglobulin, airway protection by early endotracheal intubation and, if needed, tracheostomy, IV magnesium for muscle spasm prevention, high calorie replenishment, and benzodiazepines. Due to the extreme potency of the toxin, contracting tetanus does not result in immunity (D). Tetanus immune globulin (TIG) is recommended for individuals with tetanus. Active immunization with tetanus toxoid should begin or continue as soon as the person's condition has stabilized. Tetanus is not transmittable from person to person.

Interestingly, it is the only vaccine-preventable disease that is infectious but not contagious (A). Tetanus toxoid should be given as a series of three doses in childhood for prophylaxis and as a booster dose every 10 years. It should also be given for wounds in patients with an incomplete or unknown history of the primary three doses and in those whose last dose was over 10 years ago.

20. B. As a general rule, gram-positive organisms produce exotoxins, and gram-negative organisms have endotoxins. *S. pyogenes* produces streptokinase, which acts as a fibrinolytic (A). *B. fragilis*, a gram-negative organism, does not produce an exotoxin and has defective lipopolysaccharide and lipid A. *C. tetani* produces tetanospasmin, which acts as a neurotoxin (C). *S. aureus* produces hemolysin and leukocidin, which damage plasma membranes of the host, and exfoliatin, which cleaves desmosomes (D). *C. perfringens* produces heat-labile enterotoxin causing watery diarrhea (E).

Nutrition and Metabolism 32

ERIC O. YEATES, AREG GRIGORIAN, AND CHRISTIAN DE VIRGILIO

ABSITE 99th Percentile High-Yields

I. Daily Caloric Needs and Calculations
   A. Estimated daily needs: 20 to 25 kcal/kg (approx. 50% carbohydrates, 25% protein, 25% fat)
   B. 1 g of carbs = 4 kcal, 1 g of protein = 4 kcal, 1 g of fat = 9 kcal
   C. Critically ill patients should receive 30 kcal/kg of nutritional support a day; patients who are sedated and mechanically ventilated have a lower expenditure of energy and should receive 25 kcal/kg/day; paralyzed patients should receive 20 kcal/kg/day
   D. Most critically ill patients should receive 1.2 to 2.0 g protein/kg/day; protein requirements are increased in the obese, BMI of 30 to 40 should receive 2.0 g protein/kg/day and BMI >40 should receive 2.5 g protein/kg/day as part of an overall strategy of hypocaloric feeding
   E. The presence of a 40% burn requires nutritional support with 2.5 g protein/kg/day
   F. Critically ill patients with renal failure should receive 1.25 to 1.75 g protein/kg/day, whereas patients with renal failure on continuous renal replacement therapy require 2.5 g protein/kg/day
   G. Respiratory quotient (RQ): estimates basal metabolic rate; ratio of carbon dioxide produced by the body to oxygen consumed by the body
      1. RQ > 1.0: overfeeding, can lead to difficulty weaning from ventilator due to hypercarbia
      2. RQ = 1: carbohydrate utilization
      3. RQ = 0.8 to 0.9: protein utilization (average 0.825; mixture of fat, protein, carb metabolization)
      4. RQ = 0.7: fat utilization
      5. RQ < 0.7: starvation

II. Amino Acids: Building Blocks for Proteins
   A. Essential: not made by the body, must be ingested; phenylalanine, valine, threonine, tryptophan, isoleucine, methionine, histidine, leucine, lysine
   B. Nonessential: body can produce these: alanine, asparagine, aspartic acid, glutamic acid, serine
   C. Conditional amino acids: body can produce these, but are essential in times of stress: Arginine, cysteine, glutamine, glycine, ornithine, proline, tyrosine

III. Nitrogen Balance: To Study Protein Metabolism
   A. Nitrogen balance = protein intake/6.25 – (24-hour urine nitrogen + 4 g)
   B. 4 g approximates losses via sweat and feces
   C. Positive = anabolism; negative = catabolism

IV. Starvation
   A. Certain cells (brain, red blood cells) primarily use glucose for energy (except when starving)
   B. During starvation, insulin decreases and glucagon increases, leading to an increase in glycogenolysis, lipolysis, and ketogenesis

C. Glycogen stores (glucose supply) are depleted after 1 to 2 days
D. Next, fatty acids (can't cross blood-brain barrier) are oxidized to make ketones (for brain)
E. With further starvation, muscle (protein) breaks down to provide alanine for gluconeogenesis

V. Vitamin and Mineral Deficiencies

Deficiency	Manifestation/disease
Vitamin A	Night blindness
Vitamin B_1 (Thiamine)	Wernicke's encephalopathy, Beriberi
Vitamin B_3 (Niacin)	Pellagra (diarrhea, dermatitis, dementia)
Vitamin B_6 (Pyridoxine)	Anemia, peripheral neuropathy
Vitamin B_{12} (Cyanocobalamin)	Megaloblastic anemia, peripheral neuropathy
Vitamin C	Impaired collagen cross-linking, scurvy
Vitamin D	Rickets, osteomalacia
Vitamin E	Neuropathy
Vitamin K	Coagulopathy
Chromium	Hyperglycemia, neuropathy
Copper	Anemia, leukopenia, muscle weakness
Iodine	Goiter
Phosphate	Diaphragm muscle weakness, arrhythmia, confusion
Selenium	Cardiomyopathy, weakness
Zinc	Delayed wound healing, hair loss, acne
Essential fatty acids	Dermatitis, hair loss, easy bruising, delayed wound healing
Essential amino acids	Decreased immune function

VI. Nutritional Deficiencies Associated With Surgeries/Surgical Diseases

Surgery/surgical diseases	Related nutritional deficiency
Gastric bypass	Deficiency of vitamin B12, folate, zinc, iron, copper, calcium, vitamin D
Gastric sleeve resection	Deficiency of vitamin B12, folate, zinc, iron
Carcinoid syndrome	Tryptophan deficiency (due to conversion to serotonin) causes pellagra
Blind loop syndrome	Deficiency of vitamin B12, folate, iron, vitamin E
Refeeding syndrome	Hypophosphatemia, hypomagnesemia, hypokalemia

Questions

1. A 45-year-old male is diagnosed with severe gallstone pancreatitis. It is currently hospital day 2 and he is not requiring vasopressor support or invasive mechanical ventilation. He still reports mild epigastric pain. Which of the following is true regarding the ideal management of his nutrition?

    A. He should be started on an oral diet as tolerated

    B. A nasoenteric tube should be placed with tube feeds started at a trophic rate and advanced to goal as tolerated

    C. Nasojejunal feeding is preferred over nasogastric feeding

    D. Total parenteral nutrition (TPN) is preferred over enteral nutrition

    E. Enteric feeding should not be considered until abdominal pain has resolved

2. Which of the following is true regarding immunonutrition?

    A. Alanine is a substrate in the production of nitric oxide (NO)

    B. Glutamine has been shown to reduce radiation injury to the small bowel

    C. For cancer patients undergoing surgery, immunonutrition reduces postoperative infectious complications

    D. For patients undergoing major abdominal surgery, immunonutrition reduces mortality

    E. Glutamine has been shown to decrease ventilator time in critically ill patients

3. A 55-year-old alcoholic female is admitted to the hospital for a small bowel obstruction. Her serum albumin is 1.8 g/dL (normal range is 3.4–5.4 g/dL) and prealbumin is 8 mg/dL (normal range is 15–36 mg/dL). On hospital day 5, she fails nonoperative management and undergoes an exploratory laparotomy with lysis of adhesions. She subsequently develops a postoperative ileus and is started on total parenteral nutrition on postoperative day 3. A day later, she rapidly develops weakness, altered mental status, and hypoxic respiratory failure requiring intubation. Which of the following is true regarding her condition?

    A. Thiamine deficiency is the most likely cause of her symptoms

    B. Alcoholism is not a risk factor for developing this condition

    C. This condition rarely occurs with enteral nutrition

    D. This condition could have potentially been avoided by starting TPN at a slower rate

    E. She should be given a calcium infusion

4. Which of the following amino acids can be synthesized de novo in humans in any physiologic state?

    A. Tryptophan

    B. Tyrosine

    C. Glycine

    D. Serine

    E. Any branched-chain amino acid

5. Which of the following is true regarding the use of preoperative TPN to prevent postoperative complications?

    A. It is useful even if used for as little as 3 days

    B. It is efficacious if the patient has lost more than 15% weight before surgery

    C. There is no evidence that it lowers the complication rate

    D. Slightly overfeeding for 7 days is recommended as a means to maximize replacement of caloric deficits

    E. TPN is efficacious even in mild to moderate malnutrition

6. Which of the following is true regarding nutritional deficiencies after a partial gastrectomy with a Billroth II (gastrojejunostomy) reconstruction?
   A. Calcium absorption will be minimally affected
   B. Iron deficiency anemia is more common with a Billroth I (gastroduodenostomy) than a Billroth II
   C. Vitamin B12 deficiency will present with a low mean corpuscular volume
   D. The stomach has no intrinsic absorptive ability
   E. Carbohydrate absorption is not impaired after surgery

7. Which of the following is true regarding nutrition needs and requirements?
   A. Preterm infants may need up to 2 g/kg per day of protein
   B. 1 g of fat provides 4 kcals of energy
   C. A respiratory quotient (RQ) greater than 1.0 suggests overfeeding
   D. Ventilated critically ill patients require more daily caloric intake than nonventilated critically ill patients
   E. Obese patients require less daily protein intake compared to nonobese patients

8. A 23-year-old male was admitted 7 days ago for multisystem trauma including multiple long-bone fractures, subdural hematoma, and pulmonary contusions and is still on the ventilator. Which of the following is true regarding tools for assessing nutritional status?
   A. Use of serial measurements of albumin and prealbumin is the "gold standard" for trauma patients
   B. Measurement of nitrogen balance underestimates nitrogen input
   C. The Mini Nutritional Assessment is designed specifically for hospitalized patients
   D. Creatinine height index may overestimate lean body mass in trauma patients
   E. Transferrin is the serum protein that correlates the closest to nitrogen balance

9. Which of the following is true regarding the risk of hypoglycemia following cessation of total parenteral nutrition (TPN)?
   A. It commonly occurs in patients with liver disease
   B. Tapering of TPN is recommended so as to avoid this complication
   C. This complication is relatively common
   D. It is more likely to occur in a diabetic patient
   E. It is more likely to occur in patients with renal disease

10. Which of the following is true about the pharmacologic treatment of cancer cachexia?
   A. There is no evidence that ghrelin mimetics are of benefit
   B. Cannabinoids are superior to megestrol acetate in stimulating weight gain
   C. When initiated early, megestrol acetate has been demonstrated to improve survival
   D. Megestrol is a progesterone derivative
   E. Anabolic steroids lead to improved long-term weight gain

11. Which of the following is true regarding energy homeostasis during periods of starvation?
   A. The largest source of energy after glycogen is depleted is free fatty acids
   B. Skeletal muscle has the largest store of glycogen available systemically
   C. Glucose is converted to lactate in the liver
   D. Red blood cells metabolize glucose aerobically
   E. The brain is unable to utilize ketones

12. The most important amino acid used for gluconeogenesis by the liver is:
   A. Glutamine
   B. Serine
   C. Alanine
   D. Tyrosine
   E. Asparagine

13. Poor glucose control is a manifestation of deficiency of:
   A. Zinc
   B. Copper
   C. Chromium
   D. Molybdenum
   E. Selenium

14. Which of the following is true regarding long-term TPN?
    A. Fat is considered the nutritional basis of TPN
    B. It may lead to a mucin gel matrix of cholesterol crystals and calcium bilirubinate in the gallbladder
    C. Hepatic dysfunction related to TPN is less likely to be lethal in infants than in adults
    D. It has not been shown to lead to hepatic fibrosis
    E. Carnitine supplementation has been shown to reverse TPN-related liver damage

15. Which of the following amino acids has shown potential for increasing the absorptive capability of the intestine in patients that have undergone large segment small bowel resection?
    A. Glutamine
    B. Serine
    C. Alanine
    D. Tyrosine
    E. Arginine

Answers

1. B. Though advancing to an oral diet as tolerated is recommended in mild acute pancreatitis, this is not the recommended management in moderate to severe pancreatitis (A). Instead, patients with moderate to severe acute pancreatitis should have a nasoenteric/oroenteric tube placed and enteral nutrition started in the first 1 to 2 hospital days (B). Mild epigastric pain is not a contraindication to enteric feeding (E). With regards to the level at which to feed, three randomized controlled trials showed no difference in tolerance or clinical outcomes between gastric and jejunal feeding (C). The use of parenteral nutrition rather than enteral nutrition has also been explored in multiple metaanalyses of ten randomized clinical trials. These have shown that those receiving enteral nutrition had lower infectious morbidity, shorter length of stay, fewer surgical interventions, and decreased mortality (D). Guidelines from the Society of Critical Care Medicine and the American Society for Parenteral and Enteral Nutrition now recommend consideration of probiotics in severe pancreatitis for those receiving early enteral nutrition, which is based on a 2010 metaanalysis that showed a reduction in infection and hospital LOS.

Reference: McClave SA, Taylor BE, Martindale RG, et al. Guidelines for the Provision and Assessment of Nutrition Support Therapy in the Adult Critically Ill Patient: Society of Critical Care Medicine (SCCM) and American Society for Parenteral and Enteral Nutrition (A.S.P.E.N.). *J Parenter Enter Nutr*. 2016;40(2):159–211.

2. C. Immunonutrition is the ability to modulate the immune system using specific nutrients. This strategy has most often been utilized in critically ill and surgical patients who often require exogenous nutrients through enteral or parenteral routes. The nutrients most robustly studied for immunonutrition are arginine, glutamine, omega-3 fatty acids, branched chain amino acids, and nucleotides. Arginine and glutamine, two amino acids that have been of particular interest in this field, have unique properties that may explain their mechanism of action. Arginine, via the arginine deaminase pathway, is a unique substrate for production of NO (A). Glutamine is the most prevalent free amino acid in the

human body and is also the major metabolic fuel for enterocytes and other cells within the immune system. Administration of glutamine has been shown to have no effect on reducing radiation injury (B). A number of large systematic reviews have shown benefits of immunonutrients in various subsets of surgical patients. For example, in surgical cancer patients and patients undergoing major abdominal surgery, immunonutrition reduces infectious complications and shortens length of stay, but does not decrease mortality (C, D). In burn patients, initial clinical trial data suggests that glutamine may reduce mortality, length of stay, and gram-negative bacteremia though the definitive RE-ENERGIZE trial is ongoing. However, there may be subsets of patients, like the critically ill, who may be harmed by immunonutrition. Two large multicenter randomized controlled trials of critically ill ventilated patients showed that supplementation with glutamine and/or antioxidants may increase 6-month mortality (E).

References: Calder PC. Immunonutrition. *BMJ*. 2003;327(7407):117–118.

Suchner U, Kuhn KS, Fürst P. The scientific basis of immunonutrition. *Proc Nutr Soc*. 2000;59(4):553–563.

Probst P, Ohmann S, Klaiber U, et al. Meta-analysis of immunonutrition in major abdominal surgery. *BJS*. 2017;104(12):1594–1608.

Wischmeyer PE. Glutamine in burn injury. *Nutr Clin Pract*. 2019;34(5):681–687.

Yu K, Zheng X, Wang G, et al. Immunonutrition vs standard nutrition for cancer patients: a systematic review and meta-analysis (part 1). *J Parenter Enter Nutr*. 2020;44(5):742–767.

van Zanten AR, Hofman Z, Heyland DK. Consequences of the REDOXS and METAPLUS Trials: the end of an era of glutamine and antioxidant supplementation for critically ill patients? *J Parenter Enter Nutr*. 2015;39(8):890–892.

3. D. This patient developed refeeding syndrome, which is a potentially fatal metabolic disturbance after the reinstitution of nutrition in a malnourished patient (low serum albumin and prealbumin). Prolonged starvation leads to the severe depletion of a number of minerals, though serum concentrations remain relatively normal due to compensatory intra/extracellular shifts. During refeeding, insulin is released, leading to stimulation of glycogen, fat, and protein synthesis, which requires phosphate, magnesium, and other cofactors. Phosphate, magnesium, and potassium (through the ATPase symporter) are all taken up into cells, leading to a sudden decrease in serum levels. Refeeding syndrome is caused by these depletions with hypophosphatemia being the most common and most severe disturbance (A). Some common clinical manifestations of severe hypophosphatemia are arrhythmias, metabolic acidosis, seizures, delirium, hyperglycemia, and profound weakness, sometimes manifesting as diaphragm insufficiency requiring mechanical ventilatory support. Risk factors for refeeding syndrome include anorexia nervosa, malnutrition, chronic alcoholism, cancer, recent surgery, elderly patients with comorbidities, BMI <16, recent unintentional weight loss, and recent fasting (B). Refeeding syndrome can develop with either enteral or parenteral nutrition, but may be more common with enteral nutrition due to the release of incretins (C). To prevent refeeding syndrome, it is recommended that nutrition be started at no more than 50% of normal daily requirements for those who have not eaten in 5 days (D). In patients at high-risk of refeeding syndrome, nutrition can be increased to meet full needs over 4 to 7 days. Treatment of refeeding syndrome should focus on the rapid correction of electrolyte abnormalities, with hypophosphatemia, hypomagnesemia, and hypokalemia being the most common (E).

References: McKnight CL, Newberry C, Sarav M, et al. Refeeding syndrome in the critically ill: a literature review and clinician's guide. *Curr Gastroenterol Rep.* 2019;21(11):58.

Mehanna HM, Moledina J, Travis J. Refeeding syndrome: what it is, and how to prevent and treat it. *BMJ.* 2008;336(7659):1495–1498.

4. D. Amino acids are the building blocks used for the synthesis of proteins. The nonessential amino acids are those that can be created de novo without an exogenous source. In humans, these include alanine, aspartic acid, asparagine, glutamic acid, and serine. Essential amino acids are those that cannot be synthesized and require an exogenous source: phenylalanine, threonine, tryptophan, methionine, lysine, and histidine (A–E). In addition, all the branched-chain amino acids (leucine, isoleucine, and valine [LIV]) are essential amino acids. A third category of amino acids includes those that can become essential in certain physiologic states, such as premature infants or severe states of distress. These include arginine, cysteine, glycine, glutamine, ornithine, proline, and tyrosine. Patients with phenylketonuria (PKU) need to keep their intake of phenylalanine low, and because it is the precursor to tyrosine, it can become an essential amino acid in this disease state (B, C).

5. B. Providing nutritional intervention should be limited to patients with severe malnutrition and immunologic dysfunction. In a Veterans Affairs multicenter trial, malnourished patients who lost more than 15% of their baseline body weight had decreased operative septic complications when they received preoperative nutritional intervention for 7 to 10 days (A). However, in the group stratified as having mild to moderate malnutrition, the decrease in surgical complications was more than offset by the increase in catheter-related infectious complications (E). TPN-induced hyperglycemia is likely a contributor to adverse outcomes (D).

Thus, improperly administered TPN increases the risk of catheter-related and noncatheter-related infection (C). Buzby proposed the following guidelines: (1) Postoperative TPN should be considered when oral or enteral feeding is not anticipated within 7 to 10 days in previously well-nourished patients or within 5 to 7 days in previously malnourished or critically ill patients. (2) Preoperative TPN should be considered in patients who cannot or should not eat or receive enteral feedings if the operation must be delayed for more than 3 to 5 days. (3) Preoperative TPN should be considered in the most severely malnourished surgical candidates if an operative delay is not contraindicated. In patients with only mild to moderate degrees of malnutrition, preoperative TPN is not indicated.

References: Bozzetti F, Gavazzi C, Miceli R, et al. Perioperative total parenteral nutrition in malnourished, gastrointestinal cancer patients: a randomized, clinical trial. *J Parenter Enteral Nutr.* 2000;24(1):7–14.

Buzby GP. Overview of randomized clinical trials of total parenteral nutrition for malnourished surgical patients. *World J Surg.* 1993;17(2):173–177.

6. E. The main deficiencies of clinical concern that can be seen after gastrectomy are iron (most common), calcium, and vitamin B12. Stomach acid helps reduce dietary iron from a ferric to a ferrous state, which allows it to be actively absorbed in the duodenum and jejunum. This can put patients at risk of iron-deficiency anemia following partial or total gastrectomy. It does occur more commonly with a Billroth II compared to a Billroth I (B). Calcium absorption takes place primarily in the duodenum by an active process that is regulated by vitamin D and parathyroid hormone. After gastrectomy with Billroth II reconstruction, patients are at risk for nutritional deficiencies primarily because of quicker gastric emptying and anatomically bypassing the duodenum (A). Parietal cells located in the gastric fundus and corpus are responsible for the production of intrinsic factor, which is required for the absorption of vitamin B12 in the terminal ileum. Vitamin B12 deficiency will present with a megaloblastic anemia (increased MCV) and peripheral neuropathy (C). While the stomach does not typically absorb many nutrients, it can absorb some lipid-soluble compounds such as alcohol, aspirin, and nonsteroidal antiinflammatory drugs (NSAIDs) (D). Though fatty acid absorption has been shown to be affected after gastrectomy, there is no evidence that carbohydrate absorption is impaired in any way.

References: Guyton AC, Hall JE. *Textbook of medical physiology.* 11th ed. WB Saunders; 2005.

Lee JH, Hyung WJ, Kim HI, et al. Method of reconstruction governs iron metabolism after gastrectomy for patients with gastric cancer. *Ann Surg.* 2013;258(6):964–969.

7. C. Critically ill patients should receive 30 kcal/kg of nutritional support a day. Patients who are sedated and mechanically ventilated have a lower expenditure of energy and should receive 25 kcal/kg/day (D). The daily recommended protein requirement in an adult is approximately 0.8 g/kg per day. However, this can increase in the setting of physiologic stress. Most critically ill patients should receive 1.2 to 2.0 g protein/kg/day. Burn patients' protein requirement is closer to 2 to 2.5 g/kg per day. There is also an increased demand for protein in pediatric patients because of active growth, with the largest being preterm infants who may need 3 to 4 g/kg per day (A). 1 g of fat provides 9 kcal of energy (B). Protein requirements are increased in the obese but should be part of an overall strategy of hypocaloric feeding (E). The RQ is the ratio of carbon dioxide produced to oxygen consumed, and it can be used to estimate which energy source is the primary substrate for energy production. However, it must be measured at a steady state. By knowing the RQ, you are able to determine the primary substrate being used for energy production: greater than 1 for lipogenesis (overfeeding state), 1.0 for carbohydrates, 0.8 for proteins, and 0.7 for fatty acids. This can then be extrapolated to the nutritional state of the patient by knowing what substrates are being used at various phases of fasting. A normal RQ is around 0.85 because the body is using about 50% carbohydrates and 50% fatty acids. The overfed state is predominated by conversion of glucose into fats and correlates with an RQ of more than 1. Starving patients are primarily using fatty acids as the primary fuel source and have an RQ of less than 0.7.

References: Barrett KE, Boitano S, Barman SM, Brooks HL. *Ganong's review of medical physiology.* 23rd ed. McGraw-Hill Medical; 2009.

Guyton AC, Hall JE. *Textbook of medical physiology.* 11th ed. WB Saunders; 2005.

8. D. Nutritional assessment in hospitalized patients is limited by multiple confounding factors. While there are lots of tools available for nutritional assessment, no single item has proven to be infallible in assessing a patient's nutritional status. Current Eastern Association for the Surgery of Trauma (EAST) Guidelines for nutritional assessment in the trauma patient use nitrogen balance as the "gold standard" by which all other tests are evaluated (A). Though nitrogen balance is a fairly accurate measurement of nutritional status, it is limited by the impracticality of 24-hour urine collection and the often inaccurate recording of daily nitrogen input. Nitrogen output is often underestimated and input is often overestimated (B). Of the serum proteins, prealbumin seems to correlate the closest with nitrogen balance (E). Many of the serum proteins used for nutrition assessment—albumin, prealbumin, transferrin, and retinol-binding protein—are altered in times of stress or infection, so most sources recommend including an acute phase reactant such as CRP to put these values in context. While the creatinine height index can give you an estimate of lean body mass, changes in creatinine excretion from systemic processes (e.g., trauma, renal disease, etc.) can make the results unreliable. The Mini Nutritional Assessment is specifically designed for the elderly (C).

References: Elmadfa I, Meyer AL. Developing suitable methods of nutritional status assessment: a continuous challenge. *Adv Nutr.* 2014;5(5):590S–598S.

Jacobs DG, Jacobs DO, Kudsk KA, et al. Practice management guidelines for nutritional support of the trauma patient. *J Trauma.* 2004;57(3):660–679.

Norton JA. *Essential practice of surgery: basic science and clinical evidence.* Springer; 2003.

9. D. Hypoglycemia following the abrupt cessation of TPN has been reported, though it is very rare (C). Hypoglycemia can present with diaphoresis, confusion, agitation, tachycardia, and, if severe, diabetic coma. Most patients will tolerate abrupt cessation of TPN, and tapering is generally unnecessary. Two studies published in 1995 and 2000 both showed

no difference in symptomatic hypoglycemia or serum glucose measurements between a TPN-dependent group randomized to abrupt cessation versus step-wise tapering (B). However, in the diabetic patient, and in those with poor glucose control, tapering of TPN should be considered (A–E).

References: Eisenberg PG, Gianino S, Clutter WE, Fleshman JW. Abrupt discontinuation of cycled parenteral nutrition is safe. *Dis Colon Rectum.* 1995;38(9):933–939.

Nirula R, Yamada K, Waxman K. The effect of abrupt cessation of total parenteral nutrition on serum glucose: a randomized trial. *Am Surg.* 2000;66(9):866–869.

10. D. Cancer-related cachexia/anorexia has been associated with failure of cancer treatment, delay in initiation of treatment, increased treatment toxicity, early discontinuation of treatment, and shorter survival in terminal cancer patients. It has even been implicated as a direct cause of death in 20% to 40% of cancer patients. Current National Comprehensive Cancer Network (NCCN) Guidelines recommend early screening and early treatment of this condition. Before initiation of appetite stimulation, treatable causes of anorexia such as oral candidiasis or depression should be addressed. Megestrol acetate (Megace) is the most widely studied and, so far, most efficacious medication available to help improve appetite and weight gain in this patient population. Megestrol acetate is a synthetic, orally active derivative of progesterone. It has been found to improve appetite, caloric intake, and nutritional status in several clinical trials. A study conducted in 2010 demonstrated that megestrol acetate used in combination with olanzapine was associated with improvements in weight gain, appetite, nausea, and overall quality of life when compared with megestrol acetate alone, even when corrected for improvements in depression. Unfortunately, megestrol acetate, either alone or in combination with olanzapine, has not been demonstrated consistently in the literature to improve survival (C). It is also important to note that 1 in 23 patients using megestrol acetate will have a thromboembolic event; therefore, it should be used with caution in susceptible patients. While it has been demonstrated that steroids have results equivalent to megestrol acetate, they are short-lived and patients quickly return to baseline after cessation of the drug (E). Cannabinoids have been looked at extensively in chemotherapy-related nausea and AIDS-cachexia, but studies done in the cancer population tend to show inferiority to megestrol acetate (B). Ghrelin mimetics have been demonstrated to improve lean body mass (A).

References: Nagaya N, Kojima M, Kangawa K. Ghrelin, a novel growth hormone-releasing peptide, in the treatment of cardiopulmonary-associated cachexia. *Intern Med (Tokyo).* 2006;45(3):127–134.

Navari RM, Brenner MC. Treatment of cancer-related anorexia with olanzapine and megestrol acetate: a randomized trial. *Support Care Cancer.* 2010;18(8):951–956.

Ohnuma T. Treatment of cachexia. In: Kufe DW, Pollock RE, Weichselbaum RR, et al., eds. *Holland-Frei cancer medicine review: companion to Holland-Frei cancer medicine.* 6th ed. BC Decker; 2003.

11. A. After a meal, carbohydrates are rapidly used, and any excess is stored as fatty acids or as glycogen (primarily in the liver and skeletal muscle). Though the skeletal muscle has proportionally more glycogen stored, it is not available systemically during fasting because these cells lack glucose-6-phosphatase, which is the final step needed for the creation of glucose from glycogen (B). As such, the glycogen stores are used only locally. Liver stores of glycogen are normally used within 16 to 36 hours, but it can be shorter in certain disease states. After glycogen stores are depleted, the body turns to the breakdown of skeletal muscle and lipids for energy. The largest source of energy is free fatty acids, but they are a relatively poor source of free glucose. While amino acids from protein breakdown can be used for gluconeogenesis in the liver (early in starvation) and kidney (late in starvation), most proteins serve an important role in bodily functions. Lactate and glycerol can also be used as substrates for gluconeogenesis (C). During prolonged fasting, tissues that are able to use alternate fuel sources (i.e., breakdown products of fatty acids) begin to do so, and subsequently, the breakdown of muscle slows and breakdown of body fat increases. However, gluconeogenesis never completely stops because several cells are heavily reliant on glucose as a fuel source. Red blood cells are solely reliant on the anaerobic conversion of glucose to lactate because they lack the mitochondria required for the utilization of fatty acids or for the aerobic breakdown of glucose (D). In addition, white blood cells, cells in the adrenal medulla, and peripheral nerves are all obligate glucose users. While the brain is heavily reliant on glucose as a fuel source, it can use ketones to some degree (E).

References: Brunicardi FC, Andersen DK, Billiar TR, Dunn DL, Hunter JG, Matthews JB, Pollock RE, eds. *Schwartz's principles of surgery*. 10th ed. McGraw Hill Education; 2015.

Cahill GF. Fuel metabolism in starvation. *Annu Rev Nutr*. 2006;26(1):1–22.

12. C. In humans, the main substrates for gluconeogenesis are lactate, pyruvate, amino acids, and, to a lesser extent, glycerol. This is primarily stimulated by glucagon. Alanine is the most important amino acid precursor in gluconeogenesis. When the liver has exhausted all of its alanine supply, the kidney takes over gluconeogenesis where glutamine may be used for gluconeogenesis (A). Additionally, alanine and phenylalanine are the only amino acids that increase during times of stress. Serine, tyrosine, and asparagine are not substrates for gluconeogenesis (B–D, E).

13. C. Chromium is a cofactor involved in the utilization of insulin at the tissue level, and deficiency often manifests as a sudden diabetic state in which blood sugar is difficult to control, along with peripheral neuropathy and encephalopathy. Zinc deficiency has numerous manifestations, including alopecia, poor wound healing, immunosuppression, night blindness or photophobia, impaired taste or smell, neuritis, and a variety of skin disorders (A). Copper deficiency manifests as microcytic anemia, pancytopenia, depigmentation, and osteopenia (B). Essential mineral and vitamin deficiency may occur with increased frequency in patients receiving long-term parenteral nutrition. Molybdenum deficiency is characterized by the toxic accumulation of sulfur-containing amino acids and encephalopathy (D). Selenium deficiency may result in diffuse skeletal myopathy

and cardiomyopathy, loss of pigmentation, and erythrocyte macrocytosis (E).

14. B. Glucose is considered the nutritional basis of TPN, while fat is considered the nutritional basis of peripheral parenteral nutrition (PPN) (A). Liver dysfunction is commonly observed in patients receiving TPN. It develops in 40% to 60% of infants who require long-term TPN for intestinal failure. The clinical spectrum includes cholestasis, biliary sludge (mucin gel matrix of cholesterol crystals and calcium bilirubinate), cholelithiasis, hepatic fibrosis with progression to biliary cirrhosis, and the development of portal hypertension and liver failure (D). Predisposing factors include short gut syndrome, a history of bacterial overgrowth, and recurrent sepsis or a chronic inflammatory state. Lack of enteral feeding contributes by leading to reduced gut hormone secretion, decreased bile flow, and biliary stasis. Deficiencies in particular nutrients such as carnitine, taurine, cysteine, and S-adenosylmethionine are also implicated in TPN-related liver disease. Hepatic steatosis may be improved with carnitine supplementation, but there is no evidence that it will reverse TPN-related liver damage (E). Hepatic dysfunction is more serious and lethal in infants dependent on TPN compared with adults (C). Even when enteral feeding is begun and TPN is discontinued, hepatic dysfunction may persist and may progress to cirrhosis and death. The ultimate solution is combined liver and small bowel transplantation.

Reference: Kelly D. Liver complications of pediatric parenteral nutrition: epidemiology. *Nutrition*. 1998;14(1):153–157.

15. A. In two randomized studies, patients with short gut syndrome secondary to small bowel resection were seen to have modest improvements after the administration of supplemental glutamine, exogenous growth hormone, and a modified diet with increased fiber. One study showed an improvement in calorie, protein, and carbohydrate absorption as well as a reduction in stool volume. However, the second study failed to show an increase in the absorption of macronutrients and only showed an improvement in electrolyte absorption and a reduction in delayed gastric emptying. These specific interventions seemed to exert bowel-specific trophic effects, which may influence nutritional absorption. However, it is unclear whether this is through a direct or indirect mechanism. It is important to keep in mind that these studies were done on a small number of patients, but they show some promise in patients that would otherwise be completely TPN dependent. The remaining answer choices have not been shown to improve intestinal absorption efficiency (B–E).

References: Byrne TA, Morrissey TB, Nattakom TV, Ziegler TR, Wilmore DW. Growth hormone, glutamine, and a modified diet enhance nutrient absorption in patients with severe short bowel syndrome. *J Parenter Enteral Nutr*. 1995;19(4):296–302.

Scolapio JS, Camilleri M, Fleming CR, et al. Effect of growth hormone, glutamine, and diet on adaptation in short-bowel syndrome: a randomized, controlled study. *Gastroenterology*. 1997;113(4):1074–1081.

Oncology and Tumor Biology

33

ALEXANDRA MOORE, AREG GRIGORIAN, AND CHRISTIAN DE VIRGILIO

ABSITE 99th Percentile High-Yields

I. Principles of Radiation Therapy
   A. External beam radiation therapy: high energy electrons
      1. Damages DNA during replication (M phase of mitosis) leading to apoptosis
      2. Radiation effectiveness: double-stranded DNA breaks due to oxygen free radicals
         a) Tissue hypoxia significantly reduces radiation damage and effectiveness; larger tumors are relatively hypoxic and thus more resistant to radiation compared to smaller tumors

II. Principles of Chemotherapy
   A. Most agents act during DNA replication (the S phase of mitosis)

III. Common Genetic Mutations in Specific Tumor Types
   A. RAS: colorectal, neuroblastoma, pancreas, bladder
   B. HER2/neu: breast, ovarian, stomach
   C. MYC: cervical, colon, breast, lung, gastric

IV. Monoclonal Antibodies
   A. Human epidermal growth factor receptor 2 (HER2) gene amplification:
      1. Trastuzumab: inhibits HER2-HER3 dimerization; used in HER2+ breast and stomach cancer
      2. Pertuzumab: binds extracellular HER2 domain
   B. Vascular endothelial growth factor (VEGF) inhibitor:
      1. Bevacizumab: directly binds VEGF, inhibits angiogenesis
         a) Metastatic colon cancer
         b) Side effects include hypersensitivity type-1 reaction, viscous perforation, and impaired wound healing due to inhibition of angiogenesis
   C. Epidermal growth factor receptor (EGFR) inhibitor:
      1. Cetuximab: directly binds and inhibits EGFR
         a) Metastatic KRAS wild-type colorectal cancer (no benefit in KRAS mutation), head and neck squamous cell cancer
   D. Tyrosine kinase inhibitors
      1. Imatinib: tyrosine kinase inhibitor; neoadjuvant or adjuvant use in GIST
      2. Sunitinib: tyrosine kinase inhibitors; 2nd line therapy in GIST if imatinib is ineffective; also used in unresectable neuroendocrine tumors
      3. Sorafenib: multitargeted tyrosine kinase inhibitor; used in hepatocellular and gallbladder carcinomas
   E. Immune checkpoint inhibitors:
      1. Ipilimumab: CTLA-4 checkpoint inhibitor
         a) Improves survival in unresectable, node-positive or metastatic melanoma
      2. Pembrolizumab: PD1 checkpoint inhibitor
         a) Melanoma, lung cancer

V. Systemic Biomarkers in Cancer
   A. CEA: Colon cancer. Particularly for detecting recurrence after surgery
      1. >200 ug/L before resection = poor prognosis
   B. CA 19-9: Pancreatic cancer
      1. >1000U/mL = likely metastatic disease
   C. CA-125: Epithelial ovarian cancer
   D. Inhibin-A: epithelial stroma tumors such as mucinous and endometrioid carcinoma and sex cord-stromal tumors such as granulosa cell tumor and Sertoli-Leydig cell tumor
   E. AFP: hepatocellular carcinoma (HCC), nonseminomatous germ cell tumors
   F. β-hCG: germ cell tumors
   G. Calcitonin: medullary thyroid cancer
   H. Thyroglobulin: papillary thyroid cancer; particularly for detecting recurrence after surgery and radioactive iodine therapy
   I. Chromogranin A: carcinoid tumors

Chemotherapeutic Side Effects

Agent	Side effects
Bleomycin	Pulmonary fibrosis
Carboplatin	Myelosuppression
Cisplatin	Nephrotoxicity, neurotoxicity, ototoxicity
Cyclophosphamide	Hemorrhagic cystitis (treat with Mesna), gonadal dysfunction, SIADH
Doxorubicin	Cardiac toxicity (irreversible)
Methotrexate	Nephrotoxicity, nausea (treat with folinic acid)
Oxaliplatin	Peripheral neuropathy
Taxols	Neuropathy
Trastuzumab	Cardiomyopathy (reversible)
Vinblastine	Myelosuppression
Vincristine	Peripheral neuropathy

Hereditary Cancer Syndromes

Gene	Syndrome	Associated cancers
APC	Familial adenomatous polyposis (FAP)	Colon, duodenum, gastric, thyroid, desmoid tumors
TP53	Li Fraumeni	Breast (90%), colon, lung, sarcomas, brain, adrenal
DNA Mismatch Repair (MLH1, MSH2, MSH6, PMS2, EPCAM)	Hereditary nonpolyposis colorectal cancer (HNPCC)	Colorectal, endometrial, gastric, ovarian, GU tract, hepatobiliary, small bowel, and CNS
SMAD4, BMPR1A	Juvenile polyposis	Colon, gastric
STK11	Peutz-Jeghers	Hamartomas—GI and mucocutaneous. Malignancies—breast, colon, pancreatic, gastric, ovarian, lung, small intestine, endometrial, testicular, esophageal
PTEN	Cowden	Breast, facial lesions, GI hamartomas, thyroid, endometrial
BRCA1		Breast (87% risk), ovarian (40%–60%)
BRCA2		Breast (80%), ovarian (15%–20%), prostate, pancreatic

Multiple Endocrine Neoplasia (MEN) Syndromes

Syndrome	Gene	Protein	Inheritance	MC Clinical presentation	Organs/tumors involved	What to treat first
MEN 1	11q13	Menin	Autosomal Dominant	Hypercalcemia	Pancreatic NET Pituitary Hyperparathyroidism	Hyperparathyroidism
MEN 2A	10q11.21	RET	Autosomal Dominant	Medullary Thyroid Cancer	Medullary Thyroid CA Pheochromocytoma Hyperparathyroidism	Pheochromocytoma
MEN2B	10q11.21	RET	Autosomal Dominant	Medullary Thyroid Cancer	Medullary Thyroid CA Pheochromocytoma Mucosal Neuromas Marfanoid Habitus	Pheochromocytoma

Questions

1. A 44-year-old male with a history of hypertension well controlled on medications is found to be anemic and with a positive fecal occult blood test during his yearly physical. He notes a family history that includes deaths due to colon cancer in of both his mother at age 46 and his maternal grandfather at age 51. He undergoes colonoscopy which demonstrates four adenomatous polyps in the ascending colon as well as an adenocarcinoma of the ileocecal junction. This patient is most likely to have which of the following?
   A. A mutation in the TP53 gene
   B. A mutation in the PMS2 gene
   C. A mutation in the PTEN gene
   D. A mutation in the STK11 gene
   E. A mutation in the adenomatous polyposis coli (APC) gene

2. An otherwise healthy 68-year-old woman is diagnosed with locally advanced gastric adenocarcinoma. There is no evidence of distant metastases. Her tumor is biopsied and noted to have *HER2*/neu overexpression. She is started on an appropriate chemotherapy regimen. After her second cycle, she presents with new-onset dyspnea on exertion and orthopnea. Which of the following chemotherapeutic agents is likely responsible for her symptoms?
   A. Bleomycin
   B. 5-Fluorouracil
   C. Vinblastine
   D. Trastuzumab
   E. Cisplatin

3. A 70-year-old otherwise healthy male with a history of colon adenocarcinoma that was treated with a formal resection returns two years later with a 3-cm lesion on his liver. Workup confirms a colorectal metastasis with no evidence of spread elsewhere. Which of the following is the most appropriate next step?
   A. Chemotherapy only
   B. Surgical resection only
   C. Surgical resection followed by chemotherapy
   D. Chemotherapy followed by surgical resection
   E. Surgical resection followed by radiation

4. An 87-year-old female presents to the emergency department (ED) with weight loss, vomiting, obstipation, and a distended abdomen. She has not had a bowel movement in 3 days. Past history is significant for a non-ST segment elevation myocardial infarction (NSTEMI) 6 weeks earlier. A computed tomography (CT) scan with oral contrast shows evidence of an obstructing mass in the sigmoid colon. However, the lumen does appear to be patent. Her vitals are stable. Which of the following is the best recommendation?
   A. Diverting ileostomy
   B. Diverting transverse colostomy
   C. Open sigmoid resection with proximal colostomy
   D. Colonoscopy with placement of a temporizing stent followed by elective surgery
   E. Laparoscopic sigmoid resection with proximal colostomy

5. A patient with metastatic sigmoid colon cancer is about to undergo chemotherapy, and the oncologist recommends the use of an anti-EGFR monoclonal antibody. Which of the following genetic profiles is most likely to benefit from the addition of this agent?
   A. K-ras wildtype gene
   B. BRAF mutation
   C. NRAS
   D. PIK3CA mutation
   E. K-ras mutant gene

6. Which of the following patients should be referred to a genetic counselor for BRCA testing?
   A. Family history of breast cancer in mother at the age of 55
   B. Both parents are Sephardic Jews
   C. Adopted and unknown family history, developed breast cancer at 55
   D. 55-year-old female with breast cancer in bilateral breasts
   E. 55-year-old female with an inflammatory breast cancer

7. A 55-year-old male presents to the ED with vomiting and an inability to tolerate oral intake for the last week. CT scan shows a significantly distended stomach, with a thickened mass near the pylorus. Upper endoscopy shows a large mass in the stomach that partly occludes the distal lumen. Biopsy is consistent with low-grade mucosa-associated lymphoid tissue (MALT) lymphoma. He takes proton-pump inhibitors for acid reflux. Which of the following is true regarding his condition?
   A. Triple antibiotic therapy for eradication of *Helicobacter pylori* should be started regardless of whether the patient is *H. pylori* positive or negative
   B. The patient should be given chemotherapy along with triple antibiotic therapy
   C. Gastrectomy has no role in the treatment of gastric MALT lymphoma
   D. Radiotherapy has no role in the treatment of gastric MALT lymphoma
   E. Surgery is recommended for patients who do not respond to triple antibiotic therapy

8. Which of the following is true regarding the interaction between radiation therapy and tumor cells?
   A. Radiation therapy leads to cancer cell death by directly inhibiting adenosine triphosphate (ATP) production in the mitochondria
   B. Larger tumors are more sensitive to radiation therapy
   C. As the energy used in radiation therapy increases, collateral damage to overlying skin also increases
   D. The S phase of the cell cycle is most sensitive to radiation effects
   E. Correcting anemia can increase the efficacy of radiotherapy

9. A 60-year-old male with cirrhosis presents to clinic with a newly diagnosed 4-cm hepatocellular carcinoma (HCC) in segment 6. There is no evidence of gross vascular invasion and no regional nodal or extrahepatic distant metastases. His international normalized ratio (INR) is 1.8, creatinine is 1.0 mg/dL, bilirubin is 3.1 mg/dL, and albumin is 2.6 mg/dL, and his computed tomography (CT) scan shows no evidence of ascites. Which of the following would be the best treatment option?
   A. Transarterial chemoembolization (TACE)
   B. Liver resection
   C. Radiofrequency ablation (RFA)
   D. Irreversible electroporation
   E. Liver transplantation

10. Which of the following is true regarding the development of skin cancers?
    A. Ultraviolet (UV) radiation both initiates and promotes DNA damage
    B. UVA is the ultraviolet frequency most responsible for chronic skin damage
    C. An increased level of skin melanin increases the risk of developing basal cell carcinoma
    D. UV radiation damages the DNA mismatch repair gene
    E. Mutations in the BCL-2 gene are a known mechanism for the development of skin cancer

11. A 43-year-old male is diagnosed with a high-grade right lower extremity osteosarcoma and undergoes surgical resection and adjuvant chemotherapy with MAP (methotrexate, doxorubicin, and cisplatin). After the third treatment cycle, the patient develops severe nausea, vomiting, and altered mental status. Workup reveals increased liver transaminases, a reduction in glomerular filtration rate (GFR), as well as leukopenia and thrombocytopenia. What medication can potentially reverse these effects?
    A. Cobalamin
    B. Folinic acid
    C. Folic acid
    D. Folate
    E. Omeprazole

12. Which of the following statements is true regarding patterns of metastatic spread?
    A. The most common metastatic location for breast cancer is the adrenal gland
    B. The most common metastatic location for melanoma is the small bowel
    C. Metastases to the adrenal gland most commonly originate in the lungs
    D. The most common metastatic location for colon cancer is the lungs
    E. The transverse colon is frequently the first location of metastatic spread of pancreatic cancer

13. Which of the following statements is true regarding the human protein p53?

   A. Germline mutations of the p53 gene result in Cowden Syndrome

   B. The unregulated growth seen with human papillomavirus (HPV) is partly due to binding and inactivation of the p53 protein

   C. The p53 gene suppresses the translation process in DNA sequencing and cell growth

   D. Overexpression of this gene leads to uncontrolled cell growth

   E. Mutations frequently result in benign neoplastic growth rather than malignancy

14. A 77-year-old male who resides in a subacute care facility has just finished adjuvant chemotherapy (FOLFOX and Bevacizumab) for metastatic colon cancer. Despite a normal albumin, minimal weight loss, and meticulous local wound care, his nurses have been unable to adequately treat a nonhealing sacral decubitus ulcer. The wound base looks clean, and he has no signs of systemic infection. Which of the following is true?

   A. The sacral wound should be preemptively debrided to avoid infection and facilitate wound healing

   B. Supplemental enteral nutrition will facilitate faster wound healing

   C. Rescue therapy can be attempted with leucovorin

   D. The patient should be converted to Cetuximab

   E. Barriers to healing will likely resolve in 6 months

Answers

1. B. This patient has Lynch syndrome (hereditary nonpolyposis colorectal cancer—HNPCC). The Amsterdam criteria define the criteria necessary for diagnosis. They include three or more family members who have been diagnosed with an HNPCC-associated cancer (colorectal, endometrial, gastric, ovarian, GU tract, hepatobiliary, small bowel, and CNS—but most commonly colorectal cancer), one of whom is a first-degree relative of the other two; at least two generations of family members involved; and at least one member diagnosed with colorectal cancer prior to the age of 50. In addition, no family members may have been diagnosed with FAP. HNPCC is characterized by mutations in mismatch repair genes (MLH1, MSH2, MSH6, PMS2, EPCAM), resulting in microsatellite instability (MSI), and is inherited in an autosomal dominant fashion. Additionally, there is a high frequency of cancers in HNPCC arising in the proximal colon when compared to other hereditary colorectal cancer syndromes (B). A mutation in the TP53 gene results in Li Fraumeni syndrome which is characterized by tumors of the breast (90%), colon, lung, brain, and adrenal, as well as sarcomas (A). PTEN mutations result in Cowden syndrome, in which patients develop tumors of the breast, thyroid, and endometrium as well as facial lesions and GI hamartomas (C). Peutz-Jeghers syndrome is due to a mutation in the STK11 gene and is characterized by hamartomas (both GI and mucocutaneous) as well as malignancies of the breast, colon, pancreas, stomach, ovaries, lung, small intestine, endometrium, testicles, and esophagus (D). Familial adenomatous polyposis (FAP) is due to a mutation in the APC gene and is typically characterized by the appearance of thousands of adenomatous polyps throughout the colon early in life (E).

References: Greenfield LJ, Mulholland MW, eds. *Greenfield's surgery: scientific principles & practice.* 5th ed. Lippincott Williams and Wilkins; 2010.

Mayer RJ. Lower gastrointestinal cancers. In: Jameson J, Fauci AS, Kasper DL, Hauser SL, Longo DL, Loscalzo J. eds. *Harrison's principles of internal medicine.* 20th ed. McGraw-Hill; 2018.

Morris A. Epidemiology—clinical risk factors—familial cancer syndromes. In: Greenfield LJ, Mulholland MW, eds. *Greenfield's surgery. scientific principles & practice.* 5th ed. Lippincott Williams and Wilkins; 2010.

2. D. Commonly utilized chemotherapy regimens in gastric cancer include FLOT (5-FU, leucovorin, oxaliplatin, and docetaxel) as well as capecitabine, cisplatin, and epirubicin. In cases of HER2/neu overexpression, trastuzumab may be added. Trastuzumab is a monoclonal antibody therapy used in the treatment of HER2/neu overexpressing cancers (most commonly breast and GI origins). Trastuzumab can cause reversible cardiomyopathy (D). 5-fluorouracil (5-FU) is a component of the FLOT regimen for gastric cancer, but cardiomyopathy is not a common side effect (B). Bleomycin is utilized in the treatment of lymphoma, testicular, ovarian, and cervical cancers and can cause pulmonary fibrosis (A). Vinblastine is not a typical therapeutic agent in the treatment of gastric cancer and can cause myelosuppression (C). Cisplatin is frequently utilized in the treatment of gastric cancer, but its side effects include nephrotoxicity, neurotoxicity, and ototoxicity (E).

References: Sah BK, Zhang B, Zhang H, et al. Neoadjuvant FLOT versus SOX phase II randomized clinical trial for patients with locally advanced gastric cancer. *Nat Commun.* 2020;11(1):6093.

Wagner AD, Syn NL, Moehler M, et al. Chemotherapy for advanced gastric cancer. *Cochrane Database Syst Rev.* 2017;8:CD004064.

3. C. Recent literature shows a conferred survival benefit for the resection of hepatic metastases in colorectal cancer. Multiple high-volume centers have demonstrated the 5-year survival for patients with metastatic colorectal cancer to the liver to be 25% to 58% with resection of the metastatic lesion.

Over the last two decades, the perioperative mortality associated with hepatic resection has fallen significantly, with most high-volume centers reporting a 30-day perioperative mortality of less than 2%. The presence of any of the following risk factors had a negative, and additive, effect on survival in patients with hepatic metastases from colorectal cancer: (1) node-positive primary tumor, (2) disease-free interval less than 12 months, (3) multiple liver metastases, (4) largest hepatic metastasis greater than 5 cm, and (5) serum carcinoembryonic antigen (CEA) level greater than 200 ng/mL. Those with none of these risk factors have the greatest 5-year survival at 60%. Treatment will vary depending on whether it is a synchronous or metachronous lesion. Synchronous lesions can be safely treated with combined colon and liver resection, provided the hepatic resection is limited (<3 segments). By combining the two surgeries, initiation of adjuvant chemotherapy is quicker. Interestingly, for synchronous rectal cancer (that is both nonobstructing and nonbleeding) with liver metastasis, some experts are now advocating liver resection first, followed by chemoradiation therapy (because this therapy may downstage the rectal cancer). For metachronous disease, the timing of surgery and chemotherapy is still controversial but seems to lean more heavily toward a surgery-first treatment strategy (B). Nordlinger and colleagues published the results of a large randomized trial comparing surgery alone versus perioperative chemotherapy and surgery in patients with resectable liver metastases, which showed a higher rate of complications in the preoperative chemotherapy group and no difference in survival. Many have used this to infer that preoperative chemotherapy is deleterious without conferred benefit, but the study was not powered to examine survival as a primary endpoint (D). In this potentially curable patient, surgery first is likely to confer the largest survival benefit. Patients with unresectable disease, or other poor prognostic indicators, should be considered for systemic chemotherapy, followed by restaging and consideration for surgical therapy (A). Radiation is never part of the treatment algorithm for colon cancer (E).

References: Martin RCG 2nd, Augenstein V, Reuter NP, Scoggins CR, McMasters KM. Simultaneous versus staged resection for synchronous colorectal cancer liver metastases. *J Am Coll Surg.* 2009;208(5):842–850.

Nordlinger B, Sorbye H, Glimelius B, et al. Perioperative FOLFOX4 chemotherapy and surgery versus surgery alone for resectable liver metastases from colorectal cancer (EORTC 40983): long-term results of a randomised, controlled, phase 3 trial. Lancet Oncol. 2013;14(12):1208–1215.

Yin Z, Liu C, Chen Y, et al. Timing of hepatectomy in resectable synchronous colorectal liver metastases (SCRLM): simultaneous or delayed? *Hepatology.* 2013;57(6):2346–2357.

4. D. Symptoms of obstruction are the initial presenting symptoms in up to 8% of colorectal cancers. Emergency surgery has been classically considered the treatment of choice for these patients. However, in the majority of studies, emergency colorectal surgery is burdened with higher morbidity and mortality rates when compared with elective surgery, and many patients require temporary colostomy, which deteriorates their quality of life and becomes permanent in 10% to 40% of cases. The aim of a temporizing stent is to avoid emergency surgery and plan for elective surgery (which can be laparoscopic) in order to improve surgical results, obtain an accurate tumor staging (harvesting the appropriate

number of lymph nodes), and detect the presence of any synchronous lesions. Additionally, this can allow for the medical optimization of the patient's comorbidities. Although stenting has multiple benefits, a recent prospective randomized study demonstrated no advantage to stenting over emergency surgery. However, in an 87-year-old female with a recent NSTEMI, operative risk would be prohibitive. Despite the potential immediate benefits of temporizing stents, the possible implications for the long-term results of oncologic treatment remain to be seen. However, obstruction must still be treated surgically if stenting is not possible (A–C, E).

References: Abdussamet Bozkurt M, Gonenc M, Kapan S, Kocataş A, Temizgönül B, Alis H. Colonic stent as bridge to surgery in patients with obstructive left-sided colon cancer. *JSLS.* 2014;18(4):e2014.00161.

Park SJ, Lee KY, Kwon SH, Lee SH. Stenting as a bridge to surgery for obstructive colon cancer: does it have surgical merit or oncologic demerit? *Ann Surg Oncol.* 2016;23(3):842–848.

van Hooft JE, Bemelman WA, Oldenburg B, et al. Colonic stenting versus emergency surgery for acute left-sided malignant colonic obstruction: a multicentre randomised trial. *Lancet Oncol.* 2011;12(4):344–352.

5. A. In 2012, the Food and Drug Administration (FDA) approved cetuximab, an anti-EGFR monoclonal antibody, to be used with FOLFIRI, as the first-line treatment of k-ras mutant negative (wildtype) metastatic colorectal cancer. This approval was largely based on the CRYSTAL trial, as well as two other supportive studies. A statistically significant overall survival and progression-free survival were appreciated in the cetuximab group (23.5 months versus 19.5 months). The recommended dose and schedule for cetuximab is 400 mg/m2 administered intravenously as a 120-minute infusion as an initial dose, followed by 250 mg/m2 infused over 30 minutes weekly in combination with FOLFIRI. Other studies have demonstrated the negative effects and poor response rate cetuximab has in patients with mutations in BRAF, NRAS, and PIK3CA (B–D). K-ras mutations are seen in 35% to 45% of patients with colorectal cancer, and this group of patients will not benefit from cetuximab therapy. The most common mutations are on chromosome 12 and 13. These have also been shown to predict treatment failure with cetuximab (E).

References: De Roock W, Claes B, Bernasconi D, et al. Effects of KRAS, BRAF, NRAS, and PIK3CA mutations on the efficacy of cetuximab plus chemotherapy in chemotherapy-refractory metastatic colorectal cancer: a retrospective consortium analysis. *Lancet Oncol.* 2010;11(8):753–762.

Tan C, Du X. KRAS mutation testing in metastatic colorectal cancer. *World J Gastroenterol.* 2012;18(37):5171–5180.

Van Cutsem E, Lenz HJ, Köhne CH, et al. Fluorouracil, leucovorin, and irinotecan plus cetuximab treatment and RAS mutations in colorectal cancer. *J Clin Oncol.* 2015;33(7):692–700.

6. D. In December 2013, the US Preventive Services Task Force recommended that women who have family members with breast, ovarian, fallopian tube, or peritoneal cancer be evaluated to see if they have a family history that is associated with an increased risk of a harmful mutation in one of the BRCA genes. Some risk factors that increase the likelihood of having one of these harmful genes include breast cancer before 50 years old, cancer in both breasts in the same woman, both breast and ovarian cancers in the same family, multiple breast cancers, known BRCA in the family, cases of male breast cancer, and Ashkenazi Jewish descent (B). The others listed may have an increased risk of developing breast cancer as per the GAIL model, but they have no increased risk that would necessitate genetic counseling (A, E). For adopted patients, the recommendation for genetic testing is given only if they have had breast cancer at a younger than 50 years (C).

References: U.S. Preventive Services Task Force. *Risk assessment, genetic counseling, and genetic testing for BRCA-related cancer in women: clinical summary of USPSTF Recommendation.* U.S. Preventive Services Task Force; 2013. AHRQ Publication No. 12-05164-EF-3.

7. A. Gastric MALT lymphoma is a subset of slow-growing non-Hodgkin lymphoma that typically occurs in the setting of chronic H. pylori infection. While these tumors were originally treated with surgical resection, like most lymphomas, the focus has moved away from surgery. Initially, systemic therapy mimicked that of other gastric lymphomas with good response rates to systemic chemotherapy and radiotherapy alone, as opposed to surgery. However, as the connection between H. pylori and gastric MALT lymphoma became more apparent, initial therapy has now moved toward attempted treatment with H. pylori eradication. For patients who do not respond, have a recurrence, or are metastatic at time of diagnosis, chemotherapy and radiation are recommended (B, D). Zullo et al. were even able to demonstrate treatment response in H. pylori–negative patients and advocate for a trial of eradication in all patients with gastric MALT lymphoma regardless of H. pylori status. While the role of surgical intervention is extremely limited, it remains the treatment strategy of choice in patients with complete gastric outlet obstruction who do not respond to medical therapy or those with uncontrollable bleeding (C, E).

References: Mahvi D, et al. Stomach. In: Townsend CM Jr, Beauchamp RD, Evers BM, et al, eds. *Sabiston textbook of surgery: the biological basis of modern surgical practice.* 19th ed. W.B. Saunders; 2012.

Yoon SS, Coit DG, Portlock CS, Karpeh MS. The diminishing role of surgery in the treatment of gastric lymphoma. *Ann Surg.* 2004;240(1):28–37.

Zullo A, Hassan C, Ridola L, et al. Eradication therapy in Helicobacter pylori-negative, gastric low-grade mucosa-associated lymphoid tissue lymphoma patients: a systematic review. *J Clin Gastroenterol.* 2013;47(10):824–827.

8. E. Despite longstanding use in the treatment of cancer, the complete mechanism of radiotherapy-induced cancer cell death has yet to be fully elucidated. Charged particles, usually photons, are delivered to the target cells by one of three mechanisms: external beam, brachytherapy, or as a radioactive isotope (e.g., iodine-131 in thyroid cancer). These charged particles interact with the outer layer of loosely bound electrons in normal atoms. Energy is transferred from the photon, and the electron is deflected out of orbit with a lower energy, creating a "free radical." This effect is called the Compton effect. The energy dissipated by these ionizing events leads to the disruption of chemical bonds, most importantly those in DNA. While ionizing radiation has a direct effect on DNA in certain cells, it also indirectly affects other cells by forming oxygen-free radicals (A). The most important effect seems to be the creation of double-stranded DNA breaks. While normal cells can repair this damage to some degree, tumor cells often have damaged or inhibited DNA repair mechanisms. As the energy of the photon beam increases, the penetration of tissue also increases. The skin

is spared by the production of higher-energy electrons that travel forward and achieve full intensity at a depth below the skin's surface (C). Tissue hypoxia has been shown to significantly reduce radiation damage and is one of the patient-modifiable factors that is actively being researched to improve the effectiveness of radiotherapy. The relative hypoxia within large tumor cells is one of the reasons they tend to be more resistant to radiation (B). Along this theme, systemic anemia seems to have a deleterious effect on radiotherapy and correction before radiation therapy is helpful. In regard to the cell cycle, M phase has been found to be the most vulnerable stage to radiation therapy (D).

Reference: Harrison LB, Chadha M, Hill RJ, Hu K, Shasha D. Impact of tumor hypoxia and anemia on radiation therapy outcomes. *Oncologist.* 2002;7(6):492–508.

9. E. Once the diagnosis of HCC is established, the choice of therapy must be individualized for each patient and based on tumor burden, presence of underlying liver disease, patient performance status, and the overall possibility of side effects or complications balanced with acceptable results. When feasible, anatomic resection is the treatment of choice in patients without liver disease and appears to be superior to simple wedge resection. There is a growing body of evidence suggesting that RFA may be used in select patients with similar survival benefits to surgical resection. Feng et al. randomized 168 patients with small (<4 cm) HCCs to surgical resection or RFA. There was no statistical difference in survival between the two groups, though complications were significantly lower in the RFA group. That being said, locoregional therapies (RFA, irreversible electroporation, proton beam therapy) are typically reserved for tumors that are not amenable to surgical resection or as bridge therapy to transplant (C). The best results have been seen with tumors that are less than 4 cm in size. Irreversible electroporation (Nanoknife) therapies show some promise but are still not included in the current National Comprehensive Cancer Network (NCCN) guidelines for treatment of HCC (D). Patients with liver disease and elevated bilirubin are less likely to tolerate any surgical intervention. In fact, the Barcelona Clinic Liver Cancer group identified the absence of clinically relevant portal hypertension and a normal bilirubin level as major determinants for successful liver resection (B). The only treatment modality left for cirrhotics with HCC is liver transplantation. The most widely used standard to choose appropriate patients is known as the Milan criteria, and it is used by the United Network for Organ Sharing (UNOS) to select candidates. The Milan criteria are as follows: a single tumor less than or equal to 5 cm or up to three tumors with none larger than 3 cm, and no evidence of vascular invasion, regional lymphadenopathy, or distant disease. TACE is another useful therapy for individuals not eligible for resection or regional treatment due to severity of their cirrhosis or other comorbidities (A). However, it is still contraindicated in Child class C cirrhosis or for cases in which the location precludes selective treatment. The only chemotherapy currently approved for HCC is sorafenib, which has been shown to slightly improve survival from 7.9 to 10.7 months.

References: Bruix J, Castells A, Bosch J, et al. Surgical resection of hepatocellular carcinoma in cirrhotic patients: prognostic value of preoperative portal pressure. *Gastroenterology.* 1996;111(4):1018–1022.

Mazzaferro V, Regalia E, Doci R, et al. Liver transplantation for the treatment of small hepatocellular carcinomas in patients with cirrhosis. *N Engl J Med*. 1996;334(11):693–700.

National Comprehensive Cancer Network. NCCN Clinical Practice Guidelines in Oncology: Hepatobiliary Cancers. Hepatocellular cancer current guidelines. National Comprehensive Cancer Network. 2016; Version 1.2016.

10. A. UV radiation is a known risk factor for squamous cell carcinoma, basal cell carcinoma, and possibly malignant melanoma. It acts as both an initiator and a promoter of direct DNA damage and damage of DNA repair mechanisms. The degree of risk depends on the type of UV rays and the intensity of exposure. A higher quantity of melanin in skin is protective (C). The UV portion of the electromagnetic spectrum can be divided into three wavelength ranges— UVA (320–400 nm), UVB (280–320 nm), and UVC (200–280 nm). Of these, UVB is the most significant contributor to skin damage (B). The mechanism of carcinogenicity by UVB is by formation of pyrimidine dimers in DNA (D). This damage can be repaired by the nucleotide excision repair pathway. With excessive sun exposure, it is postulated that the capacity of this pathway is overwhelmed, and some DNA that is damaged remains unrepaired. Mutations in the ras and p53 genes occur early in skin cancers, mainly at the dipyrimidine sequences. The BCL-2 gene is involved in regulating cell apoptosis (E).

References: Marcus C, et al. Tumor biology and tumor markers. In: Townsend CM Jr, Beauchamp RD, Evers BM, et al., eds. Sabiston textbook of surgery: the biological basis of modern surgical practice. 19th ed. W.B. Saunders; 2012.

Ziegler A, Leffell DJ, Kunala S, et al. Mutation hotspots due to sunlight in the p53 gene of nonmelanoma skin cancers. *Proc Natl Acad Sci U S A*. 1993;90(9):4216–4220.

11. B. Folinic acid, also known as leucovorin, is frequently given as "rescue therapy" for methotrexate toxicity. Folinic acid is a 5-formyl derivative of tetrahydrofolic acid that does not require the action of dihydrofolate reductase (DHFR) for its conversion and therefore is not affected by methotrexate's inhibitory action on DHFR. While the mechanism is not fully understood, proton pump inhibitors, such as omeprazole, delay the elimination of methotrexate and can potentially increase toxicity. These medications should be stopped during therapy, if possible (E). Folate is the natural form of vitamin B9, while folic acid is the equivalent synthetic form. Both are reliant on the DHFR for metabolism and will have no effect on methotrexate toxicity (C, D). Cobalamin, or vitamin B12, can be effective in treating megaloblastic anemia, but this will have no effect on the myelosuppression caused by methotrexate (A).

References: Jiranantakan T. Methotrexate. In: Olson KR, ed. Poisoning & drug overdose. 6th ed. McGraw-Hill; 2012.

Suzuki K, Doki K, Homma M, et al. Co-administration of proton pump inhibitors delays elimination of plasma methotrexate in high-dose methotrexate therapy. *Br J Clin Pharmacol*. 2009;67(1):44–49.

12. C. Metastatic spread to the adrenal glands is common with breast and lung cancer, with the latter being more prevalent. While breast cancer is able to spread to the brain via Batson's plexus, the most common location of metastatic disease is the lungs (A). Colon cancer spreads in a predictable pattern, starting with the corresponding nodal basin and then following the portal system to the liver. Though it is possible

for colon cancer to spread to the lungs, the liver is more common (D). Pancreatic metastases can be seen throughout the abdominal cavity, but the liver is frequently the first location following locally invasive disease (E). While the most common metastatic tumor of the small bowel is from melanoma, melanoma frequently spreads to the lungs first (B).

13. B. p53 is a protein encoded by the tumor suppressor gene TP53 that is located on the short arm of chromosome 17p13.1. It is important for cell cycle regulation, DNA replication, and apoptosis in response to DNA damage. The p53 protein binds to sequences of DNA in the promoter region of other genes to enhance or regulate transcription (C). p53 typically interacts with and enhances the effects of genes involved in the inhibition of cell growth or replication (D). Mutations in the TP53 tumor suppressor gene result in unregulated cell growth and a predisposition to the development of malignant neoplasms (E). Li-Fraumeni syndrome is an autosomal dominant, hereditary disorder characterized by a germline mutation of the TP53 tumor suppressor gene (A). However, it can also arise sporadically and is seen in more than half of all human cancers. HPV, for example, encodes the protein E6, which binds and inactivates the p53 protein. This, in part, contributes to the development of cervical dysplasia.

References: Angeletti PC, Zhang L, Wood C. The viral etiology of AIDS-associated malignancies. *Adv Pharmacol*. 2008;56:509–557.

Muller PAJ, Vousden KH. P53 mutations in cancer. *Nat Cell Biol*. 2013;15(1):2–8.

14. E. Bevacizumab (Avastin) is a humanized monoclonal antibody against vascular endothelial growth factor (VEGF). It has been shown to significantly prolong survival when added to intravenous 5-fluorouracil-based chemotherapy in first-line chemotherapy for metastatic colorectal cancer. Unfortunately, bevacizumab has numerous adverse effects, with delayed wound healing being one of the most prevalent. The inhibitory effect on VEGF receptors limits angiogenesis, which is critical in wound healing. Potentially, the most devastating complication is spontaneous bowel perforation, but this is relatively infrequent. The effects of the chemotherapy regimen on wound healing last about 6 months, with no studies showing an effect on wound healing after this time period (E). In a patient that is already showing signs of impaired wound healing, additional surgery will likely be unhelpful and potentially deleterious, especially in the absence of clinical signs of infection (A). Supplemental nutrition in the absence of proven nutritional deficit has not been shown to improve wound healing (B). Leucovorin, or folinic acid, is given in conjunction with 5-FU to reduce side effects but has no effect on bevacizumab (C). Cetuximab, a monoclonal antibody against epidermal growth factor receptor (EGFR), has shown to improve survival when used with FOLFIRI compared with bevacizumab. However, wound healing complications were found to be no different (D).

References: Heinemann V, von Weikersthal LF, Decker T, et al. FOLFIRI plus cetuximab versus FOLFIRI plus bevacizumab as first-line treatment for patients with metastatic colorectal cancer (FIRE-3): a randomised, open-label, phase 3 trial. *Lancet Oncol*. 2014;15(10):1065–1075.

Scappaticci FA, Fehrenbacher L, Cartwright T, et al. Surgical wound healing complications in metastatic colorectal cancer patients treated with bevacizumab. *J Surg Oncol*. 2005;91(3):173–180.

Pharmacology 34

ERIC O. YEATES, AREG GRIGORIAN, AND CHRISTIAN DE VIRGILIO

ABSITE 99th Percentile High-Yields

I. Pharmacology Terms
  A. Pharmacokinetics: what the body does to the drug
    1. Bioavailability: fraction of the drug that reaches the systemic circulation
    2. First-pass effect: drug gets metabolized before reaching systemic circulation (usually in liver)
       a) Sublingual/rectal drugs do not have first-pass metabolism
    3. Half-life: the time it takes concentration of the drug to be reduced by 50%
    4. Steady-state concentration: the point at which the concentration of the drug stays consistent
       a) Takes 4 to 5 half-lives to reach steady-state
  B. Pharmacodynamics: what the drug does to the body
    1. Tachyphylaxis: less effective with subsequent doses of a drug

II. Cytochrome P450 (CYPs): essential for metabolism of many medications including coumadin
  A. Inhibitors: block the metabolic activity of one or more CYP enzymes (can lead to bleeding and supratherapeutic INR in patients taking coumadin unless dose is decreased)
    1. Examples: amiodarone, cimetidine, ciprofloxacin, fluconazole, ketoconazole, metronidazole, trimethoprim/sulfamethoxazole, isoniazid, fluoxetine, verapamil, erythromycin
  B. Inducers: increase CYP activity by increasing enzyme synthesis (may prevent coumadin from working unless dose is increased)
    1. Examples: carbamazepine, phenytoin, phenobarbital, rifampin, St. John's Wort

III. List of Antidotes/Reversal Agents

Toxin/drug	Antidote/reversal agent
Benzodiazepines	Flumazenil
Opioids	Naloxone (very short half-life, will need repeat dosing/drip)
Acetaminophen	N-acetylcysteine
Cyanide	Sodium/amyl nitrite, sodium thiosulfate, hydroxycobalamin
Beta-blocker	Glucagon
Methanol/ethylene glycol	Fomepizole (preferred), ethanol
Iron	Deferoxamine
Atropine	Physostigmine, neostigmine
Warfarin	Vitamin K
Amatoxin (poisonous mushrooms)	Silibinin
Lidocaine	Intravenous lipid emulsion

IV. Antidiarrheal
   A. Loperamide: mu-opioid receptor agonist
   B. Lomotil (diphenoxylate/atropine): opioid receptor agonist

V. Adverse Reactions to Psychotropic Drugs
   A. Serotonin syndrome: altered mental status, autonomic nervous system disturbances, neurologic manifestations, hyperreflexia, clonus, mydriasis
      1. Pathophysiology: abnormal elevation in serotonin levels due to drugs that increase its release, decrease uptake/metabolism, or increase serotonin precursors; most commonly with concurrent use of multiple serotonergic agents (can also occur after initiation of single serotoninergic agents)
      2. Common inciting medications: tricyclic antidepressants, selective serotonin reuptake inhibitor, serotonin and norepinephrine reuptake inhibitor, monoamine oxidase inhibitors, triptans, nefazodone, buspirone, mirtazapine, carbamazepine, tramadol, linezolid, MDMA (ecstasy), dextromethorphan, St. John's wort, lithium, methadone, cocaine, levodopa, reserpine, and amphetamines
      3. Management: discontinue serotonergic agents, supportive care, can use benzodiazepines for agitation
   B. Neuroleptic malignant syndrome (NMS): severe muscle rigidity, hyperpyrexia (>38°C), altered mental status, autonomic instability, hyporeflexia, normal pupils
      1. Cause: dopaminergic receptor antagonism caused by antipsychotic drug use that triggers a series of homeostatic responses that result in autonomic dysregulation and hyperthermia, muscular rigidity, and altered mental status
      2. Common inciting medications: more common with atypical antipsychotics (clozapine, olanzapine, risperidone, quetiapine) than typical antipsychotics (haloperidol, chlorpromazine, prochlorperazine, fluphenazine)
      3. Management: discontinue dopaminergic antagonists, supportive care, bromocriptine, and dantrolene

Questions

1. A 75-year-old male is admitted to the hospital after blunt trauma. Two days after his trauma he develops severe agitation. He is treated with quetiapine, with little improvement in his agitation, and his dose is increased over several days. On hospital day five, he develops a high fever, profuse sweating, altered mental status, and muscular rigidity. Which of the following is true regarding this condition?
   A. This condition is more common in younger patients
   B. Typical antipsychotics are more likely to cause this condition compared to atypical antipsychotics
   C. Acute kidney failure is a complication of this condition
   D. There are no known pharmacologic treatment options
   E. It is not associated with rhabdomyolysis

2. Which of the following correctly matches the toxin and antidote?
   A. Iron and deferoxamine
   B. Warfarin and andexanet alpha
   C. Benzodiazepines and fomepizole
   D. Organophosphates and acetylcysteine
   E. Amatoxin and naloxone

3. A 35-year-old female sustains a 35% total body surface area burn. She develops respiratory distress on her second day in the hospital. An arterial blood gas demonstrates metabolic acidosis with partial respiratory compensation. Which topical antimicrobial was this patient most likely receiving?
   A. Bacitracin
   B. Silver sulfadiazine
   C. Gentamicin
   D. Collagenase ointment (Santyl)
   E. Mafenide acetate (Sulfamylon)

4. A 57-year-old Child class A cirrhotic male presents to the ED with severe left lower quadrant pain. Physical exam is concerning for peritonitis, and free air under the diaphragm is seen on chest x-ray. In the operating room (OR), he is found to have feculent peritonitis secondary to a perforated sigmoid diverticulitis and undergoes a Hartmann procedure. The following day the respiratory therapist in the ICU has difficulty ventilating and oxygenating. The patient has complete white out of both lung fields on x-ray, and the PaO2/FiO2 ratio is 180. Low tidal volume ventilation is commenced and the decision to paralyze the patient is made. Which agent should be used?
   A. Rocuronium
   B. Vecuronium
   C. Atracurium besylate
   D. Suxamethonium chloride
   E. Pancuronium

5. Which of the following is true with regards to correcting metabolic acidosis?
   A. Giving bicarbonate alone will be efficient in correcting an acidosis
   B. Correction will fix the pulmonary vasodilation seen in metabolic acidosis
   C. Administration of sodium bicarbonate can lead to hyperkalemia
   D. Sodium bicarbonate may interfere with oxygen delivery
   E. Lactic acidosis will often improve after sodium bicarbonate administration

6. A 62-year-old female with a known history of chronic pancreatitis and subtotal gastrectomy presents to the ED with abdominal pain, altered mental status, unsteady gait, and aphasia. Physical exam is significant for ophthalmoplegia on the right. The patient is confused and unable to answer any questions. Which of the following is the best treatment?
   A. Intravenous glucose
   B. Oral vitamin B12
   C. Intramuscular vitamin B12
   D. Parenteral vitamin B1
   E. Intravenous magnesium

7. Which of the following medications would lead to a patient requiring a higher warfarin dose to remain therapeutic?
   A. Ketoconazole
   B. Cimetidine
   C. Amiodarone
   D. Rifampin
   E. Allopurinol

8. Which of the following medications is associated with the development of aortic aneurysms and dissection?
   A. Cephalosporins
   B. Statins
   C. Metformin
   D. Fluoroquinolones
   E. Azithromycin

9. Which of the following is true regarding the bioavailability of medications?
   A. IV ciprofloxacin has a similar bioavailability to the oral form
   B. Drugs that are absorbed in the stomach have better bioavailability than drugs absorbed in the small intestine
   C. Hydrophobic drugs are better absorbed than hydrophilic drugs
   D. Sublingual medications have lower bioavailability than medications absorbed through the gastrointestinal tract
   E. The dose of chloramphenicol needs to be decreased in patients when given IV to decrease the chance of toxicity compared to the oral route

10. A 67-year-old female is brought into the ED in septic shock of unknown origin. She is hypotensive, diaphoretic, febrile, and found to have a leukocytosis and altered mental status. A rapid sequence intubation (RSI) is performed. On hospital day 2, the patient continues to have hypotension despite fluid resuscitation and the use of vasopressors. She is given a dose of hydrocortisone and vastly improves. Which of the following explains the patient's symptoms?
    A. Poor perfusion of the adrenal gland in the setting of shock
    B. The use of etomidate during RSI
    C. She is on steroids at home
    D. Overuse of vasopressors
    E. Pituitary dysfunction with insufficient release of adrenocorticotropic hormone (ACTH)

11. A 56-year-old male with non-Hodgkin lymphoma presents to the emergency department (ED) with mental status changes, decreased urine output, and lethargy. He recently was started on chemotherapy. Physical exam is remarkable for a newly placed implantable venous access device below the right clavicle. The port site has no evidence of erythema. Gentle tapping anterior to his external auditory canal results in contraction of his facial muscles on that side. Which of the following is true regarding this condition?
    A. Dialysis is unlikely to help
    B. The risk of this complication has decreased in the past years with the advent of newer therapy agents
    C. Alkalinization of the urine should be performed
    D. The standard initial treatment is allopurinol
    E. Laboratory exam will likely demonstrate a metabolic alkalosis

12. A 78-year-old female is recovering in the intensive care unit (ICU) from a small bowel resection due to a strangulated femoral hernia. She is known to have longstanding hearing loss. On postoperative day 2, she becomes increasingly agitated and confused. Laboratory exam and infection workup are unrevealing. She is attempting to pull out her intravenous (IV) lines. Which of the following is true regarding her condition?
    A. Lorazepam may worsen her agitation
    B. Low doses of diphenhydramine are often useful
    C. She should be placed in physical restraints
    D. It is unlikely that a hearing aid could have prevented this condition
    E. Haloperidol is contraindicated

13. Intravenous administration of Haldol should be accompanied by:
    A. A review of admission electrocardiogram (ECG) for a prolonged QT interval
    B. A review of admission ECG for Q waves
    C. Continuous ECG monitoring for development of peaked T waves
    D. Continuous O_2 saturation monitoring
    E. Serial serum creatine phosphokinase (CPK) measurements

14. Which of the following is true regarding the prophylactic role of histamine 2 (H_2) blockers and/or proton pump inhibitors (PPIs) in hospitalized patients?
    A. They have a similar rate of upper gastrointestinal bleeding
    B. Effective stress ulcer prophylaxis involves achieving an intragastric pH greater than 7
    C. Intravenous administration of PPI results in a higher intragastric pH compared with oral administration
    D. There is no difference in the rate of nosocomial pneumonia
    E. Ventilated patients that receive PPI have lower mortality rates

15. Which of the following medications is safe to give a patient who is 10 weeks pregnant?
    A. Acetaminophen
    B. Aspirin
    C. Propylthiouracil (PTU)
    D. Coumadin
    E. Lisinopril

16. Choose the medication that is correctly paired with its mechanism of action
    A. Cyclosporine—purine synthesis inhibitor
    B. Vincristine—microtubule formation and stabilization
    C. 5-Fluorouracil—thymidylate synthase inhibitor
    D. Taxol—microtubule inhibitor
    E. Infliximab—vascular endothelial growth factor (VEGF) inhibitor

17. A 52-year-old male with atrial fibrillation presents to the ED with a large biloma identified on ultrasonography 1 week after undergoing a laparoscopic cholecystectomy. He complains of abdominal pain but does not appear to be in significant discomfort. He was restarted on warfarin after the operation and his international normalized ratio (INR) is currently 2.7. The plan is to attempt CT-guided drainage the following day. How should his INR be corrected?
    A. Oral vitamin K
    B. Slow IV infusion (over 30 minutes) of vitamin K
    C. Fresh frozen plasma (FFP)
    D. Allow warfarin to autocorrect
    E. Prothrombin complex concentrate

18. A 58-year-old male postoperative patient develops a hypertensive crisis with a blood pressure of 220/100 mmHg and heart rate of 60 beats per minute. He is started on a nitroprusside drip, and the blood pressure improves. The patient subsequently develops generalized weakness and becomes unresponsive. He is immediately intubated and an arterial blood gas demonstrates a high anion-gap acidosis with a high SvO_2. His skin color appears pink, and he has the smell of bitter almonds on his breath. Which of the following should you administer next?
    A. Sodium nitrite
    B. Amyl nitrite
    C. Sodium thiosulfate
    D. Hydroxycobalamin
    E. Methylene blue

19. A 75-year-old male with stage 4 chronic kidney disease (CKD) and symptomatic peripheral arterial disease is scheduled for a catheter-based angiography. Which of the following should be administered before the study?
    A. Alkalinization of the urine with sodium bicarbonate intravenously
    B. N-acetylcysteine
    C. Aggressive fluid resuscitation with normal saline
    D. N-acetylcysteine and aggressive fluid resuscitation with normal saline
    E. Alkalinization of the urine with sodium bicarbonate intravenously, N-acetylcysteine, and aggressive fluid resuscitation with normal saline

20. Which of the following medications is paired with the correct side effect?
    A. Furosemide—nausea
    B. Metronidazole—tinnitus
    C. Spironolactone—fulminant hepatic necrosis
    D. Halothane—gynecomastia
    E. Vancomycin—cutaneous flushing

Answers

1. C. This patient most likely has neuroleptic malignant syndrome (NMS) resulting from new antipsychotic drug use. NMS is a rare condition that most often presents with high fevers, muscle rigidity, delirium, and dysautonomia. It is thought to be a result of dopaminergic D2 receptor antagonism caused by antipsychotic drug use that triggers a series of homeostatic responses that result in autonomic dysregulation and hyperthermia, muscular rigidity, and altered mental status. Atypical antipsychotics like clozapine, olanzapine, risperidone, and quetiapine cause NMS more often than typical antipsychotics like haloperidol, chlorpromazine, prochlorperazine, and fluphenazine (B). First-time usage, high dosages, changes in dosages, and parenteral administration of antipsychotics also make NMS more likely. Other risk factors include older age, polypharmacy, multiple comorbidities, and dehydration (A). NMS is a serious condition that can result in complications like aspiration and acute renal failure due to myoglobinuria and rhabdomyolysis and carries a mortality risk of approximately 10% (C, E). Most experts recommend prompt treatment by fluid resuscitation and stopping the offending agent. There is some evidence that administering bromocriptine (a dopamine agonist) is beneficial (D).

Reference: Tse L, Barr AM, Scarapicchia V, Vila-Rodriguez F. Neuroleptic malignant syndrome: A review from a clinically oriented perspective. *Curr Neuropharmacol.* 2015;13(3):395–406.

2. A. Deferoxamine is the treatment for severe iron toxicity. Andexanet alpha is the reversal agent for apixaban and rivaroxaban (B). Vitamin K reverses warfarin. Benzodiazepines can be reversed by flumazenil (C). Fomepizole is used to treat methanol and ethylene glycol poisoning. Organophosphate poisoning is treated with atropine (D). Acetylcysteine is the treatment for acetaminophen overdose. Amatoxin comes from poisonous mushrooms and can be treated with silibinin, which is made from milk thistle (E). Naloxone is used to treat opioid overdoses.

Reference: Schaper A, Ebbecke M. Intox, detox, antidotes—Evidence based diagnosis and treatment of acute intoxications. *Eur J Intern Med.* 2017;45:66–70.

3. E. There are a variety of topical regimens to treat the bacterial load within burns. Bacitracin is a commonly used topical antibiotic that can be utilized in patients with sulfa allergies, but it has notably poor eschar penetration (A). Silver sulfadiazine (Silvadene) is one of the most commonly used topical treatments for burns and is a combination of silver nitrate and the antibiotic sodium sulphadiazine. It has broad-spectrum activity but does not cover for *Pseudomonas aeruginosa.* It should not be used in patients with sulfa allergies and has the potential to cause neutropenia and thrombocytopenia (B). Gentamicin has antipseudomonal coverage and was once commonly used as a topical cream for burn dressings. It has the potential to cause ototoxicity and nephrotoxicity (C). Clostridial collagenase ointment (Santyl), typically used as an enzymatic debriding agent in wound care, has also been shown to be a safe and effective debridement

agent for burn wounds. However, it does not have any antimicrobial properties and does not cause metabolic acidosis (D). Mafenide acetate (Sulfamylon) is a topical antibiotic with broad-spectrum activity, including against *P. aeruginosa.* Due to its mechanism as a carbonic anhydrase inhibitor, it can cause metabolic acidosis, which can manifest as respiratory distress (E).

References: Barillo DJ. Topical antimicrobials in burn wound care: a recent history. *Wounds.* 2008;20(7):192–198.

Dai T, Huang YY, Sharma SK, Hashmi JT, Kurup DB, Hamblin MR. Topical antimicrobials for burn wound infections. *Recent Pat Antiinfect Drug Discov.* 2010;5(2):124–151.

Pham CH, Collier ZJ, Fang M, Howell A, Gillenwater TJ. The role of collagenase ointment in acute burns: a systematic review and meta-analysis. *J Wound Care.* 2019;28(Suppl 2):S9–S15.

4. C. In a patient with underlying liver disease, the paralytic of choice is atracurium besylate or cisatracurium. These are nondepolarizing neuromuscular blocking agents metabolized by Hoffman degradation, thereby bypassing the liver. Cisatracurium is approximately 3 times stronger than atracurium besylate and is more commonly used in this patient population. Additionally, cisatracurium does not lead to histamine release, resulting in flushing and hypotension when compared to atracurium besylate, making it a better alternative. The remaining answer choices are excreted either wholly or partly by the liver (A, B, D, E).

5. D. Persistent metabolic acidosis can lead to widespread dysfunction, but most commonly affects the cardiovascular and respiratory systems. This will result in peripheral vasodilation and pulmonary vasoconstriction in addition to enzymatic and hormone dysfunction (B). Sympathetic stimulation functions poorly because catecholamines are unable to exert their effect on tissue damaged by a low pH. Bicarbonate as an anion alone cannot be given to a patient. It is therefore paired with a hypertonic sodium solution (A). The use of sodium bicarbonate does have some adverse effects, including hypernatremia, hypokalemia, and a left shift in the oxyhemoglobin dissociation curve (C). The left shift is concerning because this can increase the affinity hemoglobin has for oxygen and leave tissue hypoxic, which in turn will lead to worsening acidosis (E). The main goal of using sodium bicarbonate is to treat patients who are persistently severely acidotic and are starting to have negative cardiovascular symptoms.

6. D. The patient is demonstrating Wernicke encephalopathy, which is caused by a deficiency in thiamine (vitamin B_1). Thiamine deficiency occurs most commonly in alcohol-dependent patients with poor diets. It may also be seen in postgastrectomy patients who are predisposed to large gastrointestinal losses and can become deficient in this vitamin, as well as hyperemesis gravidarum, prolonged malnutrition, and prolonged parenteral nutrition. Administration of thiamine quickly reverses the symptoms, particularly in the setting of acute Wernicke encephalopathy. Administering glucose before thiamine may be counterproductive because glucose oxidation is a thiamine-intensive process and may deplete any remaining thiamine that may be available (A). Magnesium may be indicated, particularly in alcoholic patients, because thiamine administration may be refractory in the setting of hypomagnesemia. However, there is no information provided in the vignette to suggest that this patient is an alcoholic (E). Vitamin B_{12} deficiency will have a more insidious onset and present with macrocytic anemia, peripheral neuropathy, and ataxic gait. Confusion, aphasia, and ophthalmoplegia are not characteristic of vitamin B_{12} deficiency (B, C).

7. D. Cytochrome P450 is a part of the superfamily of proteins containing a heme factor and is involved in the metabolism of warfarin. There are inhibitors and inducers of CYP450 that will enhance or dampen the effect of warfarin, respectively. Clinically relevant inhibitors of CYP450 include amlodipine, cimetidine, ciprofloxacin, cyclosporine, diltiazem, ketoconazole, isoniazid, and propranolol. Patients using these medications will need to decrease the dose of warfarin to maintain the same therapeutic international normalized ratio (INR). Inducers of CYP450 include barbiturates, phenytoin, prednisone, rifampin, as well as omeprazole. Patients on these medications will need to increase their warfarin dosage (A–C, E).

8. D. The FDA has issued a warning regarding the increased risk of aortic aneurysm and aortic dissection in association with the use of fluoroquinolones (A). Usage should be limited to patients with serious infections who do not have other antibiotic options. Statins have been associated with a reduced rate of aortic aneurysm growth (B). Metformin is associated with a reduced rate of aortic aneurysm development (C). There is no association between azithromycin and aortic pathology (E).

Reference: Gopalakrishnan C, Bykov K, Fischer MA, Connolly JG, Gagne JJ, Fralick M. Association of fluoroquinolones with the risk of aortic aneurysm or aortic dissection. *JAMA Intern Med.* 2020;180(12):1596–1605.

9. A. Bioavailability of a medication refers to the rate at which an administered drug is absorbed by the circulatory system. The bioavailability of a medication that is given intravenously theoretically has 100% bioavailability, but this does not always prove to be the case. Generally, the IV route provides a higher bioavailability when compared with the oral form. One notable exception is ciprofloxacin, which has similar bioavailability with either IV or oral form. Additionally, the location of absorption is important. Most drugs absorbed in the small intestine have greater bioavailability than drugs absorbed in the stomach because the bowel has 1000-fold increased surfaced area for absorption compared with the stomach (B–C). Medications absorbed by the intestines are routed to the portal circulation first and therefore are initially metabolized by the liver; this is known as "first-pass metabolism." Because of this, the medication has a lower initial bioavailability. However, this does not hold true for sublingual, rectal, intramuscular, and subdermal medications because they do not pass through the liver before their systemic spread (D). Another notable exception is chloramphenicol, an antibiotic used commonly in developing countries

but less so domestically because it can cause life-threatening aplastic anemia. This drug has better bioavailability when given orally than IV (E). Serum concentrations of IV chloramphenicol are only 70% of those achieved when compared with the oral form.

References: Drusano GL, Standiford HC, Plaisance K, Forrest A, Leslie J, Caldwell J. Absolute oral bioavailability of ciprofloxacin. *Antimicrob Agents Chemother.* 1986;30(3):444–446.

Glazko AJ, Dill WA, Kinkel AW, et al. Absorption and excretion of parenteral doses of chloramphenicol sodium succinate in comparison with per oral doses of chloramphenicol. *Clin Pharmacol Ther.* 1977;21:104.

10. B. Etomidate is the preferred anesthetic agent for RSI because it has minimal cardiopulmonary effects. It is also frequently used in the trauma population because it leads to a decreased cerebral metabolic rate and may assist in decreasing intracranial pressure. One notable disadvantage is that it can result in adrenal dysfunction because it is a known inhibitor of cortisol synthesis (11β-hydroxylase). A systematic review identified 21 studies that fit criteria evaluating the adverse effects of etomidate. It demonstrated that patients that received etomidate had an increased relative risk of 1.64 for adrenal insufficiency and an increased relative risk for mortality of 1.19. A single dose can suppress the adrenal gland for up to 72 hours. There is no information given to suggest this patient is on chronic steroids (C). Hypoperfusion of the adrenal glands in the setting of shock, overuse of vasopressors, and pituitary dysfunction are all possible, but etomidate is more likely given the use of RSI (A, D, E).

Reference: Albert SG, Ariyan S, Rather A. The effect of etomidate on adrenal function in critical illness: a systematic review. *Intensive Care Med.* 2011;37(6):901–910.

11. B. Tumor lysis syndrome (TLS) is not uncommonly seen in patients recently started on chemotherapy and primarily occurs in those with poorly differentiated lymphoproliferative diseases such as lymphomas or leukemia, but may also occur with solid organ tumors. It is commonly characterized by electrolyte abnormalities that lead to acute renal failure. Although hyperphosphatemia and hyperuricemia occur most commonly, they are often accompanied by hyperkalemia, hypocalcemia, and a metabolic lactic acidosis (E). The above patient has a physical exam sign consistent with hypocalcemia; Chvostek sign is muscle spasm with gentle tapping over the facial nerve. Newer monoclonal antibody therapies have demonstrated a decreased risk of causing TLS. Treatment includes aggressive hydration in an attempt to normalize the electrolyte abnormalities and improve renal function. Although alkalinization of urine was thought to be a useful adjunct in TLS, there are newer studies suggesting that it may contribute to renal dysfunction. This is now considered a controversial adjunct and is not widely used (C). Allopurinol is used to treat the hyperuricemia of malignancy; however, this can lead to an increased risk of xanthine and calcium phosphate crystals. Newer approaches include use of urate oxidase, which can provide effective treatment while having a safer profile. Hydration remains the best treatment modality (D). In refractory cases, dialysis can be used (A).

References: Davidson MB, Thakkar S, Hix JK, Bhandarkar ND, Wong A, Schreiber MJ. Pathophysiology, clinical consequences, and treatment of tumor lysis syndrome. *Am J Med.* 2004;116(8):546–554.

Firwana BM, Hasan R, Hasan N, et al. Tumor lysis syndrome: a systematic review of case series and case reports. *Postgrad Med.* 2012;124(2):92–101.

Howard SC, Trifilio S, Gregory TK, Baxter N, McBride A. Tumor lysis syndrome in the era of novel and targeted agents in patients with hematologic malignancies: a systematic review. *Ann Hematol.* 2016;95(4):563–573.

Jeha S. Tumor lysis syndrome. *Semin Hematol.* 2001;38(4, Suppl 10):4–8.

Marin GR, Majek E. Acute kidney injury secondary to steroid-induced tumor lysis in an adolescent with acute lymphoblastic leukemia: role of urinary alkalinisation and peritoneal dialysis. *Arch Argent Pediatr.* 2012;110(6):e118–e122.

12. A. Patients in the ICU often experience ICU delirium. It has been shown that anywhere between 20% and 80% of elderly patients in the ICU will experience delirium. The Hospital Elder Life Program (HELP) is an inpatient strategy to prevent ICU delirium and focus on primary prevention with the use of regular reorientation, encouraging proper sleep-wake cycles, meeting nutritional needs, early mobilization activities, and providing visual and hearing adaptations for patients with sensory impairments (D). Physical restraints should be avoided because they lead to decreased mobility, increased agitation, greater risk of injury, and prolongation of delirium (C). Certain patients will still require pharmacologic therapy. Benzodiazepines are not uncommonly administered to elderly patients for agitation, insomnia, and anxiety. However, they are known to have adverse and paradoxical effects so their use should be limited. Patients may experience drowsiness, depression, confusion, vertigo, insomnia, or worsened agitation. When benzodiazepines are given to patients with ICU delirium, up to 23% may experience an adverse event, including hypotension, dystonia, laryngeal spasm, malignant hyperthermia, glucose dysregulation, and urinary retention. Diphenhydramine may demonstrate a similar effect in the elderly population and should be used with caution (B). Haloperidol is often the first-line treatment in the management of an aggressive and agitated patient in the context of delirium (E).

References: Fong TG, Tulebaev SR, Inouye SK. Delirium in elderly adults: diagnosis, prevention and treatment. *Nat Rev Neurol.* 2009;5(4):210–220.

Girard TD, Pandharipande PP, Ely EW. Delirium in the intensive care unit. *Crit Care.* 2008;12(Suppl 3):S3.

Kruse WH. Problems and pitfalls in the use of benzodiazepines in the elderly. *Drug Safety.* 1990;5(5):328–344.

13. A. Elderly patients in the hospital will often experience agitation that can potentiate to aggressive behavior. In this type of situation, the patient will need to be sedated before hurting himself or others. Haloperidol (Haldol) is often the first-line treatment in the management of an aggressive and agitated patient in the context of delirium. Before the administration of haloperidol, an ECG should be performed to rule out a prolonged QT syndrome that the drug can potentiate and lead to life-threatening torsades de pointes and/or heart failure. Peaked T waves can occur with hyperkalemia, while Q waves are usually present following myocardial infarction (B, C). Continuous oxygen saturation monitoring is not required before Haldol administration (D). Serial serum CPK measurements are recommended for patients receiving continuous infusions of propofol (E).

References: Kalisvaart KJ, de Jonghe JFM, Bogaards MJ, et al. Haloperidol prophylaxis for elderly hip-surgery patients at risk for delirium: a randomized placebo-controlled study: haloperidol prophylaxis for delirium. *J Am Geriatr Soc.* 2005;53(10):1658–1666.

Kaneko T, Cai J, Ishikura T, et al. Prophylactic consecutive administration of haloperidol can reduce the occurrence of postoperative delirium in gastrointestinal surgery. *Yonago Acta Medica,* 1999;42:179–184.

14. D. Gastrointestinal stress ulceration occurs in 1% to 4% of all critically ill patients with a 50% mortality rate. The use of PPI versus H_2-blockers has been widely studied. A recent metaanalysis of eight randomized controlled trials looking at critically ill patients found no difference in the rate of nosocomial pneumonia or mortality in either group (E). However, the use of PPI may lead to an increased risk of *Clostridium difficile* infection. Additionally, the PPI group did have a decreased rate of clinically significant upper gastrointestinal bleeding (A). It has been demonstrated that achieving an intragastric pH greater than 6 results in clot stabilization and increased platelet aggregation (B). Intravenous or oral PPIs are equally effective in achieving a prophylactic intragastric pH to prevent ulcer formation when given at the same dose and frequency (C).

References: Alhazzani W, Alenezi F, Jaeschke RZ, Moayyedi P, Cook DJ. Proton pump inhibitors versus histamine 2 receptor antagonists for stress ulcer prophylaxis in critically ill patients: a systematic review and meta-analysis. *Crit Care Med.* 2013;41(3):693–705.

Barkun AN, Bardou M, Pham CQD, Martel M. Proton pump inhibitors vs. histamine 2 receptor antagonists for stress-related mucosal bleeding prophylaxis in critically ill patients: a meta-analysis. *Am J Gastroenterol.* 2012;107(4):507–520.

Barkun AN, Cockeram AW, Plourde V, Fedorak RN. Review article: acid suppression in non-variceal acute upper gastrointestinal bleeding. Aliment Pharmacol Ther. 1999;13(12):1565–1584.

Hartmann M, Ehrlich A, Fuder H, et al. Equipotent inhibition of gastric acid secretion by equal doses of oral or intravenous pantoprazole. *Aliment Pharmacol Ther.* 1998;12(10):1027–1032.

15. C. PTU has been proven to be safe during the first trimester of pregnancy to treat patients with hyperthyroidism, while methimazole has fallen out of favor because of the increased risk of congenital hypothyroidism (cretinism). ACE-inhibitors have been linked to congenital malformations and renal failure (E). Coumadin crosses the blood/baby barrier and can lead to skeletal and CNS defects (D). Aspirin and acetaminophen have both been linked to increased miscarriages and therefore should be avoided if at all possible (A, B). Acetaminophen, which had previously been thought to be safe, has now been linked to hyperkinetic and behavioral disorders such as autism. It is considered a category B drug.

References: Hackmon R, Blichowski M, Koren G. The safety of methimazole and propylthiouracil in pregnancy: a systematic review. *J Obstet Gynaecol Can.* 2012;34(11):1077–1086.

Liew Z, Ritz B, Virk J, Olsen J. Maternal use of acetaminophen during pregnancy and risk of autism spectrum disorders in childhood: a Danish national birth cohort study. *Autism Res.* 2016;9(9):951–958.

16. C. 5-Flourouracil, or 5FU, is a thymidylate synthase inhibitor that inhibits purine and DNA synthesis. When used in combination with leucovorin, it has increased activity and increased toxicity. Cyclosporine is an immunosuppressant that binds to cyclophilin proteins and inhibits genes for cytokine synthesis, particularly IL-2. Side effects of cyclosporine include nephrotoxicity, hepatotoxicity, tremors, seizures, and hemolytic uremic syndrome (A). Vincristine is a chemotherapeutic agent that works by inhibiting microtubule formation (B). Taxol is also a chemotherapeutic agent but works by microtubule formation and stabilization (D). Finally, infliximab is a monoclonal antibody against TNF-α. By binding to TNF-α, it inhibits its ability to bind to receptors and reduces the autoimmune inflammatory response. Bevacizumab is a VEGF inhibitor and has been demonstrated to improve survival in patients with metastatic colorectal cancer (E).

17. A. Reversing warfarin depends on the clinical situation. If the patient is actively bleeding, and therefore reversal is urgent, prothrombin factor concentrate is now preferred over FFP (C, E). However, in a patient that is therapeutically anticoagulated and requires an invasive intervention electively, urgent reversal is not needed. The metabolism of warfarin is regulated by diet and concomitant medications. The half-life is 48 to 72 hours, which allows the drug to continue its effects for about 4 to 6 days after cessation (D). As such, allowing warfarin to autocorrect can take up to 6 days. This patient is in no distress and there are no urgently signs to intervene, and so the correction can be done slowly with the administration of oral vitamin K. This takes up to 24 hours to have an effect and is the ideal choice for a patient undergoing CT-guided drainage the following day. IV push (over 3–5 minutes) administration of vitamin K is generally discouraged because there is a risk of thrombosis and anaphylaxis (B). However, slow IV infusion over 30 minutes is acceptable, and it usually takes 8 to 12 hours for it to have an effect.

References: DeZee KJ, Shimeall WT, Douglas KM, Shumway NM, O'Malley PG. Treatment of excessive anticoagulation with phytonadione (vitamin K): a meta-analysis. *Arch Intern Med.* 2006;166(4):391–397.

Fiore LD, Scola MA, Cantillon CE, Brophy MT. Anaphylactoid reactions to vitamin K. *J Thromb Thrombolysis.* 2001;11(2):175–183.

18. B. The patient is experiencing cyanide poisoning, which can occur following the administration of a nitroprusside drip. Nitroprusside is metabolized into nitric oxide and cyanide. The accumulation of cyanide leads to a left shift in the oxyhemoglobin dissociation curve, resulting in decreased oxygen delivery. This leads to severe lactic acidosis, which is a hallmark of cyanide poisoning. Additionally, the hemoglobin holding on to the oxygen content leads to an increase

in the SvO_2. The initial treatment is inhaled amyl nitrite followed by intravenous sodium nitrite (A). These agents are considered methemoglobin inducers, which allow for methemoglobin to reversibly bind with cyanide to make cyanomethemoglobin. Sodium thiosulfate is then administered, which helps convert cyanomethemoglobin to thiocyanate, a harmless metabolite that is renally excreted (C). Hydroxycobalamin, a form of vitamin B_{12}, is a new medication used to reverse the effects of cyanide by binding to cyanide to form cyanocobalamin, which is then excreted through the urine. Although this drug shows promise, it is not yet the standard of care (D). Methylene blue is used in the treatment of methemoglobinemia (E).

19. C. N-acetylcysteine, alkalinization of the urine, and aggressive fluid resuscitation have all been shown to have a theoretic benefit, but only intravenous fluid hydration has consistently demonstrated a clinical benefit when used in patients with CKD undergoing a contrast study (A, B, D, E). Additionally, the degree of nephrotoxicity is dose dependent and increases with ionized contrast versus nonionized contrast. In patients with normal renal function, the concept of contrast-induced nephropathy has recently come under scrutiny with several reports suggesting no harm.

References: Klima T, Christ A, Marana I, et al. Sodium chloride vs. sodium bicarbonate for the prevention of contrast medium-induced nephropathy: a randomized controlled trial. *Eur Heart J.* 2012;33(16):2071–2079.

Sun Z, Fu Q, Cao L, Jin W, Cheng L, Li Z. Intravenous N-acetylcysteine for prevention of contrast-induced nephropathy: a meta-analysis of randomized, controlled trials. *PLoS One.* 2013;8(1):e55124.

20. E. Furosemide is a loop diuretic and can result in hypocalcemia, hypokalemia, gout, ototoxicity, and tinnitus (A). Metronidazole is an antibiotic used frequently in patients in need of anaerobic coverage and can lead to intractable nausea and emesis, particularly if taken with alcohol (disulfiram-like reaction) (B). Spironolactone is a potassium-sparing diuretic that can result in hyperkalemia and gynecomastia (C). Halothane is an anesthetic agent that may rarely result in fulminant hepatic failure (D). Vancomycin will induce peripheral vasodilation resulting in cutaneous flushing, and rarely, it can cause red man syndrome.

Reference: Sivagnanam S, Deleu D. Red man syndrome. *Crit Care.* 2003;7(2):119–120.

Preoperative Evaluation and Perioperative Care

35

NAVEEN BALAN, AREG GRIGORIAN, AND CHRISTIAN DE VIRGILIO

ABSITE 99th Percentile High-Yields

I. Preoperative Medication Management

   A. In patients undergoing percutaneous cardiac intervention (PCI): most should be started on double antiplatelet therapy with aspirin and clopidogrel

     1) Balloon angioplasty—avoid surgery for 2 weeks postangioplasty; elective surgery after this period is reasonable but continue aspirin and hold clopidogrel 5 days prior

     2) Bare metal stent (BMS)—avoid surgery for 1-month post-BMS; elective surgery after this period is reasonable but continue aspirin and hold clopidogrel 5 days prior

     3) Drug-eluting stent (DES)—avoid surgery for 6-months post-DES; elective surgery after this period is reasonable but continue aspirin and hold clopidogrel 5 days prior

     4) All emergent surgical indications (e.g. peritonitis, perforated viscus with hemodynamic instability) should proceed without delay with cardiology consult, discuss risks/benefits of continuation of aspirin, and consideration of holding clopidogrel depending on risk of cardiac event versus hemorrhage

   B. Anticoagulation medication

     1) Coumadin in atrial-fibrillation patient requiring surgery: can stop without bridging with heparin, as overall risk of thrombosis is low unless CHA2DS2-VASc score ≥7, then consider bridging

       a) Age >75 (2 points), previous TIA/stroke (2 points), diabetes (1 point), previous vascular disease (1 point), hypertension (1 point), CHF (1 point), female (1 point)

     2) Novel oral anticoagulant (NOAC) drugs

       a) Direct-thrombin inhibitors

         (1) Bivalirudin, argatroban, and desirudin: parenteral administration

         (2) Dabigatran: only available oral agent; half-life is 12 to 17 hours; stop 2 days before surgery; renally metabolized so use with caution in patients with renal disease

           (a) Reversed with idarucizumab (a monoclonal antibody that binds dabigatran)

       b) Factor-Xa inhibitors (all factor-Xa inhibitors end in -xaban)

         (1) Rivaroxaban: half-life is 6 to 9 hours, and its therapeutic activity wears off after 4 to 5 half-lives; rivaroxaban should be discontinued 1 to 2 days before a surgical procedure; in patients with a reduced creatinine clearance, it should be discontinued 3 to 5 days before surgery

         (2) Apixaban: factor-Xa inhibitor, half-life of 12 hours; discontinue 2 days prior to surgery; metabolized by liver so safe for patients with renal disease

           (a) Reversed with 4-factor prothrombin complex concentrate

           (b) Andexanet alfa is a recombinant analog of factor Xa and may be considered an antidote for factor-Xa inhibitors

       c) Can restart anticoagulation 6 to 24 hours after a minor procedure, and after 2 to 3 days for major surgery (barring any perioperative bleeding)

C. Steroid therapy: chronic steroid therapy can affect the hypothalamic–pituitary–adrenal axis, leading to adrenal atrophy and a decreased capability to produce cortisol leading to a theoretical risk of hypotension in the perioperative period; however, perioperative "stress-dose" steroids are not supported by recent evidence
   1) "Stress-dose" steroids should not be routinely administered; instead, the patient should continue their home dose of steroids perioperatively
   2) Should consider additional steroids only if the patient develops refractory hypotension suggestive of adrenal insufficiency in the perioperative period

Questions

1. A 58-year-old man presents with a reducible inguinal hernia. He is not limited in his daily activities but is bothered by the appearance. He underwent percutaneous coronary intervention (PCI) with placement of a drug-eluting stent (DES) 2 months ago and is currently taking aspirin and clopidogrel. What is the most appropriate management of this patient?

   A. Schedule surgery and continue aspirin and clopidogrel
   B. Schedule surgery and Continue aspirin and stop clopidogrel 5 days prior to the operation
   C. Schedule surgery and stop aspirin and clopidogrel 5 days prior to the operation
   D. Delay surgery for an additional 4 months
   E. Delay surgery for a year post-DES

2. A 38-year-old woman develops fever, abdominal pain, and multiple loose nonbloody bowel movements following admission for perforated appendicitis. Her WBC count is 12,000 and has normal kidney function. On imaging, there is no evidence of deep space abscess or ileus and her stool tests positive for *Clostridium difficile*. This is her first episode. What is the most appropriate treatment?

   A. Fecal transplant
   B. Oral and rectal vancomycin
   C. Oral vancomycin and intravenous metronidazole
   D. Intravenous metronidazole
   E. Oral vancomycin

3. Five days after a laparoscopic Roux-en-Y gastric bypass, a patient develops fever with rigors, hypotension, tachycardia, and pain in the left shoulder. This most likely represents:

   A. Gas bloat syndrome
   B. Internal hernia
   C. Wound dehiscence
   D. Gastric volvulus
   E. Disruption of the gastric pouch–jejunal anastomosis

4. A 28-year-old woman undergoes adhesiolysis for an acute small bowel obstruction. During the course of the surgery, she requires a segmental ileal resection with primary anastomosis. On postoperative day 6, she is noted to have thick bile-colored fluid emanating from the midline wound. After IV hydration, the next step in the management should be:

   A. CT scan of the abdomen
   B. Water-soluble upper gastrointestinal series with small bowel follow-through
   C. Fistulogram
   D. Operative reexploration
   E. Octreotide

5. The most important predictor of colonic ischemia after repair of a ruptured abdominal aortic aneurysm is:

   A. Age
   B. Presence of preoperative shock
   C. Time to operation
   D. Presence of associated cardiac disease
   E. Preoperative patency of inferior mesenteric artery

6. Five days after surgery for perforated appendicitis, liquid stool emanates from the right lower quadrant wound. Which of the following is true about this condition?

   A. It is most commonly due to an unrecognized malignancy
   B. The majority will close spontaneously
   C. The patient should be placed immediately on TPN
   D. Fluid and electrolyte derangements are common
   E. The patient should be returned immediately to the operating room for surgical repair

7. Five days after a Billroth II gastric resection for a bleeding ulcer, high fever, hypotension, tachycardia, and generalized peritonitis develop in the patient. This most likely represents:

   A. Postoperative pancreatitis
   B. Acalculous cholecystitis
   C. Duodenal stump blowout
   D. Wound dehiscence
   E. Intraabdominal hemorrhage

8. Which of the following modalities is LEAST likely to assist in the prevention of postoperative pulmonary complications in a 65-year-old male smoker?
   A. Postoperative use of an incentive spirometer
   B. Postoperative deep-breathing exercises
   C. Postoperative use of continuous positive airway pressure
   D. Smoking cessation 1 week before surgery
   E. Placement of a nasogastric tube

9. Which of the following preoperative studies is most strongly associated with an increased risk of pulmonary-related postoperative complications?
   A. Blood urea nitrogen
   B. Incentive spirometry
   C. Chest radiograph
   D. Serum albumin
   E. Room air arterial blood gas

10. A 67-year-old male recovering from a pelvic exenteration secondary to locally advanced rectal cancer is started on total parenteral nutrition for prolonged ileus via a right-sided peripherally inserted central catheter (PICC) line. Several days later his arm becomes swollen. Ultrasound confirms clot in the basilic and axillary veins. What is the appropriate management of his condition?
    A. Warm compress and nonsteroidal antiinflammatory drugs (NSAIDs)
    B. Immediately remove the line
    C. Immediately remove line and then start heparin
    D. Start heparin and move the line to an alternate site
    E. Start heparin, keep the line in place, and therapeutic anticoagulation for 3 to 6 months

11. A 76-year-old diabetic male is admitted to the surgical intensive care unit after a fall. His injuries include a right femoral neck fracture and subarachnoid hemorrhage. He continues to have intermittent elevation in his intracranial pressure and is still requiring respiratory support after 2 days. Which of the following is true regarding nutritional supplementation in this patient?
    A. Postpyloric feeding may reduce his risk of developing pneumonia
    B. Gastric feeding is associated with a longer length of ICU stay
    C. Diabetic patients have better outcomes with gastric versus postpyloric feedings
    D. Postpyloric feeding more closely simulates normal physiologic feeding
    E. Gastric feeding is associated with increased total nutrition

12. A 55-year-old obese female with chronic obstructive pulmonary disease (COPD) is undergoing preoperative evaluation for ventral hernia repair. She has a 30 pack/year smoking history, though she quit 1 year ago. Her COPD symptoms are well controlled with her current medication regimen, and her last admission for COPD exacerbation was over 2 years ago. Which of the following is true regarding risk assessment for postoperative pulmonary complications in this patient?
    A. Higher ASA class is a significant risk factor
    B. Preoperative pulmonary function tests (PFTs) should be obtained
    C. A nasogastric tube should be used postoperatively to decrease pulmonary complications
    D. Upper midline and lower midline laparotomy confer similar risk for pulmonary complications
    E. A $PaCO_2$ of more than 45 mmHg is an absolute contraindication to major abdominal surgery

13. A 65-year-old woman is admitted to the hospital with a large bowel obstruction. Workup reveals a sigmoid cancer, and on hospital day 4, she undergoes laparoscopy with a plan to perform a resection with a proximal colostomy. During the operation, her end-tidal carbon dioxide suddenly drops, and she develops tachycardia to the 120s with occasional premature atrial contractions. Her systolic blood pressure is 80 mmHg. Which of the following would be most helpful in establishing the presumptive diagnosis?
    A. Electrocardiogram
    B. Cardiac enzymes
    C. Transesophageal echocardiogram (TEE)
    D. Arterial blood gas
    E. Flexible bronchoscopy

14. A 59-year-old male with a coronary artery bypass grafting 1 year prior for multivessel disease undergoes a right hip replacement surgery. His postoperative course is complicated by pneumonia requiring mechanical ventilation. Electrocardiogram shows a stable Q wave in lead II. Heart rate is 80 beats per minute and blood pressure is 116/82 mmHg. Chest radiograph shows bilateral patchy infiltrates. Laboratory exam demonstrates PaO_2 of 70 mmHg, a white blood cell count of 17,000 cells/μL, and hemoglobin of 7.4 g/dL. Which of the following is true regarding the management of his anemia?

   A. Blood transfusion will lower his risk of developing an acute coronary syndrome

   B. He should be transfused to a hemoglobin goal of 10 g/dL

   C. Red blood cell transfusion is independently associated with lower mortality

   D. Blood transfusion is not necessary at this time

   E. Hemoglobin-based oxygen carriers offer a good alternative to transfusion in this patient

15. Four days after a pancreaticoduodenectomy for pancreatic adenocarcinoma, a 65-year-old man develops a fever and tachycardia. Exam reveals tenderness, edema, and erythema over the angle of the jaw. Which of the following is true regarding this condition?

   A. It is usually due to *Staphylococcus*

   B. Massage of the area is beneficial

   C. It can be prevented with antibiotics

   D. The incidence has been increasing

   E. It can be avoided with the use of anticholinergics

16. Which of the following is true regarding venous thromboembolism (VTE) prophylaxis in surgical patients?

   A. Intermittent pneumatic compression (IPC) prevents DVT by increasing circulating tissue plasminogen activator (tPA)

   B. Thigh-high IPC is superior to knee-high IPC

   C. IPC is equivalent to pharmacologic prophylaxis in the majority of patients

   D. Unfractionated heparin (UFH) is superior to lower-molecular-weight heparin (LMWH)

   E. LMWH is superior to IPC

17. A 69-year-old patient with a tumor at the rectosigmoid junction undergoes laparoscopic sigmoid colectomy. Postoperative pain is well controlled with patient-controlled thoracic epidural anesthesia. On postoperative day 1, prophylactic anticoagulation is started with low-molecular-weight heparin (LMWH). The bladder is undergoing drainage with an indwelling Foley catheter. Which of the following is true regarding epidural anesthesia?

   A. Bladder catheterization should continue while the thoracic epidural is in place

   B. LMWH should be held for 24 hours before removal of the thoracic epidural

   C. The risk of urinary tract infection is the same regardless of whether the urinary catheter is removed on postoperative day 1 versus postoperative day 3

   D. Risk of urinary retention is not significantly higher with early removal of the Foley catheter

   E. Unfractionated heparin should not be restarted for at least 4 hours after removal of an epidural catheter

18. A 25-year-old woman develops a fever of 104°F 12 hours after an open cholecystectomy. On examination, she has foul-smelling, purulent drainage from her wound. She undergoes the appropriate treatment, and culture of the wound grows gram-positive rods. Which of the following is true regarding this patient and her condition?

   A. The causative organism is an aerobe

   B. Diabetes is not considered to be a risk factor

   C. Broad-spectrum antibiotics and fluid resuscitation resolve the majority of cases

   D. The organism produces an endotoxin

   E. Clindamycin should be included in the management

19. A 34-year-old woman undergoes a subtotal thyroidectomy for Graves disease. In the recovery room, she develops anxiety and progressive respiratory distress with stridor. Her incision is bulging and tense on exam. The most important initial step would be:

   A. Nebulized racemic epinephrine

   B. Rapid-sequence intubation

   C. Needle aspiration of the neck wound

   D. Ultrasound examination of the neck

   E. Rapidly opening the incision at the bedside

20. One day after a left colectomy for recurrent diverticulitis, a patient is noted to have an elevation of his serum creatinine. Other laboratories are unremarkable. He has a urine output of 30 to 50 mL/hour. A renal ultrasound shows no evidence of abnormalities with the exception of ascites. Computed tomography (CT) scan demonstrates discontinuity of the left ureter with contrast extravasation at the level of the pelvic brim. Which of the following about this injury is true?

    A. Immediate reoperation should not be performed
    B. Placement of ureteral stents would have prevented this complication
    C. A percutaneous nephrostomy should be placed
    D. A retrograde stent should be placed
    E. A ureteroneocystostomy will likely be the best option

21. Two days after sustaining significant crush injury to her bilateral lower extremities from a motor vehicle collision, a 32-year-old female becomes oliguric and is only producing scant dark urine. Urine dipstick reveals 4+ blood, and follow-up urinalysis shows 5 to 10 red blood cells per high power field. Prevention of acute kidney injury is best achieved by which of the following?

    A. Urgent 4-compartment fasciotomies
    B. Loop diuretics
    C. Vigorous IV fluid hydration
    D. Alkalization of urine with intravenous sodium bicarbonate
    E. Mannitol

22. Which of the following is true regarding PFTs?

    A. Total lung capacity (TLC) is generally reduced with aging
    B. A preoperative forced expiratory volume in one second (FEV_1) of less than 1.5 L is a contraindication for pulmonary lobectomy
    C. Diffusion capacity of the lungs for carbon monoxide (DLCO) will stay relatively constant with age so long as there is no intrinsic lung disease
    D. Percent-predicted postoperative FEV_1 of >40% is acceptable for a lobectomy but not for a pneumonectomy
    E. Chest wall compliance decreases with age

23. A 45-year-old male with end-stage renal disease is undergoing placement of a tunneled hemodialysis catheter. During the operation, the anesthesiologist notices a sharp decline in the continuous capnography and the calculated physiologic dead space is increased. This is followed by massive myocardial infarction and cardiac arrest. Which of the following is true regarding this condition?

    A. Electrocardiogram (ECG) will most commonly demonstrate right heart strain
    B. A congenital heart defect likely contributed to the cardiac arrest
    C. The patient should be positioned left side up
    D. Bedside transesophageal echocardiography is generally not sensitive enough to detect this complication
    E. Aspiration from the central line is usually helpful

24. A 65-year-old man with Barrett esophagus and new-onset dysphagia is being evaluated for diagnostic esophagogastroduodenoscopy (EGD), endoscopic ultrasound (EUS), and mucosal biopsy. He is on warfarin for mechanical mitral valve and has a history of embolic stroke 10 years ago. What is recommended for his anticoagulation regimen before this procedure?

    A. Hold warfarin for 3 to 5 days and bridge with low-molecular-weight heparin
    B. Hold warfarin for 48 to 72 hours, bridge with unfractionated heparin, and hold heparin 4 to 6 hours before the procedure
    C. Perform EGD and EUS while therapeutic on warfarin; if indicated, the mucosal biopsy can be performed at a later date after holding warfarin
    D. Continue warfarin without interruption
    E. Hold warfarin 3 to 5 days before procedure and restart within 24 hours after the procedure

25. A 42-year-old female with long-standing systemic lupus erythematosus (SLE) complicated by lupus nephritis and debilitating arthritis is in the ICU following an emergency bowel resection 4 days earlier. Over the next several hours, she becomes febrile, hypotensive, and complains of abdominal pain. She is given fluid boluses, but the blood pressure does not respond. Her abdominal exam is unremarkable. Laboratory values reveal a white blood cell count of 12,000 cells/L with eosinophilia, serum Na of 133 mEq/L, serum bicarbonate of 20 mEq/L, and serum K of 5.3 mEq/L. Which of the following represents the best management of this condition?

A. Two liters of normal saline followed by 4 mg of dexamethasone

B. Exploratory laparotomy

C. Vasopressin

D. Immediate administration of broad-spectrum antibiotics and 100 mg of hydrocortisone

E. Fluid resuscitation, vasopressor support, and AM cosyntropin test

26. Which of the following is true regarding the use of beta-blockers in the perioperative period for patients undergoing noncardiac surgery?

A. Starting a beta-blocker within 24 hours of surgery may increase the incidence of perioperative stroke

B. Beta-blockers should be stopped at least 1 week before surgery

C. In low- and intermediate cardiac risk patients, beta-blockers should be initiated 2 to 3 weeks before surgery

D. Beta-blockers should be avoided even in the high cardiac risk group

E. Perioperative initiation of beta-blocker decreases the 30-day mortality

Answers

1. D. The management of antiplatelet medications in patients undergoing noncardiac surgery after PCI poses a common surgical dilemma. In general, patients should be stratified by thrombotic risk based on the type and timing of PCI as well as hemorrhagic risk based on the type of surgery. Patients who underwent plain old balloon angioplasty within the past 2 weeks, bare metal stent within the past 1 month, and DES within the past 6 months are at high thrombotic risk. In general, surgery should be delayed until after this period (A–C, E). For most abdominal operations, continuing aspirin while holding clopidogrel 5 days prior to surgery is appropriate. However, in the case of time-sensitive surgery such as a colectomy in a patient with colon cancer, surgery should not be delayed and the risks/benefits of continuing double antiplatelet therapy should be discussed with the patient. Of note, there is recent literature supporting the continuation of aspirin and clopidogrel in patients with colon cancer undergoing resection, even within a couple months of DES placement.

Reference: Banerjee S, Angiolillo DJ, Boden WE, et al. Use of antiplatelet therapy/DAPT for post-PCI patients undergoing noncardiac surgery. *J Am Coll Cardiol.* 2017;69(14):1861–1870.

2. E. Infection with *C. difficile* is not an uncommon complication following antibiotic treatment. While it has been classically associated with clindamycin, it can occur following treatment with a wide variety of antibiotics. For initial episodes, infection can either be nonsevere (leukocytosis <15,000, serum creatinine <1.5), severe (leukocytosis >15,000, serum creatinine >1.5), or fulminant (shock, toxic

megacolon). Nonsevere and severe infections are treated with either PO vancomycin or PO fidaxomicin (if available) ×10d. In cases of fulminant disease, treatment should include PO vancomycin and consideration of total abdominal colectomy with end ileostomy. In cases of fulminant disease with ileus, rectal vancomycin and intravenous metronidazole should be added (B, C, D). First recurrences can be treated with PO vancomycin (usual dosing if metronidazole was used for the initial episode or a prolonged pulsed/tapered regiment if a standard PO vancomycin regimen was used for the initial episode). Alternatively, fidaxomicin may be used if a standard PO vancomycin regimen was used for the initial episode. Subsequent recurrences can be treated with antibiotics or fecal transplant (A).

Reference: McDonald LC, Gerding DN, Johnson S, et al. Clinical practice guidelines for *Clostridium difficile* infection in adults and children: 2017 Update by the Infectious Diseases Society of America (IDSA) and Society for Healthcare Epidemiology of America (SHEA). *Clin Infect Dis.* 2018;66(7):987–994.

3. E. Fever, chills, tachycardia, hypotension, and peritoneal irritation occurring together within 1 week of any surgery involving a new bowel anastomosis should immediately raise suspicion for an anastomotic disruption. Left shoulder pain is often a consequence of left diaphragm irritation and, in this case, correlates with the gastric pouch–jejunal anastomosis. Water-soluble contrast studies can aid in the diagnosis and indicate how large the leak is because contained leaks can often be managed nonoperatively. However, in this patient, hypotension and signs of peritonitis necessitate operative exploration and repair of the anastomosis. Gas-bloat syndrome results from the inability to relieve gas from the stomach after a fundoplication (A). Gastric volvulus can occur after gastric surgery; however, this is extremely rare (D). Internal hernia is less likely given the timeline (most occur beyond a month after surgery) and left shoulder pain indicative of diaphragmatic irritation (B). Wound dehiscence would be suspected if the skin is erythematous, warm, draining purulent or serous material, and has fallen apart (C).

4. A. This case represents an enterocutaneous fistula, likely resulting from either an anastomotic leak or an unrecognized intraoperative bowel injury away from the anastomosis. Management of enterocutaneous fistulas should begin with stabilizing the patient via aggressive fluid hydration and control of sepsis (if present). If the patient is manifesting signs of sepsis, prompt administration of IV antibiotics should be instituted. Sepsis, dehydration, and electrolyte/nutrient losses are the most devastating early consequences. Prompt return to the operating room is not recommended because the peritoneal cavity will likely have highly vascular adhesions, making reentry treacherous, and early attempts to reclose fistulas typically fail (D). Once the patient has been stabilized, the best initial study is a CT scan of the abdomen. This will identify whether any intraabdominal abscesses are present that might require percutaneous drainage and rule out whether there is a distal obstruction (B, C). Fistulas are loosely categorized as high and low output. High output is defined as outputs of more than 500 mL/day and low output as less than 200 mL/day. High-output fistulas are less likely to close and often cause significant fluid, electrolyte, and nutritional challenges. Factors that predict whether a fistula will close (mnemonic "FRIEND") include *f*oreign body, *r*adiation to the bowel, *i*nflammation/infection (such as inflammatory bowel disease), *e*pithelialization of the fistula tract, *n*eoplasia at the fistula site, and *d*istal obstruction. The mortality rate of enterocutaneous fistulas remains significant at 10% to 15%. Approximately 50% close spontaneously. Conservative treatment should be continued for at least 6 weeks before any reoperation is performed. Operating before 6 weeks results in higher mortality and fistula recurrence rates. Octreotide has not been shown in randomized trials to aid in earlier fistula closure but does not decrease mortality (E).

Reference: Sancho JJ, di Costanzo J, Nubiola P, et al. Randomized double-blind placebo-controlled trial of early octreotide in patients with postoperative enterocutaneous fistula. *Br J Surg.* 1995;82(5):638–641.

5. B. Colonic ischemia after repair of a ruptured abdominal aortic aneurysm occurs in 1% to 6% of operations but can occur in up to 25% of cases under certain circumstances. The greatest risk factor is the presence of prolonged hypotension preoperatively. In a patient with stable blood pressure, age, time to operation, and the presence of cardiac disease have little effect on the incidence of colonic ischemia after aortic repair (A–C, D). Patency of a patient's inferior mesenteric artery is not a good predictor of colonic ischemia because of significant avenues of collateral flow (E). Symptoms and signs of ischemia include bloody diarrhea, abdominal pain/distention, and elevated white blood cell count. If the patient has evidence of peritonitis, urgent reoperation is indicated.

Otherwise, urgent endoscopy is required to view the colonic mucosa. The majority of cases of colonic ischemia can be managed nonoperatively with bowel rest, hydration, and IV antibiotics. If the patient requires colon resection, mortality rates are as high as 75%.

6. B. This case represents a cecal fistula. The most common causes are slippage of the suture or necrosis of the remaining appendiceal stump, leading to leakage of the enteric contents into the peritoneal cavity (A). Rarely, the fistula results from unrecognized Crohn disease, malignancy, tuberculosis or distal colon obstruction. Cecal fistulas are low-output fistulas and are not associated with losses of large amounts of fluid, electrolytes, or nutrients (D). Therefore, TPN is not necessary to maintain adequate nutrition (C) and mortality rates are low in the absence of other serious complications (A). Spontaneous closure is promoted in as many as 75% of patients maintained on low-residue diets because absorption is mostly complete by the time the contents reach the cecum (B, E).

7. C. Duodenal stump blowout occurs after Billroth II operations, where back pressure on the duodenal stump results in breakdown of the stump closure, leading to abdominal sepsis and peritonitis. Acute pancreatitis is associated postoperatively with Billroth II gastrectomy and jejunostomy, in which increased intraduodenal pressure can cause backflow of activated enzymes into the pancreas but is unlikely to cause peritonitis (A). Wound dehiscence is characterized as sudden dramatic drainage of relatively large volumes of a clear, salmon-colored fluid and is apparent on physical exam (D). Acalculous cholecystitis can also occur postoperatively; however, the clinical presentation would mainly consist of right upper quadrant pain (B). Intraabdominal hemorrhage would be less likely to present with sepsis (E).

8. E. Smoking is a predictor of postoperative pulmonary complications. The respiratory epithelium is altered in smokers, and poor ciliary activity combined with the production of more viscous mucus leads smokers to be more reliant on coughing to clear secretions from their lungs. Several days after patients have stopped smoking, there may be a transient increase in sputum volume. The above reasons have typically prevented health professionals from encouraging smoking cessation in the weeks leading up to surgery. However, a metaanalysis published by the American Medical Association has concluded that the concern that stopping smoking only a few weeks before surgery might worsen clinical outcomes is unfounded and clinicians should advise smoking cessation as soon as possible (D). Postoperative lung expansion modalities (A–C) reduce postoperative pulmonary complications, although there is no added benefit from using all three. Routine use of a nasogastric tube may increase aspiration risk because the tube stents open the gastroesophageal junction. However, selective use in patients with nausea, bloating, and/or vomiting is probably protective.

References: Bluman LG, Mosca L, Newman N, Simon DG. Preoperative smoking habits and postoperative pulmonary complications. *Chest.* 1998;113(4):883–889.

Lawrence VA, Cornell JE, Smetana GW, American College of Physicians. Strategies to reduce postoperative pulmonary complications after noncardiothoracic surgery: systematic review for the American College of Physicians. *Ann Intern Med.* 2006;144(8):596–608.

Myers K, Hajek P, Hinds C, McRobbie H. Stopping smoking shortly before surgery and postoperative complications: a systematic review and meta-analysis. *Arch Intern Med.* 2011;171(11):983–989.

9. D. A serum albumin less than 3.5 g/dL is the single most important laboratory predictor of adverse pulmonary events after surgery. Blood urea nitrogen (>21 mg/dL) is also useful, although the correlation is not as strong (A). Routine spirometry for all operations does not seem to add value beyond a careful history and physical examination (B). An exception for the use of spirometry would be for lung resection. Chest radiograph and arterial blood gas are diagnostic studies that would only be predictive of postoperative complications if there were abnormal findings (C, E).

References: Lawrence VA, Cornell JE, Smetana GW, American College of Physicians. Strategies to reduce postoperative pulmonary complications after noncardiothoracic surgery: systematic review for the American College of Physicians. *Ann Intern Med.* 2006;144(8):596–608.

Qaseem A, Snow V, Fitterman N, et al. Risk assessment for and strategies to reduce perioperative pulmonary complications for patients undergoing noncardiothoracic surgery: a guideline from the American College of Physicians. *Ann Intern Med.* 2006;144(8):575–580.

10. E. Thrombosis of superficial and deep veins of the upper extremity is caused by intravenous catheters in most cases. Upper extremity DVT does pose a risk of pulmonary embolus, though less risk than pelvic and lower extremity DVT. Management begins with anticoagulation and determining the necessity for the line; in the above case, there is a continued need for TPN via a PICC line as the patient has not yet demonstrated a return of bowel function. Studies have shown that it is not necessary to remove the PICC line despite the DVT. Therapeutic anticoagulation for 3 to 6 months is recommended. Thus, removal of the catheter without anticoagulation is not acceptable because there is a risk of PE (B). Indications to remove a line include infection and a contraindication to anticoagulation. If the line is to be removed, anticoagulation is still recommended; however, the recommendation is to wait 5 to 7 days after the initiation of heparin before removing it (due to the theoretic fear that pulling the line with a fresh clot might dislodge the thrombus) (C, D). Warm compresses and NSAIDs would be appropriate for superficial thrombophlebitis (A).

Reference: Kucher N. Clinical practice. Deep-vein thrombosis of the upper extremities. *N Engl J Med.* 2011;364(9):861–869.

11. A. While there are many theoretic advantages between each method of feeding, a 2015 Cochrane review comparing postpyloric and gastric feedings showed only two significant differences: lower rates of pneumonia in the postpyloric group and some evidence for increased total nutrition delivered in the postpyloric group (E). There was no significant difference in length of ICU stay, mortality, or time on the ventilator (B). There was also no significant difference in associated complications with tube placement between the two study groups. While postpyloric feeding was associated with a longer time to initiation of tube feeding, this did not seem to affect the time it took to reach nutritional goals. Advantages of gastric feeding include a better approximation of normal physiology, ease of placement, and convenience (D). It may be a reasonable choice in patients without risk for aspiration, but patients with delayed gastric emptying

(which is common in ICU patients), diabetes, and gastroesophageal reflux should be considered for postpyloric feeds (C). In terms of timing, there is abundant evidence that earlier enteral feeding in critically ill patients results in better outcomes.

Reference: Alkhawaja S, Martin C, Butler RJ, Gwadry-Sridhar F. Post-pyloric versus gastric tube feeding for preventing pneumonia and improving nutritional outcomes in critically ill adults. *Cochrane Database Syst Rev.* 2015;(8):CD008875.

12. A. Patient-related risk factors for the development of postoperative pulmonary complications include: age more than 50 years, COPD, congestive heart failure, American Society of Anesthesiologists (ASA) class greater than 2, serum albumin less than 3.5 g/L, obstructive sleep apnea, pulmonary hypertension, and current smoking. While a preoperative $PaCO_2$ greater than 45 does increase the surgical risk, there is currently no definitive number that prohibits abdominal surgery (E). Current American College of Physicians Guidelines recommend against the routine use of preoperative chest radiography or PFT (B). Although it is important to identify patients with COPD, and some COPD patients may benefit from preoperative interventions, patients who require additional testing can be identified by history of new symptoms or physical examination findings. Thus, PFT should be restricted to those who have current symptoms or signs based on history and physical. Location of the surgical incision is an important risk factor for postoperative pulmonary complications, with incisions closer to the diaphragm inferring more risk (D). When patients have been identified as high risk for pulmonary complications, current evidence supports the use of perioperative deep-breathing exercises and incentive spirometry. Routine use of nasogastric decompression has been associated with increased rates of pneumonia and atelectasis. Current recommendations are for more selective use in patients with nausea, vomiting, or gastric distention (C).

Reference: Qaseem A, Snow V, Fitterman N, et al. Risk assessment for and strategies to reduce perioperative pulmonary complications for patients undergoing noncardiothoracic surgery: a guideline from the American College of Physicians. *Ann Intern Med.* 2006;144(8):575–580.

13. C. The differential diagnosis for a sudden drop in end-tidal CO2 in the operating room (OR) includes an obstructed airway, accidental extubation, disconnection of the circuit, cardiac arrest, and pulmonary embolism (PE). The patient described has at least three risk factors for PE including malignancy, a heart rate greater than 100, and more than 3 days of immobilization (Wells criteria). PE is estimated to occur in 1% to 2% of surgical patients in the perioperative period. While dyspnea, anxiety, tachycardia, and tachypnea are the most common findings in awake patients, physical signs of PE will be limited in patients under general anesthesia. In this situation, an astute clinician can recognize PE as presenting with hypotension, tachycardia, decreased end-tidal CO_2, and hypoxemia. In general, laparoscopic procedures have been associated with a low risk of both fatal and nonfatal PE (E). This complication is associated with 10% to 15% mortality in the perioperative period (D). Electrocardiogram changes have been shown to be present in up to 83% of patients, but they are generally nonspecific (A). Uncommonly, PE can present with a prominent S wave in lead 1, Q wave in lead 3, and inverted T wave in lead 3; this is suggestive of right heart strain. Despite potential cardiovascular consequences of massive PE, an elevated cardiac enzyme level occurs in less than 50% of cases and is not specific for PE (B). The two most sensitive tests that can be done to help diagnose PE are a TEE and calculating the physiologic dead space to look for elevations (though it can be time-consuming). TEE has been shown to yield a diagnosis in an average of 9.6 minutes with a sensitivity of 80% and specificity of 97% and is ideal in the OR setting. Although TEE is relatively poor at visualizing the PE, it is excellent at demonstrating right heart strain, which provides indirect evidence of PE. Arterial blood gas in awake patients with PE may demonstrate a low CO_2, but this may not be the case for a ventilated patient under general anesthesia (D). Flexible bronchoscopy is not helpful in diagnosing PE (E).

Reference: Desciak MC, Martin DE. Perioperative pulmonary embolism: diagnosis and anesthetic management. *J Clin Anesth.* 2011;23(2):153–165

14. D. Red blood cell transfusion has been independently associated with longer intensive care unit (ICU) and hospital stays, increased complications, and increased mortality (C). It is also an independent risk factor for multiorgan system failure and systemic inflammatory response syndrome (SIRS). Most societal guidelines agree that a liberal transfusion strategy (goal of 10 g/dL) is no better and likely worse than a more restrictive strategy (goal of 7–9 g/dL) in the majority of patients. So transfusion is needed as long as the hemoglobin remains above 7 g/dL. The Transfusion Requirements in Critical Care (TRICC) trial demonstrated that critically ill patients without active bleeding fared better with a restrictive transfusion strategy. There is also no evidence that transfusion lowers the risk of acute coronary syndromes. (A, B). While hemoglobin can improve oxygen delivery to tissues, it has not been shown to lower risk of acute coronary syndromes, decrease time on the mechanical ventilator, improve oxygen consumption, or improve outcomes in patients with adult respiratory distress syndrome or acute lung injury (A). Because of the negative effects of blood transfusion, alternative methods of managing anemia are actively being researched, including the use of recombinant human erythropoietin (EPO) and hemoglobin-based oxygen carriers. Trials designed specifically looking at administering exogenous EPO in trauma patients, the EPO-1 and EPO-2 trials showed reductions in required blood transfusions and improved mortality, respectively. While hemoglobin-based oxygen carriers show some promise, they are not currently approved for use in the United States (E).

15. A. This patient has postoperative parotitis. This most commonly occurs in elderly patients with poor oral hygiene, poor oral intake, prolonged nasogastric tube decompression, and dehydration, all leading to a decrease in saliva production. The pathophysiology involves obstruction of the salivary ducts with secondary infection and is more common in the diabetic or immunocompromised patient. Most patients will be diagnosed with parotitis 4 to 12 days postoperatively. Signs and symptoms begin with pain and tenderness over the angle of the jaw that can then progress to high fevers and

leukocytosis, as well as significant edema involving the floor of the mouth. If left undiagnosed and untreated, it can lead to life-threatening sepsis. Initial treatment is with high-dose broad-spectrum antibiotics with *Staphylococcus* coverage (most common organism) and warm compresses (B). If the patient does not improve, surgical incision and drainage are indicated. In extreme cases involving progressive airway obstruction, emergent tracheostomy may be indicated. Use of measures to stimulate salivary flow, such as sucking on candy, seems to help prevent this complication, but prophylactic antibiotics are generally not indicated (C). Within improved oral hygiene, the incidence of this rare complication is declining (D). Additionally, the use of anticholinergics will decrease salivary flow and increase the risk of developing postoperative parotitis (E).

16. E. VTE prophylaxis is generally divided into two categories: pharmacologic and mechanical. Mechanical prophylaxis includes static compression devices (like graduated compression stockings) and IPC devices. While graduated compression stockings work primarily by preventing venous stasis in the legs, IPC combines that with its effects on the intrinsic fibrinolytic system. It was originally hypothesized that intermittent compression caused the release of agents like tPA from the vascular endothelium. However, when these levels are directly measured, they seem to be relatively constant despite an increase in tPA activity. The currently proposed mechanism is related to measured decreases in plasminogen activator inhibitor-1 (PAI-1), which functions as a tPA inhibitor (A). Currently, there is no evidence that one IPC device is superior to another in preventing VTE (B). While there are relatively few contraindications to mechanical prophylaxis, traumatic injury to the extremity and evidence of ischemia secondary to peripheral vascular disease are both contraindications. Additionally, patients with confirmed DVT in the lower extremity should not be placed on IPC. Limitations of its usefulness are primarily related to interruption in treatment and improper application. Comparison between mechanical and pharmacologic VTE prophylaxis shows that in certain low-risk patients there is an equivalent reduction in the incidence of DVT and PE, though combination therapy is superior to mechanical prophylaxis alone (C). It can be considered as sole therapy in low-risk patients and patients with contraindications to pharmacologic agents. In terms of pharmacologic prophylaxis, UFH and LMWH are the two most commonly used agents. LMWH is generally regarded as more effective, especially in certain populations (e.g., trauma patients) (D).

References: Comerota AJ, Chouhan V, Harada RN, et al. The fibrinolytic effects of intermittent pneumatic compression: mechanism of enhanced fibrinolysis. *Ann Surg.* 1997;226(3):306–314.

Ho K, Tan J. Stratified meta-analysis of intermittent pneumatic compression of the lower limbs to prevent venous thromboembolism in hospitalized patients. *Circulation,* 2013;128(9), 1003–1020.

Morris R, Woodcock J. Evidence-based compression. *Ann Surg.* 2004;239(2), 162–171.

17. D. Epidural anesthesia is an excellent tool to control postoperative pain and has been shown to decrease cardiac morbidity, and as such, it has been gaining popularity in clinical practice. Routine use of urinary drainage in the setting of epidural anesthesia remains controversial. However, postoperative day 1 removal of the Foley with thoracic epidurals has been shown to significantly decrease the incidence of urinary tract infections with minimal change to the rate of urinary retention as measured by rates of recatheterization (A–C). Current recommendations for the placement and removal of epidural catheters in patients receiving prophylactic LMWH is intended to prevent an epidural hematoma and subsequent paralysis. For the placement of epidural catheters, LMWH must be held at least 24 hours before placement, and it should not be removed within 12 hours of the last dose. Prophylactic anticoagulation can be restarted 6 hours after placement and no sooner than 4 hours after removal of the epidural (B). Unfractionated heparin may be restarted after 1 hour (E).

References: FDA Safety Information and Adverse Event Reporting Program. Low Molecular Weight Heparins: Drug Safety Communication – Updated recommendations to decrease risk of spinal column bleeding and paralysis in patients on low molecular weight heparins. U.S. Food and Drug Administration; 2013. https://www.fda.gov/media/87316/download.

Hendren S. Urinary catheter management. *Clin Colon Rectal Surg.* 2013;26(3):178–181.

Horlocker TT. Regional anaesthesia in the patient receiving antithrombotic and antiplatelet therapy. *Br J Anaesth.* 2011;107 Suppl 1:i96–i106.

Townsend CM Jr, Beauchamp RD, Evers BM, Mattox KL. *Sabiston textbook of surgery: the biological basis of modern surgical practice.* 17th ed. WB Saunders; 2004.

Zaouter C, Kaneva P, Carli F. Less urinary tract infection by earlier removal of bladder catheter in surgical patients receiving thoracic epidural analgesia. *Reg Anesth Pain Med.* 2009;34(6):542–548.

18. E. Postoperative necrotizing soft-tissue infection is a rare but well-described complication. The description of "dishwater pus" is classic for a postoperative clostridial wound infection. The causative organisms are typically *Streptococcus pyogenes* or *Clostridium perfringens*. *C. perfringens* is an anaerobic gram-positive rod that produces alpha-toxin; this is a virulent exotoxin that leads to extensive tissue necrosis and cardiovascular collapse. Immunocompromised patients (diabetes, malignancy, chronic liver disease) are at increased risk (A–D). Clindamycin has been shown to limit toxin production, which decreases the virulence, slows tissue destruction, and can potentially reduce inflammatory cytokine release. Effective therapy requires rapid administration of broad-spectrum antibiotics including aerobic coverage (C) and source control via emergent operative excision of necrotic infected tissue, including fascia. Conservative management is not appropriate if a necrotizing soft-tissue infection is suspected (B).

Reference: Hakkarainen TW, Kopari NM, Pham TN, Evans HL. Necrotizing soft tissue infections: review and current concepts in treatment, systems of care, and outcomes. *Curr Probl Surg.* 2014;51(8):344–362.

19. E. Postoperative hematomas after neck surgery (thyroid, parathyroid, carotid artery) can have catastrophic consequences. Physical examination findings can be deceptively benign. Attempts at intubation may be hampered by tracheal compression and deviation (B). Furthermore, the recent neck dissection, combined with the hematoma, causes venous and lymphatic obstruction, leading to airway edema, further compromising attempts at intubation. Rapidly opening the incision at the bedside is necessary because urgent decompression is the fastest way to restore proper respiratory function. Definitive hemostasis must then be obtained in the operating room. Although ultrasonography is an important diagnostic aid for hematomas (D), clinical suspicion is sufficient in this emergent situation and the urgency of decompression does not permit waiting for an ultrasound examination. Needle aspiration would not be sufficient (C). While nebulized racemic epinephrine is used for the treatment of stridor in conditions like croup, it is not appropriate when the cause of stridor is external compression of the airway (A).

20. E. The ureters first pass medial to the psoas muscle and travel alongside the transverse processes of the lumbar vertebrae and cross anterior to the common iliac arteries near the bifurcation into the internal and external iliac arteries. The anatomic position places the ureters at risk for injury during pelvic surgery, and the situation is particularly precarious when inflammation, abscess, and/or phlegmon are present. The highest risk of ureteral injury is during an abdominoperineal resection. During mobilization of the left colon and ligation of the inferior mesenteric artery, visualization and protection of the ureter from injury are imperative. Placement of ureteral stents before the operation may help to identify the ureters and assist with identifying an injury intraoperatively, but this does not seem to correlate with a reduction in the number of injuries (B). The presence of blue dye in the operative field after intravenous administration of indigo carmine or methylene blue is diagnostic for injury to the ureter. The decision to immediately reoperate is based on the delay associated with injury recognition, the severity of the injury, and whether the patient has developed urosepsis. If discovered within a week postop, reoperation is generally recommended (A). Beyond 10 days, the inflammation present will make reoperation hazardous. In this latter case, percutaneous nephrostomy and/or retrograde drainage with a ureteral stent is indicated (C, D). The type of repair depends on the location and extent of the injury. For midureter injuries, a ureteroureterostomy is preferred. For pelvic injuries, ureteroneocystostomy is needed. If this is not possible, a psoas hitch or a Boari flap (from the bladder) may be needed.

Reference: Bothwell WN, Bleicher RJ, Dent TL. Prophylactic ureteral catheterization in colon surgery. A five-year review. *Dis Colon Rectum.* 1994;37(4):330–334.

21. C. Crush injury to the extremities causing significant muscle injury is often complicated by rhabdomyolysis, which can lead to acute renal failure. Degradation products of both hemoglobin and myoglobin are toxic to the nephron in acidic urine. Elevated serum creatine phosphokinase, hyperkalemia, and the presence of heme without a significant amount of red blood cells on urinalysis are indicative of rhabdomyolysis. Management consists of aggressive IV hydration to maintain a urine output of more than 100 mL/hour and should begin with infusion rates of at least 200 cc/hour. Myoglobin concentrates in the renal tubules precipitates when it comes in contact with Tamm-Horsfall protein. This precipitation is enhanced under acidic conditions. Routine administration of bicarbonate (D) and mannitol (E) in the prevention of acute kidney injury from rhabdomyolysis is controversial, but, theoretically, alkalinization of the urine increases the solubility of the myoglobin–Tamm-Horsfall protein P complex and should increase myoglobin washout. It also prevents lipid peroxidation and renal vasoconstriction and seems to have relatively few negative side effects if used in patients without high serum bicarbonate and without alkalosis. However, it reduces the amount of ionized calcium so should be used with caution in patients with hypocalcemia. Historical treatment of rhabdomyolysis has included forced diuresis with mannitol, but its routine use is being questioned now in the literature and may actually increase the risk of developing renal failure. A retrospective study published in *The Journal of Trauma* in 2004 looking at over 2000 patients with elevated creatine kinase showed no difference in renal failure, need for hemodialysis, or mortality in patients receiving bicarbonate and mannitol versus volume resuscitation alone. Mannitol may aid in decreasing muscle swelling and compartment pressures, but the mainstay of treatment remains decompression of muscle compartments (A). However, in the case of crush injury, normal compartment pressures would not change your strategy for preventing acute kidney injury because tissue damage alone could cause the release of myoglobin. Loop diuretics are not used in the prevention of acute kidney injury in the setting of rhabdomyolysis (B). While retrograde urethrogram would assist in the diagnosis of missed urethral injury, the urine is positive on the dipstick from myoglobin, not hemoglobin.

References: Brown CVR, Rhee P, Chan L, Evans K, Demetriades D, Velmahos GC. Preventing renal failure in patients with rhabdomyolysis: do bicarbonate and mannitol make a difference? *J Trauma.* 2004;56(6):1191–1196.

Holt SG, Moore KP. Pathogenesis and treatment of renal dysfunction in rhabdomyolysis. *Intensive Care Med.* 2001;27(5):803–811.

22. E. Pulmonary function testing generally includes three separate tests: spirometry, lung volumes, and the diffusion capacity of the lungs. Expected changes with aging include an increase in the functional residual capacity and the residual volume, with a corresponding decrease in the vital capacity. This reciprocal change generally means the TLC is preserved (A). DLCO will also decrease with age (C). Compliance of the lung can be misleading because even though the compliance of the lung tissue itself increases with age, the chest wall compliance is significantly reduced. In general, this means that the overall compliance of the pulmonary system is reduced. Preoperative pulmonary function tests are mandatory for the evaluation of potential pulmonary resection. The preoperative values to remember are FEV_1 greater than 2 L for pneumonectomy, FEV_1 greater than 1.5 L for lobectomy, FEV_1 greater than 80% predicted, and DLCO greater than 80% predicted. However, these numbers are not absolute indications, and failure to meet them simply necessitates more workup; this includes getting a ventilation/perfusion scan to determine the contribution of the predicted segment (B). If the percent-predicted postoperative FEV_1 and DLCO are greater than 60%, then the patient is a candidate for resection of the proposed segment without further testing (D). If the percent-predictive postoperative FEV_1 and DLCO are less than 60%, exercise tolerance should be tested.

Reference: Brunelli A, Kim AW, Berger KI, Addrizzo-Harris DJ. Physiologic evaluation of the patient with lung cancer being considered for resectional surgery: diagnosis and management of lung cancer, 3rd ed: American College of Chest Physicians evidence-based clinical practice guidelines. *Chest.* 2013;143(5 Suppl):e166S–e190S.

23. B. Venous air embolism is a rare and typically asymptomatic condition. Though it is often associated with the placement of central venous access catheters, it has been associated with other conditions including trauma, head and neck procedures, and neurosurgical procedures. When suspected, the patient should be immediately placed in Trendelenburg position and left lateral decubitus or right side up (Durant maneuver) (C). This maneuver is designed to trap the air embolus in the right ventricle and prevent it from going into the pulmonary arteries. Physical exam findings include jugular venous distention, millwheel murmur, and a sucking sound as air enters the venous system through a catheter. The most sensitive bedside test for diagnosis is likely transesophageal echocardiography, which can detect even small volumes of air (D). ECG suggestive of right heart strain is associated with pulmonary emboli (A). Treatment includes correct positioning as previously described, increasing inspired oxygen, mechanical ventilation, hyperbaric oxygen, and, as a last resort, closed-chest cardiac massage to try to force the air out of the pulmonary arteries and into the smaller capillaries of the lung. An attempt can be made to aspirate the air from the ventricle either through an existing central line or directly through the chest wall, but the return of air with these procedures is generally low (E). Myocardial infarction is uncommon with venous air embolism and is typically the result of the air entering the arterial system via a congenital heart defect, such as a patent foramen ovale, and occluding the coronary arteries. The volume for a fatal venous air embolism is typically estimated at 3 to 5 mL/kg injected at a rate of 100 mL/s, but these are largely based on animal studies. The volume is much lower if the air enters the arterial system.

Reference: Gordy S, Rowell S. Vascular air embolism. *Int J Crit Illn Inj Sci.* 2013;3(1):73–76.

24. D. This patient is scheduled for a low-risk endoscopic procedure and represents a high risk for thromboembolic events (mechanical valves and previous thromboembolic events), so anticoagulation should be continued without interruption. When considering endoscopic procedures for patients on anticoagulation or antiplatelet therapy, three main things need to be considered: the urgency of the procedure, the patient's risk of thromboembolic events (and in this case, the type of valve), and risk of bleeding during the proposed intervention. If the anticoagulation is temporary (e.g., treatment of venous thrombosis) or discontinuation will be safer at a later date (e.g., recent myocardial infarction [MI] with stent placement) and the endoscopy is completely elective (such as screening), the endoscopy should be delayed. The type of prosthetic valve matters too. Prosthetic mitral valves have a much higher risk of thrombosis than aortic valves (much higher flow) with cessation of anticoagulation. As such, bridging is typically not needed for aortic valves. Low-risk endoscopic procedures can safely be performed on therapeutic anticoagulation or antiplatelet therapy and these medications should be continued regardless of the intervention. Examples of these procedures are diagnostic endoscopy with mucosal biopsy, ERCP without sphincterotomy, EUS, enteroscopy, and stent deployment. In all high-risk endoscopic procedures (polypectomy, sphincterotomy, therapeutic dilation, fine-needle aspiration, endoscopic hemostasis, tumor ablation, cyst gastrostomy, and treatment of varices), anticoagulation should be discontinued with or without bridging. However, aspirin and NSAIDs can safely be continued in all endoscopic procedures. For patients on antiplatelet therapy with agents other than aspirin, they should be held 7 to 10 days before the procedure unless the thromboembolic risks are high, in which case patients may need to be switched to aspirin or, in the case of dual antiplatelet therapy, aspirin continued and the other agent discontinued. If the thromboembolic risk is low, anticoagulation can be stopped and simply restarted after the procedure. For anticoagulation with warfarin in patients with high thromboembolic risk, bridge therapy with LMWH or unfractionated heparin should be considered. Use of LMWH and mechanical valves is controversial because of reported events of fatal thromboembolism on LMWH in these patients. In general, anticoagulation can be restarted within 24 hours after the procedure (A–C, E).

Reference: ASGE Standards of Practice Committee, Anderson MA, Ben-Menachem T, et al. Management of antithrombotic agents for endoscopic procedures. *Gastrointest Endosc.* 2009;70(6):1060–1070.

25. A. Refractory hypotension in the postoperative period in patients with conditions such as SLE that are commonly treated with steroids should raise concern for acute adrenal insufficiency. When the diagnosis is suspected, treatment should begin immediately before confirmatory tests become available (E). Initial treatment consists of: volume resuscitation, laboratory studies (electrolytes, glucose, adrenocorticotropic hormone [ACTH], cortisol), and administration of either 4 mg of dexamethasone or 100 mg of hydrocortisone. Dexamethasone is preferred because it will not interfere with cosyntropin stimulation testing, which should be done the next morning to confirm the diagnosis. Glucocorticoids can then be tapered to regular maintenance doses. Routine administration of "stress-dose steroids" for patients on long-term corticosteroids is not supported by evidence. It is now recommended that patients on long-term steroids should not be given "stress-dose" perioperative corticosteroids. They should be continued on their regular maintenance dose with the consideration of additional steroids only if they develop refractory hypotension suggestive of adrenal insufficiency. While the cosyntropin stimulation test can be instrumental in detecting acute adrenal insufficiency, its usefulness as a preoperative measure for assessing risk of postoperative adrenal crisis is lacking sufficient data to support its routine use. While septic shock in the early postoperative period

is possible, this vignette provides insufficient data to point to this diagnosis (C, D). Exploratory laparotomy is not an appropriate option for the above patient (B).

References: Brunicardi FC, Andersen DK, Billiar TR, Dunn DL, Hunter JG, Matthews JB, Pollock RE. *Schwartz's principles of surgery.* 10th ed. McGraw-Hill Education; 2015.

Kelly KN, Domajnko B. Perioperative stress-dose steroids. *Clin Colon Rectal Surg.* 2013;26(3):163–167.

Marik PE, Varon J. Requirement of perioperative stress doses of corticosteroids: a systematic review of the literature. *Arch Surg.* 2008;143(12):1222–1226.

26. A. The 2008 POISE trial was a randomized controlled trial to measure the effects of perioperative initiation of beta-blockers. The control group received a placebo while the study arm was started on metoprolol on the day of surgery and received it for 30 days postoperatively. The study found that patients who received metoprolol had a lower incidence of myocardial infarction, cardiac revascularization, and clinically significant atrial fibrillation. However, patients in the study arm also had increased mortality, stroke, hypotension, and bradycardia (A, E). This increase in mortality was not seen in the previously published DECREASE trials, which also showed a reduction in myocardial infarction. However, several of these studies were retracted because of falsified data and questionable data collection techniques. Without any other large randomized trials to counter the POISE trial, it has largely become the basis for current guidelines regarding perioperative use of beta-blockers. The 2014 ACC/AHA guidelines for perioperative beta-blocker therapy can be summarized as: (1) Beta-blockers should be continued if patients are on them chronically. (2) Management of beta-blockers after surgery should be based on clinical judgment to avoid negative consequences such as hypotension or bradycardia (B). (3) Beta-blockers should not be started on the day of surgery. (4) It is unclear what the risk of starting beta-blockers is in the 2 to 45 days before surgery (C). (5) It should be considered in high-risk individuals (D).

References: POISE Study Group, Devereaux PJ, Yang H, et al. Effects of extended-release metoprolol succinate in patients undergoing non-cardiac surgery (POISE trial): a randomised controlled trial. *Lancet.* 2008;371(9627):1839–1847.

Wijeysundera DN, Duncan D, Nkonde-Price C, et al. Perioperative beta blockade in noncardiac surgery: a systematic review for the 2014 ACC/AHA guideline on perioperative cardiovascular evaluation and management of patients undergoing noncardiac surgery: a report of the American College of Cardiology/American Heart Association Task Force on practice guidelines. *J Am Coll Cardiol.* 2014;64(22):2406–2425.

Transfusion and Disorders of Coagulation

36

CAITLYN BRASCHI, JOON Y. PARK, AND ERIC R. SIMMS

ABSITE 99th Percentile High-Yields

I. Coagulation Cascade and Factors
- A. Factor I = fibrinogen, factor IA = fibrin, factor II = prothrombin, factor IIA = thrombin
- B. Intrinsic pathway of coagulation: initiated by exposed subendothelial collagen, prekallikrein, high molecular weight kininogen; also involves factors VIII, IX, XI, XII; if impaired, PTT will be elevated
- C. Extrinsic pathway of coagulation: involves factor VII; if impaired, PT/INR will be elevated
- D. Common pathway of coagulation: involves factors I, II, V, X
- E. Factor VII has the shortest half-life of all coagulation factors
- F. Protein C and S breakdown factors V and VIII
- G. Factor VIII is the only coagulation factor not made in the liver (made in the endothelium); von Willebrand factor (vWF) also made in the endothelium

II. Blood Products and Drugs for Coagulation Reversal

	Contents/mechanism of action	Indications	Notes
Fresh Frozen Plasma (FFP)	All coagulation factors, vWF, Antithrombin III (ATIII)	Warfarin reversal, DIC, TTP, liver disease, AT III deficiency, Factor V deficiency	INR of FFP is 1.4–1.6; takes 1–2 hours to thaw
Cryoprecipitate	I, VIII, XIII, vWF	DIC, vWD type III, hemophilia A, hypofibrinogenemia	Highest concentration of fibrinogen (Factor I)
Prothrombin complex concentrate (PCC)	3-factor: II, IX, X (not used in clinical practice) 4-factor: II, VII, IX, X, C, S	Warfarin reversal in life-threatening bleed (intracranial hemorrhage), reversal of direct Xa inhibitors (rivaroxaban, apixaban)	Immediate warfarin reversal
Recombinant factor VIII	VIII	Hemophilia A	Transfuse to 100% normal factor VIII levels before major surgery
Recombinant factor IX	IX	Hemophilia B	Transfuse to 100% normal factor IX levels before major surgery
Recombinant factor Xa	X	Reverse direct Xa inhibitor	Not widely available
Vitamin K	Cofactor of carboxylation of coagulation factors II, VII, IX, X, C, S	Nonurgent warfarin reversal	Warfarin reversal begins after 6–10 hours, full effect after 1–2 days
Tranexamic acid (TXA)	Binds plasmin (inhibits fibrinolysis)	Traumatic hemorrhagic shock with hyperfibrinolysis	Must be given within 3 hours of injury for benefit; if patient does not have hyperfibrinolysis, TXA increases risk for thromboembolic events

	Contents/mechanism of action	Indications	Notes
Aminocaproic acid	Binds plasmin (inhibits fibrinolysis)	tPA-associated bleed DIC	
Protamine sulfate	Binds to and inhibits heparin	Heparin overdose with associated bleed	Only partially effective against LMWH
Desmopressin (DDAVP)	V2 agonist, causes release of vWF and factor VIII from endothelium and platelets	vWD type I/II, uremia	vWD type III has absent vWF, so DDAVP ineffective

III. Anticoagulants

	Mechanism of action	Notes
Heparin	Indirect thrombin and factor X inhibitor via ATIII	Ineffective in ATIII deficiency (give FFP with heparin) Affects the intrinsic pathway (PTT)
Low-molecular-weight heparin (LMWH)	Indirect factor X inhibitor via ATIII	Superior DVT prophylaxis in cancer patients
Coumadin	Vitamin K antagonist	Contraindicated in pregnancy Extrinsic pathway (PT)
Argatroban, bivalirudin, hirudin, dabigatran	Direct thrombin inhibitors	Used in HIT (argatroban first line; bivalirudin if liver failure); Hirudin is irreversible inhibitor; Dabigatran reversal: idarucizumab
tPA, streptokinase, urokinase	Active plasminogen	Monitor fibrinogen levels
Apixaban, rivaroxaban	Direct factor Xa inhibitor	Rivaroxaban reversed with andexanet alfa

IV. Transfusion Reactions

Reaction	Clinical findings	Cause	Related products	Treatment
Febrile, nonhemolytic	Fever, pruritus, shivering as transfusion is being given; most common transfusion reaction	Cytokines from non-leukoreduced donor product	All products (rarely plasma)	Stop transfusion (although no long-term effects, need to evaluate why patient is febrile), control symptoms (antipyretics, antihistamines)
Febrile hemolytic	Fevers, chills, hypotension, chest/back pain; DIC, hematuria, renal failure	ABO incompatibility	Usually RBCs	Stop transfusion, give fluids, hemodynamic support
Urticarial	Hives	IgE reaction to product component	All products	Symptomatic treatment (antihistamines)
Anaphylactic	Hives, hypotension, wheezing, angioedema, hypoxemia	Recipient anti-IgA antibodies attack donor IgA antibodies, often in IgA-deficient patients	All products	Stop transfusion, resuscitation, epinephrine
Sepsis	Fevers, chills, hypotension, leukocytosis	Microorganism in stored product	Usually platelets (stored at room temp)	Antibiotics, hemodynamic support
Transfusion-related lung injury (TRALI)	Respiratory distress, hypoxemia, fever, *hypotension*, leukopenia, bilateral infiltrates on CXR; within 6 hrs of transfusion	"Two-hit": neutrophil sequestration and activation by donor product	All products	Stop transfusion, ventilatory support
Transfusion-associated circulatory overload (TACO)	Respiratory distress, hypoxemia, JVD, *hypertension*, pulmonary edema; 6–12 posttransfusion	Fluid overload; underlying cardiac or renal dysfunction	All products	Diuresis, ventilatory support

V. Thromboelastography (TEG)

   A. TEG is the best way to determine which blood products should be given to a bleeding patient

   B. Interpretation:

      1. R time—time to initial clot formation—if high, lacking coagulation factors -> give FFP

      2. K time—time to fibrin cross linking—if high, lacking fibrinogen -> give cryoprecipitate

      3. a angel—rate of clot formation—if low, lacking fibrinogen -> give cryoprecipitate

      4. MA (max amplitude)—maximum clot strength—if low, lacking platelets (contributes most to clot strength) -> give platelet

      5. LY30—rate of clot lysis—if high, increased fibrinolysis -> give TXA and/or aminocaproic acid

Questions

1. A 19-year-old male is evaluated in the trauma bay following a motorcycle accident. He is found to be hypotensive with an open book pelvic fracture. CT angiography of the pelvis does not demonstrate active extravasation. A thrombelastography is performed showing an elevated K time and high LY30. He has received blood products and is 5 hours post injury. Which of the following is true?
   A. Cryoprecipitate would not benefit this patient
   B. K time is a measure of the time to initial clot formation
   C. This finding is indicative of decreased fibrinogen levels
   D. FFP is indicated
   E. The patient should receive tranexamic acid (TXA)

2. The risk of posttransfusion sepsis is greatest with:
   A. Packed red blood cells
   B. Cryoprecipitate
   C. Fresh frozen plasma
   D. Platelets
   E. Whole blood

3. Which of the following is correct with regard to unfractionated heparin (UFH) and low-molecular-weight heparin (LMWH)?
   A. LMWH is contraindicated while breastfeeding
   B. UFH is associated with fewer cases of heparin-induced thrombocytopenia (HIT)
   C. Protamine is more effective in reversing LMWH compared to UFH
   D. LMWH does not need to be dose-adjusted in obese patients
   E. LMWH is considered superior in trauma patients with traumatic brain injury (TBI)

4. A 34-year-old woman with no past medical history presents with 6 weeks of left lower extremity pain and marked swelling and is found to have a left iliofemoral DVT on CT venogram. She is given a heparin bolus, and a heparin drip is started. She then undergoes catheter-directed thrombolysis (CDT). Which of the following is true?
   A. The half-life of alteplase (tPA) is 4 to 6 hours
   B. Bleeding from inadvertent overdose may benefit from administration of aminocaproic acid
   C. Bleeding risk best is best monitored by following INR
   D. The rate of intracranial bleeding following CDT is higher than systemic thrombolysis
   E. The heparin drip should be continued during CDT

5. Which of the following is true regarding the use of intraoperative blood salvage (autotransfusion)?
   A. Use of intraoperative blood salvage may lead to coagulopathy
   B. Malignancy is an absolute contraindication
   C. Autotransfusion can still be utilized if sterile water is being used in the field
   D. Most major abdominal surgeries would benefit from its use
   E. Activated clotting time (ACT) should be used intraoperatively to monitor for coagulopathy

6. A 49-year-old female with a history of von Willebrand disease type 3 presents for scheduled lobectomy for lung cancer. Which of the following is the correct perioperative management?
   A. Administer 1 unit of FFP in the preoperative holding area
   B. Transfuse recombinant factor IX to 100% normal levels prior to surgery
   C. DDAVP should be given prior to incision
   D. He can proceed without any intervention for von Willebrand type 3
   E. Preoperative von Willebrand factor concentrate should be administered

7. A 75-year-old woman with a history of atrial fibrillation on coumadin presents to the ED with a painful, enlarging bulge in her abdominal wall. She is diagnosed with a rectus sheath hematoma. Her INR is supratherapeutic at 5. She denies any recent coughing episodes or trauma. However, she reports starting a new medication. Which of the following medications could have contributed to her condition?
   A. Cimetidine
   B. Carbamazepine
   C. Rifampin
   D. Phenobarbital
   E. Phenytoin

8. Persistent life-threatening bleeding in a patient with Hemophilia A with high titers of inhibitors (factor VIII alloantibodies) is best treated with:
   A. A higher dose of factor VIII
   B. Fresh frozen plasma
   C. Cryoprecipitate
   D. Recombinant factor VIIa
   E. DDAVP (desmopressin)

9. A 76-year-old male is undergoing a laparoscopic colectomy for sigmoid colon cancer. Which of the following is the best prophylaxis for venous thromboembolic events (VTEs)?
   A. Leg compression device
   B. Unfractionated heparin (UFH) until fully ambulatory
   C. Leg compression device intraoperatively, UFH until fully ambulatory
   D. Leg compression device intraoperatively, LMWH until fully ambulatory
   E. Leg compression device intraoperatively, LMWH for 4 weeks after surgery

10. A 50-year-old male undergoes a resection of a large retroperitoneal leiomyosarcoma. There is an estimated blood loss of 750 cc. The next day, the patient is found to be anemic and is given 2 units of blood. Halfway through the first unit, the patient develops chills and his temperature increases from 37 to 39°C. Which of the following is true in regard to this patient's condition?
   A. The transfusion does not need to be stopped
   B. This occurs more commonly when given packed red blood cells versus platelets
   C. Filtration is more effective than leukocyte washing in preventing this condition
   D. Aspirin is more effective than acetaminophen in treating this condition
   E. Pretransfusion administration of acetaminophen and diphenhydramine is the most effective prevention

11. Which of the following does not affect the bleeding time?
    A. Aspirin
    B. von Willebrand disease
    C. Hemophilia A
    D. Severe thrombocytopenia
    E. Qualitative platelet disorders

12. A deficiency of which of the following factors would increase INR but not prolong the PTT?
    A. II
    B. V
    C. VII
    D. IX
    E. X

13. The most important preoperative assessment to determine the risk of abnormal intraoperative bleeding is:
    A. Bleeding time
    B. Activated partial thromboplastin time (aPTT)
    C. International normalized ratio (INR)
    D. History and physical examination
    E. Platelet count

14. Glanzmann thrombasthenia is characterized by:
    A. Normal bleeding time
    B. Treatment response to DDAVP (desmopressin) infusion
    C. Autosomal dominant inheritance
    D. Defect in platelet aggregation
    E. Prolonged INR

15. Cryoprecipitate contains a low concentration of which of following?
    A. Fibrinogen
    B. Factor VIII
    C. von Willebrand factor
    D. Fibronectin
    E. Factor XI

16. Which of the following is most likely to be useful in the treatment of bleeding in the uremic patient?
    A. Desmopressin
    B. Cryoprecipitate
    C. Fresh frozen plasma
    D. Recombinant human erythropoietin
    E. Estrogens

17. A 60-year-old man with diabetes presents with right upper quadrant pain and leukocytosis. The patient has an elevated INR of 2.5 and a prolonged PTT of 60 seconds, a low fibrinogen level, and a platelet count of 70,000 cells/µL. An ultrasound scan reveals gas in the wall of the gallbladder. The most important part in management of this patient would be:

A. Administration of fresh frozen plasma
B. Administration of cryoprecipitate
C. Checking the D-dimer assay
D. Emergent cholecystectomy
E. Administration of platelets

18. Which of the following is true in regard to von Willebrand disease (vWD)?

A. It is the second most common congenital defect in hemostasis
B. Type 1 vWD is transmitted in an autosomal recessive fashion
C. DDAVP (desmopressin) is helpful in type 3 vWD
D. Increased partial thromboplastin time (PTT) rules out vWD
E. DDAVP is ineffective for type 2B vWD

19. A 40-year-old female presents with a swollen left lower extremity, and ultrasound confirms a deep venous thrombosis (DVT). The patient is started on therapeutic heparin but despite progressively increasing the dose, the pharmacy is having difficulty achieving a therapeutic partial thromboplastin time (PTT) after 24 hours. Which of the following is the best option?

A. Convert from unfractionated heparin to low-molecular-weight heparin
B. Administer fresh frozen plasma
C. Start a direct thrombin inhibitor
D. Place an inferior vena cava filter
E. Continue to increase heparin dose as needed

20. Which of the following is true regarding prothrombin complex concentrate (PCC)?

A. Three-factor and 4-factor PCC refer to varying concentrations of factor II
B. It is thawed more rapidly than fresh frozen plasma (FFP)
C. PCC reverses warfarin to an international normalized ratio (INR) less than 1.5 within 30 minutes
D. PCC lowers INR as profoundly as recombinant factor VIIa
E. It reverses the anticoagulant effect of dabigatran

21. A 31-year-old woman in her third trimester of pregnancy presents with fever, headaches, and myalgia. She is a former intravenous drug user. She denies pruritus, but her skin appears jaundiced. Blood pressure is normal. Her laboratory exam is remarkable for elevated aspartate aminotransferase (AST) and alanine transaminase (ALT), hyperbilirubinemia as well as thrombocytopenia, anemia, and severe hypoglycemia. From which of the following conditions is she most likely suffering?

A. HELLP (hemolysis, elevated liver enzymes, low platelet count) syndrome
B. Acute fatty liver of pregnancy (AFLP)
C. Intrahepatic cholestasis of pregnancy (ICP)
D. Preeclampsia
E. Hepatitis E

22. A 35-year-old man has been in the intensive care unit sepsis due to enterocutaneous fistulas, ventilator dependence, and pneumonia for 2 weeks. He is receiving nutrition parenterally. The INR is 2.0. The aPTT is normal. The total bilirubin level is normal. The platelet count is normal. Which of the following is the most likely etiology?

A. Factor VIII deficiency
B. DIC
C. Vitamin K deficiency
D. Primary fibrinolysis
E. Chronic liver disease

23. Which of the following electrolyte abnormalities are the most likely to occur with massive blood transfusion?

A. Hypocalcemia, hypokalemia, and metabolic acidosis
B. Hypercalcemia, hyperkalemia, and metabolic alkalosis
C. Hypocalcemia, hyperkalemia, and metabolic alkalosis
D. Hyponatremia, hyperkalemia, and metabolic alkalosis
E. Hyponatremia, hyperkalemia, and metabolic acidosis

24. A 75-year-old male with a history of atrial fibrillation presents to the ED with an acute onset of left lower extremity pain and pulselessness. Heparin is started. He is found to have an occluded popliteal artery. The clot is successfully cleared with thrombolytic therapy. He remains on a heparin drip with plans to convert to warfarin. However, on hospital day 5 his platelet count drops to 160,000 u/L (from an admission level of 370,000 u/L). Which of the following is true with regard to the drop in platelet count and the concern for heparin-induced thrombocytopenia (HIT)?

    A. Because the platelet count is above 100,000 u/L, heparin can be continued
    B. The risk of recurrent thrombosis at this point is low
    C. Because the platelet count didn't drop until day 5, the concern for HIT is low
    D. HIT is less common in men
    E. Warfarin should be started

25. A 1-month-old infant with mild skeletal abnormalities suffers a cardiac arrest and passes away. On autopsy, he is found to have extensive thrombosis in his coronary arteries. Which of the following is the most likely underlying condition?

    A. Factor V Leiden mutation
    B. Prothrombin gene mutation
    C. Antithrombin III deficiency
    D. Homocystinuria
    E. Protein deficiency

26. The most common cause of transfusion-related death is:

    A. Infection
    B. ABO incompatibility
    C. Acute lung injury
    D. Delayed transfusion reaction
    E. Graft-versus-host reaction

27. A 35-year-old female develops postpartum hemorrhage and requires a transfusion of packed red blood cells and platelets. Twelve hours after transfusion, the patient abruptly develops rigors and chills. Her temperature increases to 39°C, her blood pressure drops from 110/70 to 70/40 mmHg, and her heart rate increases from 80 to 120 beats per minute. Urine output drops, although the urine is clear. Despite attempts at resuscitation, the patient expires within 24 hours. The death is most likely due to:

    A. Gram-positive sepsis
    B. ABO incompatibility
    C. Acute lung injury
    D. Anaphylaxis
    E. Gram-negative sepsis

28. A 55-year-old patient undergoes surgery, during which blood transfusions were given. One week later, skin lesions develop that appear to be purpura. The platelet count decreases from 250,000 cells/μL to 10,000 cells/μL and an upper gastrointestinal bleed develops. The patient has not been receiving any medication that could affect platelets. Which of the following is true about this condition?

    A. It is more common in middle-aged men
    B. Severe bleeding is best managed by platelet transfusions
    C. It can occur without prior antigenic exposure
    D. It is an antibody-mediated reaction
    E. Platelet counts are typically higher than with heparin-induced thrombocytopenia

29. Which of the following is true in regard to clopidogrel (Plavix)?

    A. It functionally mimics the pathophysiology of Bernard-Soulier disease
    B. It has been linked to fatal episodes of pulmonary hypertension
    C. It is recommended that clopidogrel be stopped 3 days before a major operation
    D. It inhibits platelet aggregation within 2 hours of oral administration
    E. It can inhibit the release of von Willebrand factor

30. Which of the following factors has the shortest half-life?

    A. I
    B. II
    C. VII
    D. IX
    E. X

31. A 29-year-old female is undergoing splenectomy for idiopathic thrombocytopenic purpura. Intraoperatively, the surgeon notes a significant amount of bleeding at the splenic hilum during mobilization. The surgeon would like to temporarily stop bleeding with a hemostatic agent. Which of the following would be the least effective choice for this patient?

    A. Microfibrillar collagen
    B. Oxidized cellulose
    C. Thrombin
    D. Fibrin sealant
    E. Glutaraldehyde cross-linked peptide

Answers

1. C. The use of thromboelastography (TEG) has become more common in the setting of hemorrhagic shock secondary to trauma or cirrhosis. TEG provides real-time information about clotting activity and can guide resuscitation. K time refers to the time to fibrin cross linking and an elevated K time indicates a deficiency of fibrinogen (B). Therefore, transfusion of cryoprecipitate would be indicated for this patient (A). Platelets would be indicated in the event of a low MA. R time on a TEG result refers to the time to initial clot formation, and if this is prolonged, transfusion of FFP is indicated (D). A high LY30 is consistent with hyperfibrinolysis and suggests the patient would benefit with TXA administration. Trauma patients with massive hemorrhage receiving TXA have reduced all-cause mortality. However, this benefit is only seen for patients receiving TXA within 3 hours of injury. TXA administration past the 3-hour mark is associated with worse outcomes (E).

Reference: Roberts I, Shakur H, Coats T, et al. The CRASH-2 trial: a randomised controlled trial and economic evaluation of the effects of tranexamic acid on death, vascular occlusive events and transfusion requirement in bleeding trauma patients. *Health Technol Assess.* 2013;17(10):1–79.

2. D. The risk of posttransfusion sepsis is greatest with platelet transfusion. The risk is the greatest in transfusion of pooled platelet concentrates from multiple donor versus single-donor platelet transfusion. Platelets are stored at 22°C which makes this blood product the most vulnerable to bacterial colonization and growth. If bacteria contamination of administered blood products is suspected, the transfusion should be stopped immediately and blood cultures obtained.

3. E. The rate of serious bleeding complications has been shown to be lower with the use of LMWH compared to UFH. It has also been shown to be associated with improved mortality in trauma patients with TBI. However, LMWH does not have a completely effective reversal agent available. Only 60% of the anticoagulant effect of LMWH can be reversed with the administration of protamine (C). Higher rates of major bleeding events have been shows in patients with renal insufficiency with the use of both UFH and LMWH. LMWH is renally cleared, however, and therefore should be avoided in the setting of reduced creatinine clearance. UFH undergoes excretion via the reticuloendothelial system and endothelial cells (D). Although both UFH and LMWH are associated with the development of HIT, this is more commonly seen after exposure to UFH (B). Either UFH, LMWH, or warfarin can be safely used while breastfeeding (A). Patients with obesity have a larger volume of distribution of lipophilic drugs such as LMWH and as such will require dose adjusting to reach adequate levels for thromboprophylaxis (D).

Reference: Crowther MA, Berry LR, Monagle PT, Chan AKC. Mechanisms responsible for the failure of protamine to inactivate low-molecular-weight heparin: inactivation of low-molecular-weight heparin by protamine. *Br J Haematol.* 2002;116(1):178–186.

4. B. Alteplase, a tissue plasminogen activator (tPA), is the drug most commonly used in CDT and has a very short half-life (5 minutes) (A). tPA triggers the activation of plasminogen into plasmin which then breaks fibrin cross links to dissolve clot. Aminocaproic acid is the treatment of overdose or reversal of tPA. Fibrinogen levels should be monitored closely following thrombolysis. Low levels of fibrinogen (usually less than 100 or 150 depending on clinical practice), are indicative of an increased risk of bleeding events (C). Although CDT has lower rates of intracranial hemorrhage than systemic thrombolysis (0%–1% versus 3%–6%, respectively), the patient should be monitored closely while undergoing treatment (D). Many of the same absolute contraindications to systemic thrombolysis are true for CDT including recent stroke, active bleeding, and intracranial trauma. Systemic heparin should be held during lytic therapy due to the risk of bleeding (E).

Reference: Fleck D, Albadawi H, Shamoun F, Knuttinen G, Naidu S, Oklu R. Catheter-directed thrombolysis of deep vein thrombosis: literature review and practice considerations. *Cardiovasc Diagn Ther.* 2017;7(S3):S228–S237.

5. A. Intraoperative blood salvage is recommended for clean (non-GI, noncontaminated) procedures with an estimated blood loss of 500 to 1000 mL (e.g., cardiac, liver, vascular, orthopedic cases) or more (D). This involves removing the patient's blood with a suction catheter during surgery from the operative field. The blood is then filtered, washed and returned to the patient. It has been shown to reduce the amount of allogenic transfusion required. It also theoretically increases operating room efficiency as there is less time needed to request and prepare allogenic product. Absolute contraindications include mixture with other fluids, particularly sterile water, as this hypotonic solution can lead to hemolysis (C). Malignancy is not an absolute contraindication; however, the risks and benefits should be assessed on a case-by-case basis (B). Intraoperative blood salvage only replaces red blood cells and therefore patients are at risk of coagulopathy and dilution of coagulation factors. ACT monitoring is used in the setting of systemic heparinization, not for the use of red cell salvage. Goal ACT varies by provider and procedure but 150 to 200 seconds for routine anticoagulation is commonly used (E).

References: American Society of Anesthesiologists Task Force on Perioperative Blood Management. Practice guidelines for perioperative blood management: an updated report by the American Society of Anesthesiologists Task Force on Perioperative Blood Management. *Anesthesiology.* 2015;122(2):241–275.

Carless PA, Henry DA, Moxey AJ, O'Connell D, Brown T, Fergusson DA. Cell salvage for minimising perioperative allogeneic blood transfusion. *Cochrane Database Syst Rev.* 2010;(4):CD001888.

6. E. von Willebrand disease (vWD) is the most common congenital bleeding disorder. Patients with WVD type 3 have the most severe bleeding diathesis among patients with VWD. In this type of VWD, there is an absence of von Willebrand factor (vWF). DDAVP causes release of vWF and factor VIII from endothelial stores, and therefore, patients with type 3 VWD are not responsive to DDAVP (C). The perioperative management for patients with VWD undergoing major surgery (e.g., cardiothoracic, hepatobiliary, neurologic, open vascular) includes administration of vWF (D). For patients with Hemophilia B, recombinant factor IX should be administered to a goal of 100% of normal factor IX levels preoperatively (B). FFP can be used to correct INR in the acute setting (A).

Reference: Lavin M, O'Donnell JS. New treatment approaches to von Willebrand disease. *Hematology Am Soc Hematol Educ Program.* 2016;2016(1):683–689.

7. A. This patient has a supratherapeutic INR while on coumadin. Coumadin works by interfering with the gamma-carboxylation of vitamin K-dependent coagulation factors (factors II, VII, IX, X, protein C, S), and is metabolized by the cytochrome-P450 in the liver. Several drug interactions can lead to altered coumadin metabolism. Medications that inhibit cytochrome-P450 lead to decreased coumadin metabolism and supratherapeutic INR. Inhibitors of cytochrome-P450 include cimetidine, amiodarone, several antibiotics (macrolides, fluoroquinolones, metronidazole, isoniazid, sulfonamides), voriconazole, and grapefruit juice. Conversely, inducers of cytochrome-P450 will increase metabolism of warfarin decreasing its effect. These patients may present with a new venous thromboembolism even though they have been on the same dose of warfarin for years. Examples of cytochrome-P450 include carbamazepine, rifampin, phenytoin, and phenobarbital (B–E).

8. D. Hemophilia A is a sex-linked recessive genetic condition and considered the most common coagulation disorder, accounting for 80% of all inherited coagulation disorders. With time, as many as 10% to 15% of patients with factor VIII–deficient hemophilia A develop inhibitors (alloantibodies) against factor VIII. This is usually from previous factor VIII transfusions. In situations in which life-threatening hemorrhage develops, recombinant factor VIIa is the best option. Another option is porcine factor VIII, but there is approximately a 25% cross-reactivity with inhibitors. Factor VIIa complexes with tissue factor at the site of injury, resulting in an activation of factor X, which then results in clot formation. Factor VIIa bypasses the requirement for factors VIII and IX and thus has been shown to be effective in prevention and treatment of joint hemorrhage, the treatment of life-threatening bleeding, and the prevention of surgical bleeding. Restimulation of antibodies to factors VIII and IX should theoretically be less problematic than with the use of plasma-derived products. The primary concerns with recombinant factor VIIa are the potential for inducing thrombosis (stroke, deep venous thrombosis) and the high cost. A higher dose of factor VIII would not defeat production of patient antibodies (A). Both fresh frozen plasma and cryoprecipitate contain factor VII but would be diluted with other factors including factor VIII (B, C). DDAVP would not help a patient with a coagulation defect (E). Other options that have been used but are only a temporary fix in patients with significant bleeding are plasmapheresis and immune absorption.

References: DiMichele D. *Inhibitors in hemophilia: a primer.* Treatment of Hemophilia, 2008;(7):1–4.

Kenet G, Lubetsky A, Luboshitz J, Martinowitz U. A new approach to treatment of bleeding episodes in young hemophilia patients: a single bolus megadose of recombinant activated factor VII (NovoSeven): recombinant FVIIa (NovoSeven) megadose. *J Thromb Haemost.* 2003;1(3):450–455.

9. E. Patients undergoing surgery should be assessed for VTE risk and categorized as very low, low, moderate, and high-risk patients. The Caprini score can be used to facilitate the estimation. A score of 5 or more places a patient at high risk. Age of 75 years or more = 3 points, cancer = 2 points, and major open or laparoscopic surgery longer than 45 minutes is also 2 points. As such this patient would be considered high risk. In low-risk patients, mechanical prevention (compression device) is recommended. In moderate risk, pharmacologic prophylaxis with either UFH or LMWH is recommended. High-risk patients should get both mechanical and pharmacologic prophylaxis. The drug should be administered close to surgery and continued until the patient is fully ambulatory. Recent data in high-risk patients (such as those with cancer) demonstrate enhanced VTE prophylaxis with extended LMWH for 4 weeks after surgery (A–D). Interestingly, recent data indicate that patients undergoing colectomy for inflammatory bowel disease (IBD) are also at very high risk for VTE (though IBD is not included in the Caprini score).

Reference: Vedovati MC, Becattini C, Rondelli F, et al. A randomized study on 1-week versus 4-week prophylaxis for venous thromboembolism after laparoscopic surgery for colorectal cancer. *Ann Surg.* 2014;259(4):665–669.

10. C. The patient is likely manifesting a febrile nonhemolytic transfusion reaction (FNHTR), the most common blood transfusion reaction. It occurs in 0.5% to 1.5% of all cases of blood transfusion (A). It is defined as a rise in temperature of at least 1.8°C from baseline and is not accounted for by the patient's clinical condition. However, FNHTR is a diagnosis of exclusion. As such, it is generally recommended to at least temporarily stop the transfusion and assess the patient. In particular, attention should be paid to additional symptoms and signs such as respiratory compromise, cyanosis, back pain, and hypotension; these may suggest a hemolytic reaction, TRALI, or sepsis from contaminated blood. FNHTR is more common in pregnancy and in patients with immunocompromised states (such as leukemia, lymphoma). It occurs more commonly after the transfusion of platelets but can also occur with PRBC or FFP (B). Pretreatment with acetaminophen was thought to reduce the severity of the complication. However, the only randomized controlled trial to date demonstrated no difference in the rate of FNHTR in patients that were pretreated with acetaminophen and diphenhydramine when compared to a placebo (E). The incidence of febrile reactions can be greatly reduced by the use of leukocyte-reduced blood products. Filtration removes 99.9% of the white blood cells and platelets and is more effective than washing. Leukocyte reduction prevents almost all febrile transfusion reactions. There is debate in the literature as to whether leukocyte reduction leads to a decrease in postoperative infections or mortality. Aspirin is not advised given its effects on platelets and bleeding (D).

References: Hébert PC, Fergusson D, Blajchman MA, et al. Clinical outcomes following institution of the Canadian universal leukoreduction program for red blood cell transfusions. *JAMA.* 2003;289(15):1941–1949.

Wang SE, Lara PN Jr, Lee-Ow A, et al. Acetaminophen and diphenhydramine as premedication for platelet transfusions: a prospective randomized double-blind placebo-controlled trial. *Am J Hematol.* 2002;70(3):191–194.

11. C. Bleeding time tests platelet adhesion and aggregation and will be normal in derangement of the coagulation pathways. Hemophilia A is associated with a factor VIII deficiency, which manifests as an abnormality in the coagulation cascade and presents with a prolonged PTT. Drugs that inhibit platelet function, such as aspirin (which works by inhibiting cyclooxygenase), will increase bleeding time (A). von Willebrand disease will result in prolonged bleeding time because of the qualitative or quantitative deficiency in Willebrand factor, which is required for platelet adhesion to other platelets via the IIb/IIIa receptor (B). Severe thrombocytopenia (quantitative) and platelet dysfunction (qualitative) both prolong bleeding time (D, E). Fibrinogen deficiency also prolongs bleeding time because fibrinogen is required for platelet aggregation.

12. C. The INR detects abnormalities in the extrinsic and common pathways. The extrinsic pathway is triggered by exposure of the injured vessel to tissue factor and starts with factor VII. It then merges with the intrinsic pathway at factor X (E) and is followed by activation of factors V and II and fibrinogen (factor I) (A, B). Thus, both the prothrombin time and the PTT will be prolonged in factors I, II, V, and X because they are all part of the common pathway between the intrinsic and extrinsic pathways. Factor IX is part of the intrinsic pathway and a deficiency would prolong PTT only (D).

13. D. The most important element in detecting an increased risk of abnormal bleeding before surgery is a detailed history and physical examination. A systematic review in 2008 demonstrated the poor value of using coagulation tests when it came to identifying the risk of bleeding during an operation (A–C, E). Other studies have likewise shown that routine use of laboratory testing is neither sensitive nor specific for determining increased risk of bleeding. One needs to inquire about a history of prolonged bleeding after minor trauma, tooth extraction, menstruation, and in association with major and minor surgery. In addition, one must make inquiries into medications and over-the-counter supplements that might affect hemostasis. If a careful history is negative and the planned surgical procedure is minor, then further testing is not necessary. A potential pitfall in relying solely on the history is that the history obtained might not be sufficiently thorough or the patients might not recall or recognize that they had previous abnormal bleeding after an operation. If a major operation is planned that is not a high-bleeding risk, then a platelet count, a blood smear, and an aPTT are recommended. If the history suggests abnormal bleeding or the operation is either a high bleeding–risk operation or one in which even minor bleeding may have dire consequences (neurosurgery), then a bleeding time and INR should be added and a fibrin clot to detect abnormal fibrinolysis. If there is high suspicion for a history of abnormal bleeding, a hematology consult should also be obtained.

References: Chee YL, Crawford JC, Watson HG, Greaves M. Guidelines on the assessment of bleeding risk prior to surgery or invasive procedures. British Committee for Standards in Haematology: British Committee for Standards in Haematology. *Br J Haematol.* 2008;140(5):496–504.

Chee YL, Greaves M. Role of coagulation testing in predicting bleeding risk. *Hematol J.* 2003;4(6):373–378.

Klopfenstein CE. Preoperative clinical assessment of hemostatic function in patients scheduled for a cardiac operation. *Ann Thorac Surg.* 1996;62(6):1918–1920.

Suchman AL, Mushlin AI. How well does the activated partial thromboplastin time predict postoperative hemorrhage? *JAMA.* 1986;256(6):750–753.

14. D. Glanzmann thrombasthenia is an autosomal recessive disorder that results in absence of functional glycoprotein IIb/IIIa (C). Glycoprotein IIb/IIIa is a receptor for fibrinogen and von Willebrand factor and causes platelet adhesion and aggregation. Therefore, bleeding time will be prolonged, but aPTT and INR will be normal (A–E). These patients will not respond to DDAVP because there is no quantitative defect in the endothelial release of von Willebrand factor or factor VIII (von Willebrand disease) (B). The bleeding tendency for patients with Glanzmann's is variable. Treatment is with platelets. Repeated use of platelet transfusions can induce antiglycoprotein IIb/IIIa alloimmunization, rendering the treatment ineffective. In this circumstance, recombinant factor VIIa may be useful.

References: d'Oiron R, Ménart C, Trzeciak MC, et al. Use of recombinant factor VIIa in 3 patients with inherited type I Glanzmann's thrombasthenia undergoing invasive procedures. *Thromb Haemost.* 2000;83(5):644–647.

Nurden AT. Glanzmann thrombasthenia. *Orphanet J Rare Dis.* 2006;1(1):10.

15. E. Cryoprecipitate contains all items listed as well as factor XIII. However, it contains low concentrations of factor XI (A–D). Cryoprecipitate was originally created as a treatment for hemophilia; however, it is now more often used in patients receiving massive resuscitation in conjunction with fresh frozen plasma to replenish fibrinogen levels. Factor XI deficiency is also known as hemophilia C or Rosenthal syndrome, occurs more often in the Ashkenazi Jewish population, and is treated with fresh frozen plasma (during bleeding episodes).

16. A. The etiology of abnormal bleeding in uremic patients is multifactorial, but the most important is impairment of platelet function that may be partly due to a functional defect in von Willebrand factor, which leads to impaired platelet aggregation. DDAVP (desmopressin) seems to enhance the release of von Willebrand factor by endothelial cells. A single dose of 0.3 to 0.4 mcg/kg is given intravenously or subcutaneously. It has a rapid onset and relatively short duration (4–6 hours). Dialysis is also effective in the treatment of uremic bleeding by removing toxins that cause platelet dysfunction. Cryoprecipitate has high concentrations of von Willebrand factor as well as factor VIII and fibrinogen and may also be effective; however, it should not be first-line therapy (B). Recombinant human erythropoietin (Epogen [epoetin alfa]) has been shown to help uremic bleeding in several studies as well (D). In addition to stimulating erythropoiesis, Epogen (epoetin alfa) enhances platelet aggregation. The increased red cell mass also seems to displace platelets from the center of the blood vessel and places them closer to the endothelium. Estrogens have been shown to help with bleeding in men and women. The exact mechanism is unknown, but it is theorized that they decrease arginine levels, which decreases nitric oxide. This may lead to increases in thromboxane A2 and adenosine diphosphate (E). FFP does not have high concentrations of von Willebrand factor and thus is not effective for uremic bleeding (C).

Reference: Hedges SJ, Dehoney SB, Hooper JS, Amanzadeh J, Busti AJ. Evidence-based treatment recommendations for uremic bleeding. *Nat Clin Pract Nephrol*. 2007;3(3):138–153.

17. D. This is a classic presentation of emphysematous cholecystitis complicated by sepsis, which then resulted in DIC. Elderly male diabetic patients are at higher risk of emphysematous cholecystitis, and gas in the gallbladder confirms the diagnosis. DIC leads to a dysregulation of the coagulation cascade, leading to clotting and resultant bleeding. The consumption of fibrinogen, platelets, and coagulation factors from the overactivation of the coagulation cascade results ultimately in diffuse bleeding. There is no specific test for DIC, but thrombocytopenia, hypofibrinogenemia, prolonged PT and PTT, and the presence of increased fibrin degradation products are sufficient to suggest the diagnosis of DIC (C). Fresh frozen plasma, platelets, and cryoprecipitate are all important components of the treatment, especially for an actively bleeding patient, but the most important part in the management of DIC is to identify and correct the underlying source, which in this case is by broad-spectrum intravenous (IV) antibiotics and emergent cholecystectomy (A, B, E). Without removal of the source, DIC will continue to consume transfused products. The mortality rate from DIC ranges between 10% and 50%.

Reference: Levi M, Toh CH, Thachil J, Watson HG. Guidelines for the diagnosis and management of disseminated intravascular coagulation. British Committee for Standards in Haematology. *Br J Haematol*. 2009;145(1):24–33.

18. E. The most frequent congenital defect in hemostasis is vWD (A). Laboratory tests will demonstrate increased bleeding time with a normal prothrombin time (PT). Patients may have a normal or increased PTT because von Willebrand factor (vWF) is considered a stabilizing factor for factor VIII (D). There are three types of vWD: Type I is an autosomal dominant disease characterized by a low level of vWF and considered the most common form of vWD (B). Type I is treated with DDAVP because this increases circulating vWF released from endothelial cells. Type 2 vWD is also inherited in an autosomal dominant fashion and is characterized by a qualitative defect in which there is an appropriate amount of vWF, but it does not function properly. Type 2 has multiple variants, some that can be treated with DDAVP or cryoprecipitate. Type 2b, in particular, when treated with DDAVP can induce thrombocytopenia and form platelet complexes leading to a prothrombotic state. DDAVP is contraindicated in type 2b but may be useful in other type 2 variants. Finally, type 3 is the most severe form because there is no vWF produced by endothelial cells. It is transmitted in an autosomal recessive fashion. For type 3, the recommended treatment is recombinant vWF and factor VIII because these patients

do not make any vWF and therefore DDAVP will have no effect (C).

References: Holmberg L, Nilsson IM, Borge L, Gunnarsson M, Sjörin E. Platelet aggregation induced by 1-desamino-8-D-arginine vasopressin (DDAVP) in Type IIB von Willebrand's disease. *N Engl J Med*. 1983;309(14):816–821.

Tosetto A, Castaman G. How I treat type 2 variant forms of von Willebrand disease. *Blood*. 2015;125(6):907–914.

19. B. Heparin resistance is defined as the need for more than 35,000 units in 24 hours to prolong the PTT into the therapeutic range or as an activated clotting time (ACT) less than 400 seconds despite excessive demand for heparin (>400–600 IU/kg). Heparin resistance is most commonly the result of antithrombin-III (ATIII) deficiency. Heparin binds to ATIII causing a conformational change that results in its activation. Activated ATIII then inactivates thrombin and other proteases involved in blood clotting, most notably factor Xa. ATIII deficiency can be congenital or acquired. Hereditary ATIII deficiency is rare (much less common than factor V Leiden deficiency) and can lead to venous thrombosis. Causes of acquired ATIII deficiency include pregnancy, liver disease, disseminated intravascular coagulation (DIC), nephrotic syndrome, major surgery, acute thrombosis, and treatment with heparin. For this latter reason, measurement of ATIII levels while on heparin is an inaccurate method of identifying heparin resistance. Treatment of heparin resistance consists of either administering FFP or ATIII concentrates. FFP has the highest concentration of ATIII, and therefore patients should be initially treated with FFP to replete ATIII in plasma, followed by readministration of heparin. A direct thrombin inhibitor (argatroban) is a potential alternative; however, it has the disadvantage of having no way of being reversed in the case of overdosage and bleeding (C). A disadvantage of FFP in the cardiac surgery setting is that large volumes may be required and it exposes the patient to the risks of transfusions, including transfusion-related lung injury (TRALI). Thus, in the setting of cardiac bypass, ATIII concentrate is another alternative (though it is very costly). Low-molecular-weight heparin has no effect on ATIII deficiency and should not be used in this event (A). An inferior vena cava (IVC) filter would be indicated if the patient began to bleed while on heparin but not for heparin resistance. In fact, a filter, though protective against PE, increases the risk for DVT, due to the stasis it may create (D). Most patients achieve therapeutic PTT within 6 to 18 hours of starting heparin, so simply increasing the heparin dose is not appropriate (E).

References: Kearon C, Akl EA, Comerota AJ, et al. Antithrombotic therapy for VTE disease: Antithrombotic Therapy and Prevention of Thrombosis, 9th ed: American College of Chest Physicians Evidence-Based Clinical Practice Guidelines. *Chest*. 2012;141(2 Suppl):e419S–e496S.

Spiess BD. Treating heparin resistance with antithrombin or fresh frozen plasma. *Ann Thorac Surg*. 2008;85(6):2153–2160.

20. C. PCC is an inactivated concentrate of proteins C and S, and factors II, IX, and X, with variable amounts of factor VII. PCC with normal amounts of factor VII is known as 4-factor PCC, while PCC with low levels of factor VII is 3-factor PCC (A). Since 3-factor PCC has low levels of factor VII, the addition of fresh frozen plasma is sometimes necessary for full reversal of warfarin and thus, 4-factor PCC is superior. When a nonbleeding patient on warfarin needs

INR reversal, vitamin K is given, either orally (slower acting) or intramuscularly. If a patient is bleeding with an elevated INR, vitamin K and an exogenous clotting factor formulation are given. The options are FFP, PCC, or recombinant factor VII (less often used). PPC has several advantages over FFP; it does not need to be thawed (it is lyophilized [i.e., freeze dried]), it has a more rapid correction of INR, and it can be infused faster and with less volume (this also makes it ideal for patients with congestive heart failure or chronic kidney disease) (B). Recombinant factor VIIa will lower INR faster than PCC (D). However, the concerns regarding recombinant factor VIIa include the potential for inducing thrombosis (stroke, deep venous thrombosis) as well as the high cost. PPC does not reverse the anticoagulant effect of dabigatran; this can be accomplished with idarucizumab (E).

21. B. AFLP is an uncommon but potentially fatal complication that occurs in the third trimester of pregnancy or during the early postpartum period. It typically presents with a viral prodrome characterized by fever, lethargy, malaise, and nausea and vomiting. It is thought that AFLP may be the result of mitochondrial dysfunction resulting in microvesicular fatty infiltration of hepatocytes without significant inflammation or necrosis. The mortality rate previously was very high; however, with prompt diagnosis and treatment, the maternal and perinatal mortality have decreased to 18% and 23%, respectively. Prompt delivery and intensive supportive care are the cornerstones in management of AFLP. Laboratory abnormalities in AFLP include elevations of AST and ALT (usually less than 1000 IU/L), prolongation of PT and PTT, decreased fibrinogen, renal failure, profound hypoglycemia, and hyperbilirubinemia. Laboratory studies of AFLP are similar to HELLP, but the key finding to help differentiate the two is hypoglycemia, which does not occur commonly in HELLP (A). In addition, patients with HELLP typically have preeclampsia, evidence of hemolysis, and thrombocytopenia. Preeclampsia presents with hypertension, proteinuria, and rapid weight gain and can progress to seizures (eclampsia) (D). Patients with ICP report intense pruritus most commonly in the hands and soles of the feet that is unrelieved with antihistamines (C). Hepatitis E is caused by a single-stranded RNA virus. In men and nonpregnant women, it tends to be mild. However, it can lead to severe fulminant hepatic failure in pregnant patients in the third trimester, with a mortality rate of up to 25% (particularly in developing countries) (E).

References: Ko H, Yoshida EM. Acute fatty liver of pregnancy. *Can J Gastroenterol.* 2006;20(1):25–30.

Rahman TM, Wendon J. Severe hepatic dysfunction in pregnancy. *QJM.* 2002;95(6):343–357.

Vigil-De Gracia P. Acute fatty liver and HELLP syndrome: two distinct pregnancy disorders. *Int J Gynaecol Obstet.* 2001;73(3):215–220.

22. C. Several studies have demonstrated that patients in the ICU have a high incidence of coagulopathy and that vitamin K deficiency is the most common cause (B, D, E). The differential diagnosis for an elevated INR with a normal aPTT would include a factor VII deficiency, warfarin administration, the acute phase of liver disease, and vitamin K deficiency. Vitamin K is not stable in patients receiving total parenteral nutrition; therefore, in this case, the prolonged PT correlates with vitamin K deficiency. Prolonged parenteral nutrition often leads to cholestatic liver disease, which in turn leads to the liver's inability to use vitamin K appropriately. Factors II, VII, IX, and X as well as proteins C and S all require vitamin K and will be deficient in these patients (A). Twenty percent of hospitalized patients given intravenous nutrition over a 3-week period developed elevations of INR. Vitamin K should be given at least 6 to 12 hours before a procedure in patients with adequate liver function. IM route of administration is preferred because an IV push may result in anaphylaxis. In patients with hepatocellular disease, FFP or whole blood is required. Platelets and cryoprecipitate are unrelated to prolonged prothrombin time.

References: Chakraverty R, Davidson S, Peggs K, Stross P, Garrard C, Littlewood TJ. The incidence and cause of coagulopathies in an intensive care population. *Br J Haematol.* 1996;93(2):460–463.

Crowther MA, McDonald E, Johnston M, Cook D. Vitamin K deficiency and D-dimer levels in the intensive care unit: a prospective cohort study. *Blood Coagul Fibrinolysis.* 2002;13(1):49–52.

Duerksen DR, Papineau N. Clinical research: is routine vitamin K supplementation required in hospitalized patients receiving parenteral nutrition? *Nutr Clin Pract.* 2000;15(2):81–83.

Fiore LD, Scola MA, Cantillon CE, Brophy MT. Anaphylactoid reactions to vitamin K. *J Thromb Thrombolysis.* 2001;11(2):175–183.

Shearer MJ. Vitamin K in parenteral nutrition. *Gastroenterology.* 2009;137(Suppl. 5):S105–S118.

23. C. The correct answer is hypocalcemia, hyperkalemia, and metabolic alkalosis (A, B, D, E). Severe hypocalcemia with massive blood transfusion is uncommon and does not typically manifest unless the patient is receiving more than 1 unit of packed red blood cells (PRBCs) every 5 minutes. The hypocalcemia is the result of citrate toxicity because the citrate in the transfused blood binds to circulating calcium in the patient. Because citrate is metabolized in the liver, hypocalcemia can be more severe in patients with hepatic dysfunction. Additionally, the citrate is metabolized to bicarbonate leading to metabolic alkalosis. Potassium concentration of stored PRBC is higher than human plasma potassium level. This is thought to occur as a result of red blood cell lysis during storage, releasing potassium in the supernatant. The concentration of potassium in PRBC increases linearly and is approximately equal to the number of days of PRBC storage.

Reference: Vraets A, Lin Y, Callum JL. Transfusion-associated hyperkalemia. *Transfus Med Rev.* 2011;25(3):184–196.

24. D. HIT occurs in approximately 1% to 1.2% of patients receiving heparin. A scoring system has been devised to assess risk of HIT, known as the 4 "T"s (Thrombocytopenia, Timing, Thrombosis, and other causes for Thrombocytopenia). Variables that should heighten suspicion of HIT include a platelet count drop greater than 50%, occurrence between days 5 and 10 (it takes time for antibodies to develop), nadir of platelet count greater than 20,000 (nadir below 10,000 is less likely HIT), no other reason for platelet count drop, and new skin necrosis or VTE (C). Thus, more important than the absolute nadir is the percentage drop (A). HIT is caused by antibodies that attack the heparin-platelet factor 4 (PF4) complex. Heparin-PF4 antibodies (sometimes called "HIT antibodies") in the resultant multimolecular immune complex activate platelets via their FcγIIa receptors, causing the release of prothrombotic platelet-derived microparticles, platelet consumption, and thrombocytopenia. The microparticles in turn promote excessive thrombin generation, frequently resulting in thrombosis. Patients receiving any type of heparin at any dose and by any route of administration are at risk of developing HIT antibodies. It does occur less commonly in men and occurs more frequently in the elderly. However, not all of those with HIT antibodies will necessarily develop the clinical syndrome. If this is suspected, heparin should be discontinued, and the patient should be started on a direct thrombin inhibitor (E). If anticoagulation is not initiated, the chance of another thromboembolic event is approximately 5% to 10% per day (B). Diagnosis is performed by an ELISA antibody test. If these results are equivocal, then a confirmatory serotonin release assay should be performed.

References: Ahmed I, Majeed A, Powell R. Heparin induced thrombocytopenia: diagnosis and management update. *Postgrad Med J.* 2007;83(983):575–582.

Jang IK, Hursting MJ. When heparins promote thrombosis: review of heparin-induced thrombocytopenia. *Circulation.* 2005;111(20):2671–2683.

Warkentin TE, Hayward CP, Boshkov LK, et al. Sera from patients with heparin-induced thrombocytopenia generate platelet-derived microparticles with procoagulant activity: an explanation for the thrombotic complications of heparin-induced thrombocytopenia. *Blood.* 1994;84(11):3691–3699.

Wheeler HB. Diagnosis of deep vein thrombosis. Review of clinical evaluation and impedance plethysmography. *Am J Surg.* 1985;150(4A):7–13.

25. D. Although all the answer choices can increase the risk of venous thromboembolism, homocystinuria is the most common inherited condition predisposing patients to arterial thrombosis and affects 5% to 10% of the population. It is an autosomal recessive disease. Homocystinuria is most commonly caused by a deficiency of cystathionine beta-synthase resulting in an elevated level of homocysteine in plasma and urine. The toxic effect of an elevated level of homocysteine in the brain results in mental retardation as well as seizures. Skeletal abnormalities (marfanoid habitus) may occur secondary to the interference of collagen cross-linking. Patients are at increased risk of thrombosis due to the disruption of vascular endothelium by homocysteine leading to platelet activation and aggregation. Patients identified early to have this condition will benefit with administration of pyridoxine (vitamin B6) to induce cystathionine beta-synthase activity. Factor V Leiden mutation is the most common inherited condition increasing the risk of venous thromboembolism followed by prothrombin gene mutation (A, B). Patients that do not have a response to the administration of unfractionated heparin may have antithrombin III deficiency (C). Protein C deficiency is a rare cause of venous thromboembolism (E).

References: D'Angelo A, Selhub J. Homocysteine and thrombotic disease. *Blood.* 1997;90(1):1–11.

Greico AJ. Homocystinuria: pathogenetic mechanisms. *Am J Med Sci.* 1977;273(2):120–132.

Rosendaal FR. Risk factors for venous thrombosis: prevalence, risk, and interaction. *Semin Hematol.* 1997;34(3):171–187.

26. C. The leading causes of allogeneic blood transfusion (ABT)–related mortality in the United States (in the order of reported number of deaths) include transfusion-related acute lung injury (TRALI), ABO and non-ABO hemolytic transfusion reactions, and transfusion-associated sepsis (A, B, D). Graft-versus-host reaction is not a common cause of ABT (E). Additionally, it has been demonstrated that nonleukocyte-reduced blood transfusions have been associated with increased mortality when compared with leukocyte-reduced blood transfusions.

Reference: Vamvakas E, Blajchman M. Transfusion-related mortality: the ongoing risks of allogeneic blood transfusion and the available strategies for their prevention. *Blood.* 2009;113(15):3406–3417.

27. E. Bacterial contamination of blood is the most frequent cause of death from transfusion-transmitted infectious disease and is the third most common cause of death overall in a large series (after acute lung injury and ABO incompatibility) (B, C). A key feature of ABO incompatibility (hemolytic reaction) is the development of red urine (hemoglobinuria). Patients also often complain of back pain and a sense of doom. Acute lung injury manifests with rapid onset of dyspnea and tachypnea around 6 hours after transfusion. Anaphylactic reaction rarely occurs (D). Bacterial contamination now accounts for 1 in every 38,500 cases of blood transfusion. This increase had coincided with a dramatic decrease in viral infections. The highest risk of bacterial infection is from pooled platelet transfusions because many microorganisms can live and propagate under the storage conditions of platelets (20–24°C). Gram-negative sepsis is the most lethal (A), and Yersinia is one of the most common organisms. Gram-negative sepsis can become clinically apparent within 9 to 24 hours after blood transfusion. Cytomegalovirus is the most common infectious agent transmitted, but because it is so ubiquitous, it is generally not a threat to most patients. The exception to that rule is the transplant recipient.

References: Benjamin RJ. Transfusion-related sepsis: a silent epidemic. *Blood.* 2016;127(4):380–381.

Bihl F, Castelli D, Marincola F, Dodd RY, Brander C. Transfusion-transmitted infections. *J Transl Med.* 2007;5(1):25.

Kuehnert M, Roth V, Haley N, et al. Transfusion-transmitted bacterial infection in the United States, 1998 through 2000. *Transfusion.* 2001;41(12):1493–1499.

28. D. Transfusion purpura is an uncommon cause of thrombocytopenia and bleeding after transfusion. A small minority of patients lack the HPA-1a antigen on their platelets that is present in almost all humans. Transfusion purpura requires that the patient has been previously sensitized to the HPA-1a antigen; this happens usually by a prior pregnancy or previous blood transfusion. When these patients later receive blood products that contain a small number of platelets with the ubiquitous HPA-1a, they produce alloantibodies that attack both the donor's and the patient's own platelets (C). This usually presents 5 to 12 days after a transfusion and leads to profound thrombocytopenia and bleeding that can last for weeks. Mortality occurs in 10% to 20% due to hemorrhage. Although sensitization can occur after prior blood transfusions, it has become less common with leukocyte-reduced red cells and therefore this issue is most common in women who have been pregnant (A). Diagnosis is made by demonstrating platelet alloantibodies with an absence of the corresponding antigen on the patient's platelets. Treatment is primarily with intravenous immunoglobulin (IVIG). Plasmapheresis and corticosteroids are also potential options. Treatment with platelet transfusions can exacerbate the disease process (B). The presentation can easily be confused with heparin-induced thrombocytopenia without appropriate testing. A platelet count of fewer than 15,000 cells/μL is more suggestive of transfusion purpura (E).

References: Hillyer CD, Hillyer KL, Strobl FJ, Jefferies LC, Silberstein LE, eds. *Handbook of transfusion medicine.* Academic Press; 2001:328.

Lubenow N, Eichler P, Albrecht D. Very low platelet counts in post-transfusion purpura falsely diagnosed as heparin-induced thrombocytopenia: report of four cases and review of literature. *Thromb Res.* 2000;100(3):115–125.

29. D. Clopidogrel (Plavix) irreversibly inhibits platelet aggregation within 2 hours of administration and its effects last 5 to 7 days (the half-life of platelets is 1 week) (C, D). It works by indirectly inhibiting the activation of the glycoprotein IIb/IIIa complex (E). It does this by antagonizing the ADP receptor which, when activated, inserts glycoprotein IIb/IIIa receptors on the platelet's surface. This is functionally similar to Glanzmann thrombasthenia, which is characterized by a GpIIb/IIIa receptor deficiency on platelets preventing fibrin from linking platelets together. Bernard-Soulier disease is characterized by GpIb receptor deficiency on platelets which prevents vWF from linking the platelet to exposed collagen on damaged tissue (A). Clopidogrel has been shown to decrease the rate of a combined endpoint of cardiovascular death, myocardial infarction, and stroke in patients with acute coronary syndromes. Use with aspirin increases the risk of bleeding. Clopidogrel has been associated with the development of thrombotic thrombocytopenic purpura, even with short-term use (<2 weeks). Treatment is with plasma exchange. The mortality rate is as high as 29%. It has not been associated with pulmonary hypertension (B).

30. C. Warfarin acts in the liver by blocking the vitamin K–dependent factors (II, VII, IX, and X). Of these, factor VII has the shortest half-life (A, B, D, E). A deficiency in factor VII manifests by a prolongation of the prothrombin time and the international normalized ratio. Vitamin K is critical in the γ-carboxylation of these factors that are synthesized in the liver. Patients with hepatic dysfunction would similarly display prolonged prothrombin time.

31. A. Hemostatic agents are increasingly used intraoperatively to provide a temporary measure of controlling bleeding when cautery is dangerous or inaccessible. Collagen can provide hemostasis by allowing a large surface area for platelet adherence leading to thrombus clot. However, this will not work well in patients with thrombocytopenia. Oxidized cellulose promotes red cell lysis generating an artificial clot and can even be used during endoscopic procedures. It may also have an antimicrobial effect since it decreases local tissue pH (B). Thrombin uses blood as a source of fibrinogen to create a clot (C). In contrast, fibrin sealant is composed of both fibrinogen and thrombin (D). Glutaraldehyde cross-linked peptide (commonly albumin) forms a scaffold for clot formation and can be used even on wet surfaces (E).

References: Emilia M, Luca S, Francesca B, et al. Topical hemostatic agents in surgical practice. *Transfus Apher Sci.* 2011; 45(3):305–311.

Skinner M, Velazquez-Avina J, Mönkemüller K. Overtube-assisted endoscopic application of oxidized cellulose to achieve hemostasis in anastomotic ulcer bleeding. *Gastrointest Endosc.* 2014;80(5):917–918.

Wound Healing 37

ERIC O. YEATES, AREG GRIGORIAN, AND CHRISTIAN DE VIRGILIO

ABSITE 99th Percentile High-Yields

I. Phases of Wound Healing

	Days	Cell types	Description
Hemostasis	1	Platelets	Initial transient vasoconstriction, ADP released, platelets aggregate and cause thrombosis
Inflammatory	1–10	PMNs (1–3) Macrophages (4–5) Lymphocytes (5–6) Fibroblasts (6+)	Vasodilation, PMNs phagocytose debris and bacteria, macrophages essential for wound healing and release growth factors/cytokines; nicotine is a vasoconstrictor that impairs oxygen delivery, increases platelet adhesion, and inhibits proliferation of red blood cells, fibroblasts, and macrophages, all of which impair wound healing
Proliferative	5–21	Fibroblasts	Fibroblasts deposit collagen and glycosaminoglycans, neovascularization, granulation tissue, epithelialization
Remodeling	21–365	Fibroblasts	Decreased vascularity, type III collagen replaces type I, collagen cross-linking (max strength is 80% at 8 weeks)

II. Nutrients and Wound Healing

	Function	Deficiency
Vitamin A	Increases inflammatory response in wounds, stimulates collagen synthesis, counteracts effects of steroids or radiation on wound healing (patient does NOT need to be vitamin A deficient to benefit from this)	Blindness, rash, delayed wound healing
Vitamin C	Collagen synthesis and crosslinking, angiogenesis, antioxidant, increases iron absorption; large doses may even inhibit wound healing	Scurvy (easy bruising, bleeding gums, poor wound healing)
Vitamin E	Fat-soluble antioxidant, no evidence that it improves wound healing or scar appearance	Ataxia, peripheral neuropathy, retinopathy, impaired immune response
Iron	Transports oxygen, metabolism of collagen	Fatigue, anemia, impaired wound healing
Zinc	Cofactor for collagen formation and many other enzymatic reactions in wound healing	Rash, alopecia, impaired immune function, diarrhea, delayed wound healing, reduced wound strength
Copper	Stimulates fibroblasts proliferation, upregulates collagen production	Anemia, myelopathy, neuropathy, impaired wound healing

Questions

1. Which of the following is true regarding hyperbaric oxygen therapy (HBOT) and wounds?
   A. HBOT is now widely adopted in hospitals across the United States
   B. Topical oxygen treatment (TOT) is as effective as HBOT for wounds involving bone
   C. Transcutaneous oxygen measurements (TCOM) are useful in predicting wound healing with HBOT
   D. HBOT decreases the major amputation rate in patients with diabetic foot ulcers
   E. HBOT typically takes at least 6 months to show effectiveness

2. Which of the following is true regarding diabetic foot ulcers?
   A. The lifetime risk of a patient with diabetes developing a foot ulcer is approximately 5%
   B. It is primarily due to thrombotic occlusion of distal vasculature
   C. Enzymatic debridement of diabetic foot ulcers should be avoided
   D. Sharp debridement of diabetic foot ulcers should be avoided
   E. Total-contact casts can be used in the setting of diabetic foot ulcers to promote healing

3. Which of the following is true regarding wound dressings?
   A. Honey dressings are not indicated in wounds with slough or necrotic tissue
   B. Calcium alginate dressings are ideal in wounds with a large amount of exudate
   C. Wet-to-dry dressings remain the gold standard for wound dressings in most scenarios
   D. Moisture-retentive dressings have similar rates of infection compared to gauze dressings
   E. Hydrogels with silver can be used in combination with enzymatic debriding agents

4. Which of the following is true regarding cell junctions in humans?
   A. Hemidesmosomes do not interact with intermediate filaments
   B. Tight junctions, by definition, do not allow the passage of solutes through adjacent cell membranes
   C. Connexons allow for direct communication between two adjacent cells
   D. Adherens junctions are a specialized type of tight junction
   E. Desmosomes function primarily to anchor a cell to the extracellular matrix

5. Which of the following is true regarding nutritional status and nonhealing wounds?
   A. Short periods of starvation before surgery generally have minimal effect on wound healing
   B. Malnutrition prolongs the inflammatory phase of wound healing
   C. Prealbumin will provide an accurate estimation of nutritional status over the previous several weeks
   D. Nutritional supplements have been shown to decrease interval time to complete healing of pressure ulcers
   E. Presence of granulation tissue is not predictive of adequate wound healing ability

6. A 22-year-old female with history of a gunshot wound to the abdomen requiring multiple bowel resections has been on chronic total peripheral nutrition (TPN) for short gut syndrome. She presents for a clinic follow-up stating that her hair has started to fall out, and she has developed multiple bruises over her arms and legs. In addition, she has a diffuse scaly rash and dry skin. In which following nutrients or trace elements is she likely deficient?
   A. Copper
   B. Vitamin C
   C. Linoleic acid
   D. Zinc
   E. Selenium

7. Which of the following is true regarding skin antiseptic techniques before surgery?
   A. Iodine-based preps are superior to chlorhexidine for preventing surgical site infections
   B. Chlorhexidine-based preps are safe on all body surfaces as a preoperative cleanser
   C. Preoperative bathing with chlorhexidine has been shown to reduce incidence of surgical site infections
   D. The bactericidal effect of iodine derives from its ability to form an extracellular crystal matrix and destabilize cell membranes
   E. Povidone-iodine was formulated to decrease the availability of molecular iodine

8. Which of the following is true about wound healing?
   A. Angiogenesis is the major contributor to the erythema seen in wounds
   B. Pain in the first 48 hours is secondary to newly active fibroblasts attempting to contract the wound edges
   C. At 48 hours, phagocytic cells predominate in the wound bed
   D. In the first 36 hours, macrophages are the predominate cells in the wound bed
   E. While erythema and pain can be normal, induration is typically pathologic

9. Which of the following is true regarding keloids and/or hypertrophic scars?
   A. Keloids are associated with an increased deposition of collagen
   B. Low-dose radiation is a better adjunct for treatment of hypertrophic scars
   C. Keloids can appear years after a minor injury
   D. Keloids are much more common after burn injuries than hypertrophic scars
   E. Hypertrophic scars tend to extend beyond wound borders with time

10. A severely malnourished 12-year-old boy presents with multiple pigmented spots on his bilateral thighs, bleeding gums, loose and missing teeth, and several weeping wounds. He recently arrived as a refugee from an underdeveloped country. His medical history is sparse. His diet primarily consisted of cooked grains. Which of the following is true regarding the most likely vitamin deficiency in this patient?
    A. It plays an essential step in proteoglycan synthesis
    B. Delayed wound healing is caused by failure to hydroxylate lysine and proline during collagen synthesis
    C. It does not affect iron absorption
    D. Exogenous administration has been shown in animals to have a corticosteroid-like effect on wound healing
    E. After hydroxylation by the liver and kidney, it helps with bone mineralization

11. Which of the following diseases is correctly paired with the type of collagen affected?
    A. Alport syndrome: type III collagen
    B. Ehlers-Danlos syndrome: type VII collagen
    C. Epidermolysis bullosa: type VII collagen
    D. Osteogenesis imperfecta: type II collagen
    E. Bullous pemphigoid: type I collagen

12. Which of the following is true regarding the healing of a small-bowel anastomosis?
    A. Leaks are less likely to occur with a hand-sewn anastomosis as compared with stapled
    B. There is a decreased level of collagenase when compared to healing skin wounds
    C. The serosa plays a minimal role in the healing of a small-bowel anastomosis
    D. The submucosa provides the most significant strength layer of the anastomosis
    E. Free omental flaps have been shown to improve outcomes when doing a small-bowel anastomosis

Answers

1. C. HBOT for wound healing remains incompletely adopted, likely due to cost and inconsistent efficacy in clinical trials (A). HBOT typically involves placing the patient in a pressurized chamber to around 2.0 atmospheres and administering 100% oxygen for 1 to 2 hours. These sessions can be performed once or twice daily for 2 to 4 weeks. HBOT is thought to work by delivering high arterial partial pressures of oxygen to the wound bed, as well as angiogenesis stimulation. Side effects of HBOT are rare but include claustrophobia, barotrauma, headache, and tinnitus. Though there is still debate on its efficacy, a large systematic review in 2015 suggested that HBOT improved healing rates at 6 weeks, but not at one year (E). It also did not decrease the major amputation rate compared to conventional wound care alone (D). There

is good evidence that TCOMs taken after HBOT can predict the efficacy of therapy with impressive accuracy. Specifically, diabetic foot ulcers with TCOMs >200 mmHg healed 90% of the time with HBOT (C). TOT applies 100% oxygen directly to the wound and has been studied far less than HBOT. Though there are some clinical trials suggesting efficacy in some patients, it is accepted that TOT does not penetrate to bone due to its mechanism of action (B).

References: Kranke P, Bennett MH, Martyn-St James M, Schnabel A, Debus SE, Weibel S. Hyperbaric oxygen therapy for chronic wounds. *Cochrane Database Syst Rev.* 2015;(6):CD004123.

Moon H, Strauss MB, La SS, Miller SS. The validity of transcutaneous oxygen measurements in predicting healing of diabetic foot ulcers. *Undersea Hyperb Med.* 2016;43(6):641–648.

Mutluoglu M, Cakkalkurt A, Uzun G, Aktas S. Topical oxygen for chronic wounds: a PRO/CON debate. *J Am Coll Clin Wound Spec.* 2013;5(3):61–65.

2. E. Diabetic foot ulcers are very common, with the lifetime risk of a patient with diabetes approximately 25% (A). Diabetic foot ulcers are mainly caused by peripheral neuropathy leading to scrapes/cuts of the foot that may go unnoticed for several days (B). There is also autonomic neuropathy leading to failure of sweating. This manifests as dry skin at risk for mechanical breakdown which can initiate ulcer formation. Additionally, autonomic dysregulation of the microcirculation results in poor flow to distal extremities preventing adequate wound healing. Preventative care is paramount in the prevention of diabetic foot ulcers and includes maintaining normoglycemia and daily exams for occult scrapes/cuts of the foot along with daily moisturizer use. Diabetic foot ulcers should be managed with a combination of debridement and off-loading. Sharp debridement, enzymatic debridement, biological debridement, and autolytic debridement are all acceptable methods of removing debris and necrotic tissue (C, D). Offloading is also critical to wound healing, with nonremovable total-contact casts being the gold standard. Contraindications to this type of cast are ischemia, ongoing infection, osteomyelitis, and poor skin quality.

References: Alexiadou K, Doupis J. Management of diabetic foot ulcers. *Diabetes Ther.* 2012;3(1):4.

Boulton AJM, Armstrong DG, Albert SF, et al. Comprehensive foot examination and risk assessment: a report of the task force of the foot care interest group of the American Diabetes Association, with endorsement by the American Association of Clinical Endocrinologists. *Diabetes Care.* 2008;31(8):1679–1685.

3. B. A large body of evidence supports the utilization of a moist wound environment to promote faster wound healing and less scar formation. Therefore, the wound dressing should create an ideal amount of moisture by either adding moisture to dry wounds or absorbing it from highly exudative wounds. Despite the progress made in wound dressings, many outdated strategies like wet-to-dry dressings are overly used. Wet-to-dry dressings, most often gauze, are first allowed to dry on the wound and then are removed, resulting in nonselective debridement of both slough and healthy tissue (C). Additionally, moisture-retentive dressings like hydrocolloids and transparent films have a lower infection rate than gauze dressings (D). Some wounds, despite moisture-retentive dressings, remain too dry and require supplementation. Hydrogels are useful in this case as they are hydrating to the wound bed, but care should be taken not

to use in combination with enzymatic debriding agents, as they may become inactive (E). Other wounds have a large amount of exudate which needs to be controlled in order to prevent maceration and improve wound healing. Both foam dressings and alginate dressings, which can absorb 20 times their weight, can be used in this scenario (B). Enzymatic debriding agents, like collagenase (e.g., Santyl) and medical-grade honey, are also commonly used to remove slough and necrotic tissues (A).

Reference: Niezgoda JA, Baranoski S, Ayello EA, et al. Wound treatment options. In: Baranoski S, Ayello EA, eds. *Wound care essentials.* 5th ed. Wolters Kluwer Health; 2020:184–241.

4. C. All humans have three main types of cell junctions: anchoring junctions, communicating (gap) junctions, and tight junctions. The first group (anchoring junctions) is further subdivided into desmosomes, hemidesmosomes, and adherens junctions (D). Hemidesmosomes and desmosomes both connect with intermediate filaments in the cytoskeleton, but the former connects cells to the underlying extracellular matrix, and desmosomes connect adjacent cells to one another (A, E). Adherens junctions serve the same purpose but use actin filaments as their cytoskeletal anchor. Anchoring junctions, as a whole, provide structural integrity to a tissue made up of individual cells. Communicating junctions allow direct chemical communication between adjacent cells. This is facilitated by six individual subunits, called connexins, which form a central pore, called a connexon. When two connexons from adjacent cells come in contact, a channel is formed allowing communication between the two cells. The final group, tight junctions, refers to a group of proteins that allow the selective diffusion of molecules based mainly on size, molecular charge, and polarity. These primarily act as selective barriers such as in the different layers of the skin (B).

5. B. Delayed wound healing is a multifactorial problem with many identifiable risk factors including malnutrition, vitamin deficiencies, smoking, obesity, diabetes, and hypoxemia. However, few systemic factors have been shown to speed up wound healing. Short periods of starvation can have negative effects on postoperative wound healing (A). This seems to occur primarily by prolongation of the inflammatory phase because there are inadequate building blocks for cell proliferation, protein synthesis, and creation of new DNA. The notion that malnutrition plays a key role in the development of chronic wounds led to multiple studies aimed at determining if nutritional supplementation can prevent chronic wounds or speed recovery. A Cochrane review done in 2014 looking at 23 randomized controlled trials evaluating the effect of enteral and parenteral nutrition on the prevention and treatment of pressure ulcers found no clear benefit of any intervention (D). By knowing the half-lives and current serum measurements of certain proteins, we are able to estimate the synthetic ability of the liver over a given time period. Albumin (14–20 days), transferrin (8–9 days), and prealbumin (2–3 days) all give a snapshot into someone's nutritional status but need to be combined with the entire clinical picture (C). Granulation tissue, if present, is predictive of adequate wound healing (E).

References: Greenfield LJ, Mulholland MW, eds. *Greenfield's surgery: scientific principles & practice.* 5th ed. Lippincott Williams and Wilkins; 2011.

Langer G, Fink A. Nutritional interventions for preventing and treating pressure ulcers. *Cochrane Database Syst Rev.* 2014;(6):CD003216.

Stechmiller JK. Understanding the role of nutrition and wound healing. *Nutr Clin Pract.* 2010;25(1):61–68.

6. C. A deficiency of trace elements and essential fatty acids is a relatively rare entity in patients taking food by mouth. However, it has occurred with increased frequency with the advent and widespread use of TPN, particularly in patients with a history of short gut syndrome. Copper is primarily associated with anemia resistant to iron supplementation, leukopenia, and neurologic defects (A). Vitamin C deficiency, or scurvy, causes delayed wound healing, bleeding gums, loose teeth, and abnormal bone deposition in children (B). Selenium deficiency is associated with a fatal cardiomyopathy (E). Zinc and essential fatty acid deficiency (linoleic acid and alpha-linolenic acid) have many similar features including delayed wound healing, increased infections, diarrhea, and a rash. However, the essential fatty acid rash tends to be scalier and is associated with dry skin, and the rash from zinc is primarily located in the perioral area and intertriginous skin of the fingers and toes. While alopecia and thrombocytopenia can be found with both conditions, it is more closely associated with free fatty acid deficiency. Conversely, the impaired taste, night blindness, and loss of appetite are more closely related with zinc deficiency (D).

References: Jeppesen PB, Høy CE, Mortensen PB. Essential fatty acid deficiency in patients receiving home parenteral nutrition. *Am J Clin Nutr.* 1998;68(1):126–133.

Kumar V, Fausto N, Abbas A, eds. *Robbins and Cotran pathologic basis of disease.* 7th ed. WB Saunders; 2004.

O'Leary JP, Tabuenca A, Capote LR. *The physiologic basis of surgery.* 4th ed. Wolters Kluwer Health/Lippincott Williams & Wilkins; 2008.

7. E. Surgical site infections have been shown to increase the cost of hospitalizations and length of hospital stays prompting the Surgical Care Improvement Project (SCIP) to address this major economic burden to modern health care. While preoperative bathing with antiseptic solution has been shown to decrease bacterial colonization of skin, it has not been proven to be associated with decreased rates of surgical site infections (C). Multiple preparations for preoperative skin antisepsis have been designed; however, the two most commonly in use are iodine-based and chlorhexidine-based in either an aqueous or alcohol solution. Iodine works primarily by passing through the bacterial cell membrane and replacing intracellular ions with molecular iodine and oxidizing various structures within the bacterium (D). It is also, however, toxic to normal tissues, so it is generally combined with a carrier molecule (e.g., povidone) to reduce the systemic availability of molecular iodine and reduce its toxicity. In contrast, chlorhexidine works by its ability to destabilize cellular membranes. A Cochrane review done in 2015 comparing iodine-based and chlorhexidine-based preoperative antiseptic techniques found the latter to be superior in preventing surgical site infections (A). However, it is generally not recommended for use above the chin because of ototoxicity and potential for causing damage to the cornea in higher concentrations (B).

References: Dumville JC, McFarlane E, Edwards P, et al. Preoperative skin antiseptics for preventing surgical wound infections after clean surgery. *Cochrane Database Syst Rev.* 2015;(4):CD003949.

Mangram AJ, Horan TC, Pearson ML, et al. Guideline for the prevention of surgical site infection. *Infect Control Hosp Epidemiol.* 1990;20:247–280.

8. C. Wound healing is typically divided into 3 or 4 phases: hemostasis/inflammation (combined in the 3-phase model), proliferation, and maturation (or remodeling). The hemostasis/inflammation phase is initiated with the disruption of capillaries resulting in hemorrhage. This immediately causes vasoconstriction to assist with the formation of a platelet plug. After 10 to 15 minutes, local tissue factors and platelets begin to facilitate vasodilation and increased vascular permeability. The infiltration of fluid and cells (mainly neutrophils) causes the wound to become erythematous (A). In addition, the wound is warm and edematous (induration) (E). At this point, changes in tissue pH and local tissue destruction cause the wound to be painful (B). The first cells to arrive after formation of a platelet plug are neutrophils, which don't seem to be critical to healing and mainly help with phagocytosis of bacteria and destruction of dead tissue. Neutrophil predominance persists for 48 hours, at which point they are largely replaced by macrophages, which will remain in the wound until the completion of healing (D). Macrophages are arguably the most important cell in healing because of their effects on angiogenesis, matrix deposition, and remodeling via the release of cytokines and growth factors. By day 4, the proliferative phase begins and endothelial cells and fibroblasts begin to appear in the wound. By days 5 to 7, there is no longer a significant population of inflammatory cells. The previously created matrix of type III collagen is slowly replaced with type I collagen, angiogenesis takes place, granulation tissue begins to form, and wound contraction commences. This phase persists for 3 to 4 weeks and finally gives way to the remodeling phase. At this point, vascularity decreases and collagen is continuing to be synthesized, but it is being broken down at the same rate and collagen cross-linking occurs.

References: Brunicardi FC, Andersen DK, Billiar TR, Dunn DL, Hunter JG, Matthews JB, Pollock RE. eds. *Schwartz's principles of surgery.* 10th ed. McGraw-Hill Education; 2015.

O'Leary JP, Tabuenca A, Capote LR. *The physiologic basis of surgery.* 4th ed. Wolters Kluwer Health/Lippincott Williams & Wilkins; 2008.

9. C. Hypertrophic scarring and keloid formation are both examples of pathologic excessive healing. Both are caused by the increased deposition of collagen (A). Formation of keloids has a large genetic component that is inherited in an autosomal dominant fashion. It is also more prominent in darker-skinned individuals. Hypertrophic scarring is generally caused by a delay in wound healing or by excessive tensile forces on a new wound and is at a particularly high risk of forming after burns (D). They do not spread outside of the borders of the original wound, unlike keloids (E). Hypertrophic scars tend to recede with time, but if they persist, they tend to respond better to surgical excision as compared to keloids. Excision of keloids should be performed with caution, as they tend to reoccur and become bigger. If excision is planned, it should be accompanied by an adjunctive treatment such as steroids or low-dose radiation to prevent recurrence (B). Several other adjuncts have also been shown to reduce scarring including silicone bandages, occlusive dressings, and extremity compression devices.

References: Gauglitz GG, Korting HC, Pavicic T, Ruzicka T, Jeschke MG. Hypertrophic scarring and keloids: Pathomechanisms and current and emerging treatment strategies. *Mol Med.* 2011;17(1–2):113–125.

Greenfield LJ, Mulholland MW, eds. *Greenfield's surgery: scientific principles & practice.* 5th ed. Lippincott Williams and Wilkins; 2011.

O'Leary JP, Tabuenca A, Capote LR. *The physiologic basis of surgery.* 4th ed. Wolters Kluwer Health/Lippincott Williams & Wilkins; 2008.

10. B. This patient most likely has scurvy caused by a deficiency in vitamin C and is uncommon in the modern age. It is typically seen in patients with severe malnutrition often from underdeveloped countries without access to fresh fruits and vegetables. Patients present with loose or missing teeth, open sores, pigmented spots on the extremities, bleeding mucous membranes, vague myalgias, and fatigue. It is a key cofactor in the hydroxylation of lysine and proline during collagen synthesis; as such, collagen cross-linking is extremely diminished in patients with vitamin C deficiency. It can even cause the involution of previous scars because remodeling continues, but patients are unable to synthesize new collagen. Vitamin C is also involved in iron absorption (C). Vitamin A is another essential vitamin in wound healing and assists with epithelialization, proteoglycan synthesis, and normal immune function (A). It has also been shown to reverse the effects of steroids on wound healing. Vitamin D is consumed in the diet and produced in the skin. It then undergoes activation (hydroxylation) by the liver and kidney to play an essential role in calcium metabolism (E). Exogenous vitamin E has been shown in animal trials to cause delayed wound healing via an inflammatory mechanism similar to corticosteroids (D).

Reference: O'Leary JP, Tabuenca A, Capote LR. *The physiologic basis of surgery.* 4th ed. Wolters Kluwer Health/Lippincott Williams & Wilkins; 2008.

11. C. The most common types of collagen located in the body include types I to V, though there are many more that are clinically relevant in certain diseases. Type I collagen makes up 90% of the body's collagen and is found to some degree in most tissue, including skin, bones, tendons, arterial walls, and scars. It is implicated in disease like osteogenesis imperfecta (D). Type II collagen makes up about 50% of the protein in hyaline cartilage (carTWOlidge). Type III collagen is found in bone, cartilage, and multiple types of connective tissue, and abnormalities have been found in Dupuytren contracture and the formation of aneurysms. Type IV collagen is found primarily in the basement membrane (type four

is floor) and has been associated with Alport and Goodpasture syndrome (A). Type V collagen is closely associated with type I and is in most of the same tissues but with the addition of placental tissue. While there exist clinically significant collagens outside of these main five, such as type VII (epidermolysis bullosa) and type XVII (bullous pemphigoid), they are not nearly as prevalent (E). Ehlers-Danlos is a spectrum of connective tissue disorders that can affect multiple types of collagen (B). However, the most common is type V (seen in classic type Ehlers-Danlos).

Reference: De Paepe A, Malfait F. Bleeding and bruising in patients with Ehlers-Danlos syndrome and other collagen vascular disorders: review. *Br J Haematol.* 2004;127(5):491–500.

12. D. While healing of the gastrointestinal tract goes through the same basic steps as healing of the skin, there are several key differences and unique features. Skin wounds undergo a relatively steady increase of the tensile strength of the wound over time. In contrast, the increased collagenase activity in the small bowel allows collagen breakdown to exceed collagen deposition on days 3 to 5 after an anastomosis (B). This is why anastomotic leaks in the gastrointestinal tract occur with increased frequency in this critical time period. However, the gastrointestinal tract is quicker to reach maximal tensile strength when compared with the skin. The submucosa provides most of the tensile strength for an anastomosis because of the coarse, interwoven fibers that make it up. However, the mucosa and serosa are also important, and both help provide a quick, leakproof barrier over the first several days (C). One can appreciate this effect in action by noting the relatively higher leak rates with portions of the GI tract that lack serosa such as the esophagus. Multiple adjuncts and techniques have been tried to decrease the rate of anastomotic leaks, and while there may be a trend toward fewer leaks with a stapled anastomosis in certain circumstances, there still isn't conclusive evidence that one is superior to the other in all cases (A). While omental wrapping has been shown to improve outcomes in certain situations, a devitalized "omental free flap" will necrose and will not help with the anastomosis (E).

References: Brunicardi FC, Andersen DK, Billiar TR, Dunn DL, Hunter JG, Matthews JB, Pollock RE. eds. *Schwartz's principles of surgery.* 10th ed. McGraw Hill Education; 2015.

Egorov VI, Schastlivtsev V, Turusov RA, Baranov AO. Participation of the intestinal layers in supplying of the mechanical strength of the intact and sutured gut. *Eur Surg Res.* 2002;34(6):425–431.

Thornton FJ, Barbul A. Healing in the gastrointestinal tract. *Neurosurg Clin N Am.* 1997;77(3):549–573.